*Progress in*

# Obstetrics and Gynaecology

## VOLUME 14

*Edited by*

**John Studd** DSc MD FRCOG

Consultant Gynaecologist
Fertility and Endocrinology Centre
Chelsea and Westminster Hospital and
The Lister Hospital, London, UK

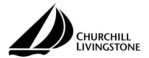
**CHURCHILL LIVINGSTONE**

EDINBURGH  LONDON  NEW YORK  PHILADELPHIA  ST LOUIS  SYDNEY  TORONTO  2000

CHURCHILL LIVINGSTONE
An imprint of Harcourt Publishers Limited

First published 2000
  Reprinted 2001

ISBN 0 443 064075
ISSN 0261 0140

**British Library Cataloguing in Publication Data**
A catalogue record for this book is available from the British Library

**Library of Congress Cataloging in Publication Data**
A catalog record for this book is available from the Library of Congress

Medical knowledge is constantly changing. As new information becomes available, changes in treatment, procedures, equipment and the use of drugs become necessary. The editors and the publishers have, as far as possible, taken care to ensure that the information given in this text is accurate and up to date. However, readers are strongly advised to confirm that the information, especially with regard to drug usage, complies with current legislation and standards of practice.

Commissioning Editor – Ellen Green
Project Editor – Michele Staunton
Project Controller – Frances Affleck
Designer – Sarah Cape
Typeset – BA & GM Haddock
Printed in China

*Progress in*

# Obstetrics and Gynaecology

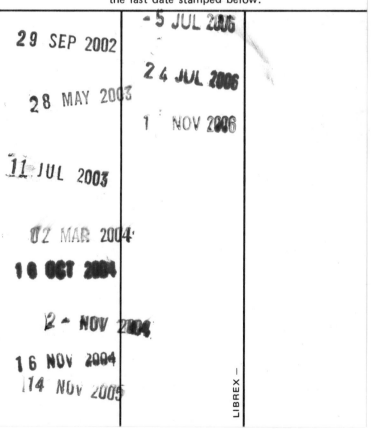

# Progress in Obstetrics and Gynaecology
*Edited by John Studd*

## Contents of Volume 13

ISBN   0 443 05868 7

# Contents

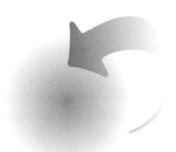

## OBSTETRICS

# Contributors

**Mohamed G.K. Abdalla** MD MSc MRCOG
Consultant in Obstetrics and Gynaecology, Wexham Park Hospital, Wexham Street, Slough SL2 4HL, UK

**S.A. Beardsworth** MRCOG
Clinical Research Fellow, Centre for Metabolic Bone Disease, Hull Royal Infirmary, Hull, UK

**Brian Beattie** MD MRCOG
Consultant in Fetal Medicine, University Hospital of Wales, Cardiff, UK

**John Bidmead** MBBS MRCOG
Research Fellow, Department of Urogynaecology, King's College Hospital, London, UK

**Iain T. Cameron** BSc MA MD FRCOG MRANZCOG
Professor of Obstetrics and Gynaecology, Princess Anne Hospital, Southampton, UK

**Linda D. Cardozo** MD FRCOG
Professor of Urogynaecology, King's College School of Medicine and Dentistry, and Consultant Gynaecologist, King's College Hospital, London, UK

**John Cason** PhD
Senior Lecturer, The Richard Dimbleby Laboratory of Cancer Virology, UMDS Guys and St Thomas' Hospital, London, UK

**Geoffrey Chamberlain** MD FRCS FRCOG FACOG
Emeritus Professor in Obstetrics and Gynaecology, Singleton Hospital, Swansea, UK

**Kevin G. Cooper** MSc MD MRCOG
Consultant Gynaecologist, Aberdeen Royal Infirmary, Aberdeen, UK

**Q. Davies** MRCOG, FRCS
Subspecialty Trainee, Department of Obstetrics and Gynaecology, City Hospital NHS Trust, Birmingham, UK

**Omer Devaja** MD MS PhD
Subspecialty Fellow, Department of Gynaecologic Oncology, Guys and St Thomas' Hospital, London, UK

**Michael P. Diamond** MD
Director, Division of Reproductive Endocrinology and Infertility, and Professor of the Department of Obstetrics and Gynecology, Wayne State University, Detroit, Michigan, USA

**T. Draycott** BSc MD MRCOG
Specialist Registrar, Department of Obstetrics and Gynaecology, Taunton and Somerset Hospital, Taunton, UK

**James Drife** MD FRCOG FRCPS FRCSE
Head, Division of Obstetrics and Gynaecology, Leeds General Infirmary, Leeds, UK

**D.L. Economides** MD FRCOG
Consultant and Senior Lecturer, University Department of Obstetrics and Gynaecology, Royal Free Hospital, London, UK

**Diaa El-Mowafi** MD
Associate Professor, Obstetrics and Gynaecology Department, Benha Faculty of Medicine, Egypt; Lecturer and Researcher, Wayne State University, Detroit, Michigan, USA

**Robert Fox** MD MRCPI MRCOG
Consultant Gynaecologist, Directorate of Obstetrics, Gynaecology and Paediatrics, Taunton and Somerset Hospital, Taunton, UK

**E. F. Nigel Holland** MD MRCOG DipVen
Consultant Gynaecologist, Warrington District General Hospital, Warrington, UK

**Jon Hyett** MRCOG
Specialist Registrar, Department of Obstetrics and Gynaecology, University College Hospital, London, UK

**Gerry J. Jarvis** MA BM BCh FRCSE FRCOG
Consultant in Obstetrics and Gynaecology, St James's University Hospital, Leeds, UK

**Richard Johanson** MA BSc MD MRCOG
Consultant Obstetrician and Gynaecologist, North Staffordshire Hospital, Stoke on Trent, UK

**Frank Johnstone** MD FRCOG
Senior Lecturer, Department of Obstetrics and Gynaecology, University of Edinburgh and Consultant, Simpson Memorial Maternity Pavilion, Edinburgh, UK

**Griff Jones** MRCOG
Fellow in Maternal Fetal Medicine, Division of Perinatology, Ottawa General Hospital, Ottawa, Canada

**C.E. Kearney** MRCOG
Clinical Research Fellow, Centre for Metabolic Bone Disease, Hull Royal Infirmary, Hull, UK

**Gautam Khastgir** MD FRCS MRCOG
Subspecialty Senior Registrar in Reproductive Medicine and Honorary
Lecturer in Obstetrics and Gynaecology, Department of Obstetrics and
Gynaecology, Imperial College School of Medicine, Chelsea & Westminster
Hospital, London, UK

**Lorin Lakasing** MRCOG
Specialist Registrar, Department of Obstetrics and Gynaecology, Northwick
Park Hospital, Harrow, Middlesex, UK

**Michelle Laybourn** MB ChB
House Officer General Surgery, Tameside General Hospital, Ashton under
Lyne, UK

**D.M. Luesley** MA MD FRCOG
Professor of Gynaecological Oncology, Department of Obstetrics and
Gynaecology, City Hospital NHS Trust, Birmingham, UK

**Anthony M. Mander** FRCOG
Consultant Obstetrician/Gynaecologist, The Royal Oldham Hospital,
Oldham, UK

**Isaac Manyonda** BSc PhD MRCOG
Consultant Gynaecologist, Department of Obstetrics and Gynaecology, St
George's Hospital, London, UK

**Michael J.A. Maresh** MD FRCOG
Consultant Obstetrician and Gynaecologist, St Mary's Hospital for Women
and Children, Manchester, UK

**Darryl Maxwell** FRCOG MRACOG
Director and Consultant Obstetrician, Fetal Medicine Unit, Guy's and St
Thomas' Hospital Trust, London, UK

**C. Jay McGavigan** MBBS
Clinical Research Fellow, University Department of Obstetrics and
Gynaecology, The Queen Mother's Hospital, Yorkhill, Glasgow, UK

**Jack Moodley** MB ChB FCOG(SA) FRCOG MD
Professor and Head, MRC/UN Pregnancy Hypertension Research Unit and
Department of Obstetrics and Gynaecology, University of Natal Medical
School, Durban, South Africa

**Andreas J. Papadopoulos** BSc MD MRCOG
Subspecialty Fellow, Department of Gynaecologic Oncology, Guys and St
Thomas' Hospital, London, UK

**Fathima Paruk** MBChB FCOG
Consultant, MRC/UN Pregnancy Hypertension Research Unit and
Department of Obstetrics and Gynaecology, University of Natal Medical
School, Durban, South Africa

**Sara Paterson-Brown** FRCS MRCOG MA
Consultant in Obstetrics and Gynaecology, Queen Charlotte's and Chelsea
Hospital, London, UK

**D.W. Purdie** MD FRCOG FRCP(E)
Head of Clinical Research, Centre for Metabolic Bone Disease, Hull Royal
Infirmary, Hull, UK

**Kankipati S. Raju** MD FRCOG
Director of Gynaecologic Oncology, Guys and St Thomas' Hospital, London, UK

**M.D. Read** MD FRCS(E) FRCOG
Consultant Obstetrician and Gynaecologist, Women's Health Directorate, Gloucestershire Royal NHS Trust, Gloucester, UK

**John Richardson** FRCS FRCOG
Consultant Gynaecologist, Directorate of Obstetrics, Gynaecology and Paediatrics, Taunton and Somerset Hospital, Taunton, UK

**David M. Semple** MRCOG
Specialist Registrar in Obstetrics and Gynaecology, Department of Gynaecology, Liverpool Women's Hospital, Crown Street, Liverpool , UK

**Nahid Siraj** MBBS MRCOG
Staff Grade, Obstetrics and Gynaecology Directorate, North Staffordshire Hospital, Stoke on Trent, UK

**John A.D. Spencer** FRCOG
Consultant, Department of Obstetrics and Gynaecology, Northwick Park Hospital, Harrow, Middlesex, UK

**Anil Sharma** MB MRCOG MRANZCOG
Senior Specialist Registrar, Directorate of Obstetrics, Gynaecology and Paediatrics, Taunton and Somerset Hospital, Taunton, UK

**John Studd** DSc MD FRCOG
Consultant Gynaecologist, Academic Department of Obstetrics and Gynaecology, Chelsea and Westminster Hospital, London, UK

**Anne Szarewski** MBBS DRCOG PhD MFFP
Senior Clinical Research Fellow in Gynaecological Oncology, Department of Mathematics, Statistics and Epidemiology, Imperial Cancer Research Fund, London and Senior Clinical Medical Officer, Margaret Pyke Centre for Study and Training in Family Planning and Reproductive Health Care, London, UK

**Ranee Thakar** MBBS MRCOG
Subspecialty Trainee in Urogynaecology, Department of Obstetrics and Gynaecology, St George's Hospital, London, UK

**Basky Thilaganathan** MD MRCOG
Senior Lecturer/Consultant and Director, Fetal Medicine Unit, St George's Hospital, London, UK

**J. Guy Thorpe-Beeston** MA MD MRCOG
Consultant Obstetrician, Chelsea & Westminster Hospital, London, UK

**B.J. Whitlow** MBBS
Clinical Research Fellow, University Department of Obstetrics and Gynaecology, Royal Free Hospital, London, UK

**Nuala Woodman** MSc
Research Assistant, Women's Health Directorate, Gloucestershire Royal NHS Trust, Gloucester, UK

*Tim Draycott  Michael D. Read*

# Training obstetricians in practical skills

'*See one, do one, teach one*' has been, for some time, the main way of teaching practical skills in obstetrics. Labour ward skills were taught by the next most senior person on the on-call rota irrespective of their abilities. This is in stark contrast to most gynaecological procedures, which are generally taught by consultants often under direct supervision. Whilst this situation may have been appropriate previously, there is an increasing requirement for more formal structured training in obstetric practical skills.

The introduction of the New Deal,[1] Calmanisation[2] and the approaching adoption of the European Working Hours Directive for junior doctors, have combined to shorten the working hours and the duration of training for junior doctors. At the same time, there is an increasing call for a greater consultant presence on the labour ward to meet the recommendations of the RCOG/RCM report.[3]

Both the recent confidential enquiries, the Confidential Enquiry Into Maternal Mortality[4] and the Confidential Enquiry Into Stillbirths and Deaths in Infancy (CESDI),[5] have highlighted the tragic consequences of substandard care, recommending improved, multi-disciplinary training. The latest CESDI report also highlighted the 'hidden' morbidity of sub-standard care for both mothers and babies. In addition, there are ever increasing patient expectations and the expectations of junior staff, who are demanding greater supervision, to be considered.

The advent of clinical governance will also have a significant impact and one must not underestimate the requirements of the Clinical Negligence Scheme for

**Mr Michael D. Read** MD FRCSEd FRCOG, Consultant Obstetrician and Gynaecologist, Women's Health Directorate, Gloucestershire Royal NHS Trust, Great Western Road, Gloucester GL1 3NN, UK (for correspondence)

**Mr Tim Draycott** BSc MD MRCOG, Specialist Registrar, Department of Obstetrics and Gynaecology, Taunton and Somerset Hospital, Taunton TA1 5DA, UK

Trusts (CNST). For units complying fully with the requirements of Level 2 of the CNST, which includes that consultants will be present on the labour ward with no other commitments for a minimum of 40 h per week, there are significant financial benefits. Underlying many of the recommendations for increased consultant presence on the labour ward, there is an expectation that the presence and more active involvement of consultants on the delivery suite will lead to a reduction in problems and subsequent litigation. This assumption has yet to be tested but there is indirect evidence from other specialties, including paediatrics,[6] general surgery[7] as well as obstetrics,[8] which suggest that there may be fewer complications with increased supervision.

It is rather unfair to give the impression that these changes are only being driven from outside the profession, as many consultants have expressed concern over the level of direct supervision the registrars have in the acute aspects of the service, which includes delivery suite, compared with the level of supervision which is available for the more elective aspects of our service including ante natal clinics, out-patient clinics and operating theatre lists. This disparity is not of anyone's deliberate choosing, but rather a reflection of the way the demands of the workload have been traditionally met and underlines the need for a significant expansion in consultant numbers.

There is certainly a need for consultants to maintain their labour ward skills, and perhaps some of the older consultants may require updating and relearning of their skills. In practice, it is likely that many units will develop their own arrangements to meet this potential need, with the younger members of the consultant team carrying a greater share of the acute obstetric load, allowing the older consultants to concentrate on other essential aspects of the day-to-day running of a department.

The working patterns of the consultant post are changing and will continue to change significantly. There is, as yet, no clear picture of the later stages of this evolution and, like any evolutionary process, different patterns will be adopted to meet local circumstances; but it is certain that the majority of future consultant posts will involve 'hands on' work in the delivery suite and so it is important that current trainees continue to develop and maintain their skills.

In this chapter, we explore a wide spectrum of approaches to training which can enhance and consolidate traditional approaches, but the important fact remains that there can be no substitute for one-to-one 'apprenticeship' training with a good quality structured approach. To many it may seem old fashioned, but in any sphere of our specialty it is, and will remain, the backbone of training.

## ANTENATAL AND INTRAPARTUM ELECTIVE PROCEDURES

### Ultrasound scanning

Over the years, the largely teach-yourself approach has led to unfortunate situations and occasional high profile media coverage of problems. Clearly, this approach is unacceptable and inexcusable and no trainee should be allowed to make executive decisions based on their own ultrasound examinations without having had adequate training to the appropriate level.

Not all trainees will have the opportunity or the desire to fulfil the criteria for the RCOG/RCR Joint Certificate in Obstetric Ultrasound. However, the possession of this certificate or recognised equivalent training will probably be a prerequisite for appointments to new consultant posts identified as having obstetric ultrasound or fetal medicine as a special interest.

Short of these stringent requirements, there is scope for a structured approach to ultrasound training for such areas as early pregnancy problems, fetal presentation and viability. Central guidelines from the RCOG and RCR would be useful, but, until then, regional training committees could agree a protocol and the individual hospitals could implement this, arranging for trainees to be released from other clinical duties for 'blocks' of intensive training. Anticipation, organisation and co-operation are all that is required to deliver this. Beyond this core foundation, individual trainees can maintain and develop their experience during their special interest sessions and some will choose to go on to certificate level training. Of necessity, this ultrasound training is essentially one-to-one.

## Amniocentesis and chorionic villus sampling

There should no longer be any role for amniocenteses being done by 'the registrar of the day'. In order to reduce the risk of pregnancy loss, unsuccessful or traumatic taps, amniocentesis should be done by experienced 'permanent' staff. Trainees undergoing intermediate level ultrasound training can be taught the technique on a one-to-one basis. Chorionic villus sampling is probably best reserved for advanced trainees only (e.g. those undertaking certificate level training).

## External cephalic version

There will be a good number of older consultants who will have seen the ECV wheel turn full cycle, from widespread use in the 1960s and early 1970s, through 20 years of exile, now to see its credibility restored and the RCOG deciding it should be discussed with all women with breech presentations and that all units should offer the facility. This resurgence of interest is only just in time, as there is a rapidly decreasing number of obstetricians who actually had significant experience of the technique previously who are around to teach the technique to the current generation of trainees.

Recent publications have confirmed that the success rate of ECV is proportional to the experience of the operator and this is another technique which should rest with selected individuals, probably those with a special interest in obstetrics.[9,10]

## Cardiotocographs

The use of continuous electronic fetal monitoring is widespread. However, interpretation, upon which clinical decisions rest, is imprecise – still more of an art than a science. There are a number of courses available to impart the fundamentals of the course organisers' views of fetal physiology, response to labour and relation to CTG traces. There is no need to continuously monitor everyone. It is not necessary and not what the patient wants.[11,12] In order to use the technique safely, regular 'in house' programmes are advisable to review

CTG traces in the context of actual cases and known outcomes. Weekly joint meetings between obstetricians and midwives – held in a reflective rather than adversarial atmosphere – can be very constructive.

## OBSTETRIC EMERGENCIES

Obstetric emergencies are, thankfully, rare but they characteristically have a high mortality and morbidity often due to 'substandard care'. They are difficult to train for, as they are sporadic and obviously cannot be 'arranged' during supervised sessions as a learning exercise which makes them very good candidates for computer simulations. The management of post partum haemorrhage (PPH) and eclampsia have repeatedly been highlighted as substandard by consecutive CEMM reports[4,13] and there are two programmes currently being piloted for these two emergencies.

Guidelines already exist for eclampsia[13] and for PPH.[13] However, these can be difficult to access, particularly in an emergency; and they are discussion documents rather than didactic instructions, which makes them difficult to use in practice. The guidelines should be modified to provide instruction sheets, flow charts and posters (similar to those already used for Cardiac Life Support) which should be regularly updated and adapted to provide a set of simple clear step-by-step instructions useful in the rapid emergency situation.

### Computer modelling

Training needs to be made available alongside these instruction sheets. The knowledge base required to accurately manage emergencies can be taught using computer aided learning (CAL) techniques prepared for Internet distribution. At first glance, the use of computers to teach practical skills appears to be rather pointless; but computer programmes have been successfully used alone, and together with mannequins, to teach practical skills for a variety of different subjects. It has been proposed that CAL systems utilise an efficient and effective method of learning.[14] Similarly, they are potentially very flexible and relatively inexpensive after the initial development costs.[15] They can be made readily accessible over a wide geographical area and easily updated to incorporate current research findings. CAL is particularly useful for individuals who initially wish to increase their theoretical knowledge of how to manage emergencies.

Knowledge alone is not enough for the effective management of emergencies, however. There is also a need for team training using simulation. The method does not need to be high-tech. Simple rehearsal using a minimum of equipment has the advantage that the method can be delivered locally so that the members of the in-house team can be trained together. Rehearsals can then occur frequently and recurrent problems analysed and amended. These 'fire drills' would be cheaper than distant courses, and reach a wider (multidisciplinary) audience. Another spin off is that team working and morale can be improved in parallel with local facilities.

### Post partum haemorrhage

A computer programme has been developed in the Northern Region for the management of PPH which requires the user to order blood, ask for help, give oxytocics, etc. and make decisions after an Examination Under Anaesthesia. The programme is based on the current RCOG/CEMM protocol for the management of post partum haemorrhage. There are a number of different scenarios available including atonic uterus, RPOCs and cervical and vaginal tears, each of which need different management strategies. The programme shows blood loss in real time with appropriate changes in the haemodynamic status of the patient depending on the fluids and oxytocics administered. There are also delays built into the programme to reproduce a life like clinical scenario. For example, the anaesthetist may take 10 min to arrive after being called and no surgical management strategies are possible until they have arrived. Cross-matched blood also taking significantly longer to arrive than either O negative blood or Group specific blood.

In a pilot evaluation in Leeds, obstetricians of varying grades were assessed using the programme. Their drill responses were compared with the departmental protocol for the management of post partum haemorrhage. Only one person treated the patient exactly following the protocol; however, all found the programme to be subjectively very useful and, after the exercise, individual feedback was given to the participants.[17]

## Eclampsia

An Internet based tutorial for the management of eclampsia has been developed. (www.swot.org.uk/simulator/titlepage) after deciding that a web based tutorial potentially offered a number of advantages over other CAL packages including the shorter learning curve required for html (the programming language on which web pages are produced) authoring programmes (e.g. MS Front Page™), platform independence and a single, generic set of browser skills would be sufficient for the target audience to use the tutorial.

The needs of the target audience were assessed using data from the Confidential Enquiry into Maternal Mortality. The most recent report identified the most common areas of substandard care for all women who died due to pregnancy induced hypertension, including eclampsia.[4]

Using the RCOG Guidelines for the Management of Eclampsia,[14] a series of linked web pages was authored by a clinician with basic computer skills. The tutorial was then evaluated in a series of multi-disciplinary workshops across the South West Region. The tutorial was successful in its primary objective to increase the knowledge base of the target audience for the management of eclampsia for 89% of the trainees. There was an improvement in some, though not all, of the areas previously identified in the Confidential Enquiry into Maternal Mortality as deficient, in particular the initial management of fitting caused confusion.

Trainees and trainers alike supported the use of the tutorial and the moderated discussion format with a tutor using the CAL programme to lead a teaching programme.

## Surgical skills

CAL programmes have also successfully been used in conjunction with mannequins. In a recent pilot of a CD ROM produced for the Royal College of

General Practitioners for the Diagnosis and Management of Minor Surgery & Skin Lesions,[18] participants preferred to use the CD ROM with the mannequins to using either CD-ROM or mannequins in isolation.[19]

## Training mannequins

Training mannequins have been demonstrated to improve retention of knowledge where incorporated into a training course[20] and to improve participants' practical skills.[21] These mannequins can vary in sophistication from the ever-present plastic pelvis and prison manufactured suede baby, through the 'Resusci-Annie' commonly used to teach the practical skills required during an arrest, right up to full scale theatre mock ups used for anaesthetic training.[22,23]

Similar mannequin technology could be used for a number of practical obstetric procedures, especially shoulder dystocia. It is widely recognised that shoulder dystocia is difficult to predict and, therefore, accurate, effective management is required at the time of presentation. Training is difficult especially because the manoeuvres needed for the management of shoulder dystocia are difficult to understand from a two dimensional book page. However, recent experience on the Management of Obstetric Emergencies & Trauma (MOET) course and Advanced Life Support in Obstetrics (ALSO) courses has demonstrated that these manoeuvres are readily understood using mannequins and models. Moreover, the use of these mannequins has been extremely popular with the participants.

More sophisticated mannequins are required and a successful model will have applications far beyond shoulder dystocia. The model could be used for training in normal deliveries, instrumental deliveries and indeed most obstetric vaginal procedures.

## Courses

Results demonstrate reduced mortality rates for patients treated by professionals who have attended training courses, as appropriate and effective treatment is provided more often and at an earlier stage.[24] There are no such standardised training schemes for obstetric emergencies in the UK, whereas they do exist for the management of major trauma, cardiac arrest and paediatric emergencies (Advanced Trauma Life Support, Advanced Cardiac Life Support, Advanced Paediatric Life Support). The American Academy of Family Physicians developed a course for the management of obstetric emergencies[25] which has been successfully used around the UK. The RCOG has also piloted a course for the management of obstetric emergencies aimed at the Management of Obstetric Emergencies & Trauma (MOET). Initial reports have been encouraging and the evaluation is currently on-going.[26]

However, the teaching methods adopted are expensive in capital outlay and very labour intensive. In addition to these financial limitations, large, centrally run courses may not have the penetration required to improve practice at the place of care, i.e. the labour ward. To ensure that best research evidence translates accurately into best practice a different model for rehearsal of obstetric emergencies is needed.

## Fire drills

The recent CESDI report[4] recommended the adoption of 'fire drills' to improve the management of rare obstetric emergencies and, whilst this umbrella term has not been defined, it may usefully be used for low-tech role play or simulation at a local level. Locally implemented drills would be cheaper than distant, expensive courses; reach a wider, more multi-disciplinary audience and also teach useful team working skills. It is important that all ward staff are involved because that is 'real life'. It is just as important for the nurse auxiliaries to complete their tasks adequately as any other member of the team – a detail missed by most courses!

A simple 'fire drill' has been developed for the management of eclampsia.[27] After the Collaborative Eclampsia Trial finished, many of the participating units continued to use the 'Trial Packs' containing the magnesium sulphate because they provided an easy to use, centralised collection of appropriate drugs for the emergency management of eclampsia[28] - a principle already utilised by the ubiquitous cardiac arrest trolleys. On this basis, an eclampsia box was developed. This contains all the drugs (anticonvulsants and antihypertensives), giving sets, venflons, etc. needed for the management of eclamptic episode, stored in an easily identifiable box on the labour ward. However, after a period of evaluation using the box for simulated eclamptic fits, a number of modifications were made and clear, didactic instructions for the management of eclampsia were included within the box.

The new, improved, eclampsia box has subsequently been evaluated and is now acceptable to all. There have been two eclamptic fits in our department since the introduction of this eclampsia box and staff who participated in the simulations all felt more confident with their subsequent management in this real-life situation. So much so that those who had not been able to attend one of the simulations all asked for more to be arranged.

Interestingly, during the evaluation in different units across the South West, the 'fire drill' revealed problems quite specific to the individual units. These have been enthusiastically addressed on an individual unit basis leading to individual solutions to their own problems but all improving the local management of eclampsia.

Although we have been unable to demonstrate a reduction in maternal mortality, the introduction of this 'fire drill' has improved staff confidence, performance levels and local facilities for the acute management of eclampsia.

## THE ROLE OF THE CONSULTANT IN THE DELIVERY SUITE

With the increasing trend for consultant sessions on the delivery suite (not merely a nominal session but a minimum of 40 h per week), there is an understandable fear that the role of the registrar will become redundant or relegated to the status of observer or supernumerary. There is also potential for midwives to be concerned that the low risk mothers who they look after in labour may be 'medicalised.

There is indeed a fine line between a consultant giving leadership by example and taking over completely the duties which have traditionally been the province of the junior staff; but, ideally, the consultant should lead the medical team on duty, delegating duties according to the experience of staff available and will draw on, support, and co-ordinate the expertise of other team members to ensure the best available patient care. Delivery suite sessions should be treated as fixed sessional commitments with no other conflicting demands on the consultant's time and the consultant should participate in the handover ward rounds at the beginning of each session. In this way, the consultant presence can strengthen the delivery suite team providing direct supervision of trainees and the flexibility to release them for other aspects of their training programmes. Observation of trainees practice will provide assessment and feedback for both trainee and training programme director. The presence of the consultant can also strengthen audit and risk management programmes. This system offers an ideal opportunity for the consultant to teach registrar and career senior house officers the practical procedures such as Caesarean section, the correct use of Ventouse and forceps and fetal blood sampling rather than relying on the traditional registrar teaching the SHO system which as been so common in the past.

It is important to recognise that this experience is two-way and, over the years, one of the authors has learned many useful tips and techniques from the registrars and very much hopes that this will continue.

When the workload demands it, the consultant would also be available to work independently; it is likely that, in future, there will be an increasing number of occasions when consultants will be working 'on the shop floor' without a registrar, particularly as the numbers of specialist registrars (NTNs) are gradually reduced to the point where, we are told by manpower meetings at the RCOG,[29] there will be only one registrar to two or three consultants.

Meetings between the midwives, consultants and registrars to review interesting labour ward cases similar to the CTG meetings described earlier, can be very useful in consolidating experience, as has been well demonstrated in Dublin[30] and France.[31]

## CONCLUSION

There is no doubt that improved supervised training is going to be required to meet the increasing demands and expectations. Following the recent high profile cases, from which our specialty is not immune, there is a definite risk of our losing the good faith and support of our patients. We must not allow this to happen. Where available, best evidence-based practice should be followed (bearing in mind that there is 'evidence' for perhaps 20% of current practice). New technologies should be embraced where they can support and enhance training but, above all, there can be no substitute for direct one-to-one supervision of training. The wholesale pursuit of the certification of every possible skill can lead to dangers of over specialisation and difficulty with maintaining a comprehensive service (as is now being experienced in some areas by our surgical colleagues), until now run by that disappearing breed of 'generalist' of whom one of the authors is an unashamed member. Rather, there is a need to rely on documented experience and honest self-assessment with agreement within departments to develop areas of interest and expertise with appropriate cross referral.

## References

1 Junior Doctors. The New Deal. London: NHS Management Executive, 1991
2 Calman K. Hospital Doctors: Training for the Future. London: Department of Health, 1993
3 Joint Working Party of the RCOG/RCM. Towards Safer Childbirth, Minimum Standards for the Organisation of Labour Wards. London: RCOG, 1999
4 Department of Health. Why Do Mothers Die? Report on Confidential Enquiries into Maternal Deaths in the United Kingdom, 1991–1993. London: Department of Health, 1998
5 Maternal and Child Health Consortium. Confidential Enquiry into Stillbirths and Deaths in Infancy. 5th Annual Report. London: Department of Health, 1988
6 Hare M J, Miles R N, Lattimore C R, Southern JP. Short report staffing in practice: five years' experience of a consultant based service in obstetrics and neonatal paediatrics. BMJ 1990; 300: 857–9
   http://wwwbiomednet.com/db/medline/90248631
7 Aitken R J, Thompson M R, Smith J A E, Radcliffe A G, Stamatakis JD, Steele R J C. Training in large bowel cancer surgery: observations from three prospective regional United Kingdom audits. BMJ 1999; 318: 702–3
8 Stewart J H, Andrews J, Cartlidge P. Numbers of deaths related to intrapartum asphyxia and timing of birth in all Wales. Perinatal survey 1993–5. BMJ 1998; 316: 657–60
9 Hofmeyer G J. External cephalic version at term. In: Neilson J P, Crowther C A, Hodnett E D, Hofmeyer G J, Keirse M J N C (eds) Pregnancy and Childbirth Module of The Cochrane Database of Systematic Reviews. Available in: The Cochrane Library, Issue 2. The Cochrane Collaboration, Oxford, Update Software
10 Van Veelen A J, Van Capellen A W, Flu P K et al. Effect of external cephalic version in late pregnancy on presentation at delivery: a randomised controlled trial. Br J Obstet Gynaecol 1989; 96, 916–21
11 MacDonald D, Grant A, Sheridan-Pereira M, Boylan P, Chalmers I. The Dublin randomized controlled trial of intrapartum fetal heart rate monitoring. Am J Obstet Gynecol 1985: 152: 524–39
12 Thacker S B, Stroup D F. Continuous electronic heart rate monitoring versus intermittent auscultation for assessment during labor. The Cochrane Library 1999; Issue 1 Page 1
13 Department of Health. Report on Confidential Enquiries into Maternal Deaths in the United Kingdom 1988–1990. London: Department of Health, 1994
14 Royal College of Obstetricians and Gynaecologists. Eclampsia Guidelines. London: RCOG 1996
15 Jelovsek F R, Adebonojo L. Learning principles as applied to computer assisted instruction. MD Comput 1993; 10: 165–72
16 Santer D, Michaelsen V E, Erkonen WE et al. A comparison of educational interventions. Multimedia textbook, standard lecture, and printed textbook. Arch Pediatr Adolesc Med 1995; 149: 297–302
17 Tomlinson A J, Simpson N A. Use of a computer programme to simulate primary post partum haemorrhage: a tool for training. Abstracts of British Congress of Obstetrics & Gynaecology. London: Blackwell, 1998
18 Kneebone R, Schofield J. Minor Surgery and Skin Lesions. London: Royal College of General Practitioners, 1988
   www.rcgp.co.uk
19 Cooper M. Using CD ROMs and mannequins together for a GP workshop. Limbs and Things, Medical and Anatomical Models. 1999
   http://limbsandthings.com
20 Kaczorowski J, Levitt C, Hammond M et al. Retention of neonatal resuscitation skills and knowledge: a randomized controlled trial. Family Med 1988; 30: 705–11
21 White J R, Shugerman R et al. Performance of advanced resuscitation skills by pediatric housestaff. Arch Pediatr Adolesc Med 1998; 152: 1232–5
   http://www.biomednet.com/db/medline/99072255
22 Norman J, Wilkins D. Simulators for anaesthesia. J Clin Monitor 1996; 12: 91–9
23 Forrest F, Taylor M. High level simulators in medical education. Hosp Med 1998; 59: 653–5

24 Williams L, Muwanga C, Worlock PH, Moran CG, Price KA. Teaching trauma management in the accident and emergency department. Arch Emerg Med 1995; 8: 205–9

25 Lewis P. The Advanced Life Support in Obstetrics course. Mod Midwife 1996; 6: 17–9

26 Johanson R B, Cox C. MOET: Management of Obstetric Emergencies and Trauma. 1998 (personal communication)

27 Draycott T, Broad G, Chidley K. The development of an Eclampsia Box and Firedrill. Br J Midwifery 2000; 8: 26–30

28 Duley L, The Eclampsia Trial Collaborative Group. Which anticonvulsant for women with eclampsia? Lancet 1995; 345: 1455–63

29 Crisis or Opportunity. Manpower Meeting. RCOG 21 April 1999

30 Impey L, Boylan P. Active management of labour revisited. Br J Obstet Gynaecol 1999; 106: 183–7

31 Draycott T. Report of the VII Meeting and Exchange of European Trainees in Obstetrics and Gynaecology. London: RCOG, 1999

*Lorin Lakasing  John A.D. Spencer*

# Clinical risk management in obstetrics

Clinical risk management (CRM) is a process of identifying and investigating cases where the perception of risk has arisen. This includes not only cases with a poor outcome, but also the 'near miss' incidents where, despite a good outcome, more effective clinical management may have prevented a potentially dangerous situation developing in the first place.[1]

CRM has been widely implemented in the US for some years and is of growing importance in the UK. This move has been largely driven by the rise in medical litigation and the subsequent cost to the Trusts.[2] CRM programmes are co-ordinated by clinical risk managers whose main role is to use the information obtained from the process to prepare the Trust against possible medico-legal action. In most units, obstetric cases form a majority of cases reported. High patient expectation, intolerance of risk and trial by media are particular problems in our specialty. Now with the practice of clinical governance,[3,4] a concept introduced in the Government's 1997 White Paper,[5] we can anticipate criticism not only from patients and the public, but also from our own colleagues.

In this chapter, we discuss the role of CRM from the perspective of the medical profession, the patient and the Trust. We also consider how CRM might affect obstetric practice in the future.

## CLINICAL RISK MANAGEMENT AND HEALTH CARE PROFESSIONALS

For CRM in obstetrics to work in practice, the programme must have the support of all maternity health care professionals. When implementing the

**Dr Lorin Lakasing MRCOG,** Specialist Registrar, Department of Obstetrics and Gynaecology, Northwick Park Hospital, Harrow, Middlesex HA1 3UJ, UK

**Mr John A.D. Spencer** FRCOG, Consultant, Department of Obstetrics and Gynaecology, Northwick Park Hospital, Harrow, Middlesex HA1 3UJ, UK

CRM protocol, the important steps to consider include identification of cases, writing CRM reports, assessment by the CRM team, feedback to staff, defining deficiencies in obstetric practice and tackling the problems. These are discussed below.

## Identification of cases

Early identification of notifiable events is recommended as it facilitates prompt investigation. Cases are identified either by staff reports or systematic screening of case notes.[6,7] Some are identified by paediatric colleagues following a poor neonatal outcome, and some follow an unexpected patient complaint. In each case, a CRM form is completed and brought to the attention of the obstetric CRM team. This usually consists of the Delivery Suite manager (a senior midwife) and a lead clinician (a consultant obstetrician). If initial review by the CRM team considers it appropriate, various individuals involved in the case are then requested to write a report regarding their role in the clinical management of the patient. In particular, emphasis is placed on their recollection of the events thought to have contributed to the outcome under investigation.

## Writing CRM reports

CRM is best conducted in a 'no blame' environment and it is important to stress that staff reports are used to ascertain the facts surrounding each case and not as a basis for personal criticism, litigation and disciplinary action.[8] The timing and sequence of events are critically important and, therefore, it is recommended that these reports are written as soon as possible following the events before memories fade or become altered by opinions expressed by others. Reports should be written in such a way that an educated but non-medical person can read them and recreate the events in his/her mind. The content of the reports should be factual and all actions by the staff involved in the care of the patient should be explained. These reports are designed to supplement the information entered into the patient's case notes. The completed reports are reviewed by the CRM team. At this point, initial feedback to staff may be appropriate particularly if clarification is required.

## Assessment by the CRM team

The Delivery Suite Manager, the Lead Obstetrician and the Clinical Risk Manager for the Trust form the core team. In some circumstances other obstetric or paediatric consultants will be involved. Regular meetings are held to discuss progress in each case. This team approach enables recurrent patterns of practice contributing to poor outcomes to be identified,[9] and highlights areas where audit and revision of guidelines are considered necessary. For each case, a summary is completed and this information entered onto a database.

## Feedback to staff

Regular staff feedback sessions are undertaken in order to elevate standards of practice and encourage commitment to the CRM process. Such feedback/

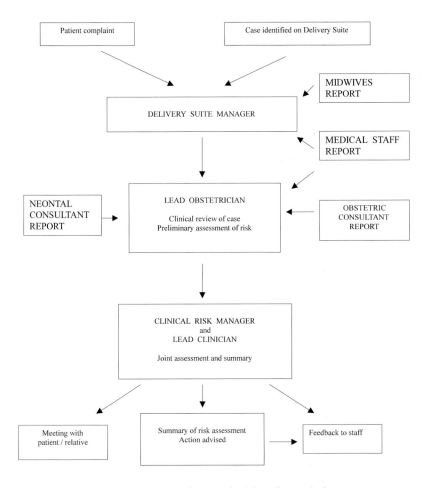

**Fig. 1** Clinical risk management protocol at Northwick Park Hospital.

teaching sessions can range from formal departmental lectures, to small groups taking part in interactive workshops. The midwifery and medical staff should be made aware of areas of deficiency in clinical practice which have been identified by CRM, and any new guidelines implemented. A schematic representation of the CRM protocol used at Northwick Park Hospital is shown in Figure 1.

## Defining deficiencies in clinical practice

Incident reporting in obstetrics is not a new concept. The Confidential Enquiries into Maternal Deaths (CEMD) established in 1952 produces triennial reports giving detailed accounts of these adverse events,[10] and more recently the Confidential Enquiries into Stillbirths and Deaths in Infancy (CESDI) established in 1995 produces annual reports.[11] Both of these have sought to identify failures in clinical management which directly contribute to adverse outcome. However, what CRM can potentially achieve is much more ambitious than this, and has the particular advantage of providing information which enables local issues specific to the unit to be highlighted.

By employing specific methods of incident analysis, we can not only focus on these direct failures, but also highlight the more subtle organisational features which adversely influence outcome. This type of detailed information is rarely available,[12] although there are notable exceptions.[13,14] One such method of incident analysis was developed by Reason to study large scale industrial accidents,[15,16] and this has been adapted for use in a medical setting.[17,18] He categorised errors in human decisions or actions as either 'active' failures or 'latent' failures.[19] Active failures include deviation from standard accepted practice, acts of omission and misinterpretation of data. These were commonly found to be the result of lack of motivation, low morale and poor examples from senior staff.[18,20] Latent failures arise from wider organisational problems and mainly result from psychological factors involved in interpersonal relationships and limited financial resources. These more subtle factors are just as important and often more difficult to address,[21,22] although attempts have been made to aid recognition of these potentially dangerous areas.[23]

At Northwick Park Hospital, a recent analysis of 195 cases reported to the CRM programme over a 3 year period between 1996–1998 has been completed.[24] In 78 (40%) cases there were potentially remediable deficiencies in clinical management. The main factors contributing to 'active' failures included errors in CTG interpretation (31%), deviations from standard practice (28%) and errors in drug administration (18%). For 'latent' failures these included inadequate communication (37%), deficiencies in staffing levels (30%) and inadequate maintenance of equipment (21%). Analysing cases in this manner highlights specific areas for attention where modification of protocols, staff education and allocation of scarce resources are needed. A schematic representation of the relationship between CRM, audit and staff education/training is shown in Figure 2.

### Tackling the problems

Defining 'safe' practice is difficult and numerous attempts have been made to put in place various systems designed to do this. The General Medical Council (GMC) provides guidance to individual doctors regarding aspects of patient care,[25] the National Institute for Clinical Effectiveness (NICE) provides more general advice, and the Royal Colleges are involved in regular review of guidelines and recommendations for maintaining excellence within each specialty. The Royal College of Obstetricians and Gynaecologists (RCOG) has recently published the Report of a Working Group outlining proposals for the setting of standards of clinical care, monitoring adherence to these standards in practice, and having mechanisms in place for when practice falls short of expectation.[26] In September 1998, The RCOG approved the setting up of a Clinical Effectiveness and Standards Board (CESB) which will produce a co-ordinated and structured programme of guidelines with auditable standards. Monitoring of these standards will be encouraged by promoting audit, clinical governance and revalidation such that doctors have to demonstrate continuing competence at fixed intervals during their careers.[27] Should standards not be

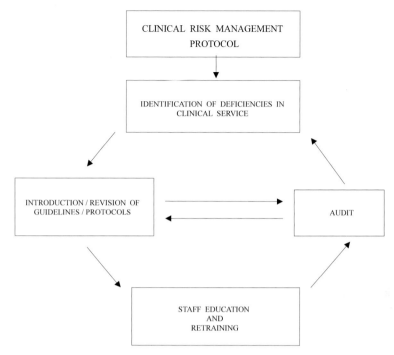

**Fig. 2** Clinical risk management, audit and education.

met, advice will be sought from a panel of senior clinicians/advisors appointed by the RCOG. The RCOG is also likely to set up a mechanism for mediation in disputes between clinicians and managers.

Intrapartum clinical management has always been a priority, and the recent RCOG Report of a Joint Working Party entitled *Towards Safer Childbirth – Minimum Standards for the Organisation of Labour Wards*, detailed recommendations which apply to all maternity units.[28] These include the need for the following: (i) consultant involvement on the Delivery Suite, especially out-of-hours;[29,30] (ii) adequate training and supervision of junior doctors; (iii) guidelines/protocols to be reviewed and up-dated regularly; (iv) formal handovers between medical teams at the start of each shift; (v) good communication with colleagues; (vi) good communication with patients and obtaining informed consent;[31] (vii) continuity of care; (viii) regular maintenance of equipment; and (ix) detailed documentation in case notes.[32] In maternity care there is no difference in workload with respect to time of day[33] and, therefore, these recommendations apply in all circumstances. Studies have shown that errors are more likely to occur when health care professionals work irregular shifts,[34] and this is an area which needs to be addressed.

Whilst these national guidelines are undoubtedly important, problems still need to be tackled at a local level. Specific recommendations will vary from one unit to another, and this is where CRM is potentially of greatest value. For example, in our own unit, after the second annual review of obstetric risk management cases, it was noted that there were several cases of unrecognised uterine hyperstimulation with subsequent fetal distress following augmentation of labour with oxytocin. As a result, the intravenous oxytocin regimen was re-written with particular emphasis on the different doses and different time increments for administration of this drug in primagravid compared with multigravid patients. In addition, new guidelines for the administration of intravenous tocolysis in the treatment of uterine hyper-stimulation were drawn up. Another example from our unit is the recent modification of the protocol for the management of shoulder dystocia. When the CRM reports of these cases were reviewed, it became apparent that the existing guidelines caused considerable confusion. These were subsequently revised and two practical workshops organised to allow feed-back from midwifery and medical staff alongside practical training in the management of this condition.

Problem areas can only be addressed effectively if senior medical and midwifery staff are committed to elevating standards of care. Junior midwives and doctors often feel unduly criticised whilst other senior colleagues within the unit may be unwilling to change their practice. Tact, discretion, team support and dedication to training are essential for a CRM programme to be of benefit in the long-term.

## CLINICAL RISK MANAGEMENT AND THE PATIENT

Patients may encounter numerous problems following an adverse event. Some are particularly upset not by the outcome of their cases so much as the lack of opportunity for discussion with the staff involved in their care such that they can improve their understanding of the clinical events.[35] Long delays in processing and addressing complaints add to their anger and frustration, and many feel that vital information is being withheld.[36] Some will seek advice from the Community Health Council (CHC), a locally appointed lay body whose role it is to ensure that health care standards are maintained. Others will receive support from organisations such as the Association for Victims of Medical Accidents (AVMA) which represent the interests of NHS consumers and help patients to seek financial compensation.

It is well recognised that most disputes arise from misguided allegations[37,38] and much time and money are wasted unnecessarily.[39] If complaints are dealt with efficiently using the information obtained by a CRM programme, patients and their relatives will be better informed and may feel that their concerns are being addressed in an honest and objective manner. An admission that care has been substandard is appreciated by patients, as is the knowledge that all appropriate steps were taken despite a poor outcome.[40] Every opportunity should be taken to create a relaxed atmosphere where patients feel able to question various aspects of their management and, in some cases, more than one meeting may be required. Occasionally, a framework for the management in a future pregnancy is drawn up, and patients may feel that their bad experience has at least in some way been constructive.

In cases where legal action is justified, the CRM programme should provide support and information without hesitation. Recognition of a serious error in management does not alter the initial approach to patient feedback. In equivocal cases, the Clinical Risk Manager for the Trust may recommend outside advice and an external expert opinion may be sought. If the grounds for concern are confirmed, then the patient should be advised to seek legal assistance. This type of independent review is encouraged to show lack of bias or collusion. In our unit, we have assisted in the rapid recognition of a need for financial aid and achieved agreement regarding ongoing management in a recent case.

## CLINICAL RISK MANAGEMENT, THE TRUST AND MEDICAL LITIGATION

Litigation in obstetrics is high and continues to increase.[41] The NHS Litigation Authority deals with claims where large payments are involved and recent data show that obstetric cases account for 24% of claims, but 54% of the cost in terms of payments. Cerebral palsy cases form the majority of claims cases and payments vary between £750,000 and £1.5 million or more depending on the life expectancy. There has been a recent settlement in excess of £3 million. Therefore, for financial reasons, it is in the interest of every NHS Trust to reduce the number of medico-legal claims made against it. Many Trusts perceive the CRM team as being instrumental in this process by virtue of their role in promoting good practice, thought to be the cornerstone of avoidance of litigation.[42] In reality, how much of a direct effect CRM has on reducing future incidents remains unknown.[43]

Attempts have been made to set national minimum standards for risk management practice in order to protect NHS Trusts from the financial consequences of clinical negligence. The Clinical Negligence Scheme for Trusts (CNST) offers financial incentives to those NHS Trusts which meet these standards through discounted contributions.[44] Additional discounts are offered to NHS Trusts which meet not only the minimum standards (level 1), but other optional standards (levels 2 or 3). This scheme has been operational since 1 April 1995 and is constantly being updated as more information from CRM programmes becomes available. NHS Trusts become members of the CNST following an initial assessment, and in subsequent years members who have met the criteria for a given level, may apply for a further assessment if they subsequently satisfy the standards for the next level. At present 98.5% of NHS Trusts are CNST members but over 25% have failed to reach any standards. Of those that have, 67% have met level 1 standards, 5% have met level 2 standards and none have met level 3 standards. NHS Trusts which have benefited from discounted contributions are subject to random CNST assessments to ensure that they continue to maintain the necessary level of compliance. At present the average maternity unit pays £200,000 *per annum* and estimates suggest that these contributions are set to almost double each year. A summary of Risk Management Standard Number 11 pertaining to maternity services from the most recent CNST report is shown in Table 1. These standards are due to be updated in late 1999.

Unfortunately, despite every attempt to elevate standards of care and communicate effectively with patients, it is inevitable that adverse incidents will still occur. A proportion of these will result in justifiable legal action. Medical law is a rapidly evolving area and numerous changes have occurred in the last few years. Until recently, the legal profession applied the Bolam test in the judgement of most medical cases.[45] This focused on adherence to guidelines for clinical practice, and if there was sufficient evidence that an

**Table 1** CNST standards for maternity care

| CNST number | Standard | Level 1 | Level 2 | Level 3 |
|---|---|---|---|---|
| 11.1.1 | The professional responsible for antenatal care clearly identified | * | | |
| 11.1.2 | The professional responsible for intrapartum care is clearly identified | * | | |
| 11.1.3 | There are detailed multi-disciplinary policies for the management of all key conditions on labour ward, e.g. diabetes, pre-eclampsia, shoulder dystocia | * | | |
| 11.1.4 | Senior midwives can refer cases directly to consultants without involvement from junior doctors | * | | |
| 11.1.5 | There is personal handover of care when medical and midwifery shifts change | * | | |
| 11.2.1 | There is a named consultant responsible for Labour Ward matters | | * | |
| 11.2.2 | There are clear guidelines for the transfer of care during the intrapartum period | | * | |
| 11.3.1 | A doctor of 12 months' obstetric experience is on Labour Ward at all times, or available within 5 minutes A doctor of 3 years' obstetric experience is available within 30 minutes | | | * |
| 11.3.2 | The delivery interval in CS for fetal distress is subjected to an annually audited standard | | | * |
| 11.3.3 | There is personal handover to obstetric locums by post holder or senior member of team, and vice-versa | | | * |

individual or group of individuals had deviated from practice widely accepted as being safe by a responsible body of medical opinion, they were held accountable. The NHS Trust they were employed by was then committed to bear the financial burden involved. Over recent years, there has been much criticism about this test of medical competency[46] and, in particular, the credibility of expert witnesses. Some have argued that consideration should be given to negotiated or mediated settlement which may expedite resolution, especially where small claims are involved.[47–49] Others have called for a change in the law and, as a result, the situation has been reviewed by the House of Lords. Over the last 5 years, the new reformed Civil Procedures Rules have been drawn up and these laws were implemented on 26 April 1999.[50] This new system aims to encourage the settlement of disputes prior to formal litigation proceedings in an attempt to avoid unacceptably long delays and large financial losses with the inevitable emotional consequences of these to patients, relatives and health care professionals alike. It is hoped that his approach will be less adversarial, more objective and more efficient at reaching settlements.

# CLINICAL RISK MANAGEMENT IN OBSTETRICS AND THE FUTURE

Maternity care has changed considerably in recent years. The UK Government report *Changing Childbirth*[51] recommended giving women more choice in their care. These changes occurred in response to pressure from consumer groups and midwives. However, as obstetricians, we know that many aspects of maternity care offered to women are of questionable benefit. Routine antenatal visits are of dubious value,[52,53] prenatal diagnosis and obstetric ultrasound imaging is fraught with difficulties of risk evaluation and counselling,[54-56] intrapartum electronic fetal monitoring in plagued by subjective interpretation,[57,58] vaginal delivery (especially if instrumental) is complicated by damage to maternal tissues in a significantly larger number of cases than previously thought,[59] and the Caesarean section rate has been rising steadily,[60,61] with little sign of abating.[62] Even after delivery, despite a well developed community midwifery service, much postnatal morbidity goes unrecognised.[63] Indeed every aspect of pregnancy and childbirth has a degree of risk associated with it. Since almost all women put safety at the top of their list of priorities, it is therefore sensible to assume that their choices reflect the options they consider to have the least associated risk to themselves and/or their babies.

The conflict between patient choice and expectation versus medical judgement is not always easy to resolve. In the late 1980s, Thornton showed that many women were willing to opt for medical intervention and delivery by Caesarean section at lower levels of risk than obstetricians had thought,[64] and more recently some women are requesting delivery by elective Caesarean section on the basis that this is 'safer' for themselves and their babies, a belief which has, in part, been endorsed by the medical profession.[65] Should such a request be refused by the clinician whose care a woman is under, she is free to seek a second opinion. Should she agree to labour and develop a complication which could have contributed to a poor outcome, she may feel she has even more valid grounds for complaint. Should she be delivered by Caesarean section and have a complication as a result of that, she may be fearful that her case be viewed less sympathetically by health care professionals and even lawyers because this was the mode of delivery she elected to have. A similar situation can arise with the woman who refuses intervention which a clinician deems necessary, e.g. the recent protracted debate regarding Caesarean section.[66,67] This raises the issue of 'informed consent' which is a veritable minefield.[68] Women who consider themselves to have been adequately informed experience a greater degree of satisfaction with their choice.[69] Some complain that they are given too little information,[70] whilst others are often overwhelmed by the number of options offered to them and ask their clinician what they would do in their situation. Some clinicians will admit that encouraging patients to make decisions on various aspects of clinical management absolves them, at least in part, of taking full responsibility for their care. This enforced choice is surely every bit as undemocratic as the dogmatic style of patient management that brought about the need for change in the first place.

If CRM is implemented without careful consideration, it could be potentially destructive. Lack of support and fear of recrimination may lead us to practice defensive medicine often apportioning blame to 'the system', other colleagues or the patient herself. Recent changes in postgraduate medical training such as the reduction of junior doctors' hours, the introduction of shift systems and the breakdown of the firm structure only serve to compound the problem. Guidelines and protocols can incorrectly be perceived as a substitute for clinical acumen and judgement, and health care professionals may be less concerned about clinical outcomes than about how they will justify their actions to inappropriately critical colleagues. This type of pressure causes individuals a great deal of stress and ultimately leads to a poor morale in the workplace, which in turn encourages poor practice.

CRM will undoubtedly be of increasing importance in all medical specialties in the future. It is potentially of enormous benefit in maternity care but will only operate effectively if it is implemented in a positive atmosphere with support from health care professionals and the Trust. It is likely that in the future there will be an increased separation between the legal/financial aspects of CRM and those aspects concerned directly with patient safety. Some Trusts are considering employing a claims manager with a distinct job separate to that of the clinical risk manager. Also, it is hoped that health care professionals will be less reliant on claims for information gathering and be more proactive about seeking deficiencies in service provision before adverse events arise. In order to obtain the maximum benefit from risk management, health care providers will be encouraged to look at other institutions, e.g. airline companies, who have more experience in this field.

---

**KEY POINTS FOR CLINICAL PRACTICE**

- CRM is used to achieve different objectives which relate to the perspective from which it is viewed.
- For health care professionals, CRM is used to aid in the recognition of aspects of practice which give rise to poor clinical outcomes, to monitor standards of care by clinical audit, for the modification of guidelines and for continuing education.
- For the patient, CRM may represent an opportunity to have individualised review of care, to question practice and receive explanations so as to improve understanding of the clinical outcome.
- For the Trust, CRM can help assess the financial risk involved in individual cases and provide information used to prepare to defend or settle litigation claims as appropriate.

---

### References

1 van der Schaaf T W. Development of a near miss management system at a chemical process plant. In: van der Schaaf TW, Lucas DA, Hale AR (eds) Near Miss Reporting as a Safety Tool. London: Butterworth-Heinemann, 1991
2 Fenn P, Hermans D, Dingwall R. Estimating the cost of compensating victims of medical negligence. BMJ 1994; 309: 389–391
3 Scally G, Donaldson L J. Clinical governance and the drive for quality improvement in the new NHS. BMJ 1998; 317: 61–65

4 Clinical Governance. Making it happen. London: The Royal Society of Medicine Press, 1999

5 Secretary of State for Health. The New NHS. London: HMSO, 1997

6 Beard R W, O'Connor A M. Implementation of audit and risk management: a protocol. In: Vincent C. (ed), Clinical Risk Management. London: BMJ Publishing Group, 1995

7 Lindgren O, Secker-Walker J. Incident reporting systems: early warnings for prevention and control of clinical negligence. In: Vincent C. (ed) Clinical Risk Management. London: BMJ Publishing Group, 1995

8 O'Connor A M. The attitude of staff towards clinical risk management. Clin Risk 1996; 2: 119–122

9. Drife J. Reducing risk in obstetrics. In: Vincent C. (ed) Clinical Risk Management. London: BMJ Publishing Group, 1995

10 Why mothers die. Report on Confidential Enquiries into Maternal Deaths in the United Kingdom 1994–1996. London: Department of Health, 1998

11 Maternal and Child Health Research Consortium. Confidential enquiry into stillbirths and deaths in infancy: 5th annual report. London: Department of Health, 1998

12 Leape L L. Error in medicine. JAMA 1994; 272: 1851–1857

13 Cooper J B, Newbower R S, Kitz R J. An analysis of major errors and equipment failures in anesthesia management considerations for prevention and detection. Anesthesiology 1984; 60: 34–42

14 Vincent C. The study of errors and accidents in medicine. In: Vincent C, Ennis M, Audley R J. (eds) Medical Accidents. Oxford: Oxford University Press, 1993

15 Reason J T. Understanding adverse events: human factors. In: Vincent C. (ed) Clinical Risk Management. London: BMJ Publishing Group, 1995

16 Reason J T. Human Error. Cambridge: Cambridge University Press, 1990

17 Bogner M S. Human Error in Medicine. New Jersey: Lawrence Erlbaum Associates, 1994

18 Eagle C J, Davies J M, Reason J T. Accident analysis of large scale technological disasters applied to an anaesthetic complication. Can J Anaesth 1992; 39: 118–122

19 Vincent C, Clements R V. Clinical risk management – why do we need it? Clin Risk 1995; 1: 1–4

20 Cook R I, Woods D A. Operating at the sharp end: the complexity of human error. In: Bogner M S. (ed) Human Error in Medicine. New Jersey: Lawrence Erlbaum Associates, 1994

21 Vincent C, Bark P. Accident investigation: discovering why things go wrong. In: Vincent C. (ed) Clinical Risk Management. London: BMJ Publishing Group, 1995

22 Anonymous Medical Accidents. Oxford: Oxford Medical Press, 1993

23 Stanhope N, Vincent C, Taylor-Adams S E, O'Connor A M, Beard R W. Applying human factors methods to clinical risk management in obstetrics. Br J Obstet Gynaecol 1997; 104: 1225–1232.

24 Lakasing L, Chapman E J, Spencer J A D. Lessons from clinical risk management in obstetrics. J Obstet Gynaecol 1999; 19: S19

25 General Medical Council. Maintaining Good Medical Practice. London: GMC, 1998

26 Report of a Working Group. Maintaining Good Medical Practice in Obstetrics and Gynaecology. The Role of the RCOG. London: RCOG Press, 1999

27 Parboosingh J. Revalidation for doctors. BMJ 1998; 317: 1094–1095

28 Report of a Joint Working Party. Towards Safer Childbirth. Minimum Standards for the Organisation of Labour Wards. London: RCOG Press, 1999

29 Stewart J H, Andrews J, Cartlidge P H T. Numbers of deaths related to intrapartum asphyxia and timing of birth in all Wales perinatal survey, 1993–5. BMJ 1998; 316: 657–660

30 MacFarlane A. Variations in numbers of births and perinatal mortality by day of week in England and Wales. BMJ 1978; ii: 1670–1673

31 Elstein M. Containment of litigation in obstetrics and gynaecology: prevention. J Med Defence Union 1987; 3: 19–20

32 UKCC. Guidelines for Record Keeping. London: UKCC, 1998

33 British Postgraduate Medical Federation. Patterns of Hospital Medical Staffing in Obstetrics and Gynaecology. London: HMSO, 1991

34 Gold D R, Rogacz S, Bock N, Tosteson T D, Baum T M, Spiezer F E. Rotating shift work, sleep and accidents related to sleepiness in hospital nurses. Am J Public Health 1992; 82: 1011–1014

35  Vincent C, Young M, Phillips A. Why do people sue doctors? A study of patients and relatives taking legal action. Lancet 1994; 343: 1609–1613.
36  Simanowitz A. Standards, attitudes and accountability in the medical profession. Lancet 1985; ii: 546
37  Neale G. Clinical analysis of 100 medicolegal cases. BMJ 1993; 307: 1483–1487
38  Ward C J. Analysis of 500 obstetric and gynaecological malpractice claims: causes and prevention. Am J Obstet Gynecol 1991; 165: 298–300
39  Hawkins C, Paterson I. Medicolegal audit in the West Midlands region: analysis of 100 cases. BMJ 1987; 295: 1533–1536
40  Allsopp K M. Saying sorry. J Med Defence Union 1986; 2: 2
41  Chamberlain G, Orr C. How to avoid medico-legal problems in obstetrics and gynaecology. London: RCOG, 1990
42  Clements RV. Litigation in obstetrics and gynaecology. Br J Obstet Gynaecol 1991; 98: 423–426
43  Clements R V. Anonymous Safe Practice in Obstetrics and Gynaecology: a Medico-Legal Handbook. Avon: The Bath Press, 1994
44  Clinical Negligence Scheme for Trusts (CNST): Risk Management Standards and Procedures, 1997(CNST, Department C, Granary Warf House, Water Lane, Leeds LS11 5PY)
45  Bolam vs Frien Hospital Management Committee. All England Law Reports, 1957
46  Maynard vs West Midland Regional Health Authority. All England Law Reports, 1984
47  B-Lynch C, Coker A, Dua J A. A clinical analysis of 500 medico-legal claims evaluating the causes and assessing the potential benefit of alternate dispute settlement. Br J Obstet Gynaecol 1996; 103: 1236–1242
48  De Witt Wijnen O L O. ADR: the civil law approach. J Chartered Inst Arbitrators 1995; 61: 38–42
49  Morgan R. Medical negligence disputes: alternatives to litigation. Br J Obstet Gynaecol 1994; 101: 185–187
50  Woolfe H. Access to Justice: Final Report to the Lord Chancellor on the Civil Justice System in England and Wales. London: HMSO, 1996
51  Department of Health. Changing Childbirth. London: HMSO, 1993
52  Chamberlain G. Organisation of antenatal care. BMJ 1991; 302: 647–650
53  Hall M. Is routine antenatal care worthwhile? Lancet 1980; ii: 78–80
54  Abuelo D N, Hopmann M R, Barsel-Bowers G, Goldstein A. Anxiety in women with low maternal serum alpha-fetoprotein screening results. Prenat Diagn 1991; 11: 381–385
55  Khalid L, Price S M, Barrow M. The attitudes of midwives to maternal serum screening for Down's syndrome. Public Health 1994; 108: 131–136
56  Layng J. Screening for nuchal translucency. Counselling should be considered an integral part of screening programmes. BMJ 1998; 317: 749–749
57  Murphy K W, Johnson P, Moorcraft J, Pattinson R, Russell V, Turnbull A. Birth asphyxia and the intrapartum cardiotocograph. Br J Obstet Gynaecol 1990; 97: 470–479
58  Spencer J A D. Deaths due to intrapartum asphyxia. BMJ 1998; 316: 640
59  Sultan A H, Kamm M A, Hudson C N, Thomas J M, Bartram C I. Sphincter disruption during vaginal deliveries. N Engl J Med 1993; 329: 1905–1911
60  Dermon R, Patel N B, Thiery M. Implications of increasing rates of Caesarean section. In: Studd J. (ed), Progress in Obstetrics and Gynaecology. Edinburgh: Churchill Livingstone, 1988; 175
61  Wilkinson C, McIlwaine G, Boulton-Jones C, Cole S. Is a rising Caesarean section rate inevitable? Br J Obstet Gynaecol 1998; 105: 45–52
62  What is the right number of Caesarean sections [editorial]? Lancet 1997; 349: 844
63  Glazener C M A, MacArthur C, Garcia J. Postnatal care: time for a change. Contemp Rev Obstet Gynaecol 1993; 5: 130–136
64  Thornton J G. Measuring patients' values in reproductive medicine. Contemp Rev Obstet Gynaecol 1988; 1: 5–12
65  Al-Mufti R, McCarthy A, Fisk N M. Obstetricians' personal choice and mode of delivery. Lancet 1996; 347: 544

66 Draper H. Women, forced Caesareans and antenatal responsibilities. J Med Ethics 1996; 22: 327–333

67 Mould T, Chong S, Spencer J A D, Gallivan S. Women's involvement with the decision preceding their caesarean section and their degree of satisfaction. Br J Obstet Gynaecol 1996; 103: 1074–1077

68 Lescale K B, Inglis S R, Eddleman K A, Peeper E Q, Chervenak F A, McCullough L B. Conflicts between physicians and patients in nonelective cesarean delivery: incidence and adequacy of informed consent. Am J Perinatol 1996; 103: 171–176

69 Feldman G B, Freiman J A. Prophylactic Caesarean section at term? N Engl J Med 1985; 312: 1264–1267

70 Vincent C A, Martin T, Ennis M. Obstetric accidents: the patient's perspective. Br J Obstet Gynaecol 1991; 98: 390–395.

**3**

*Mohamed G. K. Abdalla    R. Bryan Beattie*

# Ultrasound markers of chromosomal abnormalities

Most fetuses with chromosomal abnormalities have either external or internal defects which can be recognised by detailed ultrasonographic examination. Studies from tertiary referral centres have found that nearly all fetuses with trisomy 13, 77–100% of fetuses with trisomy 18 and 33–50% of fetuses with Down's syndrome have significant sonographic signs which may be detected by a second trimester scan.[1-4] Trisomy 21, or Down's syndrome, is by far the most common chromosomal abnormality and an important cause of perinatal death and infant handicap. It occurs in 1/660 births[5] and its incidence is related to increasing maternal age (Table 1).[6]

## SCREENING FOR CHROMOSOMAL ABNORMALITIES

Until a decade ago, pre-natal karyotyping was usually restricted to women of 35 years or older, but screening based on this criterion identified only 20% of all trisomy 21 fetuses. Screening protocols combining maternal age, α-fetoprotein and free β-human chorionic gonadotrophin (β-hCG) have improved detection rates up to 69% with a 5.2% false positive rate in the second trimester.[7]

Before the introduction of serum screening, 140 amniocenteses would have been required to identify one case of Down's syndrome based on a maternal age of more than 35 years. This figure has been reduced to one in 60 amniocenteses after the introduction of serum screening.[8] The use of serum screening has enabled prenatal karyotyping to be focused on pregnancies at highest risk for chromosomal abnormalities.

**Mr Mohamed G.K. Abdalla** MD MSc MRCOG, Specialist Registrar in Obstetrics and Gynaecology, Wexham Park Hospital, Wexham Street, Slough SL2 4HL, UK (for correspondence)

**Mr Robert Bryan Beattie** MD MRCOG, Consultant in Fetal Medicine, University Hospital of Wales, Heath Park, Cardiff CF4 4XW, UK

**Table 1** Trisomy 21, age-related risk at birth

| Age | Age-related risk |
| --- | --- |
| 20 | 1/1527 |
| 21 | 1/1507 |
| 22 | 1/1482 |
| 23 | 1/1448 |
| 24 | 1/1406 |
| 25 | 1/1352 |
| 26 | 1/1286 |
| 27 | 1/1206 |
| 28 | 1/1113 |
| 29 | 1/1008 |
| 30 | 1/895 |
| 31 | 1/776 |
| 32 | 1/659 |
| 33 | 1/547 |
| 34 | 1/446 |
| 35 | 1/356 |
| 36 | 1/280 |
| 37 | 1/218 |
| 38 | 1/167 |
| 39 | 1/128 |
| 40 | 1/79 |
| 41 | 1/73 |
| 42 | 1/55 |
| 43 | 1/41 |
| 44 | 1/30 |

Modified from Snijders and Nicolaides.[6]

There is still room for improvement since we still perform 59 amniocenteses on chromosomally normal fetuses to diagnose each case of trisomy 21. Given the inherent procedure related loss rate attributed to invasive testing, which is 1 in 200 with amniocentesis[9] and 1 in 100 for chorionic villous sampling (CVS), one normal fetus may be lost as a complication of amniocentesis for every 3–4 fetuses identified with trisomy 21. It is important, therefore, that the selection policy of women for amniocentesis or CVS is continually improved.

An alternative, and possibly complementary, method of screening for fetal chromosomal abnormalities is ultrasonography, which is non-invasive and has no inherent procedure related loss.

## ULTRASOUND MARKERS

Several ultrasonographic features have been described in the second trimester that could possibly assist in the detection of fetuses with trisomy 21. These can be classified into two categories. The first category comprises major fetal structural abnormalities that are associated with Down's syndrome, namely congenital heart defects, ventriculomegaly and doudendal atresia.[10,11] The other category comprises many minor sonographic appearances, 'soft markers', which may be present in normal fetuses, but have been found in association with abnormal karyotypes.

The main reason for distinguishing these two categories is that some clinicians feel that the presence of major structural abnormalities such as heart defects are significant ground for offering diagnostic amniocentesis or CVS.

**Table 2** Ultrasound soft markers of chromosomal abnormalities

| Common markers | Less discriminatory markers |
| --- | --- |
| Nuchal translucency | Sandal gap |
| Hyperechogenic bowel | Short ear length |
| Choroid plexus cysts | Cerebral ventricular dilatation |
| Renal pelvi-calyceal dilatation | Fifth digit mid-phalanx hypoplasia |
| Cardiac echogenic foci | Increased iliac length |
| Short femur or humerus | Short frontal lobe |

The presence of a soft marker, which is not in itself an abnormality, however needs to be considered with other factors before offering an amniocentesis or CVS.

## SOFT MARKERS

Soft markers are minor, usually transient ultrasound features which may indicate a risk of serious fetal anomaly but which in themselves are probably inconsequential.[12] The most commonly described soft markers are: nuchal fold thickness, pyelectasis (dilatation of renal pelvis), hyper-echogenic bowel, choroid plexus cysts, short femur or humerus length and cardiac echogenic foci (golf balls). The other soft markers which are substantially less discriminating and less commonly described include borderline cerebral ventricular dilatation, ear length, fifth digit mid-phalanx hypoplasia, sandal gap, increased iliac length and short frontal lobe (Table 2).[13–18]

Ultrasound imaging has improved vastly in resolution, and for this reason, and because first and second trimester scans are now performed more often, the frequency with which soft markers are observed has risen correspondingly. Some markers may well have disappeared by the time of the 'routine' scan at 18–20 weeks. The presence of two or more markers makes the possibility of abnormal karyotype more likely, although some markers, such as nuchal translucency, have a significant association with chromosomal anomalies even when they occur alone.[19] On the other hand, absence of these markers in a high-risk population could reduce the prior risk of chromosomal abnormalities by up to 50%, and many tables have been calculated to adjust the risk according to the presence or absence of these markers.

## NUCHAL FOLD THICKNESS

Nuchal folds and cystic hygromas have been described as markers for aneuploidy since 1966. The incidence of aneuploidy has ranged from 22% to more than 70% in various series.[19] However, development of nuchal membranes could be a transient observation that may represent normal development of the lymphatic system and can be observed in some normal fetuses in the early and mid first trimester with high-resolution ultrasound. The persistence of nuchal membranes later in gestation may represent a delayed or abnormal development of the lymphatic system, suggesting aneuploidy. A simple membrane may be more representative of a delayed development in a normal fetus, thus the lower rate of aneuploidy, whereas septated membranes may

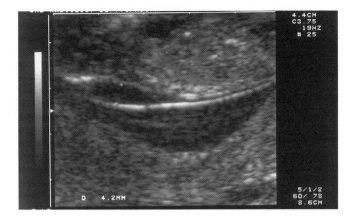

**Fig. 1** Increased nuchal translucency thickness at 12 weeks' gestation.

represent an abnormal lymphatic development that coincides with a higher rate of aneuploidy.

Much confusion has arisen from the literature because of inconsistency with definition and reporting of the ultrasonographic findings as regards nuchal translucency. However, when a posterior neck fluid collection is visualised, it is considered abnormal and called nuchal membrane or nuchal fold, when the thickness is more than 3 mm before 15 weeks gestation (Fig. 1), and more than 5 mm thereafter.[19] A thickness of $\geq 6$ mm at 18–20 weeks has been used in other studies.[4] This should be described as simple or with septation, as the risk of aneuploidy is greatest in the presence of septation.

A literature review showed an overall risk for aneuploidy with abnormal nuchal findings of 32% in 1649 cases in 21 series. A risk which is clearly high enough to warrant karyotypic evaluation, even when such abnormality presents in isolation, and regardless of gestational age at diagnosis.[19] However, measurement of nuchal translucency has now been refined to the point where risk can be calculated with some precision when the test is performed between 10–14 weeks of gestation, taking maternal age, gestational age and the degree of nuchal thickness into consideration.[20]

Traditionally, Turner's syndrome (45,X) was the anomaly associated with nuchal folds or membranes. Although its incidence is high (8%), Down's syndrome (trisomy 21) is the most common aneuploidy reported (13%).[19] However, Turner's syndrome is the most common aneuploidy rated in the group with septated membranes, with the highest rate found in the late mid-trimester (35%).[21]

When counselling patients, clinicians must remember that, even with a normal karyotype, an association between nuchal membranes and other syndromes has been noted, such as Noonan's syndrome, Robert's syndrome, distichiasis lymphoedema syndrome and lethal pterygium syndrome. These syndromes have different pattern of inheritance, many being autosomal dominant.[19]

An important part of evaluation of nuchal membrane is the evaluation of the subtle signs of hydrops fetalis. Even in the presence of a normal karyotype, perinatal outcome is extremely poor in the presence of fetal hydrops.[22-26] Also, hydrops with a cystic hygroma carries a poor prognosis, often ending in intra-uterine fetal death.[27] If the patient decides to continue the pregnancy, serial ultrasonography is warranted to monitor the progression or resolution of the nuchal membrane and to evaluate the development or progression of hydrops.

In cases without underlying aneuploidy, nuchal membranes may be indicative of, or result from, cardiac anomalies. The fluid collection may represent very early signs of cardiac failure,[24] and fetal echocardiogram is recommended in such cases, as detection of cardiac defects by the standard four chamber view is poor even in experienced hands (detection rate about 50%).[28] These anomalies associated with Down's syndrome include aterioventricular canal defects, ventricular septal defects, complete transposition of great vessels and tetralogy of fallot.[29] The ultrasound identification of these defects could, however, be improved by the use of colour flow mapping and Doppler.

Resolution of an isolated nuchal membrane or nuchal fold has been reported in fetuses with normal karyotypes and no evidence of hydrops. Most of these fetuses have a normal phenotype at birth.[25,30–32] Extreme maternal anxiety is however generated by reporting an increase in nuchal translucency measurement.

## CHOROID PLEXUS CYSTS

The choroid plexus produces cerebrospinal fluid and is seen prominently in the posterior horn of the lateral ventricle in second trimester ultrasound scans. Choroid plexus (CP) cysts are echolucent, well-circumscribed structures found in the choroid plexus (Fig. 2), and it is generally believed that they represent normal neuro-epithelial folds that subsequently fill with cerebrospinal fluid and cellular debris.[33,34] These cysts almost always resolve later in pregnancy, usually between 22–26 weeks' gestation, and they are not usually associated with any other central nervous system problems or neurological sequelae.[35] Very rarely, symptomatic cysts have been described in infants, young children and adults.[36,37] CP cysts are found in approximately 1% of routine second trimester ultrasound examinations,[38], and 50% of all autopsy studies across all age groups.[33]

Many researchers have examined the relationship of CP cysts with aneuploidy, especially trisomy 18 and 21. In one study,[39] it was found that up

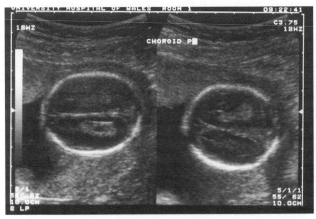

**Fig. 2** Choroid plexus cyst in a routine scan at 18 weeks' gestation.

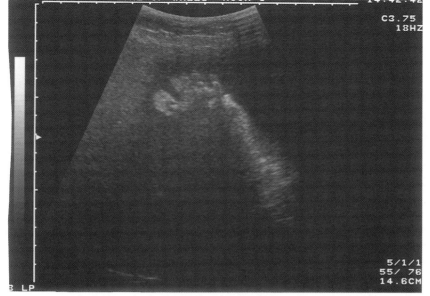

**Fig. 3** Sandal gap. One of the subtle ultrasonic markers of chromosomal abnormalities.

to 71% of fetuses with trisomy 18 have CP cysts. Trisomy 18 is however, usually associated with additional sonographic abnormalities, and the detection of CP cysts should alert the sonographer to search for additional anomalies, including subtle ones such as overlapping fingers, micrognathia, club foot,[40] and sandal gap (Fig. 3).

A dilemma arises when no other specific features apart from CP cysts are detected ante-natally. A review of the literature showed that the presence of apparently isolated CP cysts increases an individual's prior risk of trisomy 18 by a factor of 9, while the mid-trimester maternal age related or serum screening risk of Down's syndrome remains unchanged.[40] These risks increase substantially in the presence of other sonographic abnormalities and with advanced maternal age. The prior risk of trisomy 18 in the presence of other ultrasonic anomalies increases by a factor of almost 1800,[40] and hence karyotyping should be offered irrespective of maternal age.

Maternal age remains the main factor that determines the magnitude of the adjusted risk, and should be used in deciding whether or not to offer fetal karyotyping when isolated CP cysts are detected on mid-trimester scan (Table 3). For example, the age-related risk for trisomy 18, in a 31 year old woman is 1 in 2385, increasing to 1 in 264 in the presence of an isolated CP cyst.[40] If a cut-off point of 274 is used as an accepted threshold for amniocentesis, this means that amniocentesis should be offered for women over 31 years who show apparently isolated CP cysts on mid-trimester scan.

Also, the level of ultrasound expertise within individual units should be taken into consideration as a factor when deciding whether to offer amniocentesis or not in fetuses with isolated CP cysts. The more detailed the antenatal ultrasound, the more likely it is that another abnormality will be detected in a fetus with trisomy 18, and the lower the rate of trisomy 18 fetuses with apparently isolated CP cysts.

**Table 3** Maternal age-related risk and adjusted risk for trisomy i8 at mid-trimester in fetuses with isolated CP cysts

| Maternal age (years) | Age-related (prior) risk | Isolated CP cysts |
|---|---|---|
| 20 | 1/4576 | 1/506 |
| 21 | 1/4514 | 1/499 |
| 22 | 1/4435 | 1/491 |
| 23 | 1/4333 | 1/479 |
| 24 | 1/4204 | 1/465 |
| 25 | 1/4045 | 1/447 |
| 26 | 1/3850 | 1/426 |
| 27 | 1/3619 | 1/400 |
| 28 | 1/3351 | 1/371 |
| 29 | 1/3050 | 1/337 |
| 30 | 1/2724 | 1/301 |
| 31 | 1/2385 | 1/264 |
| 32 | 1/2046 | 1/226 |
| 33 | 1/1721 | 1/190 |
| 34 | 1/1420 | 1/157 |
| 35 | 1/1152 | 1/127 |
| 36 | 1/921 | 1/102 |
| 37 | 1/727 | 1/80 |
| 38 | 1/567 | 1/63 |
| 39 | 1/439 | 1/49 |
| 40 | 1/338 | 1/37 |

Modified from Gupta et al.[40]

There is no evidence that the incidence of chromosomal abnormalities in the presence of CP cysts is associated with location of the cysts (unilateral or bilateral), morphology of the cyst (simple or complex), size of the cyst, gestational age at diagnosis, gestation of cyst resolution or, sex of the fetus.[40] Finally, a large prospective controlled study is necessary in order to have uniform recommendations and solve the existing controversy.

## HYPERECHOGENIC FETAL BOWEL

The clinical significance of ultrasonographically demonstrated fetal hyperechogenic bowel is not yet clearly established. This finding has been described as normal variant,[41–43] but may also be associated with cystic fibrosis,[44–48] meconium peritonitis,[49] trisomy 21[4,50] or cytomegalovirus (CMV) infection.[51–53].

Normal intestinal echogenicity varies with gestational age and between patients. Because the intestine has no characteristic structural features, the examination is subjective. Fetal bowel is considered hyperechogenic if its echogenicity is grossly similar to, or greater than, that of the surrounding bone, regardless of the shape of the echogenic mass, which is either round and well defined or has the sinuous appearance of an intestinal loop. Some studies used the fetal iliac crest as a reference of echogenicity and scored the degree of bowel echogenicity accordingly (Fig. 4).[54]

Because of the relatively low prevalence of hyperechogenic bowel, studies to date have involved small populations, although it was found that hyperechogenic bowel is a physiological and normal variant in many instances (approximately 67% of cases).[41,42] Its association with increased risk of cystic fibrosis, meconial ileus, trisomy 21, CMV infection and adverse fetal outcome like

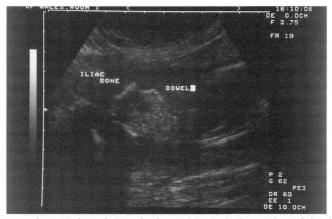

**Fig. 4** Hyperechogenic bowel. Bowel echogenicity is similar to that of the iliac bone.

intra-uterine growth retardation (IUGR) and intra-uterine fetal death (IUD) warrants further investigations.

Diagnosis of cystic fibrosis is based on amniotic fluid deoxyribonucleic acid mutation analysis by PCR, but only 87% of cystic fibrosis in the UK are due to common known mutations. Immunoreactive trypsin assay and sweat testing confirm the diagnosis post-natally. Some regions in the UK, such as Wales, have universal maternal screening for cystic fibrosis based on the heel-prick test at about one-week old.

Screening for infectious diseases should be implemented routinely when hyperechogenic bowel is identified, otherwise the true incidence of fetal infection is likely to be underestimated.[55] This can be performed by testing for maternal IgG and IgM, or fetal CMV PCR analysis of amniotic fluid. The higher fetal loss rate from cordocentesis for fetal CMV IgG and IgM analysis is not justified. In any case the fetal immune system may not mount a sufficient response prior to 24 weeks of gestation, such that false negatives may occur by using cordocentesis.

Karyotyping for aneuploidy, particularly trisomy 21, is part of the diagnostic work-up,[4,50] and should be offered. Also careful search for other ultrasonic anomalies is always recommended. When all previous investigations reveal no abnormality, ultrasonographic follow-up remains crucial because IUGR (8%) and IUD (23%) are frequent associations.[55]

## CARDIAC ECHOGENIC FOCI

Increasing use of high resolution ultrasound and the incorporation of the four chamber view into routine pre-natal ultrasound examination have increasingly identified cardiac echogenic foci, or the so-called golf balls. They were first described by Schechter et al[56] in 1987. They are defined as hyperechogenicity located in the chordae tendineae not attached to the ventricular walls and moving simultaneously with the aterioventricular valves (Fig. 5).

The clinical significance of golf balls is unclear and, although most of these echogenic foci resolve spontaneously and the neonates are born normal,[56–59] several reports[60,61] recently indicated an association with chromosomal trisomies, particularly that of trisomy 21.

When identified in a second trimester scan, their number, size and site (right or left ventricle) is described, followed by a careful search for other anomalies.

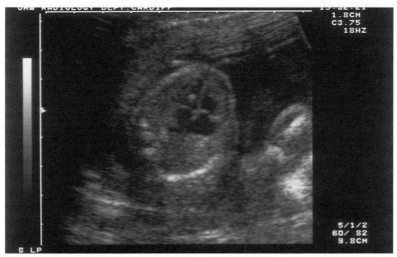

**Fig. 5** Cardiac echogenic focus or golf ball.

Fetal echocardiography may be recommended in such cases to rule out other cardiac anomalies, especially those associated with Down's syndrome, which are still difficult to detect in the four chamber view.

To evaluate the association of cardiac echogenic foci with chromosomal abnormalities, a review of the English language literature was done by Achiron et al in 1997[62]; in which they found 489 cases with fetal heart echogenic foci among 37,498 fetuses screened. Among these 489 fetuses with echogenic foci, 6 cases were identified as having trisomy 21. The calculated risk of trisomy 21 was found to be 1 in 500 (0.002%).

This risk is obviously far lower than the risk of a procedure related loss from amniocentesis, which is 1 in 200 (0.5%), and is lower than the risk of trisomy 21 in a 35-year-old woman (0.27%), based on maternal age, which is a widely accepted threshold for amniocentesis. Therefore, it was concluded that the finding of isolated fetal heart echogenic foci in the general, low risk population under 35 years of age is not associated with increased risk of Down's syndrome.

## PELVI-CALYCEAL DILATATION (PCD)

Fetal pyelectasis or renal pelvic dilatation is diagnosed when the antero-posterior diameter of the renal pelvis is $\geq 4$ mm before 33 weeks' gestation, and $\geq 7$ mm thereafter.[63] Others use 3 mm or 5 mm limits at 18–20 weeks' scan (Fig. 6). It was originally thought that PCD is strongly associated with chromosomal abnormalities, particularly Down's syndrome.[64] This association holds when PCD is found with other markers,[65] like short femur or structural cardiac malformations. However, when isolated, i.e. not associated with any other abnormalities or markers, the risk of Down's syndrome is small. One study[8] showed that isolated PCD has a sensitivity of only 1.8% and a false positive rate of 2%. Therefore, it does not seem to increase the risk for trisomy 21; however, Snijders et al[66] have calculated a 1.6-fold increased risk for Down's syndrome in an analysis of prospectively collected data on isolated PCD.

The major benefit of prenatal diagnosis of fetal PCD is to identify fetuses who are at increased risk of developing renal disease in the future, and to

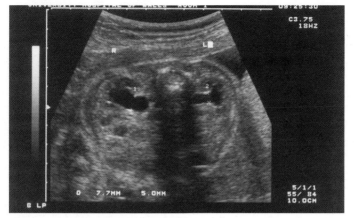

**Fig. 6** Bilateral renal pelvi-calyceal dilatation.

detect clinically silent lesions that may manifest themselves later in life. Those fetuses will require neonatal urological investigation, antibiotic prophylaxis and follow-up.

The clinical significance of fetal PCD is unclear. Although some investigators believe that an antero-posterior diameter of the renal pelvis less than 10 mm is physiological and does not require any post-natal investigations,[67] others have recommended post-natal follow-up if the diameter is ≥ 4 mm before 33 weeks or ≥ 7 mm after 33 weeks.[68] Following these criteria, one study[69] showed that approximately two-thirds of fetuses with persistent pyelectasia beyond 28 weeks of gestation were found to have urinary tract anomalies at birth, with uretero-pelvic junction obstruction (37%) and vesico-ureteric reflux (33%) being the most common.

Post-natal ultrasonographic evaluation is usually done on the first week of life to avoid any false-negative or false-positive results because of the relative state of dehydration in the infant after birth and the muscle relaxing effect of progesterone-like hormones on the fetal upper urinary tract.[70,71] Ultrasonic evaluation is, however, warranted in the first day of life in a male baby, with bilateral PCD and big bladder because of the possibility of posterior urethral valve (PUV). In the majority of the cases with mild hydronephrosis, there is no need for immediate surgery and most of these infants are managed expectantly with close assessment of pathological features of the urinary tract.[72] They will usuallybe given antibacterial prophylaxis, especially in the presence of vesico-ureteral reflux, to decrease the incidence of urinary infection.[70–72]

The presence of unilateral versus bilateral pyelectasis may be considered as a potential prognostic indicator for post-natal renal pathology. One study showed that bilateral PCD is more likely to regress *in utero* with advancing gestation. Moreover, fetuses that do have persistent bilateral PCD have a significantly lower risk of urinary tract pathology at birth compared to those with unilateral involvement.[69]

## LONG BONE BIOMETRY

Current evidence suggests that fetuses with Down's syndrome are more likely to exhibit shortened long bone measurements compared with the normal population.[73] Whether or not these differences are sufficient to justify routine screening has been a subject of many debates in the literature.

Femur and humerus length has been used in most studies performed to identify the risk of Down's syndrome and to adjust this risk according to the presence or absence of shortening. Limb length is usually compared with biparietal diameter (BPD) rather than menstrual age due to the uncertainty of the menstrual history. The BPD is measured in a transverse plane, from the outer edge to the inner edge of the skull at the level of the thalami, while long bones are measured with a standard method that includes the diaphyseal portion of the shaft. In one study when the regression coefficient was calculated and various cut-off points examined, it was found that the tenth percentile of BPD to femur length provided optimal sensitivity and specificity,[74] but this approach identifies 10% of all babies as being high risk. Abnormal fetal long bone biometry is defined as the presence of one or more abnormally short bones. It is important to be aware that regression coefficients of long bones may vary between institutions due to systematic differences in measurement methods and differences in population. Therefore, each institution should establish its own data, and cut-off values for defining 'shortness' of a particular bone.

In one study,[73] either short humerus or short femur was found in 31.1% of fetuses with Down's syndrome, compared with 7.5% of normal fetuses (relative risk = 4.1). Furthermore, fetuses with both short humeri and short femurs carry an 11-fold greater risk of Down's syndrome (relative risk = 11.1). Currently, tables are available to adjust the risk of trisomy 21 according to presence or absence of long bone shortening (Table 4).[74]

If the currently accepted risk (1 in 274) of a 35-year-old woman is used as an indication for offering genetic amniocentesis, amniocentesis would not be

**Table 4**  Trisomy 21, mid trimester risk based on maternal age and long bone biometry

| Maternal age (years) | Age-related risk (mid-trimester) | Adjusted risk (short femur) | Adjusted risk (short humerus) |
|---|---|---|---|
| 20 | 1/1231 | 1/769 | 1/375 |
| 21 | 1/1145 | 1/715 | 1/349 |
| 22 | 1/1065 | 1/665 | 1/324 |
| 23 | 1/1000 | 1/625 | 1/305 |
| 24 | 1/942 | 1/588 | 1/287 |
| 25 | 1/887 | 1/554 | 1/270 |
| 26 | 1/842 | 1/526 | 1/257 |
| 27 | 1/798 | 1/499 | 1/243 |
| 28 | 1/755 | 1/472 | 1/230 |
| 29 | 1/721 | 1/451 | 1/220 |
| 30 | 1/685 | 1/428 | 1/209 |
| 31 | 1/650 | 1/406 | 1/198 |
| 32 | 1/563 | 1/352 | 1/172 |
| 33 | 1/452 | 1/283 | 1/138 |
| 34 | 1/352 | 1/220 | 1/108 |
| 35 | 1/274 | 1/172 | 1/84 |
| 36 | 1/213 | 1/133 | 1/65 |
| 37 | 1/166 | 1/104 | 1/51 |
| 38 | 1/129 | 1/81 | 1/31 |
| 39 | 1/100 | 1/63 | 1/31 |
| 40 | 1/78 | 1/49 | 1/24 |

Modified from Vintzileos et al.[74]

justified in the presence of normal long bone biometry except in women of 40 or more years old.[74] This ultrasound risk adjustment may lead to better selection of candidates for amniocentesis, with higher yields of positive amniocentesis results and reduced procedure related losses of normal fetuses. The main advantage of this approach is that great expertise is not usually required for identifying and measuring a long bone.

## DEBATE

### Second trimester ultrasonogram as a screening tool

Despite the lack of clear evidence on the performance of second trimester ultrasound screening for chromosomal abnormalities, it is now becoming common practice to offer such screening. It is carried out in two ways – either by automatic inclusion of ultrasound markers in the routine anomaly scan at 18–20 weeks or, by doing so in women with a positive serum screening result to adjust their risk according to the presence or absence of ultrasound markers. Both approaches are subject to criticism.

### Automatic inclusion of markers in 18–20 weeks anomaly scan

When the association between different ultrasound markers and chromosomal abnormalities, particularly trisomy 21, were evaluated by reviewing the literature, widely different estimates for both the detection and false positive rates were found. The best ultrasound marker seems to be nuchal translucency (NT) measurement, yielding a 38% detection rate for 1.3% false positive rate for estimates of detection rate varying from 8–75% and estimates of the false positive rate ranging from 0–8.5%.[75] The other markers are substantially less discriminating (Table 5).

Using the ultrasonographic signs of structural abnormalities, such as heart defects, to identify the risk of chromosomal abnormalities, a maximum detection

**Table 5** Summary estimates of screening performance of different ultrasound markers in mid-trimester

| Ultrasound markers | No. of studies | Detection rate (%) | False positive) rate ( % |
|---|---|---|---|
| Nuchal translucency (NT) | 16 | 38 | 1.3 |
| Hyperechogenic bowel | 3 | 11 | 0.7 |
| Renal pelvi-calyceal dilatation | 4 | 19 | 2.4 |
| Femur length (comparing observed with expected) | 10 | 34 | 5.9 |
| Femur length(ratio of biparietal to femur length) | 4 | 22 | 5.9 |
| Humerus length (comparing observed with expected | 6 | 37 | 5.3 |
| Femur length and humerus length combined | 3 | 36 | 3.7 |

Modified from Wald et al.[75]

rate of 45–50% of viable Down's syndrome pregnancies is possible with a false positive rate of at least 0.7%.[75] Fetal karyotyping is usually offered whenever cardiac defects are identified sonographically, regardless of the presence of other markers, as the prevalence of chromosomal abnormalities in such cases is 5–10%.[75]

Both detection rates – 38% for second trimester nuchal translucency and 45% for structural heart defects – are substantially less than the detection rate achievable with serum screening (69%).[7] In addition, given the lack of information on the significance of some of the markers, clinicians are faced with difficult decisions on what action, if any, they should take. Therefore, the use of second trimester ultrasound as a primary screening method for trisomy 21 is not yet justified.

The performance of screening could be improved by producing a risk estimate for trisomy 21 based on the presence or absence of a combination of ultrasound markers. The problem with this approach is that this combination has the potential of increasing the false positive rates (estimated at 10–18%). In addition, information on the extent to which these markers are independent variables in both affected and unaffected pregnancies must be obtained.

## Marker scans after high Down's risk on serum screening

One or more sonographic anomalies were detected in 50% of fetuses with trisomy 21, compared with only 7.2% of normal fetuses.[76] Detection of one or more ultrasonographic markers in pregnancies that are serum screen positive could increase the risk of trisomy 21 by 5- to 8-fold[76,77] (likelihood ratio of 41)[77] and their absence could decrease this risk by 5-fold (likelihood ratio 0.2).[77]

Tables were calculated in which a prior risk of both high and low risk women were adjusted according to the sonographic findings and, therefore, would allow clinicians to improve their ability to counsel individual patients about their risk of having an affected fetus (Table 6). This should, in turn, lead to a more accurate selection of patients for invasive testing, and minimise the loss of unaffected fetuses, in addition to significant reduction in costs.[78]

It is suggested that a combination of maternal age, serum biochemical screening, and subsequent second trimester ultrasound could provide a better mechanism for selection of pregnancies to undergo invasive testing. Currently, many women found to be at increased risk of carrying a fetus with trisomy 21 by biochemical testing are wanting further confirmation before having amniocentesis, especially if their serum screening is borderline. Equally, some women with advanced maternal age might seek reassurance by a normal ultrasound examination after having a negative serum screen, before deciding not to have invasive testing.

However, some caution must be exercised. First, the observations are based on a small number of affected fetuses. Second, the two screening methods of biochemical markers and ultrasonographic signs used in combination is reliant on the tests being independent of each other; although this seems to be the case, further confirmation is necessary. Thirdly, it must be realised that the detection of these features depends on the expertise available at different centres and that the likelihood ratios may differ between separate units. In addition, about 50% of trisomy 21 fetuses will not demonstrate any ultrasonographic markers.

**Table 6** Trisomy 21, age-related risk and adjusted risk at birth, according to presence or absence of different soft markers

| Age | Age-related risk | Soft markers/adjusted risk | | | | | |
|---|---|---|---|---|---|---|---|
| | | Non 0.5 | CP cysts 1.5 | PC dilatation 1.5 | FL < 5th centile 2.5 | Echogenic bowel 5.5 | NT > 6 mm 10 |
| 20 | 1/1527 | 1/3054 | 1/1018 | 1/1018 | 1/661 | 1/278 | 1/153 |
| 21 | 1/1507 | 1/3014 | 1/1005 | 1/1005 | 1/603 | 1/274 | 1/151 |
| 22 | 1.1482 | 1/2964 | 1/988 | 1/988 | 1/593 | 1/269 | 1/148 |
| 23 | 1/1448 | 1/2896 | 1/965 | 1/965 | 1/579 | 1/263 | 1/145 |
| 24 | 1/1406 | 1/2812 | 1/937 | 1/937 | 1/562 | 1/256 | 1/141 |
| 25 | 1/1352 | 1/2704 | 1/901 | 1/901 | 1/541 | 1/246 | 1/135 |
| 26 | 1/1286 | 1/2572 | 1/857 | 1/857 | 1/514 | 1/234 | 1/129 |
| 27 | 1/1206 | 1/2412 | 1/804 | 1/804 | 1/482 | 1/219 | 1/121 |
| 28 | 1/1113 | 1/2226 | 1/742 | 1/742 | 1/445 | 1/202 | 1/111 |
| 29 | 1/1008 | 1/2016 | 1/672 | 1/672 | 1/403 | 1/183 | 1/101 |
| 30 | 1/895 | 1/1790 | 1/597 | 1/597 | 1/358 | 1/163 | 1/90 |
| 31 | 1/776 | 1/1552 | 1/517 | 1/517 | 1/310 | 1/141 | 1/78 |
| 32 | 1/659 | 1/1318 | 1/439 | 1/439 | 1/264 | 1/120 | 1/66 |
| 33 | 1/547 | 1/1094 | 1/365 | 1/365 | 1/219 | 1/99 | 1/55 |
| 34 | 1/446 | 1/892 | 1/297 | 1/297 | 1/178 | 1/81 | 1/45 |
| 35 | 1/356 | 1/712 | 1/237 | 1/237 | 1/142 | 1/65 | 1/36 |
| 36 | 1/280 | 1/560 | 1/187 | 1/187 | 1/112 | 1/51 | 1/28 |
| 37 | 1/218 | 1/436 | 1/145 | 1/145 | 1/87 | 1/40 | 1/22 |
| 38 | 1/167 | 1/334 | 1/111 | 1/111 | 1/67 | 1/30 | 1/17 |
| 39 | 1/128 | 1/256 | 1/85 | 1/85 | 1/51 | 1/23 | 1/13 |
| 40 | 1/97 | 1/194 | 1/65 | 1/65 | 1/39 | 1/18 | 1/10 |

Therefore, patients should also be counselled that, with this approach of adjusting the risk, some cases with trisomy 21 might still be missed. Finally, these observations are valid for pregnancies with positive serum biochemistry and cannot be used for general obstetric population or for women with negative serum biochemical screening.

Recent studies have shown that the proportion of women at high risk of Down's syndrome who prefer to have a marker scan as a first option rather than amniocentesis has increased (55.2% in one study).[78] In the University Hospital of Wales (UHW), 74% of women who are high risk prefer to have a marker scan as a first option, 60% of these will proceed to amniocentesis, while in women who do not have a marker scan, 90% will proceed to amniocentesis.

## COUNSELLING

The problem with soft markers is that, even when karyotypic abnormalities are excluded, the parents as well as the obstetrician may remain in doubt as to their significance.[12] The psychological sequelae of false positive results of routine prenatal screening tests are considerable; numerous studies have reported high levels of parental anxiety and worry even after subsequent normal test results.[79] Furthermore, this anxiety has been reported up to 12 months after false positive results of screening.[80]

In the case of ultrasound screening, these psychological costs may be exacerbated by the visual imagery, which is an integral part of the procedure.[81]

It is not easy to convey to couples the idea that an indicator of abnormality that can be visualised is probably inconsequential. Women whose fetuses are deemed to be at an increased risk of chromosomal abnormality on the basis of an ultrasound examination might interpret this result quite differently to those receiving a report of similar risk as a result of maternal serum screening.

Information about ultrasonographic markers is relatively new. Many of the background data came from referral units and are, therefore, biased, making counselling difficult in many situations. Sometimes, the disclosure of the presence of a soft marker does more harm than good and the anxiety caused as a result may far outweigh the potential gain. It has been suggested, therefore, that specialist counselling methods need to be developed and further research is needed into methods of pre-screening counselling.[82]

It is always forgotten that the second trimester anomaly scan is optional and patients should be given an informed choice whether to have it done or not. They need to understand that the aim of this scan is to detect structural abnormalities, which may require intervention in the form of termination, intra-uterine treatment, or early neonatal correction. When the choice is to have the scan performed, the possibility of detecting soft markers which may be associated with chromosomal abnormalities, but at the same time could be inconsequential, should be explained and discussed. Again, patients should be given the choice of whether to disclose this information about soft markers or not.

### Comparison between first trimester ultrasound screening and second trimester serum screening for chromosomal abnormalities:

Ultrasound in the first trimester has been increasingly used in recent years to identify pregnancies at risk of Down's syndrome. Nuchal translucency (NT) measurement in the first trimester seems highly discriminatory and its performance has improved by adjusting its measurement for gestational age. Nicolaides et al[83] reported a detection rate for trisomy 21, in routine screening, of 84% for a false positive rate of 5.8% using a risk cut-off point of 1:300. This risk has been calculated on the basis of maternal age and NT adjusted for gestational age based on crown-rump length.

All the serum markers used or considered in the second trimester screening have been assessed in Down's syndrome and unaffected pregnancies during the first trimester. Two serum markers stand out as being useful in screening at 10–14 weeks' gestation-namely, free β-subunit human chorionic gonado-trophin (β-hCG), and pregnancy associated plasma protein-A (PAPP-A). In trisomy 21, free β-hCG is higher and PAPP-A is lower when compared with chromosomally normal fetuses. At a risk cut-off point of 1 in 300, the screening performance of free β-hCG and PAPP-A is 63% for a false positive rate of 5.5%.[84] This screening performance is comparable with second trimester serum screening by the triple test (β-hCG, α-fetoprotein, and oestradiol).

The relationship between first trimester serum screening utilising β-hCG or PAPP-A and first trimester NT measurement in chromosomally normal and abnormal fetuses has been examined. It was found that they are independent variables (i.e. no significant association). Therefore, a combination of both is estimated to have a positive predictive value of 90% for Down's syndrome and 5% false positive rate.[85]

It is clear that NT measurement in the first trimester, whether used alone or in combination with serum β-hCG or PAPP-A, is highly discriminatory and has a higher positive predictive value for chromosomal abnormalities (84% and 90%, respectively), when compared with serum screening in the second trimester (69%), without concomitant increase in the false-positive rate (nearly 5% for both).

NT measurement in the first trimester also has the advantage of early identification of the pregnancies at high risk of aneuploidy and the option of early intervention. Surgical termination of pregnancy in the first trimester by suction curettage is undoubtedly technically easier than termination by the prostaglandins in the second trimester. It is also associated with fewer complications, lower cost implications and is less traumatic emotionally for the mother. It has therefore social, medical, emotional and economic advantages.

There are, however, several potential problems with NT measurement in the first trimester as a screening tool for chromosomal abnormalities. First, the majority of the reported studies have been performed on selected populations at high risk of aneuploidy either based on older maternal age, or because of family history of chromosomal abnormality. Therefore, these results can not be extrapolated to the unselected or low risk populations. Implementation of first trimester NT measurement in unselected populations in Frimley Park and St Peter's General Hospitals (6000 deliveries per year), did, however, show a similar screening performance to its use in women at high risk.[86]

Secondly, there is heterogeneity between the published estimates of screening performance of first trimester NT measurement, so one can not be sure that results in one centre can be replicated in another. However, this heterogeneity can be reduced by specifying a standard technique that can be adopted at all centres and by better training of the staff providing the service. Validation and quality control are, therefore, vitally important.

Another criticism is that NT measurement requires highly skilled operators and is prone to inter- and intra-observer variation. However, all sonographers performing fetal scans should be capable of measuring reliably the crown-rump length and obtaining a proper sagittal view of the fetal spine. For such sonographers, it is easy to acquire within few hours the skill to accurately measure the NT without additional costs or significantly increasing the scanning time. Inter- and intra-observer variations have been studied; it was found that NT measurement is highly reproducible when measured by well-trained operators. The repeatability was unrelated to the size of the NT and when the mean of two measurements was used, 95% of the time inter- and intra-observer variability was 0.62 mm and 0.54 mm, respectively[87]. Also, by combining the trans-abdominal (TA) and transvaginal (TV) approach, repeatability coefficients were 0.4 mm and 0.2 mm, respectively.[88]

Failure to measure NT is another potential problem. Failure rates vary between 10–40% in different studies.[89,90] This seems to be gestational age related to some extent. Success rate increases with increasing gestational age. Eleven weeks' gestation is considered the optimum.[89] Also, combination of TA and TV scans increases success and reduces failure.[88]

A number of studies have demonstrated an increase in miscarriage rates in fetuses with increased NT measurement in the first trimester irrespective of their chromosomal pattern (normal or abnormal).[91–94] These studies have clearly demonstrated that screening for aneuploidy using NT measurement will inevitably identify a proportion of fetuses destined to die in late first or early second trimester. The implications of this are: the estimated 84% positive predictive value of NT measurement in the first trimester could be an overestimate for live births at term; and, therefore, more parents may need to make the difficult decision to terminate a pregnancy which would have otherwise been lost spontaneously. The estimated spontaneous loss rate is about 25% in fetuses with Down's syndrome between 10–15 weeks' gestation.[95,96] However, there is no published data about how women view the difference between spontaneous and induced miscarriage in the presence of an abnormality, and whether one is more distressing than the other.

A further criticism of NT measurement in the first trimester is that early identification of women at increased risk of aneuploidy entails the invasive diagnostic procedure of CVS. CVS is less widely available, and associated with a higher miscarriage rate (2 in 100), when compared with amniocentesis (0.5–1%). In addition, it is more expensive and has a false positive rate of about 2%, as a result of placental mosaicism.

First and second trimester screening should be fully evaluated quantitatively in the same pregnancy and this is the basis of SURUSS study which should report in the year 2001. The final assessment should be determined mainly on the basis of efficacy, safety and cost.

## SUMMARY

Ultrasound scan markers were introduced as a screening test for chromosomal abnormalities with the aim of reducing the number of amniocentesis in high risk pregnancies and increasing the detection rate for chromosomal abnormalities. In our current practice more chromosomal abnormalities are now detected on the basis of scanning than on serum screening.

With the advent of high resolution machines, not only major structural abnormalities become identifiable, but also a wide range of minor defects which could be associated with chromosomal abnormalities, but at the same time could be inconsequential. These minor defects are called soft markers.

Using second trimester marker scan as an alternative to serum screening cannot be justified at present as the detection rate of chromosomal abnormalities achievable by second trimester scans in isolation is substantially less than that achievable by serum screening. Using second trimester ultrasound screening in low risk pregnancies is compounded with the problem of the need for ultrasound and counselling expertise, which is not widely available, and consumption of radiology resources. Also there is a potential for increasing false positive rates when so many markers are used.

Also, the use of ultrasound markers in high risk pregnancies as complementary to serum screening to adjust the risk of chromosomal abnormalities according to the presence or absence of ultrasound markers, makes important assumptions about these two screening tools being independent variables. Although this seems to be the case, this assumption needs further confirmation. Also the adjusted risk tables are based on data derived from a small number of affected pregnancies came from tertiary referral centres, which make these data mostly biased, in addition to the fact that the likelihood ratios may differ between separate units.

High level of specialist counselling before and after screening for chromosomal abnormalities using ultrasound markers is required as the anxiety and psychological costs may be tremendous and out-weigh the potential gain.

Further research is required in this fascinating and interesting area as it has the potential of being a useful screening and diagnostic tool for fetal chromosomal abnormalities, with potentially higher detection rates, lower false positive rates and less procedure related losses from diagnostic testing. Certainly the recent work by Howe et al[97] who found a 68% detection rate for Down's syndrome for a 6.6% amniocentesis rate using 2nd trimester ultrasound would support this view.

## References

1 Benacerraf B R, Gelman R, Frigoletto F D. Sonographic identification of 2nd trimester fetuses with Down syndrome. N Engl J Med 1987; 317: 1371–1376
2 Benacerraf B R, Miller W A, Frigoletto F D. Sonographic detection of fetuses with trisomies 13 and 18: accuracy and limitations. Am J Obstet Gynecol 1988; 158: 404–409
3 Benacerraf B R, Nadel A, Bromley B. Identification of second trimester fetuses with autosomal trisomy by use of sonographic scoring index. Radiology 1994; 193: 135–140
4 Nyberg D A, Resta R G, Lathy D A, Hickok D A, Mahony D S, Hirsch J H. Prenatal sonographic findings of Down syndrome. Review of 94 cases. Obstet Gynecol 1990; 76: 370–377
5 Bilardo C. Second trimester ultrasound markers for fetal aneuploidy. Early Hum Dev 1996; 47 (Suppl): S31–S33
6 Snijders R J M, Nicolaides K H. (eds). Ultrasound Markers for Fetal Chromosomal Defects. London: Parthenon, 1996; 184
7 Spencer K, Carpenter P. Prospective study of prenatal screening for Down's syndrome with free beta human chorionic gonadotrophin. BMJ 1993; 307: 764–769
8 Vintzileos A M, Egan J F X. Adjusting the risk for trisomy 21 on the basis of second trimester ultrasonography. Am J Obstet Gynecol 1995; 172: 837–844
9 Simpson J L. Genetic counselling and prenatal diagnosis. In: Gabbe S G, Niebyl J R, Simpson J L. (eds) Obstetrics: Normal and Problem Pregnancies. New York: Churchill Livingstone, 1996; 215–248
10 Benacerraf B R. The second trimester fetus with Down's syndrome: detection using sonographic features. Ultrasound Obstet Gynecol 1996; 7: 147–155
11 Nicolaides K, Shawwa L, Brizot M, Snijders R. Ultrasonographically detectable markers of fetal chromosomal defects. Ultrasound Obstet Gynecol 1993; 3: 56–69
12 Whittle M. Ultrasonographic 'soft markers' of fetal chromosomal defects. BMJ 1997; 314: 918
13 Bahado-Singh R O, Goldstein I, Uerpairojkit B, Copal J A, Mahoney M J, Baumgarten A. Normal nuchal thickness in the mid-trimester indicates reduced risk of Down syndrome in pregnancies with abnormal triple screen results. Am J Obstet Gynecol 1995; 173: 1106–1110
14 Toi A, Simpson G F, Filly R A. Ultrasonically evident fetal nuchal thickening: is it specific for Down syndrome? Am J Obstet Gynecol 1987; 157: 150–153
15 Lettieri L, Rodis J F, Vintizileos A M, Feeney L, Ciarleglis L, Craffey A. Ear length in second trimester aneuploidy fetuses. Obstet Gynecol 1993; 81: 57–60
16 Benacerraf B R, Harlow B L, Frigoletto F D. Hypoplasia of the middle phalanx of the fifth digit. J Ultrasound Med 1990; 9: 389–394
17 Abuhamad A Z, Kolm P, Mari G. Ultrasonographic fetal iliac length measurement in the screening for Down syndrome. Am J Obstet Gynecol 1994; 171: 1063
18 Bahado-Singh R O, Wyse L, Dorr M A, Copel J A, O'Connor T, Hobbins J C. Fetuses with Down syndrome have disproportionately shortened frontal lobe dimensions on ultrasonographic examination. Am J Obstet Gynecol 1992; 167: 1009–1014

19 Blandwehr J B, Johnson M P, Hume R F, Yaron Y, Sokol R J, Evans M I. Abnormal nuchal findings on screening ultrasonography: aneuploidy stratification on the basis of ultrasonographic anomaly and gestational age at detection. Am J Obstet Gynecol 1996; 175: 995–999

20 Pandya P P, Snijders S J M, Johnson S P, de Lourdes Brizot M, Nicolaides K I I. Screening for fetal trisomies by maternal age and nuchal translucency thickness at 10 to 14 weeks of gestation. Br J Obstet Gynaecol 1995; 102: 963–969

21 Abramowicz J S, Warsof S L, Doyle D L, Smith D, Levy D L. Congenital cystic hygroma of the neck diagnosed prenatally: outcome with normal and abnormal karyotype. Prenat Diagn 1989; 9: 321–327

22 Chervenak F A, Isaacson G, Blakemore K J et al. Fetal cystic hygroma. N Engl J Med 1983; 309: 822–825

23 Gembruch U, Hansmann M, Bald R, Zerres K, Schwanitz G, Fodisch H J. Prenatal diagnosis and management in fetuses with cystic hygromata colli. Eur J Obstet Gynecol Reprod Biol 1988; 29: 241–255

24 Nadel A, Bromley B, Benacerraf B R. Nuchal thickening or cystic hygromas in first and early second trimester fetuses : prognosis and outcome. Obstet Gynecol 1993; 82: 43–48

25 Bronshtein M, Bar-Hara I, Blumenfeld I, Bejar J, Toder V, Blumenfeld Z. The difference between septated and non-septated nuchal cystic hygroma in the early second trimester. Obstet Gynecol 1993; 81: 683–687

26 Mostello D J, Bofinger M K, Siddiqi T A. Spontaneous resolution of fetal cystic hygroma and hydrops in Turner syndrome. Obstet Gynecol 1989; 73: 862–865

27 Hyett J, Moscoso G, Papapanagiotou G, Perdu M, Nicolaides K H. Abnormalities of the heart and great arteries in chromosomally normal fetuses with increased nuchal translucency thickness at 11–13 weeks of gestation. Ultrasound Obstet Gynecol 1996; 7: 245–250

28 Copel J A, Cullen M, Green J J, Mahoney M J, Hobbins J C, Kleinman C S. The frequency of aneuploidy in prenatally diagnosed congenital heart disease: an indication for fetal karyotyping. Am J Obstet Gynecol 1998; 158: 409–413

29 Rotmensch S, Liberati N, Bronshtein M et al. Prenatal sonographic findings in 187 fetuses with Down's syndrome. Prenat Diagn 1997; 17: 1001-1009

30 Schulman L P, Emerson D S, Felker R F, Philips O P, Simpson J L, Elias S. High frequency of cytogenetic abnormalities in fetuses with cystic hygroma diagnosed in the first trimester. Obstet Gynecol 1992; 80: 80–82

31 Johnson M P, Johnson A, Holzgreve W et al. First trimester simple hygroma: cause and outcome. Am J Obstet Gynecol 1993; 168: 156–161

32 Podobnik M, Singer Z, Podobnik-Sarkanji S, Bulic M. First trimester diagnosis of cystic hygromata using transvaginal ultrasound and cytogenetic evaluation. J Perinat Med 1995; 23: 283–291

33 Shuangshoti S, Netsky M G. Neuroepithelial (colloid) cysts of the nervous system. Further observations on pathogenesis, location. I Incidence and histochemistry. Neurology 1966; 16: 887–903

34 Shuangshoti S, Roberts M P, Netsky M G. Neuroepithelial (colloid) cysts. Pathogenesis and relation to choroid plexus and ependyma. Arch Pathol 1965; 80: 214–224

35 Morcos C L, Platt L D, Carlson D E, Gregory K D, Greene N H, Korst L M. The isolated choroid plexus cyst. Obstet Gynecol 1998; 92: 232–236

36 Andreussi L, Cama A, Cazzutto C, Gianbartolomei G, Grossi G. Cyst of the choroid plexus of the left lateral ventricle. Surg Neurol 1979; 12: 53–57

37 Fakhry J, Schechter A, Tenner M S, Reale M. Cysts of the choroid plexus in neonates: documentation and review of the literature. J Ultrasound Med 1985; 4: 561–563

38 Platt L D, Carlson D E, Medeoris A L, Walla C A. Fetal choroid plexus cysts in the second trimester of pregnancy: a cause for concern. Am J Obstet Gynecol 1991; 164: 1652–1656

39 Fitzsimmons J, Wilson D, Pascoe-Mason J, Shaw CM, Cyr D R, Mack L A. Choroid plexus cysts in fetuses with trisomy 18. Obstet Gynecol 1989; 73: 257–260

40 Gupta J K, Khan K S, Thornton J G, Lilford R J. Management of fetal choroid plexus cysts. Br J Obstet Gynaecol 1997; 104: 881–886

41 Manco L G, Nunan F A, Sohnen H, Jacobs E J. Fetal small bowel simulating an abdominal mass at sonography. J Clin Ultrasound 1986; 14: 404–407

42 Fakhry J, Reiser M, Shapiro L R, Schechter A, Pait L P, Glennon A. Increased echogenicity in the lower fetal abdomen: a common normal variant in the second

trimester. J Ultrasound Med 1986; 5: 489–492

43 Parulekar S G. Sonography of normal fetal bowel. J Ultrasound Med 1991; 10: 210–211

44 Muller F, Frot J C, Aubry M C, Boue J, Boue A. Meconium ileus in cystic fibrosis fetuses. Lancet 1984; ii: 223

45 Schwimer S R, Vanely G T, Reinke R T. Pre-natal diagnosis of cystic meconium peritonitis. J Clin Ultrasound 1984; 12: 37–39

46 Lince D M, Pretorius D H, Manco-Johnson M L, Manchester D, Clewell W H. The clinical significance of increased echogenicity in the fetal abdomen. AJR 1985; 145: 683–686

47 Goldstein R B, Filly R A, Callen P W. Sonographic diagnosis of meconium ileus *in utero*. J Ultrasound Med 1987; 6: 663–666

48 Caspi B, El Chalal U, Lancet M, Chemke J. Pre-natal diagnosis of cystic fibrosis: ultrasonographic appearance of meconium ileus in the fetus. Prenat Diagn 1988; 8: 379–382

49 Blumenthal D H, Rushovich A M, Williams R K, Rochester D. Pre-natal sonographic findings of meconium peritonitis with pathologic correlation. J Clin Ultrasound 1982; 10: 350–352

50 Bromley B, Doubilet P, Frigoletto F, Krauss C, Estroff J, Benacerraf B. Is fetal hyperechoic bowel on second trimester sonogram an indication for amniocentesis? Obstet Gynecol 1994; 83: 647–651

51 Pletcher B A, Williams M K, Mulivor R A, Barth D, Linder C, Rawlinson K. Intra-uterine cytomegalovirus infection presenting as fetal meconium peritonitis. Obstet Gynecol 1991; 78: 903–905

52 Forouzan I. Fetal abdominal echogenic mass: an early sign of intra-uterine cytomegalovirus infection. Obstet Gynecol 1992; 80: 535–537

53 Dechelotte P J, Mulliez N M, Bouvier R J, Vanlieferinghen P C, Lemery D J. Pseudo-meconium ileus due to cytomegalovirus infection – a report of three cases. Pediatr Pathol 1992; 12: 73–82

54 Slotnick R N, Abuhamad A Z. Prognostic implications of fetal echogenic bowel. Lancet 1996; 347: 85–7

55. Muller F, Dommergues M, Aubry M et al. Hyperechogenic fetal bowel: an ultrasonographic marker for adverse fetal and neonatal outcome. Am J Obstet Gynecol 1995; 175: 508–513

56 Schechter A G, Fakhry J, Shapiro L R, Gewitz M H. *In utero* thickening of the chordae tendineae: a cause of intra-cardiac echogenic foci. J Ultrasound Med 1987; 6: 691–695

57 Levry D W, Mintz M C. The left ventricular echogenic focus: a normal finding. AJR 1988; 150: 85–86

58 How H Y, Villafane J, Parihus J A, Spinnato J A. A small hyperechoic foci of the fetal cardiac ventricle: a benign sonographic finding? Ultrasound Obstet Gynecol 1994; 4: 205–207

59 Petrikovsky B M, Challenger M, Wyse L J. Natural history of echogenic foci within ventricles of the fetal heart. Ultrasound Obstet Gynecol 1995; 5: 92–94

60 Sepulveda W, Cullen S, Nicolaides P, Hollingsworth J, Fisk N M. Echogenic foci in the fetal heart: a marker of chromosomal abnormality. Br J Obstet Gynaecol 1995; 102: 490–492

61 Bromley B, Lieberman E, Laboda L, Benacerraf B. Echogenic intracardiac focus: a sonographic sign for fetal Down syndrome. Obstet Gynecol 1995; 86: 998–1001

62 Achiron R, Glaser J, Gelernter I, Hegesh J, Yagel S. Extended fetal echocardiographic examination in detection of cardiac malformation in low risk women. BMJ 1992; 304: 671–674

63 Corteville J E, Gray D L, Grane J P. Congenital hydronephrosis: correlation of fetal ultrasonographic findings with infant outcome. Am J Obstet Gynecol 1991; 165: 384–388

64 Benacerraf B R, Mandell J, Estroff J A, Harlow B L, Frigoletto F D. Fetal pyelectasis; a possible association with Down syndrome. Obstet Gynecol 1990; 76: 58–60

65 Snijders R J M, Farrias M, Von Kaisenberg C, Nicolaides K H. Fetal abnormalities. In: Snidjers R J M, Nicolaides K H. (eds) Ultrasound Markers for Fetal Chromosomal Defects. Carnforth: Parthenon, 1996; 1–62

66 Snidjers R J, Sebire N J, Nicolaides K H. Assessment of risks. In: Snidjers R J M, Nicolaides K H. (eds) Ultrasound Markers for Fetal Chromosomal Defects, London: Parthenon, 1996; 63–120

67 Grignon A, Filion R, Filiatrault D et al. Urinary tract dilatation *in utero*: classification and clinical applications. Radiology 1996; 160: 64–67

68 Corteville J E, Gray D L, Crane J P. Congenital hydronephrosis: correlation of fetal ultrasonographic findings with infant outcome. Am J Obstet Gynecol 1991; 165: 384–388

69 Adra M A, Mejides A A, Dennaoui M S, Beydoun S N. Fetal pyelectasis: is it always 'physiologic'? Am J Obstet Gynecol 1995; 173: 126–126

70 King L R. Fetal hydronephrosis: what is the urologist to do? Urology 1993; 42: 229 231

71 Laing F C, Burke V D, Wing V W, Jeffrey R B, Hashimoto B. Post-partum evaluation of fetal hydronephrosis: optimal timing for follow-up sonography. Radiology 1984; 152: 423–424

72 Blachar A, Blachar Y, Livne P M, Zurkowski L, Pelet D, Mogilner B. Clinical outcome and follow-up of pre-natal hydronephrosis. Pediatr Nephrol 1994; 8: 30–35

73 Nyberg D A, Resta R G, Luthy D A, Hickok D E, Williams M A. Humerus and femur length shortening in the detection of Down's syndrome. Am J Obstet Gynecol 1993; 168: 534–538

74 Vintzileos, A M, Egan J F X, Smulian J C, Campbell W A, Guzman E R, Rodis J F. Adjusting the risk for trisomy 21 by a simple ultrasound method using fetal long bone biometry. Obstet Gynecol 1996. 87: 953–958

75. Wald N, Kennard A, Hackshaw A, McGuire A. Ultrasound markers at 15–22 weeks of pregnancy. Health Technol Assess 1998; 2: 41–48

76 Nyberg D A, Luthy D A, Cheng E Y, Sheley R C, Resta R G, Williams M A. Role of prenatal ultrasonography in women with positive screen for Down's syndrome on the basis of maternal serum markers. Am J Obstet Gynecol 1995; 173: 1030–1035

77 Verdin S M, Economides D L. The role of ultrasonographic markers for trisomy 21 in women with positive serum biochemistry. Br J Obstet Gynaecol 1998; 105: 63–67

78 Vintzileos A M, Guzman E R, Smulian J C, McLean D A, Anath C V. Choice of second trimester genetic sonogram for detection of trisomy 21. Obstet Gynecol 1997; 90: 187–190

79 Marteau T M, Cook R, Kidd J et al. The psychological effects of false-positive results in prenatal screening for fetal abnormality; a prospective study. Prenat Diagn 1992; 12: 205–214

80 Tymstru T. False positive results in screening tests: experience of parents of children screened for congenital hypothyroidism. Fam Pract 1986; 3: 92–96

81 Marteau T M. Screening in practice: reducing the psychological costs. BMJ 1990; 301 : 26–28

82 Royal College of Obstetricians and Gynaecologists. Report of the RCOG Working Party on Ultrasound Screening for Fetal Abnormalities. London: RCOG, 1997

83 Nicolaides K H, Sebire N J, Snijders R, Johnson S. Down's syndrome screening in the UK. Lancet 1996; 347: 906-907

84 Wald N J, Kennard A, Hackshaw A K. First trimester serum screening for Down's syndrome. Prenat Diagn 1995; 15: 1227-1240

85 Snijders R J M, Pandya P, Brizot M L, Nicolaides K H. First trimester nuchal translucency. In: Snijders R J M, Nicolaides K H. (eds) Ultrasound Markers for Fetal Chromosomal Defects. London: Parthenon, 1996; 121–156

86 Pandya P P, Goldberg H, Walton B et al. The implementation of first trimester scanning at 10–13 weeks' gestation and the measurement of fetal nuchal translucency thickness in two maternity units. Ultrasound Obstet Gynaecol 1995; 5: 20-25

87 Pandya P P, Allman D, Brizot M L, Peltersen H, Nicolaides K H. Repeatability of measurement of fetal nuchal translucency thickening. Ultrasound Obstet Gynaecol 1995; 5: 334–337

88 Ecomomides D L, Braithwaite J M, Armstrong M A. First trimester fetal abnormality screening in low risk population. Proceedings of the British Congress of Obstetrics and Gynaecology, Dublin 1995; 455

89 Roberts L J, Bewley S, MacKinson A M, Rodeck C H. First trimester fetal nuchal translucency: problems with screening in the general population 1. Br J Obstet Gynaecol 1995; 102: 381–385

90 Kornman L H, Morssink L P, Beekhuis J R, deWolf B T H M, Heringa M P, Mantingh A. Nuchal translucency cannot be used as a screening test for chromosomal abnormalities in the first trimester of pregnancy in a routine ultrasound practice. Prenat Diagn 1996; 16: 797–805

91 Bewley S, Roberts L J, MacKinson A M, Rodeck C H. First trimester fetal nuchal translucency: problems with screening in the general population 2. Br J Obstet Gynaecol 1995; 102: 386–388

92 Szabo J, Gellen J, Szemere G. First trimester ultrasound screening for fetal aneupolidies in women over 35 and under 35 years of age. Ultrasound Obstet Gynecol 1995; 5: 161–163

93 Pandya P P, Kondylios A, Hilbert L, Snijders R J M, Nicolaides K H. Chromosomal defects and outcome in 1015 fetuses with increased nuchal translucency. Ultrasound Obstet Gynaecol 1995; 5: 15–19

94 Hyett J A, Sebire N J, Snijders R J M, Nicolaides K H. Intrauterine lethality of trisomy 21 fetuses with increased nuchal translucency thickness. Ultrasound Obstet Gynaecol 1996; 7: 101–103

95 Macintoch M C M, Wald N J, Chard T, Hansen J, Mikkelsen M, Therkelsen A J et al. Selective miscarriage of Down's syndrome fetuses in women aged 35 years and older. Br J Obstet Gynaecol 1995; 102: 798–801

96 Macintoch M C M, Wald N J, Chard T, Hansen J, Mikkelsen M, Therkelsen A J et al. The selective miscarriage of Down's syndrome from 10 weeks of pregnancy (letter). Br J Obstet Gynaecol 1996; 103: 1172–1173

97 Howe D T, Gornall R, Wellesley D, Boyle T, Barber J. Six year survey of screening for Down's syndrome by maternal age and mid-trimester ultrsound scans. BMJ 2000; 320: 606–610

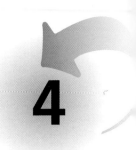

**4**

*B. J. Whitlow   D. L. Economides*

# Screening for fetal anomalies in the first trimester

One child in 55 will be born with a major structural abnormality.[1] Such abnormalities can contribute up to 15% of perinatal deaths and a similar number of deaths in the first year of life.[1] Whilst fetal abnormalities are more common in certain high risk groups (e.g. insulin-dependent diabetes mellitus, epileptics on anticonvulsants and those with a positive family history), the vast majority of fetal abnormalities will not be anticipated. It is, therefore, important to screen for fetal abnormalities in the general obstetric population. This will maximize the chance of detecting fetal anomalies, although it may prove more expensive. Fetal structural defects are at least twice as common as chromosomal abnormalities, and the most common reasons for terminating a fetus with a serious anomaly are neural tube defects followed by chromosome abnormality.[2]

Antenatal care should allow the clinician to reduce maternal and perinatal mortality while preserving maternal satisfaction with the pregnancy. The antenatal detection of fetal malformations has been shown to reduce perinatal mortality (PMR) by allowing elective termination of malformed fetuses.[3] Indeed, once a serious abnormality such as anencephaly or Down's syndrome has been diagnosed, parents will electively choose to terminate such a pregnancy in 80–90% of cases.[4] It is not just for terminations that prenatal diagnosis is useful. It has profound implications on antenatal and intrapartum management. Certain malformations can be treated *in utero* (e.g. diaphragmatic hernia) or postnatally (e.g. certain cardiac defects), so early diagnosis can facilitate decision making regarding mode and place of delivery, especially if neonatal resuscitation and immediate surgery are required.

**Mr B.J. Whitlow** MB BS, Clinical Research Fellow, University Department of Obstetrics and Gynaecology, Royal Free Hospital, Pond Street, London NW3 2QG, UK

**Mr D.L. Economides** MD FRCOG, Consultant and Senior Lecturer, University Department of Obstetrics and Gynaecology, Royal Free Hospital, Pond Street, London NW3 2QG, UK (for correspondence)

It would be preferable to perform the suction termination of pregnancy in the first trimester as it is safe, can be performed as a day case and is less traumatic for the patient than a second trimester termination. Current guidelines from The Royal College of Obstetricians and Gynaecologists recommend an ultrasound examination at 18–20 weeks.[5] Should fetal abnormalities be detected at this stage, a second trimester termination maybe necessary and this is associated with marked psychological sequelae in around 25% of cases.[6] It is assumed that if prenatal diagnosis is made earlier then a safer first trimester termination could be achieved.[7–9]

Technological advances in prenatal ultrasound and the introduction of trans-vaginal sonography (TVS) have enabled detection of fetal malformations in the first trimester. This chapter will focus on the exciting new potential of first trimester sonography for the detection of fetal anomalies.

## GENERAL USES OF SONOGRAPHY IN THE FIRST TRIMESTER

It is important to accurately date a woman's pregnancy in order to provide good obstetric care. When gestational age is confirmed in this manner, induction rates may be reduced by nearly 40%.[10] By using crown-rump length, it is possible to accurately predict gestational age to within 7 days in the first trimester. Viability of a pregnancy can also be determined when the crown-rump length is 6 mm or more and/or the mean gestational sack diameter is 20 mm or more. If there is absence of cardiac activity in the presence of the aforementioned criteria, then the pregnancy can be diagnosed as being non-viable. Determination of chorionicity in multiple pregnancies can be more easily detected in the first trimester, as the lambda sign (suggesting dichorionicity) becomes obliterated at later gestations. Early ultrasound may re-assure those mothers with increased anxiety (especially those who have had a previous ectopic pregnancy or those that suffer from recurrent early miscarriages).[11] Indeed, the presence of a viable fetus at 12–13 weeks' gestation may be associated with a live birth in over 98% of cases.

A significant proportion (2.2%) of pregnancies at 11–14 weeks will have failed and the detection of such missed abortions will enable a planned evacuation of the uterus, avoiding emergency surgery and the physical and emotional trauma of unexpected vaginal haemorrhage. The earlier in the first trimester the scan is performed, the greater the incidence of failed pregnancies. In a recent study of pathological examination of terminated pregnancies for social reasons of up to 9 weeks' gestation, 19% had a structural abnormality and it was estimated that 34% would have ended in a failed pregnancy.[12] In the case of chromosomal abnormalities diagnosed at 11–14 weeks, it is estimated 46% of trisomy 21 and 83% of trisomy 18 and 13 will end up as intra-uterine deaths, although this will depend on the severity of the structural defects present. The other problem of diagnosing structural anomalies early is that pathological confirmation is technically more difficult, time consuming and impossible if suction termination is performed. Although medical evacuation of the uterus using mifepristone or misoprostol is possible,[13] the majority of patients in our unit choose to have suction termination. However, it might be possible to confirm some diagnoses by using embryoscopy prior to the terminations.

**Table 1** Earliest gestation when fetal structures are visualised using transvaginal sonography

| Structures | Gestation when visualised | | | | | |
|---|---|---|---|---|---|---|
| | 8 | 9 | 10 | 11 | 12 | 13 |
| Extremities | ———————————————————————— | | | | | |
| Digits | | | | ———————————— | | |
| Cord insertion | | | ————————————————— | | | |
| Diaphragm | | ———————————————————— | | | | |
| Fetal spine | | ———————————————————— | | | | |
| Choroid plexi | ——————————————————————— | | | | | |
| Cerebellum | | | | ————————————— | | |
| Ventricles | | ———————————————————— | | | | |
| Orbits | | ——————————————————— | | | | |
| Stomach | | | ————————————————— | | | |
| Bladder | | | | ————————————— | | |
| Kidneys | | | ————————————————— | | | |

## Feasibility of examining fetal anatomy in the first trimester

Interpretation of fetal anatomy in the first trimester requires comprehensive understanding of embryological development. Quashie et al[14] investigated visualisation of fetal anatomy with increasing gestation using transvaginal sonography (TVS). The gestation times when various organs are first visualised are shown in Table 1.

## Feasibility of TAS

Green and Hobbins, using TAS, commented that with the greater resolution of modern-day ultrasound the ventricular system, mid-line structures, thalami, cerebellum and choroid plexus could all be well delineated by 12 weeks.[15] Also the spine, although often seen completely at 10 weeks in the sagittal plane, could not be adequately visualised in the coronal plane until 12 weeks. Fetal face, including ears, mandible, maxilla, and orbits could all be defined at 10–11 weeks. The fetal limbs including elbows and knees were visible by 10 weeks and by 12 weeks all the fetal long bones as well as fetal digits could usually be clearly seen. They concluded that detailed fetal anatomy could be visualised with TAS in the first trimester.

## Advantages of TAS

Probe manoeuvrability is superior with transabdominal sonography (TAS) compared to TVS. Orientation and training is quicker and easier with TAS. It also takes less time to perform, is less invasive and does not require the presence of a chaperone.

## Advantages of TVS

TVS in general has superior resolution over TAS, although this will depend in part on the frequency of the probe (the higher the frequency, the better the resolution). Also TVS will give better quality images in patients with a high

**Table 2** Criteria necessary for complete anatomical survey of the first trimester fetus (Braithwaite et al[38])

| Organ | Criteria necessary for adequate visualisation |
|---|---|
| Brain | Complete cranium, septum pellucidum, thalamus, choroid plexi, cerebellum and ventricles |
| Spine | Complete vertebrae seen in both transverse and coronal planes with normal overlying skin |
| Face | Correct position of mandibles, maxillae and orbits |
| Lungs | Normal shape, echogenicity and hypoechoic interface between abdomen and thoracic cavities |
| Heart | Four chamber view, symmetrical ventricles and atria |
| Abdomen | Normal cord insertion and abdominal wall |
| GI tract | Single, hypoechoic structure in left upper abdomen |
| Kidneys | Visualisation of cortex and pelvis of both kidneys and hypoechoic structure anteriorly and in the midline of the pelvis (bladder) |
| Extremities | Visualisation of the long bones, correct posture of the hands and feet |

body mass index (BMI) and/or with retroverted uterus. The acceptability of TVS for examining the fetus in uncomplicated pregnancies has been investigated recently by Braithwaite et al. TVS was acceptable to the majority (88.1%) of these women, and of those undergoing TVS, 99% would be have been happy to have the procedure in a future pregnancy. Indeed, bladder filling for TAS was found to cause marked discomfort in 4.9%. whilst marked discomfort with TVS was found in only 0.7%.[16]

## TAS versus TVS

Achiron and Tadmor concluded that TVS was more sensitive than TAS in the detection of first trimester anomalies.[17] Conversely, Cullen concluded that TVS was better used to complement, not replace TAS examination for the visualisation of the first trimester fetus. One problem with both of these studies was that criteria to define organ visualisation were not stated clearly in either study.[18]

Braithwaite et al examined fetal anatomy by scanning 264 women between 12–13 weeks' gestation with both TAS and TVS.[19] A maximal anatomical survey was attempted with each scan mode, the criteria of which were clearly stated (Table 2) and were comparable to those normally applied in the mid-trimester. It was noted that a high BMI resulted in the inability to visualise certain organs such as the heart, kidneys and bladder with TAS, and TVS was the preferred scan mode in such patients. TVS, however, took longer than TAS, with the mean scan time for a complete anatomical survey being 11 min for TAS and 16 min for TVS. Visualization was consistently superior for every fetal organ with TVS compared to TAS. Complete anatomical surveys were performed in 72% by TAS and 82% by TAS, and in 95% using a combination of both scan modes. Fetal anatomy not seen with one scan type was more easily seen with the other, since the probes approach the fetus from almost opposite angles. Thus, the two scan modes were found to be complimentary.

## The unique appearance of fetal organs in the first trimester

There is a clear need to recognise the normal anatomical structures in the first trimester, and it is important to have a good understanding of the embryological basis of when and how defects develop. The appearance of the brain in the first trimester is somewhat different to later gestations. The choroid plexi completely fill the lateral borders of the posterior and anterior ventricles,[20] and this in turn occupies most of the hemisphere; thus, hydrocephalus can be potentially difficult to diagnose in the first trimester. Certain anomalies in the first trimester have a uniquely different appearance compared to the second trimester. A notable example is the diagnosis of anencephaly. In the first trimester, anencephalic fetus neural tissue can be seen but the cranium is absent, giving rise to the so-called 'Mickey Mouse' appearance, which is different from the 'frogs' eyes' seen in the second trimester.[21] False positive diagnoses of exomphalos can be made if the sonographer is not familiar with first trimester anomaly scanning. Since the bowel is present in the umbilical cord in early embryonic development, an omphalocoele should not be considered as abnormal unless the crown-rump length of the fetus is $\geq 46$ mm.[22]

The heart is difficult to visualize in detail in the first trimester, as the atrial and ventricular septi are small (approaching the upper limit of resolution of the ultrasound machine). Most investigators would accept a 4 chamber view of the heart as sufficient detail. However, Dolkart et al assessed the 4 chamber view including the major outlet vessels and found that by 12 weeks some 90%, and by 13 weeks 100%, of cardiac views were satisfactory.[23] It was commented that the ability to detect the 4 chamber view of the fetal heart is the most important view since, if this is normal, then it would exclude most congenital heart abnormalities, and scanning to examine the major vessels at this gestation would take up to 50 min, thus making such screening impractical.

Fetal kidneys form as early as 5 weeks in the embryonic phase of development and can be visualised from 9 weeks via TVS. The kidneys' appearance changes with gestation, being very echodense at 9–10 weeks and becoming more sonolucent at 11 weeks as excretory function begins. One should be careful not to confuse the adrenals with the kidneys in the first trimester, as the adrenals have a dense medulla in contrast to the kidneys.[24] The ability to view the fetal kidneys was assessed by Bronshtein et al using TVS.[25] They concluded that by 11, 12 and 13 weeks the kidney could be seen in 30%, 80% and 100% of cases, respectively. Since excretory function only occurs after 11 weeks, major renal tract anomalies are unlikely to be visualised before this time.

The hands are often open in the first trimester, thus making it easier to count the digits and examine for polydactyly, whereas the hand is often closed in the second trimester. However, postural deformities become easier to visualize as the musculo-skeletal system of the fetus develops and shortening of the long bones (such as campomelic dysplasia) becomes more obvious in the mid-trimester.

# NUCHAL TRANSLUCENCY MEASUREMENT

Nuchal oedema, or nuchal translucency (NT) as it is now more commonly known, is measured from a sagittal view of the fetus and is the maximum thickness of subcutaneous translucency between the skin and soft tissues overlying the cervical spine (Fig. 1). The association between a thickened nuchal region and Down's syndrome in the first trimester is now well established. It should be noted that nuchal translucency is quite distinct from nuchal skin fold thickness, a term that is applied to fetuses in the second trimester and has quite different implications.

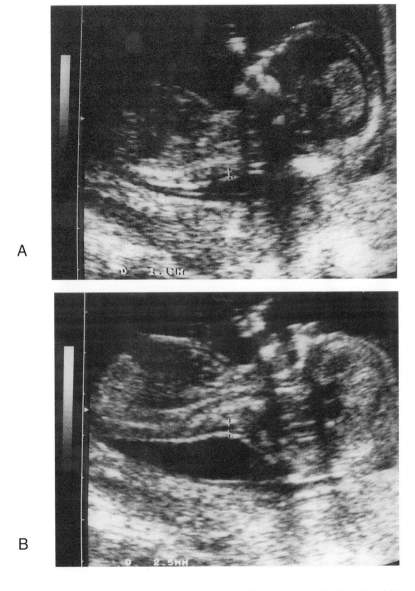

A

B

**Fig. 1** Nuchal translucency measurement in sagittal plane in (A) flexed and (B) extended positions.

## Pathophysiology of nuchal translucency

The pathophysiology of nuchal translucency is not fully understood. Some investigators have proposed a theory of transient cerebral hyperperfusion, with associated diffusion of fluid across a primitive atlanto-occipital membrane in the first trimester, and this might explain the transient nature of NT.[26] Other theories proposed have suggested that cardiac abnormalities (particularly at the aortic isthmus) and heart failure may be a determining factor in increased nuchal translucency along with collagen defects.[26–28]

If NT screening is to be successful, it is imperative that NT can be accurately and consistently obtained by all examiners. It has been shown that NT can be measured in 90% and 92% of fetuses using TVS and trans-abdominal sono-graphy (TAS), respectively, and in 100% of fetuses when using a combination of both techniques.[29] Trans-vaginal sonography is particularly useful in women with an increased BMI or retroverted uteri. Measurement of NT should also be accurately reproducible and consistent. Indeed, it has also been demonstrated that satisfactory repeatability in NT measurements for both TAS and TVS can be attained when viewed by experienced observers; the repeatability using TVS was proved to be superior.[30] In addition, Braithwaite et al have described a training regimen and set the standards required for a potential sonographer to be considered trained to measure NT, and this is usually achieved after 80–100 supervised scans.[30]

## Standardising nuchal translucency measurement

### Position

Most studies examining NT in the first trimester will measure the NT in the midline sagittal plane and measure only the sonolucent (black) area between the fetal spine and skin at 38–83 mm crown-rump length. It has also been suggested that the image size of the fetus should be 75% of the size of the screen in order to accurately position the callipers.[31] On the other hand, other workers have found that image magnification does not contribute to the repeatability of calliper placing.[32] However, recently, the effect of fetal neck position on nuchal translucency measurement has been examined with the fetal neck in the extended, neutral and flexed positions.[33] On average, the extended NT was 0.59 mm greater than the neutral NT value. The flexed NT was on average 0.40 mm less than the neutral position NT value (Fig. 1). Repeatability of measurements was more accurate with the fetal neck in the neutral position. These findings may prove to have important implications for clinicians using nuchal translucency to screen the general obstetric population. The repeatability of the measurement is also dependent on the mode of scanning (0.22 mm and 0.40 mm for TAS and TVS, respectively).[29] Other groups have found that the fetal umbilical cord can be positioned around the neck in 8.23% of fetuses at 10–14 weeks' gestation, and that this can add a mean of 0.8 mm to the NT measurement, if one is not careful to exclude it.[34] Recently, a software tool has been developed for eliminating this bias in a semi-automatic way, thus attempting to improve the reproducibility of the method, although this has not yet been fully evaluated.[35]

### Cut-off values/upper limits of normal

After the initial studies by Szabo and Gellen,[36] many other observers also reported a strong relationship between nuchal oedema and chromosomal abnormalities in a high-risk population (i.e. women > 35 years of age). Nicolaides et al demonstrated that the number of trisomies with an NT less than 2.5 mm was approximately 5 times less than expected on the basis of maternal age, and with an NT of 3 mm and ≥ 3 mm, it was 5 times and 24 times greater than expected, respectively.[37] Charts were constructed to derive the probabilities of a fetus being affected by a chromosomal abnormality on the basis of maternal age combined with NT measurement. Using this method, an 85% sensitivity for the detection of fetal chromosomal abnormality was predicted with a false positive rate of 5%. Investigators have since found that measurement of NT increases with gestation to a peak at 13$^{+2}$ weeks, after which it decreases (Fig. 2).[38] Consequently, the use of a single NT threshold value for all gestations (10–14 weeks) is incorrect. Using such reference ranges for NT with respect for fetal crown-rump length may improve the sensitivity and specificity of chromosomal abnormality detection.[38] Thus centiles for each individual gestation can be constructed and the operator can decide on the 95th or 99th centile to use as an upper limit. False positives can be further improved by combining maternal age with the given NT value at a given gestation (as risk of trisomy will increase with increasing maternal age and decreasing gestational age) and software packages are now available to calculate individual risk figures based on the afore-mentioned criteria.[31]

### Nuchal translucency in unselected populations

Until recently, there were no large studies investigating the usefulness of NT screening in unselected populations (Table 3). Pandya et al investigated the implementation of NT screening in two maternity units.[39] The introduction of the additional NT screening between 10–13 weeks' gestation required intensive initial training of staff, but not an increase in sonographers or scan machines. In contrast, Bewley et al, in a study of 1,368 women, reported that only 2 of 5 affected fetuses had increased NT.[40] However, that particular study has been widely criticised, as the ultrasonographers were instructed not to take extra time

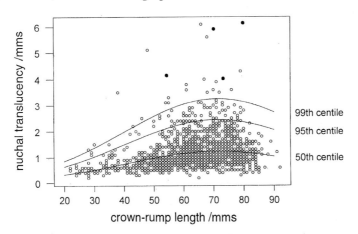

**Fig. 2** Variation in nuchal translucency measurement with increasing gestational age.

**Table 3** Studies screening for fetal aneuploidy using nuchal translucency in low risk populations

| Reference | No. patients | NT | Gestation (weeks) | Sensitivity |
|---|---|---|---|---|
| Bewley et al 1995[40] | 1127 | ≥ 3 mm | 8–13 | 40% |
| Hafner et al 1995[68] | 1972 | ≥ 2.5 mm | 10–13 | 73% |
| Pandya et al 1995[39] | 1763 | ≥ 2.5 mm | 10–13 | 75% |
| Kornman et al 1996[69] | 923 | ≥ 3 mm | 10 | 40% |
| Taipale et al 1997[70] | 10,010 | ≥ 3 mm | 10–15.9 | 62% |
| Economides 1998[41] | 2281 | ≥ 99th centile & structural anomalies | 11–14 | 81% |
| Snijders et al 1998[42] | 96,127 | > 95th centile | 10–14 | 77% |
| Total | 114,203 | ≥ 2.5–3 mm/ 95–99th centile | 8–15.9 | 70% |

beyond that for a normal dating scan to measure the NT and NT measurements were not attempted in an unspecified number of subjects. Therefore, patience and motivation of sonographers are important when measuring NT.

The authors have recently published a study comprising ultrasonographic examination of the first trimester fetal anatomy, including the fetal neck.[41] This has been shown to be an effective method of screening for chromosomal abnormalities. Without taking maternal age into consideration and using either the 99th centile for nuchal translucency or the presence of a structural abnormality as indications for karyotyping, we were able to diagnose 81% of chromosomal abnormalities and 75% of cases of trisomy 21 at 11–14 weeks. The detection rate is similar to a nuchal translucency screening programme where nuchal translucency measurement in combination with maternal age and the 95th centile for gestational age has been demonstrated to detect 77% of cases of trisomy 21.[42] This is the largest UK multicentre trial (96,127 women) involving NT to date. They found that on average, 30 invasive tests would be required to identify one affected fetus.

## Sonographic markers for chromosomal abnormalities in the first trimester

The significance of 'soft' ultrasound markers for the detection of chromosomal abnormalities in the first trimester is unknown, although ultrasonographic markers for aneuploidy in the second trimester have been studied widely. A study examining the significance of echogenic foci in the fetal heart ('golf-ball' sign) was conducted by Achiron et al on 2,214 low risk women at 13–16 weeks. They concluded that these foci were not significantly associated with trisomy 21.[43] The authors have recently carried out the first prospective study in an unselected population of 5,287 patients to determine the significance of so called 'soft' ultrasound markers in the first trimester. Patients were scanned at 11–14[+6] weeks and then rescanned at 18–20 weeks; the presence of choroid plexus cysts, 'echogenic foci in the left ventricle' and pyelectasis (> 3 mm) were recorded. Choroid plexus cysts were seen to be more common in the first than the second trimester (2.2% versus 1.4% ). 'Echogenic foci in the left ventricle' (0.7%) and pyelectasis (0.9%) had a similar incidence in the two trimesters.[44] Fetuses with markers in the first trimester were not necessarily the same fetuses with markers in the second trimester. Pyelectasis and 'echogenic foci in the left ventricle' in the first trimester appeared to be associated with aneuploidy but choroid plexus cysts did not. So whilst early data may suggest that isolated echogenic foci and pyelectasis are statistically significant markers of chromosomal abnormalities, larger data sets will be required to confirm these initial findings. Otherwise this may generate inappropriate anxiety in pregnant women.[44] The presence of two or more such markers should stimulate the clinician to discuss invasive karyotyping with the patient in the first trimester.

Martinez et al combined nuchal translucency with umbilical Doppler velocimetry for detecting fetal trisomies in the first trimester of pregnancy. Using the 95th centile and 3 mm as the cut offs for UAPI and NT, respectively, in 553 cases, the detection rate for all chromosomal anomalies was 84.2%, with a false positive rate of 6.6%, a positive predictive value of 31.3%, and a negative predictive value of 99.4%.[45] The number of cases studied was small, however, and these conclusions are tentative and preliminary.

## Outcome of fetuses with enlarged nuchal translucency and a normal karyotype

Whilst the number of fetuses with an increased NT will have an abnormal karyotype in 34% of cases overall,[46] this figure will vary depending on the maternal age, degree of increased NT and gestation at diagnosis. Should the karyotype be normal, the patient may well ask what is the prognosis for such a child. Souka et al, in a study of over 4000 such cases, found that a live birth can be expected in 94.4%.[47] Structural abnormalities can be expected in 10–17% of cases.[46,48] Equally, genetic syndromes and single gene disorders can be expected in an additional 12% of fetuses. Additionally, Sebire et al found that NT values in monochorionic twins > 95th centile were significantly more likely to develop twin–twin transfusion syndrome.[49] Therefore, in addition to detecting chromosomal abnormalities, increased NT may also have a role in screening for a number of other abnormalities. Thus the chances of taking home a normal baby in the presence of an increased NT is around 34% (when chromosomal, structural, genetic syndromes and miscarriages are considered together).[46]

## Nuchal translucency and cardiac abnormalities

Increased NT is also associated with cardiac system abnormalities; the greater the measurement of NT, the more severe the abnormality.[27,28] It was demonstrated that the incidence of major cardiac defects was 17 per 1000 live-births in cases where first trimester nuchal translucency was > 2.5 mm. The incidence of major cardiac defects was also found to increase with increasing NT. It was, therefore, concluded that karyotypically normal fetuses with increased NT should have mid-trimester fetal echocardiography.

## Nuchal translucency and cost-effectiveness

In the practice of medicine today, screening tests must be cost-effective and this applies to NT screening. Vintzileos has addressed this issue and found that first-trimester sonography using NT for the detection of Down's syndrome was found to be beneficial if the overall sensitivity for detecting Down's syndrome was greater than 70%, and, even then, the cost-benefit ratio depended on the corresponding false-positive rate.[50] Thus, they concluded that the benefits of first-trimester sonography for the detection of Down's syndrome depend on its diagnostic accuracy, but it has the potential for annual savings of $22 million in the US.

Screening for Down's syndrome using nuchal translucency was given a grade B recommendation by The Royal College of Obstetricians and Gynae-cologists working party report, as was serum screening at 9–13 weeks. There are, however, still questions regarding cost-effectiveness of such an early scan, and Neilson has argued that a randomised trial of first trimester versus second trimester screening will need to be completed before nuchal translucency is implemented fully on a wider scale.[51]

## Maternal first trimester serum biochemical screening

There have been a number of studies recently describing the use of first trimester maternal serum biochemistry in screening for chromosomal abnormalities. Wald et al measured free $\beta$-hCG and PAPP-A at 8–14 weeks' gestation and found that the respective multiple of the median values in those pregnancies affected by Down's syndrome were on average 1.79 and 0.43, respectively.[52] The combination of these two markers were shown to be 63% sensitive and 94.5% specific. Other markers – $\alpha$-fetoprotein ($\alpha$-FP), unconjugated oestriol, total hCG, free $\alpha$-hCG and dimeric inhibin A – were also examined in this study, but were found not to be of clinical significance. Other investigators studied $\alpha$-FP, free $\beta$-hCG and PAPP-A at 10–13 weeks and demonstrated a sensitivity of 66% for detecting chromosomal abnormalities.[53] Haddow et al investigated the use of such markers on a selected population (where 82% of whom were 35 years of age or older) and the rates of detection of Down's syndrome for the serum markers were: 17% for $\alpha$-FP, 4% for unconjugated estriol, 29% for hCG, 25% for the free $\beta$ subunit of hCG, and 42% for pregnancy-associated protein A, at false positive rates of 5%. When used in combination with the serum concentration of pregnancy-associated protein A and maternal age, the detection rate was 63% for hCG.[54]

Nuchal translucency and first trimester biochemical markers are not related, and so they can be combined in screening for aneuploidy. In a study of 2,010 singleton pregnancies between $9^{+0}$ and $13^{+4}$ maternal dried whole-blood specimens were collected and a subset of 744 pregnancies underwent ultrasound nuchal translucency measurement. It was reported that Down's syndrome was detected by biochemistry in 61%, by nuchal translucency in 73% and in 87% by combining both methods for a 5% false-positive rate.[55] Thus by combining nuchal translucency with first trimester biochemical screening and maternal age, detection rates for fetal aneuploidy can be improved, and this agrees with other investigators.[56] Future maternal biochemical screening may involve blood being taken at initial ultrasound visit (11–14 weeks) and results being available by the end of the scan, thus improving efficiency and giving the mother one single risk figure rather than one risk for maternal age, one for NT and one for biochemical screening.

Thus it would appear that combining maternal age, first trimester serum biochemistry and nuchal translucency measurement could improve the detection rate of chromosomal abnormalities. However, in the presence of fetal structural abnormalities or a nuchal translucency measurement of greater than or equal to the 99th centile, fetal karyotyping should be performed irrespective of maternal age or maternal serum biochemistry.

## The optimal gestational age to perform the first trimester scan

There is a need for healthcare professionals to know when to organise the first trimester scan. A study was carried out by the authors to answer this question.[57] A total of 1,288 women were studied from an unselected population. Visualisation of fetal anatomy was found to improve with increasing gestational age from 6%, 75%, 96%, 98% at 10, 11, 12 and 13 weeks of gestation and was similarly high (98%) at 14 weeks. The ability to measure nuchal translucency was similar from weeks 10 to 13 (100%, 98%, 98%, 98%), but could only be measured in 90% of fetuses at 14 weeks. The need for transvaginal sonography steadily decreased with increasing gestational age, being 100%, 42%, 21%, 15% and 11% at 10, 11, 12, 13 and 14 weeks, respectively. Thus the optimal gestational age to examine fetal

**Table 4** Visualisation of fetal anatomy by anatomical systems and gestational age (Whitlow & Economides[57])

| Organ | Gestation (weeks) | | | | |
|---|---|---|---|---|---|
| | 10 | 11 | 12 | 13 | 14 |
| Brain visualised | 21% (11/53) | 90% (132/147) | 99% (464/465) | 100% (458/458) | 100% (151/151) |
| Spine visualised | 25% (13/53) | 92% (135/147) | 99% (461/465) | 100% (458/458) | 100% (151/151) |
| Face visualised | 58% (31/53) | 95% (139/147) | 99% (463/465) | 100% (458/458) | 100% (151/151) |
| Lungs visualised | 85% (45/53) | 96% (141/147) | 99% (463/465) | 99% (457/458) | 100% (151/151) |
| Heart (4 chamber view) visualised | 9% (5/53) | 83% (122/147) | 96% (447/465) | 98% (450/458) | 98% (148/151) |
| Abdomen visualised | 89% (47/53) | 97% (145/147) | 100% (465/465) | 100% (458/458) | 100% (151/151) |
| GI tract visualised | 74% (39/53) | 97% (143/147) | 99% (463/465) | 99% (457/458) | 100% (151/151) |
| Kidneys visualised | 45% (24/53) | 86% (126/147) | 97% (453/465) | 99% (454/458) | 99% (150/151) |
| Extremities visualised | 91% (48/53) | 99% (146/147) | 100% (465/465) | 100% (458/458) | 100% (151/151) |

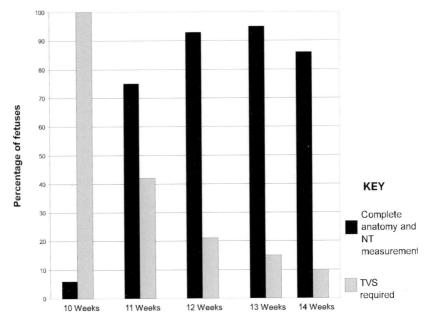

**Fig. 3** Ability to visualise fetal anatomy and nuchal translucency at 10–14 weeks.

anatomy and measure nuchal translucency in the first trimester was found to be at 13 weeks (Table 4 & Fig. 3).[57]

### First trimester detection of fetal structural abnormalities

Detection of fetal abnormalities in the first trimester using TVS has been described by Rottem et al.[58] In this study, 141 pregnant women at high-risk of fetal abnormalities due to previous pregnancy complications were examined between 9–12 weeks' gestation. Four structural abnormalities in three fetuses within the study group were diagnosed: (i) at 9.5 weeks' gestation an anencephalic fetus with an open spina-bifida; (ii) at 9.5 weeks' gestation, a cystic hygroma; and (iii) at 11.5 weeks' gestation a cystic hygroma and generalised fetal oedema was seen. In this small study, the feasibility of first trimester ultrasonographic diagnosis of developmental abnormalities was established for the first time.

In a subsequent study on 1652 patients at 9–16 weeks using TVS, Rottem and Bronshtein diagnosed 61 malformations in 40 fetuses (2.6%), although formal assessment of first and early second trimester diagnostic sensitivity was not performed in this study.[59]

Bronshtein et al investigated the merits of TVS in a larger study on 4,878 fetuses scanned by TVS at gestations between 9–16 weeks in a mixture of high and low-risk patients: 229 anomalous fetuses were detected but 104 (39%) of these abnormalities such as hydronephrosis and choroid plexus cysts were transient.[60] Karyotyping performed because of these anomalies detected 14 dyskaryotic fetuses and interestingly in 7 (50%) of these the anomaly for which the amniocentesis was performed had resolved by the time of the traditional 18–20 week sonogram. It was concluded that performing the first ultrasound

**Table 5** Studies detecting fetal structural defects in the first trimester

| Reference | Low risk? | No. patients | Gestation (weeks) | Scan mode (TVS or TAS) | Anomalies detected |
|---|---|---|---|---|---|
| Rottem et al 1989[58] | No | 141 | 9–12 | TVS | 3 |
| Cullen et al 1990[24] | No | 622 | 8–13 | TVS | 32 |
| Rottem & Bronshtein 1990[59] | No | 1652 | 9–16 | TVS | 40 |
| Bronshtein & Blumenfeld 1991[60] | No | 4878 | 9–16 | TVS | 229 |
| Achiron & Tadmor 1991[17] | No | 800 | 9–13 | TVS | 12 |
| Hernadi et al 1997[71] | Yes | 3991 | 12 | TVS | 43 |
| Economides & Braithwaite 1998[19] | Yes | 1632 | 12–13 | TAS & TVS | 17 |

at a later gestational age would miss transient anomalies associated with chromosomally abnormal fetuses, and suggested that screening in the early mid-trimester be offered to everyone.

## Screening low-risk populations for structural anomalies

Most studies to date have concentrated on screening high-risk groups for fetal abnormalities using TVS (Table 5 & Fig. 4), but few studies have assessed the sensitivity and specificity of the technique. We have preliminarily investigated the performance of anomaly scanning in a low-risk population, between 11–14 weeks' gestation.[61] Patients were initially scanned using TAS, and TVS was additionally performed if visualization of fetal anatomy was incomplete with

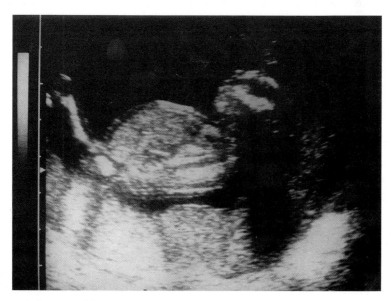

**Fig. 4** Sonogram of fetus with anencephaly at 13 weeks.

**Table 6** Structural abnormalities diagnosed by trimester and anatomical system

| System | 1st trimester | 2nd trimester | Postnatal |
|---|---|---|---|
| Central nervous system | 88% (15/17) | 12% (2/17) | 0% (0/17) |
| Face | 0% (0/2) | 50% (1/2) | 50% (1/2) |
| Neck | 100% (12/12) | 0% (0/12) | 0% (0/12) |
| Cardiovascular | 37% (3/8) | 13% (1/8) | 50% (4/8) |
| Lung | 33% (1/3) | 33% (1/3) | 33% (1/3) |
| GI tract | 100% (6/6) | 0% (0/6) | 0% (0/6) |
| Renal | 75% (3/4) | 25% (1/4) | 0% (0/4) |
| Skeletal | 0% (0/4) | 75% (3/4) | 25% (1/4) |

TAS. A total of 5,616 patients have been studied so far. The abnormality rate was found to be 0.8% (47/5,616). Thirty-two of these abnormalities were diagnosed in the first trimester (68% sensitivity), with a specificity of 99.9%.

Fetal abnormalities from all the major systems have been diagnosed in the first trimester. Certain abnormalities are more easily detectable at 11–14 weeks than others. First trimester sonography was found to be particularly good for diagnosing central nervous system defects, neck anomalies, gastrointestinal and renal defects.[61] However, spina-bifida, heart anomalies and limb defects are more difficult to detect (Table 6 & Fig. 5). Of course, these are the anomalies that can also be difficult to diagnose in the second trimester. In the two cases of spina-bifida, the spinal lesion was a closed defect and very difficult to visualise even at the second trimester scan. The diagnosis was aided by the presence of cranial signs (banana shaped cerebellum and lemon shaped cranium). Recently, the presence of a lemon shaped skull in the first trimester has been described and this may prove to aid diagnosis of spina-bifida.[62] The detection of cardiac abnormalities in the first trimester in this study was below

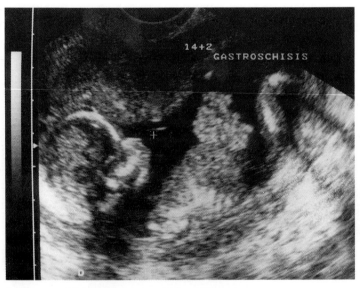

**Fig. 5** Sonogram of fetus with gastroschisis at 13 weeks.

what one might expect when compared to the second trimester scan (i.e. 38% versus 69%). This may be due to the fetal heart being of relatively small size in the first trimester and, even with high resolution TVS, small defects will always be very difficult to diagnose.

Eight out of 47 anomalies were detected at the second trimester scan, including three heart defects (two ventricular septal defects and one Fallot's tetralogy), two cases of spina-bifida, three limb abnormalities (absent fibula and distal forearm and one talipes). This is in agreement with other investigators, who found that some 17% of abnormalities not detected at 13–16 weeks were subsequently detected at the 18–20 week scan.[63] The anomalies not diagnosed by the combination of first and second trimester scans are mainly heart and limb defects. This is comparable to the other mid-trimester studies. However, the detection of heart anomalies may improve by the measurement of NT in the first trimester. Thus, in karyotypically normal fetuses with increased NT, there maybe a place for mid-trimester fetal echocardiography at 22–24 weeks' gestation when the cardiovascular system can be better visualised. Interestingly, 3/8 cases with cardiac abnormalities in the study group had a nuchal translucency above the 95th centile for gestational age.

Some abnormalities, however, develop as a transitory finding in the first trimester and may not be present at later gestations (e.g. cystic hygromas and nuchal translucency). Other fetal anomalies may present at varying times throughout gestation, for example talipes, hydrocephalus and obstructive uropathy. Certain abnormalities may be regarded as unstable anomalies, such that they may be initially present then disappear, only to re-appear a few days later, such as exomphalos and megacystis. Other fetal abnormalities such as arachnoid cysts tend to present late in gestation and are not detectable in the first trimester. Thus the sonographer should be aware of the chronological order of development of specific malformations. Therefore, a single scan in pregnancy will not detect all fetal malformations.

The introduction of routine first trimester scanning will have important implications for the second trimester scan. Certainly, if the majority of chromosomal abnormalities are being detected in the first trimester, then there will be a smaller number of fetuses with chromosomal abnormality in the population having second trimester scans. Therefore, the presence of sonographic soft markers will be of lesser significance. Thus, in the second trimester scan, there should be more emphasis on diagnosing the more difficult anomalies by concentrating on the heart, spine and limbs.

One concern voiced by many clinicians is that diagnosis of fetal anomalies may be easier to visualise at 18–20 weeks and that there may be a significant false positive diagnosis in the first trimester. The false positive rate is low and comparable with the second trimester scan. The main reason for this is physiological bowel herniation into the cord that does occur up to 11 weeks, and can be mistaken for exomphalos. There is a need for the sonographer to have a sound knowledge of the embryological development and different appearances of certain organs in the first trimester.

## The psychological aspects first trimester scanning

It is important that every woman undergoing a first trimester scan is fully

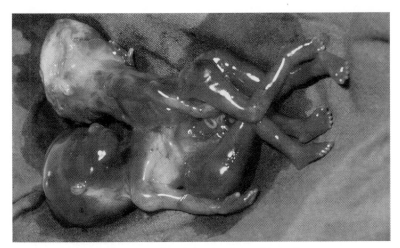

**Fig. 6** Postmortem confirmation of conjoined twins at 14 weeks.

informed of the possible abnormalities and consequences of having such a scan. Some women maybe happy to have a first trimester scan, but, for ethical or religious reasons, may not wish to have their baby's nuchal translucency measured. It has been shown that the level of psychological morbidity following termination for fetal abnormality in the second trimester is similar to that following spontaneous perinatal loss and is of the order of 25%.[64] Whilst first trimester termination of pregnancy maybe easier for health professionals to cope with,[65] there is, as yet, no firm evidence that it is psychologically advantageous for a woman to undergo a first trimester termination of pregnancy versus second trimester termination of pregnancy for fetal abnormality. Indeed, later termination may facilitate mourning, if the baby is seen and held and the parents are provided with a photograph of the baby (Fig. 6).[8]

### Financial implications of screening for fetal anomalies in the first trimester

The financial implications of introducing an extra routine scan for all pregnant women are considerable and the cost-effectiveness of such a programme needs to be assessed before becoming routine practice. Assuming the cost of a single first trimester scan is £33, (which might be different in other obstetric units) then we have estimated that the detection of one single anomalous fetus in the first trimester will cost £3955, for trisomy 21 £15,491 and for any aneuploidy £6885 (Fig. 7). In a recent study, the incidence of anomalous fetuses detected in the first trimester was 0.9%.[61] This figure is 5 times greater than the projected number of potential anomalies that were estimated to be detected in the first trimester by The Royal College of Obstetricians and Gynaecologists working party report for screening for fetal anomalies.[66] It will be difficult to estimate the life-long costs of caring for individuals with different congenital abnormalities, but it is estimated that the yearly cost of one Down's syndrome individual would be £6811–29,665.[67] There will also be significant reductions in in-patient costs for women undergoing day-case suction termination of pregnancies. A suction termination was performed in 66% of cases in our study. In a first trimester

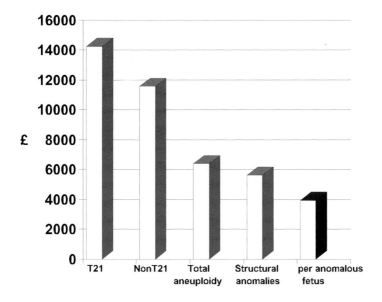

**Fig. 7** Cost of screening in the first trimester.

screening programme, there should not be any significant change in the karyotyping rate and we have not experienced this in our unit. Thus, in conclusion, we have found that first trimester sonography at 11–14 weeks could detect the majority of fetal structural defects (68%) and chromosomal defects (79%), at an estimated cost per abnormality of £6885 for detecting fetal aneuploidy, £5809 per case for structural defects and £3955 per anomalous fetus.

## CONCLUSIONS

Nuchal translucency screening for Down's syndrome has been given a grade B recommendation by the RCOG working party, as has serum screening at 9–13 weeks. In addition, as a result of advances in a ultrasound technology, visualization of the first trimester fetus has markedly improved. By examining fetal anatomy and measuring NT at 11–14 weeks' gestation, the majority of structural (68%) and chromosomal (79%) abnormalities can be diagnosed in early pregnancy. However, significant abnormalities can be missed, e.g. heart and spine defects; therefore, the mid-trimester scan will be needed as a supplement to the first trimester scan, although the role of the former needs to be redefined.

### References

1 OPCS. London: HMSO, 1994
2 Northern Regional Survey Steering Group. Fetal abnormality: an audit of its recognition and management. Arch Dis Child 1992; 67: 770–774
3 Butcher H C, Schmidt J G. Does routine ultrasound scanning improve outcome in pregnancy? Meta-analysis of various outcome measures. BMJ 1993; 307: 13–17
4 EUROCAT Working Group, Part 1. 1995; 36
5 Royal College of Obstetricians and Gynaecologists Working Party. Routine Ultrasound Examination in Pregnancy. London: RCOG Press, 1984

6  Zeanah C H, Dailey J V, Rosenblatt M, Saller D N. Do women grieve after terminating pregnancies because of fetal abnormalities? A controlled investigation. Obstet Gynecol 1993; 82: 270–275

7  Grimes P A, Cates W. Complications from legally induced abortion: a review . Obstet Gynecol Survey 1979; 34: 177–191

8  Leon I G. Pregnancy termination due to fetal anomaly: clinical considerations. Infant Ment Health J 1995; 16: 122–126

9  White-van Mourik M, Connor I, Ferguson-Smith M. The psychological sequelae of a second trimester termination of pregnancy for a fetal abnormality. Prenat Diagn 1992; 12: 189–204

10  Neilson J P. Routine ultrasound in early pregnancy. In: Neilson J P, Crowther C H, Hodnett E G, Hofmeyr G J, Kierson M J N C (eds) Pregnancy in Childbirth: Module of the Cochrane Database of Systematic Reviews. London: BMJ Publishing Group, 1996

11  Campbell S, Reading A E, Cox D N et al. Ultrasound scanning in early pregnancy; the short term psychological effects of early real time scans. J Psychosom Obstet Gynaecol 1982; 1: 57–61

12  Blanch G, Quenby S, Ballantyne E S, Gosden C M, Neilson J P. Embryonic abnormalities at medical termination of pregnancy with mifepristone and misoprostol during first trimester: observational study. BMJ 1998; 316: 1712–1713

13  Spitz I M, Bardin C W, Benton L, Robbins A. Early pregnancy termination with mifepristone and misoprostol in the United States. N Engl J Med 1998; 338: 1241–1247

14  Quashie C. Weiner S. Bolognese R. Efficacy of first trimester transvaginal sonography in detecting normal fetal development. Am J Perinatol 1992; 9: 209–213

15  Green J J, Hobbins J C. Abdominal examination of the first trimester fetus. Am J Obstet Gynecol 1988; 159: 165–175

16  Braithwaite J M. Economides D L. Acceptability by patients of transvaginal sonography in the elective assessment of the first-trimester fetus. Ultrasound Obstet Gynecol 1997; 9: 91–93

17  Achiron R, Tadmor O. Screening for fetal anomalies during the first trimester of pregnancy: trans-vaginal verses trans-abdominal sonography. Ultrasound Obstet Gynecol 1991; 1: 186–191

18  Cullen M T, Green J J, Reece E A, Hobbins J C. A comparison of transvaginal and abdominal ultrasound in visualising the first trimester coceptus. J Ultrasound Med 1989; 8: 565–569

19  Braithwaite J M, Armstrong M A, Economides D L. The assessment of fetal anatomy at 12–13 weeks using transabdominal and transvaginal sonography. Br J Obstet Gynaecol 1996; 103: 82–85

20  Blaas H G, Eik-Ness S H, Kiserud T, Hellevik L R. Early development of the forebrain and midbrain: a longitudinal study from 7 to 12 weeks of gestation. Ultrasound Obstet Gynecol 1994; 4: 183–192

21  Chatzipapas I K, Whitlow B J, Economides D L. The diagnosis of anencephaly in early pregnancy: the 'Mickey-Mouse'ˆ sign. Ultrasound Obstet Gynecol; 1999; 13: 196–200

22  Snijders R J M, Brizot M L, Faria M, Nicolaides K H. Fetal exomphalos at 11-14 weeks of gestation. J Ultrasound Med 1995; 14: 569–574

23  Dolkart L A, Reimers F T. Transvaginal fetal echocardiography in early pregnancy: normative data. Am J Obstet Gynecol 1991; 165: 688–691

24  Cullen M T, Green J, Whetham J, Salafia C, Gabrielli S, Hobbins J C. Transvaginal ultrasonographic detection of congenital anomalies in the first trimester. Am J Obstet Gynecol 1990; 163: 466–476

25  Bronshtein M, Yoffe N, Brandes J M, Blumenfeld Z. First and early second trimester diagnosis of fetal urinary tract anomalies using transvaginal sonography. Prenat Diagn 1990; 10: 653–666

26  Moscoso G. Fetal nuchal translucency – a need to understand the physiological basis. Ultrasound Obstet Gynecol 1995; 5: 6–8

27  Hyett J, Moscoso G, Papapanagiotou G, Perdu M, Nicolaides K H. Abnormalities of the heart and great arteries in chromosomally normal fetuses with increased nuchal translucency thickness at 11–13 weeks of gestation. Ultrasound Obstet Gynecol 1996; 7: 245–250

28  Hyett J A, Perdu M, Sharland G K, Snijders R J M, Nicolaides K H. Increased nuchal translucency at 10–14 weeks of gestation as a marker for major cardiac defects.

Ultrasound Obstet Gynecol 1997; 10: 242–246

29 Braithwaite J M, Economides D L. The measurement of nuchal translucency with transabdominal and transvaginal sonography – success rates, repeatability and levels of agreement. Br J Radiol 1995; 68: 720–723

30 Braithwaite J M, Kadir R A, Pepera T P, Thompson P T, Economides D L. Nuchal translucency measurement – training of potential examiners. Ultrasound Obstet Gynecol 1996; 8: 192–195

31 Nicolaides K H. Oral presentation, Fetal Medicine Foundation Course. London, June, 1997

32 Herman A, Maymom R, Dreazen E, Caspi E, Bukovsky I, Weinraub Z. Image magnification does not contribute to repeatability of caliper placement in measuring nuchal translucency thickness. Ultrasound Obstet Gynecol 1998; 11: 266–270

33 Whitlow B J, Chatzipapas I, Economides D L. The effect of fetal neck position on nuchal translucency measurement. Br J Obstet Gynaecol 1998; 105: 872–876

34 Schaefer M, Laurichesse-Delmas H, Ville Y. The effect of nuchal cord on nuchal translucency measurement at 10–14 weeks. Ultrasound Obstet Gynecol 1998; 11: 271–273

35 Bernardino F. Cardoso R. Montenegro N. Bernardes J. de Sa J M. Semiautomated ultrasonographic measurement of fetal nuchal translucency using a computer software tool. Ultrasound Med Biol 1998; 24: 51–54

36 Szabo J, Gellen J. Nuchal fluid accumulation in trisomy 21 detected by vaginography in the first trimester. Lancet 1990; i: 1133

37 Nicolaides K H, Brizot M L, Snijders R J. Fetal nuchal translucency: ultrasound screening for fetal trisomy in the first trimester of pregnancy. Br J Obstet Gynaecol 1994; 101: 782–786

38 Braithwaite J M, Morris R W, Economides D L. Nuchal translucency measurements: frequency distribution and changes with gestation in a general population. Br J Obstet Gynaecol 1996; 103: 1201–1204

39 Pandya P P, Goldberg H, Walton B et al. The implementation of first-trimester scanning at 10–13 weeks' gestation and the measurement of fetal nuchal translucency thickness in two maternity units. Ultrasound Obstet Gynecol 1995; 5: 20–25

40 Bewley S, Roberts L J, Mackinson A M, Rodeck C H. First trimester fetal nuchal translucency: problems with screening the general population, 2. Br J Obstet Gynaecol 1995; 102: 386–388

41 Economides D L, Whitlow B J, Kadir R, Lazanakis M L, Verdin S. First trimester sonographic detection of chromosomal abnormalities in an unselected population. Br J Obstet Gynaecol 1998; 105: 58–62

42 Snijders R J M, Noble P, Sebire N, Souk A, Nicolaides K H. UK multicentre project on assessment of risk of trisomy 21 by maternal age and fetal nuchal translucency thickness at 10–14 weeks of gestation. Lancet 1998; 351: 343–346

43 Achiron R, Lipitz S, Gabbay U, Yagel S. Prenatal ultrasonographic diagnosis of fetal heart echogenic foci: no correlation with Down syndrome. Obstet Gynecol 1997; 89: 945–948

44 Whitlow B J, Lazanakis M S, Kadir R A, Chatzipapas I K, Verdin S M, Economides D L. The significance of choroid plexus cysts, echogenic heart foci and renal pyelectasis in the first trimester. Ultrasound Obstet Gynecol 1998; 12: 385–390

45 Martinez J M, Borrell A, Antolin E et al. Combining nuchal translucency with umbilical Doppler velocimetry for detecting fetal trisomies in the first trimester of pregnancy. Br J Obstet Gynaecol 1997; 104: 11–14

46 Bilardo C M, Pajkrt E, De Graaf I, Mol B W, Bleker O P. Outcome of fetuses with enlarged nuchal translucency and normal karyotype. Ultrasound Obstet Gynecol 1998; 11: 401–406

47 Souka A P, Snijders R J M, Novakov A, Soares W, Nicolaides K H. Defects and syndromes in chromosomally normal fetuses with increased nuchal translucency thickness at 10–14 weeks of gestation. Ultrasound Obstet Gynecol 1998; 11: 391–400

48 Van Vugt J M G, Tinnemans B W S, Van Zalen-Sprock R M. Outcome and early childhood follow-up of chromosomally normal fetuses with increased nuchal translucency at 10–14 weeks gestation. Ultrasound Obstet Gynecol 1998; 11: 407–409

49 Sebire N J, D'Ecrole C, Hughes K, Carvalho M, Nicolaides K H. Increased nuchal translucency thickness at 10–14 weeks of gestation as a predictor of severe twin-to-twin

transfusion syndrome. Ultrasound Obstet Gynecol 1997; 10: 86–89

50  Vintzileos A M. Ananth C V. Fisher A J. Smulian J C. Day-Salvatore D. Beazoglou T. An economic evaluation of first-trimester genetic sonography for prenatal detection of Down syndrome. Obstet Gynecol 1998; 91: 535–539

51  Neilson J P. Assessment of fetal nuchal translucency test for Down's syndrome. Lancet 1997; 350: 754–755

52  Wald N J, George L, Smith D, Densem J W, Petterson K. Serum screening for Down's syndrome between 8 and 14 weeks of pregnancy . Br J Obstet Gynaecol 1996; 103: 407–412

53  Zimmerman R, Hucha A, Savoldelli G, Binkert F, Ascherman B, Grudzinskas J G. Serum parameters and nuchal translucency in first trimester screening for fetal chromosomal abnormalities . Br J Obstet Gynaecol 1996; 103: 1009–1014

54  Haddow J E, Palomaki G E, Knight G J, Williams J, Miller W A, Johnson A. Screening of maternal serum for fetal Down's syndrome in the first trimester. N Engl J Med 1998; 338: 955–961

55  Orlandi F, Damiani G, Hallahan T W, Krantz D A, Macri J N. First-trimester screening for fetal aneuploidy: biochemistry and nuchal translucency. Ultrasound Obstet Gynecol 1997; 10: 381–386

56  Brizot M L, Snijders R J M, Butler J, Bersinger N A, Nicolaides K H. Maternal serum hCG and fetal nuchal translucency thickness for the prediction of fetal trisomies in the first trimester of pregnancy. Br J Obstet Gynaecol 1995; 102: 127–132

57  Whitlow B J, Economides D L. The optimal gestational age to examine fetal anatomy and measure nuchal translucency in the first trimester. Ultrasound Obstet Gynecol 1998; 11: 258–261

58  Rottem S, Bronshtein M, Thaler I, Brandes J M. First trimester trans-vaginal diagnosis of fetal anomalies. Lancet 1989; i: 844–845

59  Rottem S, Bronshtein M. Transvaginal sonographic diagnosis of congenital anomalies between 9 weeks and 16 weeks menstrual age. J Clin Ultrasound 1990; 18: 307–314

60  Bronshtein N, Blumenfeld Z. Trans-vaginal sonography – detection of findings suggestive of fetal chromosomal abnormalities in the first and early second trimesters. Prenat Diagn 1991; 12: 587–593

61  Whitlow B J, Chatzipaps I K, Lazanakis M S, Kadir R A, Economides D L. The value of first trimester sonography in the detection of fetal abnormalities in an unselected population. Br J Obstet Gynaecol 1999; 106: 929–936

62  Sebire N J, Noble P L, Thorpe-Beeston J G, Snijders R J M, Nicolaides K H. Presence of the 'lemon' sign at the 10–14 week scan. Ultrasound Obstet Gynecol 1997; 10: 403–405

63  Yagel S, Achiron R, Ron M, Revel A, Anteby E. Transvaginal ultrasonography at early pregnancy cannot be used alone for targeted organ ultrasonographic examination in a high-risk population. Am J Obstet Gynecol 1995; 172: 971–975

64  Zeanah C H, Dailey J V, Rosenblatt M, Saller D N. Do women grieve after terminating pregnancies because of fetal abnormalities? A controlled investigation. Obstet Gynecol 1993; 82: 270–275

65  Kaltreider N B, Goldsmith S, Margolis A J. The impact of midtrimester abortion techniques on patients and staff. Am J Obstet Gynecol 1979; 135: 235–238

66  Grudzinskas J G, Ward R H T. Screening for Down Syndrome in the First Trimester (32nd RCOG study group). London: RCOG Press, 1997; 354

67  Goldstein H. One year of health and social services for adolescents with Down's syndrome. A calculation of costs in a representative area of Denmark. Soc Psychol Psychiatr Epidemiol 1989; 24: 30–34

68  Hafner E, Schuchter K, Philipp K. Screening for chromosomal abnormalities in an unselected population fetal nuchal translucency. Ultrasound Obstet Gynecol 1995; 6: 330–333

69  Kornman L H, Morssink L P, Beekhuis J R, DeWolf B T H M, Heringa M P, Mantingh A. Nuchal translucency cannot be used as a screening test for chromosomal abnormalities in the first trimester of pregnancy in a routine ultrasound practice. Prenat Diagn 1996; 16: 797–805

70  Taipale P, Hiilesmaa V, Salonen R, Ylostalo P. Increased nuchal translucency as a marker for fetal chromosomal defects. N Engl J Med 1997; 337: 1654–1658

71  Hernadi L, Torocsik M. Screening for fetal anomalies in the 12th week of pregnancy by trans-vaginal sonography on a non-selected population. Prenat. Diagn 1997; 17: 753–759

*Geoffrey Chamberlain*

# Antenatal corticosteroids

Many innovations in science are attributed to serendipity, the facility for making fortuitous discoveries. Serendip was the former name of Ceylon now Sri Lanka. Horace Walpole in his 1754 fairy story *The Three Princes of Serendip* really implied a slightly more focused meaning - his princes were 'always making discoveries by the sagacity of things they were not in quest of'. The sagacity or acuteness of their mental discernment led them to see the relevance of these chance findings, they were using trained minds. Such a prepared mind was possessed by Mont Liggins, the New Zealand obstetrician and physiologist, when in the 1960s, he was working on preterm labour using sheep as his model. There are many variations of hormones involved in the initiation and maintenance of uterine contractions and these differ in various species. Liggins was using glucocorticoid steroids in an attempt to prevent labour.[1] He also found, however, that the functional maturation of the lamb's lungs 'was accelerated by the steroids' and wondered if this could be a possible way to reduce the effects of the respiratory distress syndrome (RDS) which seems to result from pulmonary immaturity in the human lung. Liggins suggested that steroids caused premature liberation of surfactant from the alveoli, perhaps by induction of an enzyme concerned with the biosynthesis of surfactant.[2]

Liggins went on with Howie, a paediatrician, to perform a controlled trial of betamethazone in humans.[3] Some 280 women, admitted in preterm labour between 24 and 36 weeks from 1969 to 1971, agreed to enter the trial. A series of randomly issued, identical ampoules were prepared by the pharmacist who himself held a key for identification but the contents were blind to the observers. Some contained 6 mg of betamethazone and the others contained 6 mg of cortisone, a steroid which had only about 1/70th of the potency of betamethazone. In the final outcome, of the 213 women who went into

**Prof. Geoffrey Chamberlain** MD FRCS FRCOG FACOG, Emeritus Professor in Obstetrics and Gynaecology, Singleton Hospital, Swansea SA2 8QA, UK

spontaneous premature labour, the early neonatal mortality was 3.2% in the treated group and 15% in the controls (*P* = 0.01) with no deaths from RDS in the treated group. RDS occurred less often in treated babies than controls (9% versus 25.8%, *P* = 0.0003). Among the babies under 32 weeks' gestation who were treated for at least 24 h, the RDS rates were 11.8% for the treated and 69.6% for the control babies (*P* = 0.02). No hazards of the steroids in the puerperium were noted. In this, the original Auckland study, only one course of steroids were given.

Liggins and Howie continued this series and reported over the years at Cambridge,[4] Ross Laboratories[5] and an RCOG scientific meeting of The Royal College of Obstetricians and Gynaecologists in 1977,[6] always showing the benefits of a single course of corticosteroids on respiratory maturation without serious side effects. Others did research which consolidated the original work,[7-11] and these results are well analysed by Crowley in her updated meta-analysis in the Cochrane Data Base (Fig. 1).[12] Gradually, workers started to publish not just on the medical respiratory improvement but the economic savings in the reduction of intensive neonatal care – not only in expensive maintenance regimens with exogenous surfactant and extra-corporial oxygenation, but in total time in intensive care neonatal units which are so skilled-labour intensive.

Undoubtedly, neonatal morbidity and mortality from RDS has been reduced and the need for intensive care is lessened by the use of antenatal steroids provided they are given at the right time and have sufficient time to work.

## HOW DO THEY WORK?

The air–liquid surface of the alveolus is under surface tension to retract. Any reduction in surface tension helps it to relax and stay open so presenting a wider interface for oxygen exchange. Surfactants reduce surface tension and stabilise the alveolus against such collapse so helping to maintain the residual volume promoting expansion on inspiration and reducing the compliance; this lessens the work of breathing. A surfactant-deficient alveolus leads to reduced lung volume with stiff or decreased compliance.

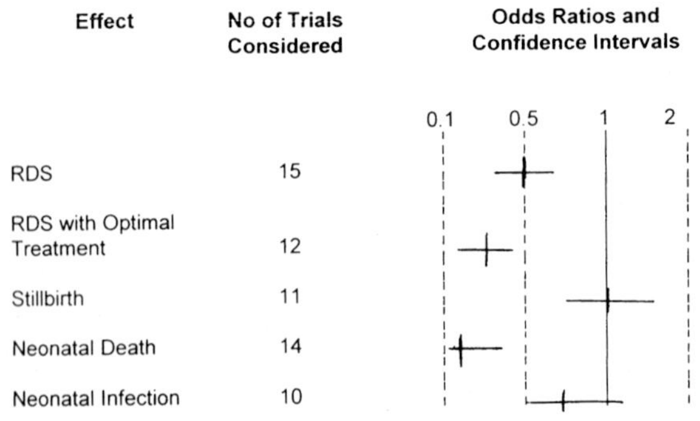

**Fig. 1** Outcomes after antenatal steroids compared with no treatment in selected randomised controlled trials. After Crowley 1998.[12]

The surfactant is mostly lipid, consisting in half of dipalmitoyl phosphatidyl choline (DDPC) and a quarter of unsaturated phosphatidyl cholines. The DPPC accumulates at the air–liquid interface and helps to reduce surface tension. There are three specific apolipoproteins associated with surfactant which act in a synergistic way to destabilise it and so enable it to spread rapidly on the air–liquid interface. DPPC is mostly synthesised in the type II pneumocytes which are in the epithelium of the alveolus; these cells cover only about 10% of the alveolar surface area, being frequently situated at the corners of the alveoli. Their cytoplasm contains granules which store surfactant, each cell having about 150 granules. These cells also synthesise apolipoproproteins which catalyse the release of surfactant. This process is regulated by a number of pharmacological stimuli including steroids which are known to have an action on transcriptional modification of surfactant and normally act alongside other hormonal influences (such as thyroxine) from about 24–26 weeks of gestation in the human. At about this time, the fetal adrenal cortex increases rapidly in size and production of corticosteroids is greatly boosted. Probably exogenous steroids act in the same way, on the cells so stimulating surfactant production and release.

It has been known for a long time that babies that die with RDS have a reduced mean weight of their adrenal glands by as much as 20%.[13] Anencephalic fetuses with congenitally hypoplastic adrenal cortices also have a very greatly reduced numbers of granules in the type II pneumocytes. Corticosteroids pass across the placenta relatively easily and so maternal administration of these hormones could be a method of exposing the fetus to higher levels of corticosteroid activity. What is not known is whether having stimulated a burst of activity in surfactant production and kick-started the granules into action, does this effect then go on or is further boosting of corticosteroid levels in the fetal blood required to continue the activity?

Morphologically, the pneumocyte type II epithelial cells on the surface epithelium in the lung which has been treated with corticosteroids are identical to the mature type II cells of the adult lung. It would seem that the reduction in RDS associated with antenatal steroids is not statistically significant in the sub-group of babies delivered more than 7 days after a single course of treatment. Hence, the practice has arisen of repeating course of treatment at weekly intervals for women who do not go into labour but remain at risk for a preterm delivery. This administration of repeated steroids has never been subjected to proper randomised trials and we have no evidence that multiple doses of steroids are more effective than a single dose. One of the problems is that the fetus is growing older by the week and various other in-built mechanisms of lung maturation are coming into action.

The timing of therapy is critical. The best neonatal respiratory results come after a complete course of two doses of betamethazone 12 mg, 24 h apart or four doses of dexamethasone 6 mg, hours apart. Delivery 3–7 days after this completed course is ideal. Many obstetricians use tocolytes to delay labour so that the steroids can act fully. However, even if this time cannot be gained, it is still better to give the steroids, because infants born within 24 h of the steroid course or even before the course is completed show a treatment benefit which is, however, non-significant.

## SINGLE COURSES OF CORTICOSTEROIDS

### Methods of administration

The steroids used are usually dexamethasone or betamethasone. They are identical biologically and readily cross the placenta. They have little mineral cortico-activity and are relative weak in immune suppression. Biological action is of longer duration than methoprednisilone or cortisol and seems to be best at imitating the fetal adrenal gland in providing antenatal corticosteroids.

Usually two doses of 12 mg betamethazone are given intramuscularly 1 day apart or four doses of 6 mg dexamethasone are given intramuscularly 12 h apart. Originally, these regimens were arbitrarily selected by Liggins and Howie, but they have shown to provide concentrations that are correct for the maturation of the fetal respiratory system. It is possible that they also provide an induction of activity at receptor mediators of other fetal target organs. Higher doses of steroids do not increase the benefits to the respiratory tract and could increase the likelihood of side effects. There is little doubt that between 28 and 34 weeks of gestation, the use of antenatal steroids reduces significantly the incidence, morbidity and mortality of RDS. Before this time, steroids may reduce the severity of the condition but numbers of cases in proper trials are not great. It is, however, common practice now to offer mothers these drugs in those earlier times. Before 24 weeks, however, there would be little point for the type II pneumocytes are not sufficiently formed to release any surfactant. After 34 weeks, the risk of RDS is low and its severity is usually less. There is, thus, little improvement in the outcome for such babies; whilst the official bodies do not recommend it, individual obstetricians in consultation with their neonatal colleagues still use corticosteroids up to 36 weeks.

These recommendations are in line with the National Institutes of Health Consensus of Statement of March 1994. This American method of deciding scientific matters involves bringing together a large number of experts, hearing them all out, thrashing out a combined opinion and then publishing it. In addition, similar advice comes from two influential bodies that govern most Western obstetricians. The American College of Obstetricians and Gyneco-logists and The Royal College of Obstetricians and Gynaecologists published, respectively, a *Committee Opinion Number 147* in 1995[15] and *Guideline Number 7*.[16] These were mostly in line with the recommendations of the NIH Consensus Statement. Interestingly, both stressed the point that there was no evidence that repeated doses of corticosteroids after 7 days, should the woman had not delivered, were not useful and urged further research to show if this was so.

### Indications

It has now become accepted wisdom in the Western world that women who are at risk of preterm labour or with spontaneous rupture of the membranes before labour between 28 and 34 weeks of gestation should be given antenatal steroids in line with the preceding paragraphs. In the UK, this seems to be the case with 201 out of 206 obstetric units responding to a recent survey[17] reporting that they gave corticosteroids to women at risk of producing a very immature baby. Indeed, only one unit out of 206 never prescribed any antenatal corticosteroids to women perceived to be at risk of a preterm delivery. There is considerable variation within European countries.[18] Conversely, work published from South Africa in 1995, showed that only 20% of relevant mothers received antenatal corticosteroids, the major reason for not giving it was that labour was progressing too fast.[19] In the US, the NIH Consensus Statement confirmed that only 12–18% of women who delivered infants from 1501–2500 g birth-weight were treated with antenatal corticosteroids.[20] In the US, there were many physicians who were not treating women because of concerns about the efficacy of the corticosteroids and their potential complications; also labour came on too fast so overtaking the time needed to let the steroids work Since the scientific community seems to have come out in favour of the use of antenatal corticosteroids for most fetuses at risk for early preterm delivery, perhaps both the professionals (midwives, obstetricians and paediatricians) and the public themselves need education on this matter further. In countries with a fee-for-service basis of medical care, there maybe a financial disincentive for giving steroids but this does not apply in most of the European health services.

## Contra-indications

There are few contra-indications to giving antenatal steroids. The general background fears about steroids and infection apply and perhaps even more among women with premature rupture of the membranes in mid-pregnancy. Here infection could be very serious for the fetus and so many obstetricians could be concerned about the giving of steroids that might amplify this. The NIH Consensus Group, making a compromise, recommended a reduced steroid therapy from an upper limit of 34 weeks to 30 weeks in such women,[20] although the RCOG Guidelines did not.[16] It is a question of relative risks and steroids should be given if, after full consideration, an obstetrician together with a neonatal paediatrician think that the enormous improvement in respiratory function of the fetus, who might be delivered prematurely, can be weighed against a smaller risk of infection of the mother. Caution, however, should be used in women who present with membranes ruptured for over 24 h; here the risks of infection are much higher.

The original controlled study of Liggins[2] found that there is an excess of fetal deaths amongst the treated group of women who had severe pregnancy induced proteinuric hypertension. This has not been found in subsequent studies[9] and, on balance, it is probable that the risks of neonatal RDS are that much greater than the risk of giving the mother steroids. It is now recommended that hypertensive women should be treated in the same way as other women.

Diabetic mothers give rise to a problem, particularly when the diabetic control has been poor. Steroid administration not only increases the risk of infection but does result in an instability of diabetic control which, in itself, has a detritus adverse effect on fetal respiratory maturation. Few diabetic mothers have entered into the randomised trials so far; but, again, after full consideration, the view of most clinicians is that the benefits of steroids to the fetus outweigh the disadvantage to diabetic women. One should give the steroids to help the fetus and after that look to the fine tuning of diabetic control with insulin which may follow from this short dose of steroids.[21]

The position with twin pregnancies is complicated by a very practical problem; most women bearing a multiple pregnancy will deliver early and almost a fifth will do so before 34 weeks. In a review of 325 twin pregnancies recently,[22] some 18% were delivered at less than 34 weeks and so would have qualified for antenatal steroids; but, of these, 70% were delivered within 24 h of presentation at the hospital. Examination of the data showed that 31% received no steroids because it was believed that delivery was imminent. In fact, 50% of this subset did deliver within 24 h with only 19% delivering more than 24 h later. Hence, the benefits of steroids for such a group would be limited by the speed of oncoming events.

Tuberculosis is unusual in the UK but still common in other parts of the world. This, in itself, might mitigate against the use of antenatal steroids. Clinicians must make individual judgement here, remembering that the risks of RDS to the fetus in the early days of the third trimester is very great. Balanced against this is a theoretical risk of a flare of tuberculosis. This could be covered by the newer, more rapid acting anti-tuberculosis drugs, if available.

Beyond these, there are few contra-indications to antenatal steroids given for fetal reasons, provided that one remembers that all the evidence produced so far is based upon a single course of treatment and there is little work published in the form of statistically powerful, randomised, controlled trials that show the side effects or contra-indications of repeated dosage.

### Long-term effects

There would seem to be no long-term effects on the mother from any of the studies that were followed-up. Long-term results in the infant have been published up to 3 years in the US Collaborative Group Trial 1994,[23] to 6 years in the Auckland trial reported in 1982[24] and up to 12 years in the Amsterdam trial reported in 1990.[25] In none of these long-term observational follow-ups, which started with a single course of antenatal corticosteroids, was any effect on the infants' growth or health noted. There was no evidence, in particular, of any differences in the scores achieved by a battery of psychometric tests and the concurrence of the results for these three follow-up studies would seem to give strength to the idea that the infants are unharmed for a single corticosteroid course.

## MULTIPLE COURSES OF CORTICOSTEROIDS

Built on the idea that exogenous steroids given to the mother and passed to the fetus might only have a short-term effect, people became concerned about those women who threatened early preterm labour, but did not actually deliver, going on with their pregnancy. It was feared that, after a week with no labour and having received a course of steroids more than 7 days before, the effect would wear off despite the evidence of maturation in the morphology of type II pneumocytes. On the grounds that if one dose is good, two must be better, obstetricians were led into giving repeated doses of corticosteroids to the mother in the subsequent weeks. Indeed, there are reports of as many as 10

**Table 1** Maturity and early respiratory outcomes by various dosage regimens of corticosteroids administered (% of those in treatment groups in brackets). After French et al.[26]

|  | No Steroids<br>$n = 311$ | 1 course<br>$n = 125$ | 2 courses<br>$n = 20$ | 3 or more courses<br>$n = 23$ |
|---|---|---|---|---|
| Death | 75 (25%) | 14 (11%) | 1 (5%) | 2 (9%) |
| Severe RDS | 70/257 (27%) | 12/121 (9.9%) | 3/15 (16.7%) | 3/22 (13.6%) |
| Chronic lung diseases later | 55 (18%) | 29 (24%) | 3 (15%) | 6 (26%) |
| Severe chronic lung disease later | 27 (9%) | 13 (11%) | 2 (10%) | 6 (26%) |

doses of weekly steroids having been given to women in middle pregnancy. There is, however, no evidence from properly conducted or powerful enough studies that this has improved the outcome to the fetus. In a recent paper published from Western Australia,[26] the relevant data (included in Table 1) show the great improvement in respiratory function after one course of antenatal steroids over those who had no steroids, but there is no improvement among those women who had two or three or more courses at weekly intervals. Polypharmacy is always to be discouraged as, although the risks of repeated steroids to the mother are small, they will increase with each dose.

Reports of harmful effects to the mother are not common but, for example, there was a preliminary report[27] at a meeting of the Society for Feto-Maternal Medicine in January 1999 from Columbus, OH, USA. The administration of multiple courses of antenatal betamethazone resulted in a diminished response of the mother's adrenal glands to ACTH stimulation, an indication of decreased steroid stores and adrenal cortical atrophy which could have potentially serious later maternal ramifications.

There have been several papers published on the long-term problems of multiple doses of steroids to the fetus. These started with animal work, mainly in sheep. In experiments performed in Western Australia in one series, sheep were given weekly injections of betamethazone up to four doses and the results were compared the result with control animals that had saline injections. The three or four dose betamethazone animals had a reduction of 27% in birth-weight of their lambs.[28] There was also a dose-dependant improvement in immediate postnatal lung function, but this should be weighed against the expense of the effects on birth-weight. Work of a similar nature on sheep has shown that the optic nerves in the lambs subjected to repeated antenatal steroids have been affected.[29] Examination by electron microscopy showed significant delay in myelinisation of the axons. The longer-term implications of this are not yet known and no similar work exists in humans.

More recently, observational studies have been published on the human. Again from Western Australia came a study which showed that three years after the giving of steroids in various doses to 477 mothers bearing single infants who

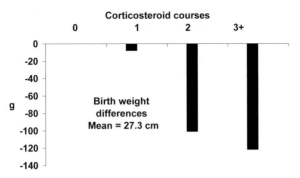

**Fig. 2** Estimated birth weight difference reduction associated with various doses of corticosteroids – multivariant analysis of variance after controlling for maternal age, parity, maturity, sex, socio-economic class, aboriginal origin, cigarette smoking and pregnancy complications. After French et al (1999)[29]

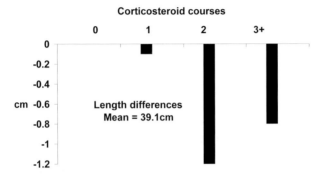

**Fig. 3** Estimated mean length difference reduction associated with various doses of corticosteroids – multivariant analysis of variance after controlling for maternal age, parity, maturity, sex, socio-economic class, aboriginal origin, cigarette smoking and pregnancy complications. After French et al (1999)[29]

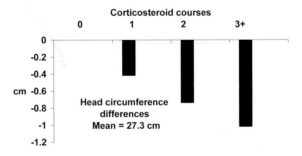

**Fig. 4** Estimated mean head circumferencereduction associated with various doses of corticosteroids – multivariant analysis of variance after controlling for maternal age, parity, maturity, sex, socio-economic class, aboriginal origin, cigarette smoking and pregnancy complications. After French et al (1999)[29]

were born before 33 weeks of gestation, the birth-weight ratio decreases were associated with an increased number of doses.[27] The results of birth-weight difference, head circumference difference and length of fetus difference are shown in Figures 2–4. Of these infants, 36% had been exposed to a full course of antenatal steroids. As might be expected, those who had more than three courses started their exposure earlier in uterine life. There is a significant decrease in the birth-weight ratio (the birth-weight standardised for gestational age and sex) with an increasing number of corticosteroid courses. A series of multiple regression analyses of variance was performed to produce the results seen in Figures 2–4. It is noticeable that, whilst both the incidence of severe RDS was greatly reduced among those who had steroids – whether it was one dose or more – there was 'no significant gains for those infants whose mothers received additional courses of corticosteroids beyond the first'. The incidence of chronic lung disease was not influenced by the additional courses either.

Some 81% of these babies survived to 3 years; follow-up information was obtained in 92% of these, with 85% having clinical assessments. Multivariant analysis of weight, height and head circumference ratios at this stage showed no differences with the number of courses of antenatal corticosteroids that had been given antenatally.

These results come from an observational study which covered probably most of the births that occur in a large area of a sparsely populated country, but they are not a randomised controlled trial. They do, however, give grounds for concern.

## The next step

The use of repeated antenatal steroids is fast becoming established practice and soon obstetricians and paediatricians will think it is the right thing to do because it has 'always been done'. This is the conventional pattern of prescribing in medicine. However, many who have thought about the subject and the regulatory bodies of obstetricians in the UK and US (the RCOG Guidelines and the ACOG Committee Guidance) are asking for a proper randomised control study to examine the effects of multiple steroids compared with a single course. No one doubts that the single course regimen greatly improves the chance of the immature child, but most thinking obstetricians are concerned about the multiple doses; there is no evidence that it does any good, whilst there is an accumulating body of evidence that it may do some harm to the growth and to those areas of development of tissues that has been examined. Further, there is a concern amongst the public about the giving of drugs to pregnant women. This is an increasing lobby and, whilst it should not be the only motivation, scientists would do well to listen to public demands and pressures and ensure their therapies are based on sound evidence not just clinical nouse.

A group of interested obstetricians and workers at the National Perinatal Epidemiology Unit in Oxford, UK have started to work on a randomised controlled trial of this.[17] In late 1997, a questionnaire was posted to each of the 279 delivery units in the UK with reminders a month later; 208 were returned (75% of those contacted). Only one unit never prescribed any antenatal steroids for women thought to be at risk for preterm labour. Of the remainder, five never prescribed repeated courses but the rest did, at least on some occasions; 80% of units did not prescribe corticosteroids earlier than 24 weeks and 63% no later than 34 weeks. Dexamethasone was used by 60% and betamethazone by 36%. Both drugs were given in 7 units according to consultant's opinion (4%). Mostly, the standard regimens applied, but in 25 units (7%) the dose varied with indication.

**Table 2** Indications for which repeated causes of antenatal steroids would be considered. Note these categories are not mutually exclusive. After Brocklehurst et al.[17]

|  | n | % |
| --- | --- | --- |
| Prelabour SROM before 32 weeks | 169 | 86.7 |
| Suspected preterm labour | 164 | 84.1 |
| Recurrent APH | 125 | 64.1 |
| Moderate/severe pre-eclampsia | 122 | 62.9 |
| Triplet or higher order birth | 116 | 59.5 |
| Previous preterm delivery | 109 | 55.9 |
| Placenta praevia | 72 | 36.9 |
| Cervical cerclage | 40 | 20.5 |
| Uncomplicated twin delivery | 26 | 13.3 |
| Chronic hypertension | 19 | 9.7 |
| Previous recurrent miscarriage | 18 | 9.2 |
| Bacterial vaginosis | 4 | 2.1 |
| Other indications | 20 | 10.4 |

Those who used steroids to help mature the immature fetal respiratory tract were asked if they would be prepared to participate in a proposed randomised trial; 70% were firmly in favour, while a further 17% were unsure as yet and wished to see the details first.

The indications being used in these units for repeat courses of antenatal steroids are shown in Table 2. Most considered use in preterm rupture of the membranes before 32 weeks or suspected preterm labour when the woman did not labour. Since most units did not prescribe after 34 weeks, it may be assumed that the preterm labours under examination were mostly before that time. It is interesting that an intermediary group of indications have arisen where there are complications of pregnancy such as recurrent antepartum haemorrhage, pre-eclampsia or triplets. The only other indication which predominated in this survey is proven placenta previa; in addition, a fifth of women who had had cervical cerclage would also be so considered. This indicates the ideas of UK obstetricians at the moment and should act as an incentive to find out what the answer to repeated steroid usage really is.

The NPEU group will be mounting a multi-centre study with random-isation based upon Oxford. When contacted by telephone, they would allocate women, who had been recruited and properly informed about the study, to one of two groups. The former would receive steroids of standard dosage at weekly intervals until 34 weeks or delivery, whichever came first; the latter would have an injection of a placebo. Information on the methods of resus-citation and maintenance of respiration (including ECMO) and surfactant, postnatal steroids and the use of high frequency oscillation or nitrous oxide would also be collected. Measures of outcome would include perinatal death and post neonatal death, the diagnosis of RDS, or intracranial bleeding diag-nosed by ultrasound. Birth-weight, head circumference and maternal post-partum infection data would be included; infant infection in the first 48 h after birth and necrotising enteritis would be examined.

A long-term follow-up study would also be mounted at 2 years when the blood pressure and growth of the baby would be measured and chronic lung disease and respiratory symptoms noted. Individual domain scores on the

Griffith's Scale would also be obtained. Of those babies who died, autopsies would be performed by a perinatal pathologist. Because of the suspected concern that repeated doses of steroids may have an affect on brain maturation, sections of the brains of the infants would be examined by an expert consultant neuropathologist.

The prepilot of this study has been started in three clinical units in the UK with the agreement of the Local Ethical Research Committees. The figures, so far, are small and not reportable at the moment, but it is hoped to collect enough data inside 2 years of the full study starting to allow an answer to this question to be given. Funding has recently been awarded for the large pilot study, starting in 1999.

## CONCLUSIONS

It is essential that questions about the need, efficacy and safety of repeated antenatal steroids is answered. If it is not done in the next 2–3 years, the opportunity will be gone and repeated steroids will be given to everybody. The next move will be that the lawyers will jump on the act and start asking questions about those babies who have respiratory problems of prematurity and judges will start making *obiter dicta* that the steroids are an essential part of modern treatment. We live in an age where research must not be motivated because of fear of medicolegal reasons, but it may be stimulated by legal enquiry. Here is a good example of where we need an answer on the repeated dose of steroids.

Liggins and Howie in their original research showed that a single course of steroids was beneficial. Others have proved it and it has entered clinical use with great effect. The NIH Consensus Statement of 1994 concluded with:

> *The use of antenatal corticosteroids for fetal maturation is a rare example of a technology that yields substantial cost savings in additional to improving health*

---

**KEY POINT FOR CLINICAL PRACTICE**

- All women between 26 and 33 weeks' gestation who show signs of labour or have premature membrane rupture should receive antenatal corticosteroids to help maturation of the fetal respiratory tract and so reduce the incidence and severity of RDS in any baby born in the period. There is good evidence for this action and side effects of a single course seem minimal. The same cannot be said of repeated doses where a body of observational data is developing which shows no increased protection but detriment to fetal growth and development.

---

*References*

1 Liggins G. The fetal role in the initiation of parturition of the ewe in fetal autonomy. In: CIBA Foundation Symposium, London, Churchill Livingstone, 1969; 142

2  Liggins G. Premature delivery of fetal lambs infused with gluco-corticoids. J Endocrinol 1969; 45: 515–521

3  Liggins G, Howie R. A controlled trial of antepartum glucocorticoid treatment: for the prevention of the respiratory distress syndrome in premature infants. Pediatrics 1972; 50: 515–525

4  Liggins G, Howie R, Beard R. (Eds) Prevention of respiratory distress syndrome by antepartum corticosteroids following the proceedings of the Joseph Bancroft Centenary Symposium on Fetal and Neonatal Physiology. Cambridge: Cambridge University Press, 1973; 613–617

5  Liggins G. Prenatal cortico-steroid treatment: prevention of respiratory distress syndrome. In: Moore T. (ed) 70th Ross Conference on Paediatric Research. Ross Laboratories, 1976: 97–103

6  Howie R, Liggins G. Clinical trial of antepartum betamethazone therapy in prevention of respiratory distress in preterm labour. In: Anderson A, Beard R, Dunn T. (eds) Preterm Labour. London: RCOG, 1977; 281–289

7  Carcarachv Botetf Sentis J, Carmonas N. A multicentre prospective and randomised study of preterm rupture of the membranes. Proceedings of the 13th World Congress of Obstetrics and Gynaecology (FIGO) Singapore, 1991: 262

8  Doran T, Sawyer P, Murrey B et al. Results of a double blind controlled study for the use of betamethazone in the prevention of respiratory distress syndrome. Am J Obstet Gynecol 1980; 136: 313–320

9  Gamsu H, Mullinger B, Donnai P, Dash C. Antenatal administration of betamethazone to prevent respiratory distress syndrome in preterm infants: report of a UK multicentre trial. Br J Obstet Gynaecol 1989; 96: 401–410

10  Garite T, Rumney P, Briggs G et al. A randomised placebo-controlled trial of betamethazone for the prevention of respiratory distress syndrome at 24–28 weeks gestation. Surg Gynecol Obstet 1993; 176: 37

11  Kari M, Akino T, Hallman M. Prenatal dexamethazone treatment before preterm delivery and rescue therapy of exogenous surfactant – surfactant components and surface activity in airway specimens. In: Proceedings of the 14th European Congress of Perinatal Medicine, Helsinki, 1994; 486

12  Crowley P. Corticosteroids prior to preterm delivery. Pregnancy and childbirth module of the Cochrane Database of Systematic Reviews Issue 1 Oxford: Updated software 1998

13  Naeye R, Harcke H, Blanc W. Adrenal gland structure and the development of hyline membrane disease. Pediatrics 1971; 47: 650

14  Snyder J, Johnston J, Mendelson C. Differentiation of type II cells of human fetal lung in vitro. Cell Tissue Res 1981; 220: 17–25

15  American College of Obstetricians and Gynecologists Committee Opinion Number 147. Antenatal cortico-steroid therapy for fetal maturation. Int J Gynaecol Obstet 1995; 18: 340–342

16  Royal College of Obstetricians and Gynaecologists. Antenatal corticosteroids to prevent respiratory distress syndrome. London: RCOG, 1996; Guideline Number 7

17  Brocklehurst P, Gates S, McKenzie-McHarg K, Alfiravic Z, Chamberlain G. Are we be prescribing multiple courses of antenatal corticosteroids? A survey of practice in the UK. Br J Obstet Gynaecol 1999; 106: 977–980

18  Alfiravic Z, Elborne D. Thyrotrophin releasing hormone and corticosteroids prior to preterm labour: a survey of current practice in nine European countries. Eur J Obstet Gynaecol Reprod Biol 1986; 68: 43–45

19  Ballot D, Ballot N, Rothberg A. Reasons of failure to administer antenatal corticosteroids in preterm labour. S Afr Med J 1995; 85: 1005–1007

20  NIH Consensus Statement. Effect of corticosteroids for fetal maturation on perinatal outcome. 1994; 12

21  Farrag O. Prospective study of three metabolic regimes in pregnant diabetes. Aust N Z J Obstet Gynaecol 1987; 27: 69–74

22  Hulmes R, Wardal P, Tuohy J. Antenatal steroid administration in twin pregnancies. Contemp Rev Obstet Gynaecol 1996: 8: 181–184

23  Collaborative Group of Antenatal Steroid Therapy. The effects of antenatal dexamethazone administration on infant long term follow up. J Pediatr 1984: 104: 259–267

24  MacArthur B, Howie R, Dezoet J, Elkins J. School programme and cognitive development of 6 year old children whose mothers were treated antenatally with betamethazone. Pediatrics 1982: 20: 99–105

25  Smolders-De Haas H, Neupal J, Schmand B, Treffers P, Koppe J, Hoeks J. Physical development and medical history of children who were treated antenatally with corticosteroids to prevent respiratory distress syndrome: a ten to twelve year follow up. Pediatrics 1990; 86: 65–70

26  French N, Hagan R, Evans S, Godfrey N, Newham J. Repeated antenatal corticosteroids: size of birth and subsequent development. Am J Obstet Gynecol 1999; 180: 114–121

27  MacKennar D, Wittber G, Samuels P. The effects of repeated doses of antenatal corticosteroids on maternal adrenal function. Am J Obstet Gynecol 1999: 180: 515

28  Ikegami M, Jobe A, Newnham J, Pulk D, Willet K, Sly P Repetitive prenatal gluco-cortico-steroid affects lung function and growth in preterm lambs. Am J Respir Crit Care 1997; 156: 178–184

29  Dunlop S, Archer M, Wuinlivan J, Beasley L, Newnhan J. Repeated prenatal corticosteroids delay myelinization of the ovine central nervous system. J Matern Fetal Med 1997; 6: 309–313

*Griff Jones Darryl Maxwell*

# Cervical ultrasound in pregnancy

The uterine cervix undergoes considerable physiological, biochemical and anatomical changes during the transition between the antenatal and intra-partum periods. In 1969, Anderson and Turnbull reported that, in primi–parous women, cervical dilatation and effacement were related to the time in gestation at which labour started.[1] However, they also pointed out that dilatation of the internal os after the 28th week of gestation did not invariably predict either preterm birth or neonatal risk. Unfortunately, digital examination of the cervix is subjective and has considerable inter-observer variability.[2] Furthermore, only that portion of the cervix below the anterior vaginal wall is assessed. Techniques for measuring cervical length have been compared in non-pregnant women undergoing hysterectomy.[3] Digital examination consistently underestimated length by more than 13 mm. In contrast, ultrasonographic measurements correlated well with those obtained using a ruler on the postoperative specimen.

## EARLY WORK

### Transabdominal ultrasound

Work in the 1980s suggested that transabdominal ultrasound could allow repeated cervical assessment throughout pregnancy. Varma et al[4] initially reported data on 30 low-risk pregnancies scanned serially and found the average cervical length to be between 35–40 mm. Up to 6 mm of dilatation at the internal os was 'normal' with no significant cervical change seen from the 10th to the 36th week of gestation.

**Mr Griff Jones** MRCOG, Fellow in Maternal Fetal Medicine, Division of Perinatology, Ottawa General Hospital, 501 Smyth Road, Ottawa K1H 8L6, Canada (for correspondence)

**Mr Darryl Maxwell** FRCOG MRACOG, Director and Consultant Obstetrician, Fetal Medicine Unit, Guy's and St Thomas' Hospital Trust, 15th Floor, Guy's Tower, London SE1 9RT, UK

The same group subsequently studied 115 women with risk factors for cervical incompetence.[5] Patient management was largely based on clinical (as opposed to ultrasound) findings. Those women who had no ultrasonic evidence of cervical weakness (i.e. cervical length $\geq 2$ cm and cervical canal width $\leq 8$ mm) did not undergo cerclage. All delivered at term, regardless of whether or not there was clinical suspicion of cervical abnormality. Of the women with evidence of moderate cervical weakness on ultrasound, one-third were found to have clinically normal cervices. With expectant management, 75% delivered before 34 weeks' gestation. Most of the remaining two-thirds, in whom digital cervical examination was suspicious, underwent cerclage with 25% delivering before 34 weeks. Twenty patients had evidence of severe cervical deficiency with membranes prolapsing down the cervical canal. Where cerclage was used, only 25% delivered before 34 weeks; without the figure was 67%. A further report by the same group describes 4 primigravid patients who were found to have widening of the internal cervical os on ultrasound.[6] In all, progression to membrane herniation and subsequent abortion occurred.

Riley et al[7] also report a 50% risk of preterm birth in women co-incidentally found to have cervical shortening and membrane funneling on transabdominal scanning. Although some of the women had no preceding risk factors for early delivery, a variety of non-randomised treatments were used, masking the absolute predictive ability of the test. Michaels et al[8] describe the outcomes of high risk women managed according to the transabdominal cervical ultrasound findings. They felt that simple observation was not ethical, as they had found mid-trimester loss to occur in this situation. Of 25 women with ultrasound-based evidence of cervical weakness who underwent cerclage, 20% delivered preterm with no mid-trimester losses.

## Transvaginal ultrasound

Brown et al[9] were the first to suggest that adequate cervical images were more likely to be obtained by transvaginal scanning. This was re-iterated by Andersen[10] who reported that 86% of cervices could be seen transabdominally when the bladder was partially-full, falling to only 46% when it was empty. In contrast, the cervix could be visualised transvaginally 99% of the time. When transabdominal and transvaginal cervical length measurements from the same woman were compared, transabdominal measurements were on average 5 mm longer, presumably secondary to bladder filling. Mason and Maresh[11] systematically studied the effects of bladder volume on cervical appearance. Of 30 women, 29 demonstrated an increase in cervical length with increasing bladder volume, which occurred throughout the bladder volume range, not just with over-distension. Confino et al[12] also reported cases in which quantified bladder filling or manual pressure exerted via the transducer led to significant reductions in internal os dilatation in patients with suspected incompetence (Fig. 1A,B). Indeed, it has been reported that deliberate bladder over-distension is a useful 'no-touch' technique for the reduction of prolapsing membranes prior to rescue or emergency cerclage.[13]

The transvaginal approach yields clearer and more detailed images due to both the close proximity of the ultrasound probe to the cervix and the higher transducer frequencies used. However, the maternal bladder should still be

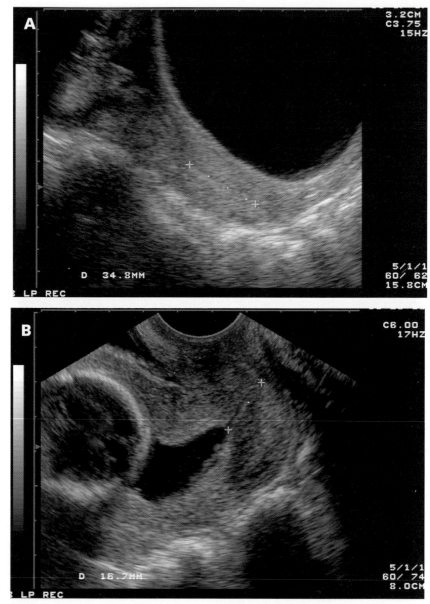

**Fig. 1** **(A)** Transabdominal cervical scan at 20 weeks' gestation with the cervix appearing long and closed. **(B)** Transvaginal ultrasound 11 min later showed significant cervical shortening with dilatation at the internal os and funneling.

empty. Okitsu et al[14] showed that, even using transvaginal scans, bladder filling elongated the cervix and could cause a dilated internal os to appear closed.

As mentioned, digital examination only assesses that portion of the cervix below the vaginal wall. Goldberg et al[15] found the mean cervical lengths in 43 pregnant women measured by transvaginal ultrasound (39 mm) to be over twice as long as those measured digitally (19 mm) by experienced examiners. Similarly, Sonek et al[16] found that digital measurement of cervical length showed a poor correlation with vaginal ultrasonography. There is also evidence that cervical dilatation starts at the internal os, farthest away from the examiners' finger. High-lighting the importance of this, Okitsu et al[14] reported that two-thirds of women with a dilated internal os on transvaginal scan appeared normal on digital examination. Others have reported similar findings.[5,17]

## Safety and acceptability

Adequate views of the cervical canal are obtained with the transvaginal probe introduced only a few centimeters into the vagina. It has been shown that the angle between the long axis of the vaginal probe and that of the cervical canal is such that the probe should never pass through the external os.[18] Supporting this, bleeding provoked by transvaginal scanning in cases of placenta praevia has not been reported. The introduction of pathogens is another area of concern. However, providing a sterile technique is employed, no increase in infectious morbidity has been reported after transvaginal scanning in the presence of ruptured membranes.[19,20]

The full bladder necessary for transabdominal scanning not only leads to false measurements but is associated with significant maternal discomfort. However, pregnant women report transvaginal cervical ultrasound to be less uncomfortable than digital examination.[21] Heath et al[22] questioned 100 consecutive women about the acceptability of a transvaginal scan at 23 weeks' gestation: 94% experienced no, or minimal, discomfort only and 98% reported no or only mild embarrassment. Half of the women found it to be less uncomfortable than a speculum examination, with only 15% finding it more uncomfortable.

## Normal values for cervical length

Initial reports concentrated on the 'normal' cervical length, as measured by transvaginal scanning in the general obstetric population with singleton pregnancies. There appears to be no clinically significant difference between the mean cervical lengths of primiparous and multiparous women.[23,24] Mean cervical lengths have been variously reported as 45 mm (largely Hispanic), 43 mm (Italian), 37 mm (Nebraska, USA) and 36–38 mm (Japan).[14,23,25–27] Several groups commented that shortening was often seen from the beginning of the third trimester onwards.[14,23,26,27]

It is possible that ethnic differences in cervical length exist. Heath et al[22] found a statistically significant difference in cervical length at 23 weeks gestation between Caucasians and Afro-Caribbean women. However, as this amounted to only 2 mm (39.5 mm versus 37.4 mm), it is unlikely on its own to be of clinical significance.

Most normative data were obtained in low-risk women. The work of the National Institute of Child Health and Human Development Maternal-Fetal Medicine Unit Network has shown a short cervix ($\leq 25$ mm) to be significantly more common in high risk women.[28] Heath at al[22] confirmed this in a multiple regression analysis of their own data. Iams et al,[29] in a fascinating study in high risk women, related cervical length in the current pregnancy to the gestation at delivery in their first preterm birth. They argued that the gestational age of a prior preterm birth should indicate indirectly the relative competence of a patient's cervix and be reflected in its measured length. Although interpretation of the results is confounded by the high use of cerclage, they found that the two were significantly correlated in a continuous manner. In other words, the earlier a previous preterm birth occurred, the shorter the cervical measurement was likely to be in the next pregnancy.

## DIAGNOSTIC ROLE

### Preterm labour

The diagnosis of preterm labour is notoriously difficult, with up to half of patients receiving placebo in randomised trials of tocolytic therapy delivering at term.[30] Murakawa et al[27] studied 32 women presenting with threatened preterm labour. None of the 15 women with cervical lengths greater than 30 mm delivered preterm. If the cervix was less than 30 mm, 65% delivered preterm and all early births were identified. All women with a cervical length below 20 mm delivered preterm. However, only 25% of such early births met these more stringent criteria. Iams et al[31] reported their findings in 60 women in preterm labour, although they 'muddied the waters' by including 12 twin pregnancies. They also found a cervical length greater than 30 mm to be invariably associated with term birth with shorter cervices carrying a 55% risk of preterm delivery. Gomez et al[32] reported more detailed cervical ultrasound findings on 59 women in suspected preterm labour who were less than 3 cm dilated. They developed the term 'cervical index' to include information about endocervical length and funnel length in a single figure. The 'cervical index' is calculated as (funnel length + 1)/(endocervical length). The '+ 1' allows an index to be calculated when funneling is absent. No significant relationship was found between cervical effacement, as assessed clinically, and cervical length on ultrasound. Funneling was present in 58% of women and associated with a nearly 3-fold increase in the risk of preterm birth. A complex statistical analysis suggested that a cervical index $\geq 0.52$, cervical length < 18 mm, funnel length > 9 mm and funnel width > 6 mm were all significantly associated with preterm birth. The cervical index performed best, increasing the relative risk of early birth by 6.4. Women with a high cervical index or shortened cervix had a median admission-to-delivery interval of 13 days compared to 40 days if either sign was absent. Timor-Tritsch et al[33] simply used the presence or absence of funneling in their risk assessment of 70 patients presenting with threatened preterm labour. Women with funneling had shorter cervical lengths (17 versus 32 mm) and delivered sooner (5.7 versus 9.8 weeks). Funneling was present in 54% of patients, of whom over half delivered preterm. All the patients who delivered preterm had a funnel present. Unfortunately, they did not explore further the relationship between cervical length and funneling. Rizzo et al[34] scanned 108 women in threatened preterm labour. They report a cervical index of > 0.5 or a cervical length of < 20 mm to correctly predict 65–70% of preterm births while incorrectly identifying approximately 1 in 5 women who subsequently delivered at term. The positive predictive value of either sign was 70%. The presence or absence of funneling was a less reliable predictor.

One important omission in these studies of women presenting with threatened preterm labour is that no account is taken of gestational age at the time of the assessment. It is known that cervical length decreases as gestation advances, particularly in the early third trimester. In other words, it is less unusual to have a short cervix at 32 weeks' gestation than at 26 weeks' gestation. Accuracy may be improved by quoting results of cervical length as percentiles within each gestational age. History of previous spontaneous prematurity and ethnic origin may also have to be taken into account.

Three of the studies compared the cervical ultrasound findings with digital vaginal examination.[31,32,34] In patients without advanced cervical change, cervical dilatation and effacement as assessed by digital examination, had no ability to predict preterm birth. The benefits of improved diagnostic accuracy with ultrasound may include a reduction in both tocolytic use and in-patient admissions.[35]

## Cervical anatomy

The ability to diagnose (or exclude) placenta praevia is one of the main benefits ascribed to antenatal ultrasound. However, the relationship of the internal os to the placental edge, particularly when situated on the posterior uterine wall, can be difficult to define transabdominally. Transvaginal scanning allows placenta praevia to be diagnosed safely and with greater accuracy.[18,36,37] Provided that the placental edge is at least 20 mm from the internal os, a vaginal birth appears safe.[38] The transvaginal approach also allows a detailed inspection of pelvic masses, such as cervical and lower segment fibroids, that may later interfere with parturition.

## Cervical incompetence

Classical cervical incompetence has remained difficult to diagnose either on history or examination. The uterus is an unreliable witness (Fig. 2A,B). Michaels et al[39] investigated 23 patients with a history of *in utero* exposure to diethylstilbestrol (DES), a known risk factor for uterine anomalies and cervical abnormality. Weekly transabdominal ultrasound scans were performed from 14 weeks' gestation and 5 patients (22%) were found to develop a combination of cervical shortening and membrane funneling. In contrast, El-Azeem et al[40] did not find transvaginal cervical scanning to be a useful predictor of spontaneous prematurity in 28 women with a history of DES exposure, despite 10 preterm deliveries. They suggest that other mechanisms may be responsible. Cervical conization may iatrogenically predispose to cervical incompetence. Westgren and Sjoberg report a woman who had two term deliveries followed by a cone biopsy and subsequent 29 week preterm birth.[41] Transabdominal scanning in her next pregnancy demonstrated gradual dilatation and shortening of the cervical canal from 22 weeks' gestation onwards. Unable to perform cerclage because of a deficient cervix, she was treated with bed-rest and tocolytics. Despite this, she delivered at 28 weeks' gestation. More recently, El-Azeem et al[42] scanned 81 women with a past history of conization and found a significant difference in cervical length between those delivering preterm or at term. Wong and Ludmir[43] reported that 1 in 5 asymptomatic women with a past history of unexplained mid-trimester rupture of the membranes developed prolapsing membranes on transvaginal scan. In 75% of cases, this was before any change was detectable on clinical examination.

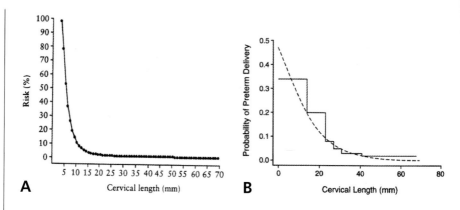

**Fig. 2** **(A)** The risk of spontaneous preterm birth < 32 weeks' gestation for various cervical lengths measured at 23 weeks' gestation.[45] Reprinted with permission of Parthenon Publishing. **(B)** The risk of spontaneous preterm birth < 35 weeks' gestation for various cervical lengths measured at 24 weeks' gestation.[24] Reprinted with permission of the Massachusetts Medical Society.

Very preliminary data on three-dimensional ultrasound of the cervix have appeared.[44] This technique could theoretically allow assessment of cervical and/or funnel volume and possibly detect defects within the cervical substance, particularly laterally.

## MANAGEMENT ROLE

### Assessment of risk of preterm birth

*Cervical length*
Could cervical length measured by transvaginal scanning in asymptomatic women be a useful screening test for spontaneous preterm birth? Three large screening studies have now been published, each involving several thousand predominantly low-risk women.[24,45,46]

In the first, nearly 3000 women of mixed-risk were screened at both 24 and 28 weeks of gestation in 10 inner city centres in the US.[24] Of the study population, 63% were black. Results were blinded from clinicians unless there were 'prolapsed membranes or advanced cervical dilatation', but the numbers of such women and their subsequent outcome were not reported separately. The mean cervical length was approximately 35 mm and the overall incidence of spontaneous preterm birth ≤ 35 weeks' gestation was 4.3%. There was a clear inverse relationship between cervical length and risk of preterm birth. One-third of births before 35 weeks' gestation occurred in women whose cervix measured below the 10th centile (25 mm) at 24 weeks' gestation, a 6-fold increase in relative risk. Cervical shortening between the two scans, particularly when > 5 mm, was also associated with prematurity. A later publication broke down the value of cervical scanning by prior maternal obstetric history.[47] A short cervix (≤ 25 mm) was associated with an 8% probability of spontaneous preterm delivery ≤ 35 weeks gestation in low-risk parous women. In high-risk women, this probability climbed to 31% with the same cervical measurement.

The second study was carried out at a single inner city centre in the UK.[45] Results from cervical scans at 23 weeks' gestation were blinded unless the length was less than 16 mm. In 2505 women, the median cervical length was 38 mm and 1.7% had a cervical length ≤ 15 mm. It should be noted that although Afro-Caribbeans made up 48% of the study population, they accounted for 84% of 'short cervices'. The overall incidence of spontaneous preterm birth ≤ 34 weeks' gestation was 2.3% and 38% of these births were identified by a short cervix (≤ 15 mm) at 23 weeks. However, the primary endpoint chosen in this study was spontaneous delivery before 32 weeks' gestation. A cervical length of ≤ 15 mm at 23 weeks' gestation carried a risk of spontaneous delivery ≤ 32 weeks of 50% and correctly identified 58% of these births. Their work also shows the importance of individualising risk assessments when counselling patients. This risk increases gradually as the length falls below 15 mm and even more dramatically when it is less than 10 mm (Fig. 2A). At 15 mm, the risk of spontaneous delivery ≤ 32 weeks was 4%, at 10 mm the risk was approximately 15% and at 5 mm, it was 78%. Similar data are available from the multicentre American study (Fig. 2B).[24]

The third study was from a well-defined geographical area in Helsinki, Finland with a 99% white population.[46] Results were blinded from clinicians with 3694 women scanned between 18–22 weeks' gestation. The overall incidence of spontaneous preterm birth ≤ 35 weeks' gestation in this population was only 0.8%. The mean cervical length was just over 40 mm and a short cervix was defined as one ≤ 29 mm, corresponding to the 3rd centile. In their population, a short cervix correctly predicted 19% of subsequent deliveries ≤ 35 weeks but had a positive predictive value for the individual of only 6%. Nonetheless, considering the very low background prevalence, this corresponds to an 8-fold increase in risk

All three studies confirm the ability of transvaginal cervical ultrasound to reliably stratify women by risk of spontaneous preterm birth. However, they used different definitions of a short cervix and different timings for both the initial scan and the clinical endpoint. It is clear that the shorter the interval between the scan and the endpoint, the better the predictive ability. The sensitivity of a 'short' cervix at 23 weeks for predicting spontaneous births ≤ 28, ≤ 30, ≤ 32 and ≤ 34 weeks' gestation progressively fell from 86% to 82%, 58% and then 38%.[45] From a different perspective, the sensitivity of a short cervix for predicting births ≤ 35 weeks' gestation was nearly 50% at 28 weeks compared to 37% at 24 weeks.[24]

Even more importantly, the background or pre-test risk of spontaneous preterm birth must be taken into account when interpreting cervical sonograms. The absolute positive predictive value in a low-risk parturient remains low. For every 100 low-risk women with a cervical length of ≤ 25 mm at 24 weeks' gestation, at least 92 will progress beyond 35 weeks' gestation,[24] a time when perinatal morbidity and mortality is very low. The risks of any potential treatments must be balanced against this.

### Membrane funneling

Strict criteria for the diagnosis of funneling do not yet exist. Berghella et al[17] reported on 43 patients who had funneling of the membranes at the internal os detected in the mid-trimester; 35% had no risk factors for preterm birth and

74% had a long, closed cervix on digital examination. If the funnel length was greater than the length of closed cervix below it, 75% of patients delivered before 37 weeks' gestation. A funnel width exceeding 15 mm was another risk factor. In the Helsinki study,[46] less than 1% of women were found to have dilatation of the internal os ≥ 5 mm at 18–22 weeks' gestation but this carried a 28-fold increase in risk of spontaneous delivery ≤ 35 weeks. In the large American multicentre study of the Iams et al,[24] a funnel protruding 3 mm or more into the cervical canal was seen in 6% of women and was associated with a 5-fold increase in relative risk of early birth. It is difficult to separate the effects of cervical dilatation with subsequent funneling from shortening of the cervical canal. Indeed, one group has suggested that dilatation is not seen without shortening,[48] while another group report that serial scans always demonstrate cervical shortening before the appearance of funneling.[49] Heath et al[22] found that all women with a cervical length ≤ 15 mm exhibited funneling compared to only one-third of those with a cervical length of 16–25 mm. It remains unclear whether a 20 mm cervix without funneling carries an identical risk to a 20 mm cervix with 10 mm of funneling above.

### Dynamic changes

Parulekar and Kiwi[50] observed changes in cervical dilatation during the course of a single transabdominal ultrasound examination in more than 25% of a group of 56 patients with a diagnosis of cervical incompetence. These dynamic changes were all associated with the finding of a long, closed cervix at some time during the examination. Outcome details are unfortunately inadequate, as no comment was made about the use of cerclage. Sonek[51] subsequently reported the same phenomenon in women not believed to have cervical incompetence, using transvaginal scanning. He went on to state that the funneling could be accentuated or brought on by gentle manual pressure on the uterine fundus and advocated this as an 'internal os stress test'. Hertzberg et al[52] detected dynamic cervical change on 27 women scanned for a variety of indications of whom 75% delivered preterm. As reported previously, there was an inverse relationship between the maximum funnel width and funnel length and gestation at birth. Similarly, as the length of closed cervix below the funnel increased, so did the gestation at birth. The absolute magnitude of change between maximum and minimum values had no predictive value.

Guzman et al[53] systematically studied the effects of transfundal pressure on cervical appearance in pregnancy. None of 150 low-risk women showed any response to transfundal pressure when scanned once transabdominally between 16–24 weeks' gestation. There were 2 mid-trimester miscarriages and 7 preterm deliveries between 32–37 weeks' gestation in this group. Thirty-one women with suspected cervical incompetence were serially scanned transvaginally and half showed a response to fundal pressure. The combined second trimester loss and preterm delivery rate was the same as the responders as in the group with no response. However, almost all the responders had cervical cerclage placed, except one who aborted at 22 weeks. It was impossible to know if this was because the cerclage improved outcome or because the response to fundal pressure is not a good marker (and led to unnecessary cervical surgery). The same group later reported on 10 patients who had a positive response to fundal pressure but a normal pelvic examination.[54] Management was initially conservative. Within an average of 7 days, all showed further shortening of the cervix to the point where it was felt that cerclage was indicated. In two-thirds of cases, the membrane funnel reached the external os. It is unclear how many of these cervices would have been classified as abnormal with simple observation only, as the pre-fundal pressure lengths ranged from 7–36 mm. It has been the authors' personal experience that fundal pressure usually only accentuates a previously suspected abnormality. Furthermore, we have found that suprapubic pressure, elevating the presenting part away from the internal os, sometimes reveals funneling not seen in response to fundal pressure.

At present, transfundal pressure cannot be standardised. More recently, reports have appeared advocating the use of a postural challenge, with the cervix being scanned first while the mother is supine and then when upright. This is theoretically attractive, as the stressor is standardised (gravity) and there is natural therapy in bed-rest and restricted activity. Guzman et al[55] reported that fundal pressure was better than postural change in detecting cervical change. However, their use of a surrogate endpoint (cervical length < 26 mm) with subsequent cerclage confuses test interpretation. Wong et al[56] found that there was no cervical shortening in response to a postural challenge in 24 low-risk women. In high-risk women, 40% showed cervical shortening of ≥ 33 % on standing. Over 85% of these 'responders' delivered preterm (mean gestation 31 weeks) compared to less than 5% of high-risk 'non-responders' (mean gestation 38 weeks) with significantly longer NICU stays and a trend towards more perinatal deaths. Once again, this study was unblinded and intervention advised on the basis of the ultrasound findings. Nonetheless, the negative predictive value appears high, especially since the one false-negative test had a resting cervical length of less than 20 mm.

## Cervical cerclage

### Timing

The final report of the MRC/RCOG Multicentre Randomised Trial of Cervical Cerclage suggested benefit in only 4% of cases with prior clinical uncertainty.[57] Detailed inspection revealed that cerclage improved outcome only after three or more previous very early deliveries. Clearly, better techniques for assessing when the operation may or may not be appropriate are needed. Fox et al[58] used serial ultrasound to detect cervical change in high risk women before undertaking cerclage. All patients had a normal cervical length (> 40 mm) at 14 weeks' gestation. One-third showed no cervical change throughout the study, avoided surgical treatment and delivered at term. Twelve women developed cervical change and had McDonald sutures inserted. One patient delivered at 20 weeks' gestation with chorioamnionitis but the rest went on to term. Guzman et al[59] reported on 29 high risk women who underwent emergency cerclage after the ultrasonic finding of membrane funneling. In just under half of the cases, the membranes were at or beyond the external os. Nearly 50% of the women delivered before 36 weeks' gestation. Interestingly, the mean interval between cerclage removal and delivery was 2.3 weeks. As these cases all had clearly demonstrated ultrasonographic cervical change, the implication is that prompt delivery after suture removal is not mandatory for the diagnosis of cervical incompetence, as suggested by Quinn (Fig. 3A,B).[60] A recent

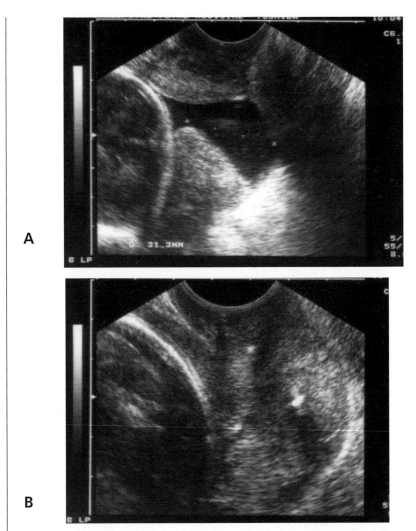

**Fig. 3** (**A**) Transvaginal ultrasound at 23 weeks' gestation showing funneling extending beyond the external os in a primiparous woman. Speculum examination confirmed bulging membranes in the upper vagina. Amniocentesis was performed to exclude infection. (**B**) Postoperative ultrasound showing a McDonald cerclage in the middle third of the cervix. The suture was removed at 38 weeks' gestation and the patient laboured spontaneously 12 days later. After 14 h, narcotics and an epidural for analgesia and oxytocin augmentation, a vaginal delivery was achieved.

publication from the same group compared the outcomes after elective cerclage based on history alone and selective cerclage performed for ultrasound-detected cervical change.[61] No difference in obstetric outcome was found. However, the study was non-randomised and there were important demographic differences between the two groups. Furthermore, it failed to truly compare a policy of elective versus selective cerclage, as the outcomes of the women scanned but not operated upon are not included. As the authors suggest, only 1 in 4 high-risk women require cerclage, it is conceivable that a policy of selective cerclage could lead to improved overall outcomes. We have followed 22 women with a history of cerclage in a previous pregnancy using transvaginal scanning and similarly found only 25% needed a repeat suture.[62] A recent publication from the King's College group has heightened interest in the role of cerclage in treating an ultrasonographically-diagnosed short cervix.[63] According to which clinician was responsible for patient care, 43 women with cervical lengths of ≤ 15 mm at 23 weeks' gestation either received a Shirodkar-type cerclage or expectant management. The rate of spontaneous delivery ≤ 32 weeks gestation in the cerclage group (5%) was significantly lower than the 52% rate observed in the expectant management group. Although these results are striking, it should be remembered that the vast majority of these women were Afro-Caribbean, the treatment allocation was not randomised and no special treatment or advice was given to the women managed expectantly. The same group is now undertaking a randomised trial of cerclage in the same circumstances.

### Cerclage placement

Fox et al[58] found that McDonald cerclage closed a funneled upper cervix in all cases even though the stitches were at least 1 cm away from the level of the internal os. This has not always been our experience.[64] Both Andersen et al[65] and Quinn[60] reported all the McDonald sutures in their series to be in the middle third of the cervix. The optimal placement of a suture was obtained in the single patient that was treated with a Shirodkar-type cerclage, involving preliminary dissection of the anterior vaginal wall. (Fig. 4) Guzman et al[59] also found that 80% of their McDonald sutures were in the middle section of the cervix. Gibb reported a comparison of suture location in the three main types of cerclage procedure, using ultrasonic assessment.[66] Only 25% of McDonald cerclages were in the upper third of the cervix compared with 87% of Shirodkar sutures and 100% of transabdominal procedures. Furthermore, the mean distance of the suture from the internal os was 12 mm, 7 mm and 4 mm, respectively. Although surgeons strive for anatomical perfection, there is no strong evidence that

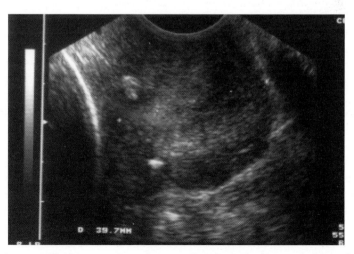

**Fig. 4** A transvaginal scan at 17 weeks' gestation showed a large membrane funnel in this woman with a history of 4 first trimester therapeutic abortions since her first term delivery. By the time of cerclage 2 days later, the membranes were visible at the external os. The post-operative ultrasound shows the Shirodkar-type cerclage situated close to the internal os.

cerclage position influences outcome. Lysikiewicz et al[67] specifically investigated the relationship of suture position and gestation at delivery. Only a small number of women were studied, but they found that suture position did not influence success rates. Although the surgical technique is not described, two-thirds of their sutures were in the distal half of the cervix, close to the external os. They and ourselves[64] have hypothesised that cerclage may act by mechanisms other than simply retention of the pregnancy within the uterus. Guzman et al[59] also comment that there was no apparent correlation between suture site and gestation at delivery in their study.

Ludmir et al[68] used transabdominal ultrasound to help them undertake cervical cerclage in 5 cases with gross cervical deficiencies. It aided dissection into the region of the supravaginal cervix and directed sutures to the level of the internal os. All the patients delivered at term.

### Post-cerclage follow-up

Rana et al[69] used transabdominal ultrasound to serially follow-up women who underwent first trimester elective cerclage for suspected cervical incompetence. If the internal os remained closed, no patient delivered preterm. Between 25–30% of patients developed funneling above the cerclage. In the first part of the study, these women were simply observed. Clinical evidence of cervical change only appeared 4–9 weeks after ultrasonographic evidence and the women with funneling delivered preterm, at 24 weeks, 29 weeks and 35 weeks, respectively. In the second part of the study, women with funneling on ultrasound were admitted to hospital and given oral ritodrine. Seven of the eight cases delivered at term, suggesting that intervention based on cervical change could lead to improved outcomes. Using transvaginal scanning, Quinn[60] followed up 21 women who underwent elective cerclage for suspected cervical incompetence; 20% of pregnancies developed funneling in the second trimester and all delivered within 4–7 weeks. However, there were 6 other women who delivered preterm with no preceding ultrasound evidence of cervical change. Closer inspection of their details reveals that one was a twin pregnancy and that three others had a past history of term deliveries followed by a change of partner and the onset of second trimester losses. It is conceivable that a different pathophysiology was acting in these cases. Andersen et al[65] performed serial transvaginal scans in 32 women who underwent elective cerclage. Results were made available to clinicians and a variety of non-randomised treatments subsequently used. Eight patients had significant membrane funneling develop with less than 10 mm of closed cervix between the funnel and the suture; 75% of this group delivered before 34 weeks' gestation. Only one of the 24 women with no significant cervical change delivered this early. Subsequent correspondence in the same journal revealed that in 6 women the funnel reached the level of the suture with 5 of these pregnancies ending preterm.[70] Wong et al[56] suggest that cervical shortening in response to standing identifies those women who are at high risk of preterm birth despite cerclage. Fox et al[58] only performed cerclage when cervical change was documented on serial scanning. Twelve patients underwent cerclage but seven subsequently developed further evidence of progressive cervical change. These women underwent a repeat cerclage and all delivered at term.

## Twin pregnancies

Although making up only approximately 1% of all pregnancies, multiple gestations account for 10% of very preterm births and neonatal intensive care admissions. Michaels et al[71] managed 53 twin pregnancies with serial transabdominal cervical ultrasound scans from the mid-trimester onwards. Cervical weakness was diagnosed on the basis of cervical shortening, dilatation and membrane funneling but specific criteria were not given. Cervical cerclage was undertaken in 14% of patients on the basis of cervical scans. Three delivered before 34 weeks' gestation and 4 women went beyond 36 weeks. They compared their patients to 153 consecutive control twin pregnancies managed without cervical scanning by other doctors at the same hospital and provided evidence suggesting a reduction in prelabour rupture of the membranes, extremely preterm birth and perinatal mortality. Kushnir et al[72] were the first to report transvaginal ultrasound measurements of the cervix in twin pregnancy. In 25 women, who all delivered at term, significant shortening was observed from 20 weeks' gestation onwards (mean cervical lengths: 20–25 weeks 39 mm, 26–31 weeks 33 mm, 32–37 weeks 28 mm). More importantly, when compared to cervical length measurements in singleton pregnancies,[23] cervical length was significantly shorter in each gestational age group.

Goldenberg et al[73] scanned 147 twin pregnancies at 24 and 28 weeks' gestation. A cervical length of less than 25 mm was twice as common in twin pregnancies as in singletons and became more common as gestation advanced, occurring in 18% of women at 24 weeks and 33% at 28 weeks. Of women with a short cervix at 24 weeks, 27% delivered within the next 8 weeks compared to only 5% of those whose cervix measured > 25 mm. Both this group and others[74] have commented on the lack of association between traditional risk factors for prematurity in singleton pregnancies when applied to multiple pregnancy.

## Cervical ultrasound and routine antenatal care

Lorenz et al[48] compared serial transabdominal cervical scans with vaginal examinations in patients at risk of prematurity and found no evidence to support the use of ultrasound. However, their study was very small with only 57 patients in total. When Andersen et al[75] investigated the prediction of preterm delivery using cervical ultrasound, they found that transvaginal measurements of cervical length were significantly predictive of early birth while simultaneously taken transabdominal measurements were not. Although Zalar[76] suggested that knowledge of transvaginal cervical ultrasound measurements can lead to a reduction in spontaneous low birth-weight deliveries, it cannot yet be concluded that cervical ultrasound has a place in routine antenatal care in low-risk pregnancies.

## Preterm prelabour rupture of the membranes

Carlan et al[19] randomised 92 women with preterm prelabour rupture of the membranes (PPROM) to either weekly transvaginal assessments of cervical length or no transvaginal scans. They found that the use of transvaginal sonography was not associated with either an increased rate of infectious

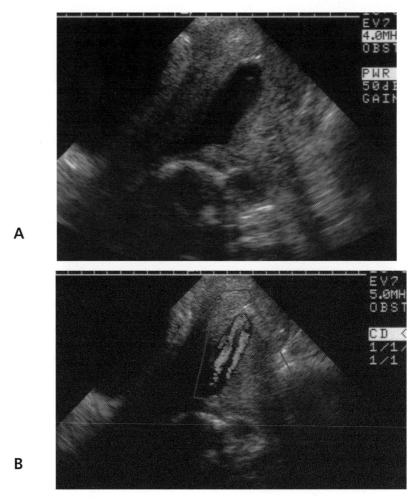

**A**

**B**

**Fig. 5** (**A**) Transvaginal scan at 23 weeks' gestation in a woman with PPROM demonstrating funneling. (**B**) The addition of Power Doppler revealed the 'funnel' to be a loop of cord. The cord appeared suddenly at the vulva 3 days later. The scan had allowed difficult management decisions to be made outside of the acute situation.

morbidity or a shortening of the latency period before labour. It is of concern that all 3 perinatal deaths occurred in the ultrasound group, although all appeared to be related to pulmonary immaturity. They were unable to demonstrate a significant relationship between cervical length and the number of days to spontaneous labour. Rizzo et al[20] measured cervical length transvaginally in 92 women presenting with PPROM. A cervical length of ≤ 20 mm was associated with a significant reduction in the time interval from admission to delivery (median 2 days versus 6 days). Unfortunately, the knowledge of such a small change in latency before labour is unlikely to be clinically useful. Furthermore, some patients with cervical lengths > 20 mm delivered within 24 h. Although there is evidence that cervical ultrasound can be safely used in the setting of PPROM, there is little evidence to suggest any clinical benefit. However, both Carlan et al[19] and ourselves have detected occult cord prolapse in this situation (Fig. 5A,B).

# TECHNIQUES FOR CERVICAL SCANNING

## Transabdominal

As mentioned previously, cervical images are best obtained transabdominally with a full bladder. Unfortunately, this is associated with artificial lengthening of the cervix and potential closure of a dilated internal os. Therefore, it will lead to false reassurance in some cases. The external os can also be difficult to identify transabdominally. In the studies of Varma et al,[4] an inflated Foley catheter balloon was placed against it to overcome this problem.

## Transvaginal

This remains the gold standard for cervical imaging. Adequate images have been obtained with a variety of transducers. Although Sonek et al[16] have advocated the use of a probe with a 240° scanning field, this would appear to be unnecessary. No variation in measurement according to the ultrasound machine used has been reported by one group.[29] Inter-observer variation is reported as 4–13%[25,29,32,34] with intra-observer error between 5–9%.[25,32,34] This is due to both calliper placement and variations in obtaining the image.[22] As discussed earlier, scanning should be performed with the maternal bladder empty. Pressure on the cervix can falsely increase the measured length and obscure funneling at the internal os.[77] Failing to appreciate that not all cervical canals follow a straight line can lead to underestimates of length (Fig. 6). The most authoritative description of technique comes from Iams et al.[24] Pressure artefacts are avoided by withdrawing the probe until the image is blurred and then re-applying it sufficiently to restore the image. Burger et al[78] have recommended that the width of the anterior and posterior cervical lips should appear equal on the image used, reflecting the fact that the cervical canal is normally central. At least 3 measurements should be taken and the shortest

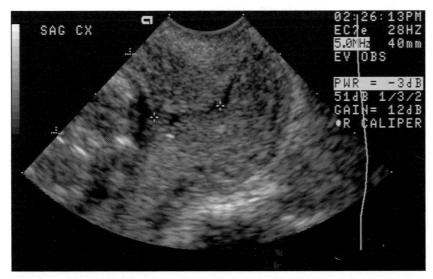

**Fig. 6** This transvaginal cervical scan was falsely reported as 13 mm. The upward angulation of the canal was not appreciated and the true cervical length was 25 mm.

(not the average) used. Most authors advise scanning over approximately 5 min to detect dynamic changes. The presence of a funnel should be noted and funnel width and length recorded. Some authors have reserved the term 'funnel' for membrane protrusions greater than 5 mm down the endocervical canal, referring to anything less as 'nippling'. The use of videotapes facilitates both teaching and quality control.

### Transperineal scanning

Women at high-risk of prematurity are usually happy to undergo serial trans-vaginal scans to assess the cervix.[58,60] The same may not be true of women at low-risk of early birth, who may find it invasive and uncomfortable and incorrectly perceive it to carry some risk. Several groups have reported experience with the technique of transperineal cervical scanning.[52,79,80] A glove-covered 3.5 MHz or 5 MHz sector or curvilinear transducer is applied to the perineum to visualise the cervix. It is reportedly easily tolerated by patients,[79] but is best performed before digital or speculum examination which, by introducing air into the vagina, produce artefact. Gas in the rectum may cause similar problems. It is definitely a more technically difficult technique to master compared to transvaginal scanning. Nevertheless, Kurtzman et al[81] have shown an excellent correlation between cervical measurements obtained both transvaginally and transperineally, provided a period of in-house training is undertaken. In our experience, the technique has been particularly useful in cases of prolapsing membranes when cerclage is not being undertaken. The contrast provided by the funnel of membranes usually allows excellent visualisation and serial monitoring. Transperineal ultrasonography may prove to be an acceptable mass screening technique.

## OTHER WORK

### Induction of labour

Paterson-Brown et al[21] attempted to replace the traditional Bishop score for cervical assessment prior to labour induction with measurements obtained by transvaginal scan. Unfortunately, most parameters showed no correlation with induction outcome. A recent report from Japan studied the endocervical mucosa, as seen with transvaginal sonography.[82] They found a strong correlation between the presence of an endocervical mucosal layer and a traditional Bishop score. They hypothesised that this mucosa represented cervical glands, which disappear during the process of cervical ripening. There may be other useful information, in addition to measurements of length which can be obtained from cervical ultrasound.

### Intrapartum use

In a fascinating study, Zilianti et al[80] used the transperineal approach to study the cervix during term labour. During the process of cervical effacement, there was progressive cervical shortening along with membrane funneling. The relevance of this to previous studies investigating cervical change and preterm labour is difficult to ignore. It has also been suggested that this technique may allow more accurate assessment of descent of the presenting part in labour.[83]

## CONCLUSIONS

The traditional obstetric view has been that cervical incompetence either exists or does not. As proposed by Iams et al,[29] ultrasound imaging suggests cervical competence to be a continuous variable. This continuum may reflect a patient's ability to resist a variety of triggers or stimuli to preterm birth. Not only does the risk of preterm delivery increase with decreasing cervical length, but also the shortness of the cervix reflects the actual gestation at the time of preterm birth. Infection has attracted considerable interest as one of the most important aetiologies behind preterm labour and delivery. A weak or short cervix could offer less resistance to ascending infection. Romero et al[84] studied 33 women presenting with asymptomatic cervical dilatation in the mid-trimester. Half had positive amniotic fluid cultures, representing advanced ascending infection. Iams et al[85] have recently reported that a cervical length of less than 25 mm at 24 weeks' gestation is strongly associated with subsequent perinatal infection. The risk of ascending infection may be related not only to the magnitude of the cervical barrier but also to the virulence of the organisms within the genital tract and to other factors, such as sexual intercourse. Bacteria can ascend the genital tract attached to motile sperm. Antibiotics may play just as important a role as cervical cerclage in preventing prematurity. Indeed, when advanced cervical changes are seen, it may be safest to assume that infection of the membranes and/or decidua is present. As prostaglandins are implicated in the process of cervical ripening, non-steroidal anti-inflammatories such as indomethacin may have a role for ultrasonographic cervical change, at least before 28 weeks' gestation. Just as preterm birth is a heterogeneous group of disorders, many different therapies may have to be employed, either alone or in combination. Cervical ultrasound undoubtedly allows a far better assessment of risk than clinical examination. Some studies referred to in this review have suggested that intervention on the basis of cervical scans may lead to improved outcomes. What is needed is the scientific evaluation of these various therapies in formal randomised and controlled trials.

*References*

1  Anderson A B M, Turnbull A C. Relationship between length of gestation and cervical dilatation, uterine contractility and other factors during pregnancy. Am J Obstet Gynecol 1969; 105: 1207–1214

2  Phelps J Y, Higby K, Smyth M H, Ward J A, Arredondo F, Mayer A R. Accuracy and interobserver variability of simulated cervical dilatation measurements. Am J Obstet Gynecol 1995; 173: 942–945

3  Jackson G M, Ludmir J, Bader T J. The accuracy of digital examination and ultrasound in the evaluation of cervical length. Obstet Gynecol 1992; 79: 214–218

4  Varma T R, Patel R H, Pillai U. Ultrasonographic assessment of cervix in normal pregnancy. Acta Obstet Gynecol Scand 1986; 65: 229–233

5  Varma T R, Patel R H, Pillai U. Ultrasonic assessment of 'at risk' patients. Acta Obstet Gynecol Scand 1986; 65: 147–152

6  Varma T R, Patel R H, Pillai U. Ultrasonic assessment of cervix in 'at risk' patients. Int J Gynecol Obstet 1987; 25: 25–34

7  Riley L, Frigoletto F D, Benacerraf B R. The implications of sonographically identified cervical changes in patients not necessarily at risk for preterm birth. J Ultrasound Med 1992; 11: 75–79

8  Michaels W H, Montgomery C, Karo J, Temple J, Ager J, Olson J. Ultrasound differentiation of the competent from the incompetent cervix: prevention of preterm delivery. Am J Obstet Gynecol 1986; 154: 537–546

9  Brown J E, Thieme G A, Shah D M, Fleischer A C, Boehm F H. Transabdominal and transvaginal endosonography: evaluation of the cervix and lower uterine segment in pregnancy. Am J Obstet Gynecol 1986; 155: 721–726

10  Andersen H F. Transvaginal and transabdominal ultrasonography of the uterine cervix during pregnancy. J Clin Ultrasound 1991; 19: 77–83

11  Mason G C, Maresh M J A. Alterations in bladder volume and the ultrasound appearance of the cervix. Br J Obstet Gynaecol 1990; 97: 457–458

12  Confino E, Mayden K L, Giglia R V, Vermesh M, Gleicher N. Pitfalls in sonographic imaging of the incompetent uterine cervix. Acta Obstet Gynecol Scand 1986; 65: 593–597

13  Scheerer L J, Lam F, Bartolucci L, Katz M. A new technique for reduction of fetal membranes for emergency cervical cerclage. Obstet Gynecol 1989; 74: 408–410

14  Okitsu O, Mimura T, Nakayama T, Aono T. Early prediction of preterm delivery by transvaginal ultrasonography. Ultrasound Obstet Gynecol 1992; 2: 402–409

15  Goldberg J, Newman R B, Rust P F. Interobserver reliability of digital and endovaginal ultrasonographic cervical length measurements. Am J Obstet Gynecol 1997; 177: 853–858

16  Sonek J D, Iams J D, Blumenfeld M, Johnson F, Landon M, Gabbe S. Measurement of cervical length in pregnancy: comparison between vaginal ultrasonography and digital examination. Obstet Gynecol 1990; 76: 172–175

17  Berghella V, Kuhlman K, Weiner S, Texeira L, Wapner R J. Cervical funneling: sonographic criteria predictive of preterm delivery. Ultrasound Obstet Gynecol 1997; 10: 161–166

18  Timor-Tritsch I E, Yunis R A. Confirming the safety of transvaginal sonography in patients suspected of placenta praevia. Obstet Gynecol 1993; 81: 742–744

19  Carlan S J, Richmond L B, O'Brien W F. Randomised trial of endovaginal ultrasound in preterm premature rupture of the membranes. Obstet Gynecol 1997; 89: 458–461

20  Rizzo G, Capponi A, Angelini E, Vlachopoulou A, Grassi C, Romanini C. The value of transvaginal ultrasonographic examination of the uterine cervix in predicting preterm delivery in patients with preterm premature rupture of membranes. Ultrasound Obstet Gynecol 1998; 11: 23–29

21  Paterson-Brown S, Fisk N M, Edmonds D K, Rodeck C H. Preinduction cervical assessment by Bishop's score and transvaginal ultrasound. Eur J Obstet Gynecol Reprod 1991; 40: 17–23

22  Heath V C F, Southall T R, Souka A P, Novakov A, Nicolaides K H. Cervical length at 23 weeks of gestation: relation to demographic characteristics and previous obstetric history. Ultrasound Obstet Gynecol 1998; 12: 304–311

23  Kushnir O, Vigil D A, Izquierdo L, Schiff M, Curet L B. Vaginal ultrasonographic assessment of cervical length changes in normal pregnancy. Am J Obstet Gynecol 1990; 162: 991–993

24  Iams J D, Goldenberg R L, Meis P J et al. The length of the cervix and the risk of spontaneous prematurity. N Engl J Med 1996; 334: 567–572

25  Zorzoli A, Soliani A, Perra M, Caravelli E, Galimberti A, Nicolini U. Cervical changes throughout pregnancy as assessed by transvaginal sonography. Obstet Gynecol 1994; 84: 960–964

26  Smith C V, Anderson J C, Matamoros A, Rayburn W F. Transvaginal sonography of cervical width and length during pregnancy. J Ultrasound Med 1992; 11: 465–467

27  Murakawa H, Utumi T, Hasegawa I, Tanaka K, Fuzimori R. Evaluation of threatened preterm delivery by transvaginal ultrasonographic measurement of cervical length. Obstet Gynecol 1993; 82: 829–832

28  Goldenberg R L, Iams J, Mercer B et al. The preterm prediction study: the value of new versus standard risk factors in predicting early and all spontaneous preterm births. Am J Public Health 1998; 88: 233–238

29  Iams J D, Johnson F F, Sonek J, Sachs L, Gebauer C, Samuels P. Cervical competence as a continuum: a study of ultrasonographic cervical length and obstetric performance. Am J

Obstet Gynecol 1995; 172: 1097–1106

30 Canadian Preterm Labor Investigators Group. Treatment of preterm labor with the beta-adrenergic agonist ritodrine. N Engl J Med 1992; 327: 308–312

31 Iams J D, Paraskos J, Landon M B, Teteris J N, Johnson F F. Cervical sonography in preterm labor. Obstet Gynecol 1994; 84: 40–46

32 Gomez R, Galasso M, Romero R et al. Ultrasonographic examination of the uterine cervix is better than cervical digital examination as a predictor of the likelihood of premature delivery in patients with preterm labor and intact membranes. Am J Obstet Gynecol 1994; 171: 956–964

33 Timor-Tritsch L E, Boozarjomehri F, Masakowski Y, Monteagudo A, Chao C R. Can a 'snapshot' sagittal view of the cervix by transvaginal ultrasonography predict active preterm labor? Am J Obstet Gynecol 1996; 174: 990–995

34 Rizzo G, Capponi A, Arduini D, Lorido C, Romanini C. The value of fetal fibronectin in cervical and vaginal secretions and of ultrasonic examination of the uterine cervix in predicting premature delivery for patients with preterm labor and intact membranes. Am J Obstet Gynecol 1996; 175: 1146–1151

35 Rageth J C, Kernen B, Saurenmann E, Unger C. Premature contractions: possible influence of sonographic measurement of cervical length on clinical management. Ultrasound Obstet Gynecol 1997; 9: 183–187

36 Timor-Tritsch I E, Monteagudo A. Diagnosis of placenta praevia by transvaginal sonography. Ann Med 1993; 25: 279–283

37 Smith R S, Lauria M R, Comstock C H et al. Transvaginal ultrasonography for all placentas that appear to be low-lying or over the internal cervical os. Ultrasound Obstet Gynecol 1997; 9: 22–24

38 Oppenheimer L W, Farine D, Ritchie J W, Lewinsky R M, Telford J, Fairbanks L A. What is a low-lying placenta? Am J Obstet Gynecol 1991; 165: 1036–1038

39 Michaels W H, Thompson H O, Schreiber F R, Berman J M, Ager J, Olson K. Ultrasound surveillance of the cervix during pregnancy in diethylstilbestrol-exposed offspring. Obstet Gynecol 1989; 73: 230–239

40 El-Azeem S, Samuels P, Iams J D. Cervical ultrasound length and outcome in pregnancies complicated by in utero exposure to diethylstilbestrol. Am J Obstet Gynecol 1997; 176: S51

41 Westgren M, Sjoberg N. Surveillance of the cervix by ultrasonography at cervical incompetence. Acta Obstet Gynecol Scand 1986; 65: 655–657

42 El-Azeem S, Samuels P, Iams J. Cervical ultrasound length and outcome in patients with prior history of cervical conization. Am J Obstet Gynecol 1997; 176: S50

43 Wong G, Ludmir J. Sonographic evaluation of the cervix in patients with unexplained second trimester rupture of membranes in previous pregnancies (PROM). Ultrasound Obstet Gynecol 1996; 8: 74

44 Chan L, Uerpairojkit B, Gomez F L, Reece E A, Ludomirski A. Three dimensional assessment of cerclage placement and cervical incompetence. Am J Obstet Gynecol 1996; 174: 427

45 Heath V C F, Southall T R, Souka A P, Elisseou A, Nicolaides K H. Cervical length at 23 weeks of gestation: prediction of spontaneous preterm delivery. Ultrasound Obstet Gynecol 1998; 12: 312–317

46 Taipale P, Hiilesmaa V. Sonographic measurement of uterine cervix at 18–22 weeks gestation and the risk of preterm delivery. Obstet Gynecol 1998; 92: 902–907

47 Iams J D, Goldenberg R L, Mercer B M et al. The Preterm Prediction Study: recurrence risk of spontaneous preterm birth. Am J Obstet Gynecol 1998; 178: 1035–1040

48 Lorenz R P, Comstock C H, Bottoms S F, Marx S R. Randomized prospective trial comparing ultrasonography and pelvic examination for preterm labor surveillance. Am J Obstet Gynecol 1990; 162: 1603–1610

49 Joffe G M, Del Valle G O, Izquierdo L A et al. Diagnosis of cervical change in pregnancy by means of transvaginal ultrasonography. Am J Obstet Gynecol 1992; 166: 896–900

50 Parulekar S G, Kiwi R. Dynamic incompetent cervix uteri. Sonographic observations. J Ultrasound Med 1988; 7: 481–485

51 Sonek J. Cervical length may change during ultrasonographic examination. Am J Obstet Gynecol 1990; 162: 1355–1357

52 Hertzberg B S, Kliewer M A, Farrell T A, DeLong D M. Spontaneously changing gravid cervix: clinical implications and prognostic features. Radiology 1995; 196: 721–724

53 Guzman E R, Rosenberg J C, Houlihan C, Ivan J, Waldron R, Knuppel R. A new method using vaginal ultrasound and transfundal pressure to evaluate the asymptomatic incompetent cervix. Obstet Gynecol 1994; 83: 248–252

54 Guzman E R, Vintzileos A M, McLean D A, Martins M E, Benito C W, Hanley M L. The natural history of a positive response to transfundal pressure in women at risk for cervical incompetence. Am J Obstet Gynecol 1997; 176: 634–638

55 Guzman E R, Pisatowski D M, Vintzileos A M, Benito C W, Hanley M L, Ananth C V. A comparison of ultrasonographically detected cervical changes in response to transfundal pressure, coughing and standing in predicting cervical incompetence. Am J Obstet Gynecol 1997; 177: 660–665

56 Wong G, Levine D, Ludmir J. Maternal postural challenge as a functional test for cervical incompetence. J Ultrasound Med 1997; 16: 169–175

57 MRC/RCOG Working Party on Cervical Cerclage. Final report of the Medical Research Council/Royal College of Obstetricians and Gynaecologists Multicentre Randomised Trial of Cervical Cerclage. Br J Obstet Gynaecol 1993; 100: 516–523

58 Fox R, James M, Tuohy J, Wardle P. Transvaginal ultrasound in the management of women with suspected cervical incompetence. Br J Obstet Gynaecol 1996; 103: 921–924

59 Guzman E R, Houlihan C, Vintzileos A, Ivan J, Benito C, Kappy K. The significance of transvaginal ultrasonographic evaluation of the cervix in women treated with emergency cerclage. Am J Obstet Gynecol 1996; 175: 471–476

60 Quinn M J. Vaginal ultrasound and cervical cerclage: a prospective study. Ultrasound Obstet Gynecol 1992; 2: 410–416

61 Guzman E R, Forster J K, Vintzileos A M, Ananth C V, Walters C, Gipson K. Pregnancy outcomes in women treated with elective versus ultrasound-indicated cervical cerclage. Ultrasound Obstet Gynecol 1998; 12: 323–327

62 Jones G, Maxwell D. Once a cerclage, always a cerclage? Ultrasound Obstet Gynecol 1998; 12: P87

63 Heath V C F, Souka A P, Erasmus I, Gibb D M F, Nicolaides K H. Cervical length at 23 weeks of gestation: the value of Shirodkar suture for the short cervix. Ultrasound Obstet Gynecol 1998; 12: 318–322

64 Jones G, Clark T, Bewley S. The weak cervix: failing to keep the baby in or infection out? Br J Obstet Gynaecol 1998; 105: 1214–1215

65 Andersen H F, Karimi A, Sakala E P, Kalugdan R. Prediction of cervical cerclage outcome by endovaginal ultrasonography. Am J Obstet Gynecol 1994; 171: 1102–1106

66 Gibb D M F. Transvaginal ultrasound imaging of cervical cerclage. Ultrasound Obstet Gynecol 1996; 8: 231

67 Lysikiewicz A, Canterino J, Robinson R P, Tejani N. Ultrasonographic follow-up of cervical cerclage placement. Am J Obstet Gynecol 1996; 174: 414

68 Ludmir J, Jackson M, Samuels P. Transvaginal cerclage under ultrasound guidance in cases of severe cervical hypoplasia. Obstet Gynecol 1991; 78: 1067–1072

69 Rana J, Davis S E, Harrigan J T. Improving the outcome of cervical cerclage by sonographic follow-up. J Ultrasound Med 1990; 9: 275–278

70 Quinn M. Ultrasonographic diagnosis of 'cervical incompetence'. Am J Obstet Gynecol 1995; 172: 1953–1954

71 Michaels W H, Schreiber F R, Padgett R J, Ager J, Pieper D. Ultrasound surveillance of the cervix in twin gestations: management of cervical incompetency. Obstet Gynecol 1991; 78: 739–744

72 Kushnir O, Izquierdo L A, Smith J F, Blankstein J, Curet L B. Transvaginal sonographic measurement of cervical length. Evaluation of twin pregnancies. J Reprod Med 1995; 40: 380–382

73 Goldenberg R L, Iams J D, Miodovnik M et al. The preterm prediction study: risk factors in twin gestations. Am J Obstet Gynecol 1996; 175: 1047–1053

74 Berkowitz G, Lapinski R, Berkowitz R. Risk factors for spontaneous preterm birth in twin gestations. Am J Obstet Gynecol 1994; 170: 380

75 Andersen H F, Nugent C E, Wanty S D, Hayashi R H. Prediction of risk for preterm delivery by ultrasonographic measurement of cervical length. Am J Obstet Gynecol 1990; 163: 859–867

76 Zalar R W. Transvaginal ultrasound and preterm labor: a non-randomized intervention study. Obstet Gynecol 1996; 88: 20–23

77 Ben-Shlomo I, Weiner E, Lahav D, Shalev E. Transvaginal evaluation of cervical incompetence: should pressure be applied through the transducer. Ultrasound Obstet Gynecol 1996; 8: 107

78 Burger M, Weber-Rossler T, Willmann M. Measurement of the pregnant cervix by transvaginal sonography: an interobserver study and new standards to improve the interobserver variability. Ultrasound Obstet Gynecol 1997; 9: 188–193

79 Richey S D, Ramin K D, Roberts S W, Ramin S M, Cox S M, Twickler D M. The correlation between transperineal sonography and digital examination in the evaluation of the third-trimester cervix. Obstet Gynecol 1995; 85: 745–748

80 Zilianti M, Azuaga A, Calderon F, Pages G, Mendoza G. Monitoring the effacement of the uterine cervix by transperineal sonography: a new perspective. J Ultrasound Med 1995; 14: 719–724

81. Kurtzman J T, Goldsmith L J, Gall S A, Spinnato J A. Transvaginal versus transperineal ultrasonography: a blinded comparison in the assessment of cervical length at midgestation. Am J Obstet Gynecol 1998; 179: 852–857

82 Sekiya T, Ishihara K, Yoshimatsu K, Fukami T, Kikuchi S, Araki T. Detection rate of the cervical gland area during pregnancy by transvaginal sonography in the assessment of cervical maturation. Ultrasound Obstet Gynecol 1998; 12: 328–333

83 Barbera A, Pombar X, Perugino G et al. A new method to assess fetal head descent in labor with transperineal ultrasound. Ultrasound Obstet Gynecol 1996; 8: 95

84 Romero R, Gonzalez R, Sepulveda W et al. Infection and labor. VIII. Microbial invasion of the amniotic cavity in patients with suspected cervical incompetence: prevalence and clinical significance. Am J Obstet Gynecol 1992; 167: 1086–1091

85 Iams J D, NICHD MFMU Network. The preterm prediction study: cervical length and perinatal infection. Am J Obstet Gynecol 1997; 176: S6

*Fathima Paruk   Jack Moodley*

# Treatment of severe pre-eclampsia/eclampsia syndrome

Pre-eclampsia/eclampsia is an unpredictable, multi-organ disorder unique to human pregnancy. It is associated with significant maternal and fetal morbidity and mortality world-wide. Treatment of this disorder remains a challenge to even the most experienced obstetrician, mainly because the exact aetiology is unknown. Changes such as increased sensitivity to vasopressors, reduced plasma volume, altered proximal tubular function and activation of the coagulation system antedate overt hypertension and suggest that hypertension may not be central to the pathogenesis of pre-eclampsia. Consequently, management is directed towards detection of the disorder at an early stage and to effect, or at least ameliorate its progression in an attempt to achieve fetal maturity while preventing maternal complications.[1]

## DEFINITION

A number of classifications for hypertensive disorders in pregnancy have been proposed.[1,2] The International Society for the Study of Hypertension in Pregnancy (ISSHP) currently defines pre-eclampsia as the occurrence of hypertension in combination with proteinuria, developing after 20 weeks' gestation in a previously normotensive non-proteinuric patient.[2] The ISSHP is, however, reviewing its definition of hypertension in pregnancy as concepts have changed in the last decade. Further, based on recent evidence,[3] the ISSHP has agreed that the Korotkoff V (K5) sound be used as a measure of diastolic blood pressure. The K4/K5 difference is smaller in hypertensive than in

**Dr Fathima Paruk** MBChB FCOG, Consultant, MRC/UN Pregnancy Hypertension Research Unit and Department of Obstetrics and Gynaecology, University of Natal Medical School, Private Bag 7, Congella 4013, South Africa

**Prof. Jack Moodley** MB ChB FCOG(SA) FRCOG MD, Head, MRC/UN Pregnancy Hypertension Research Unit and Department of Obstetrics and Gynaecology, University of Natal Medical School, Private Bag 7, Congella 4013, South Africa

**Table 1** Criteria for severe pre-eclampsia

| | |
|---|---|
| 1. | Systolic blood pressure greater than 160 mmHg or diastolic blood pressure greater than 110 mmHg on 2 occasions, at least 6 h apart |
| 2. | Proteinuria exceeding 5 g/24 h |
| 3. | Oliguria (urine output below 400 ml/day) |
| 4. | Neurological symptoms or signs: headaches scotomata visual blurring altered consciousness |
| 5. | Pulmonary oedema/cyanosis |
| 6. | Epigastric pain |
| 7. | Deranged liver function tests |
| 8 | Liver rupture/subcapsular liver haematoma |
| 9. | Thrombocytopenia below 100,000/mm$^3$ |
| 10. | HELLP syndrome |

normotensive pregnant women, and K5 is closer to the actual intra-arterial pressure, is more reliably detected and is reproducible. The universal adoption of K5 is recommended.[4]

The criteria for the diagnosis of severe pre-eclampsia are listed in Table 1. In pregnancy, a diastolic blood pressure of 110 mmHg or greater constitutes a hypertensive crisis as it has been found that young women may develop encephalopathy with diastolic blood pressures of 120 mmHg.[4,5] Systolic hypertension, however, is as dangerous as diastolic hypertension and persistent systolic values of greater than 170 mmHg are associated with significant risks of complications.

It is important to emphasise that pre-eclampsia is a multisystem disorder, but which organ system is going to be affected predominantly, cannot be predicted. Thus hypertension is only one sign, albeit the commonest one, of pre-eclampsia. The concept of 'normotensive pre-eclampsia' is well recognised. Approximately 20% of eclamptic patients and 15% of patients with the 'haemolysis, elevated liver enzymes and low platelets' (HELLP) syndrome are normotensive.[6]

Eclampsia is defined as the occurrence of generalised convulsion(s) associated with signs of pre-eclampsia during pregnancy, labour, or within 7 days of delivery and not caused by epilepsy or other convulsive disorders. In the absence of a high blood pressure or if the convulsion occurs after day 7 postpartum, the condition is referred to as atypical eclampsia.

## TREATMENT OF SEVERE PRE-ECLAMPSIA

Once the diagnosis of severe pre-eclampsia is established, the only cure is termination of pregnancy. In many patients, however, a delay in delivery may be in the interest of the mother, the fetus, or both. It is thus of paramount importance to evaluate each patient individually and weigh the benefits of delivery against the potential risks of continuing the pregnancy. Although the hypertension of pre-eclampsia is a secondary feature, it is associated with significant morbidity and maternal mortality from cerebrovascular accidents.

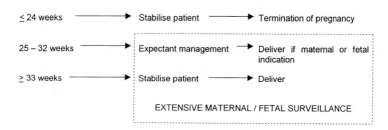

**Fig. 1** Suggested management of severe pre-eclampsia at various gestational stages.

Therefore, good control of high blood pressure is mandatory. Blood pressure control involves short-term control and maintenance of this control long enough until after delivery, when the risk of complications recede.

The objectives in management are as follows:

1. *Prevention of complications such as pulmonary oedema, renal failure, cardiovascular accidents and abruptio placentae.*

2. *Prevention of convulsions as this is associated with a 10 times increased risk in maternal mortality as well as increased risk of perinatal mortality.*

3. *Delivery of a healthy neonate with minimal maternal morbidity.*

The principles of management of severe pre-eclampsia are illustrated in Figure 1.

### Patients presenting at 34 weeks' gestation and greater

It is universally accepted that all patients with severe pre-eclampsia beyond 33 weeks of gestation and where there is evidence of fetal lung maturity, should be delivered. It is important to obtain diastolic blood pressure levels of 95–105 mmHg and to subsequently induce labour (provided there exists no contra-indication to an induction of labour). This approach to management avoids maternal and fetal complications that could arise with conservative manage-ment. Each case, however, needs to be managed on an individual basis.

### Patients presenting before 24 weeks' gestation

It is generally believed that termination of pregnancy is the management of choice at this gestational age. Odendaal et al[7] reported that there were no fetal survivors in 11 such pregnancies at less than 24 weeks' gestation. Sibai et al, from Tennessee, also found that the perinatal survival rate is low in severe pre-eclampsia developing before 25 weeks' gestation compared to that developing after 25 weeks' gestational age — 3% versus 24%, respectively.[8] Similarly, Moodley et al,[9] from Durban, found no fetal survivors in 12 pregnancies at this gestational age. Thus, in patients with severe pre-eclampsia presenting before 24 weeks' gestation, termination of pregnancy is recommended. The preferred mode of delivery is induction of labour provided the high blood pressure is reasonably controlled and the patient does not have a 'toxic' clinical appearance.

## Patients presenting between 24 and 32 weeks' gestation

The management of severe pre-eclampsia in the mid-trimester is indeed a challenge. Aggressive management with delivery may result in a high neonatal mortality whilst conservative management may be associated with an increase in maternal complications. It is clearly evident from the literature that expectant management of patients in this group, in highly specialised units, with the necessary maternal and fetal surveillance facilities, can result in improvement fetal survival without an increase in maternal complications.[7,8]

Odendaal et al studied 38 severe pre-eclamptics: 20 were treated aggressively (control of high blood pressure, betamethasone for 48 h followed by elective delivery); and 18 treated expectantly (betamethasone therapy, delivery indicated by maternal or fetal jeopardy).[10] All patients had severe pre-eclampsia between 28 and 34 weeks' gestation and were randomly assigned to either group of management. Expectant management when compared to aggressive management resulted in a statistically significant prolongation of gestational age by a mean value of 7.1 days, a reduction in neonatal ventilation (11% versus 33%), a reduction in total neonatal complications (33% versus 75%) and no increase in maternal mortality. In a similar study, Sibai et al reported on 109 patients with severe pre-eclampsia diagnosed at or before 27 weeks' gestation of whom 84 patients were between 24 and 27 weeks.[11] All were counselled for conservative management; 30 patients were delivered immediately because of refusal of conservative management either by the patient or the attending physician. Conservative management in the remaining 54 patients was associated with an average prolongation of gestational age by 2 weeks and perinatal morbidity and mortality improved significantly. A perinatal survival rate of 94% was found with expectant management compared to 35.5% in the group that underwent immediate delivery. Maternal morbidity was not increased in the group of patients managed expectantly. Thus, in pregnancies between 28 and 32 weeks, it is suggested that expectant management together with antenatal steroid administration and appropriate maternal and fetal surveillance be recommended. Pregnancy is continued until a maternal or fetal indication for delivery arises. There are some severe pre-eclamptic patients in this group, however, who will require expedited delivery (within 48 h period, regardless of gestational age). This category of patients may be characterised by one or more of the following: (i) thrombocytopenia of less than $50 \times 10^9/l$; (ii) AST/ALT more than twice the normal value; (iii) epigastric pain; (iv) persistent headaches, visual disturbances; (v) pulmonary oedema; (vi) rapidly deteriorating renal function tests; (vii) impending eclampsia; (viii) uncontrollable hypertension; (ix) oliguria not resolving to fluid administration; (x) severe fetal growth impairment and gestation; and (xi) fetal heart rate abnormalities.

It should be noted that appropriate patient selection for expectant management is of paramount importance in severe pre-eclamptic patients.

## IMPORTANT ISSUES

The following issues need to be taken cognisance of in the treatment of severe pre-eclampsia.

## Role of admission

Traditionally, the management of patients suspected of having pre-eclampsia has been to admit such patients in order to confirm the diagnosis, evaluate maternal and fetal condition and to manage the patient as an in-patient until recovery post-delivery. This still holds true for patients with severe pre-eclampsia as such management optimises strict bed rest and appropriate intensive feto–maternal surveillance by a multi-disciplinary team which includes the nursing staff, obstetrician, obstetric anaesthesiologist and neonatologist. Recently, the role of day-care assessment visits and out-patient management of patients with hypertensive disorders of pregnancy has received much attention and research is increasingly being channelled towards these issues.[12] The majority of these studies are numerically restricted and have been based on aproteinuric hypertensive patients. Furthermore, they are conducted in affluent societies with high literacy rates, accessibility to health care facilities and availability of feto–maternal surveillance facilities. In general, results have been positive with respect to maternal and perinatal outcome and cost containment. A Canadian trial which focused on mild pre-eclampsia demonstrated that maternal and perinatal morbidity was not altered.[11] In addition, there was a substantial cost-saving due to reduction in duration of hospital stay. It thus appears that there may be a role for out-patient management of a select subset of mild pre-eclamptic patients in certain select populations.

## Fluid management and cardiovascular monitoring

Plasma volume and cardiac output are usually decreased in severe pre-eclampsia. The state of low oncotic pressure and 'leaky blood capillaries' predispose patients to pulmonary oedema with injudicious use of volume expanders. Thus appropriate cardiovascular monitoring is extremely important. Although the place of central venous and pulmonary capillary pressure monitoring is controversial, central venous pressure (CVP) monitoring is useful to correct any hypovolaemia with Ringer's lactate solution prior to parenteral antihypertensive therapy. The optimal fluid, viz. crystalloid versus colloid, remains a debatable issue. The use of crystalloid alone may decrease oncotic pressure, whilst colloid use might lead to an increase in the CVP and result in pulmonary oedema. Crystalloids are administered at 1 ml/kg/h and titrated to achieve an acceptable CVP reading. The use of colloids should be individualised.

The CVP reflects on right ventricular function and systemic vascular compliance whilst the use of the Swan Ganz catheter (SGC) provides information of left ventricular functions. Thus, the SGC may have a role in patients with uncontrollable hypertension, pulmonary oedema, severe oliguria not responding to appropriate fluid administration or multi-organ failure. However, it must be borne in mind that pulmonary artery catheterisation is associated with maternal morbidity and mortality. In addition to the complications which can arise with a CVP line insertion, the SGC is also associated with cardiac arrhythmias, pulmonary haemorrhage and pulmonary infarction. Pulmonary infarction may be prevented by appropriate care and handling of the catheter and its removal within 72 h of insertion.

## Blood pressure control

The blood pressure is very labile in both severe pre-eclamptics and eclamptics and appears to be particularly sensitive to rapid-acting antihypertensives. Marked hypotension and/or hypoxia may follow over-enthusiastic lowering of high blood pressure. Nonetheless, it is important to lower high blood pressure promptly but slowly, and in a gradual fashion.[13] It is suggested that the diastolic blood pressure not be lowered by more than 30 mmHg or the mean arterial pressure by 25% to achieve diastolic pressures of between 100–110 mmHg. Drugs should be administered in small intermittent doses, or by controlled infusion. Combinations of hypotensive agents should be avoided since they may have a compound effect. Postural hypotension would have a similar result, therefore patients should be nursed on their sides or tilted with the aid of a pelvic wedge.

Dihydralazine, a vasodilator, remains the preferred antihypertensive agent for the treatment of hypertensive crisis of pregnancy. It is easy to administer, being a parenteral agent. The drug is used most frequently in the form of intermittent boluses of low doses of 5 mg. It may also be administered as a continuous infusion, but this is not popular because of its significant delay in action of 20–30 min and its long half-life. The drug also has considerable side-effects. It works by directly inhibiting the contractile activity of smooth muscle of both venules and arterioles. In the cerebral circulation, it does this by initially dilating the capacitance vessels causing an increase in intracranial blood pressure. This probably accounts for the side-effect of severe headache and may mimic impending eclampsia or result in further increases in intracranial pressure in women with eclampsia. Subsequently, the cerebral resistance vessels dilate and cerebrovascular flow increases. A marked tachycardia almost always occurs probably due to increased cardiac output, resulting in increased venous return. This, in addition to the release of noradrenaline, could explain the anxiety, restlessness and hyper-reflexia, which also mimic impending eclampsia.[13]

It is not surprising that the indices of the uteroplacental flow are not improved by the use of dihydralazine as it releases noradrenaline, a potent vasoconstrictor of the uteroplacental circulation. In fact, signs attributable to fetal distress have been reported by Vink et al,[14] who suggested that the risk of abnormal fetal heart rate patterns detected by electronic fetal heart rate monitoring is reduced by correction of hypovolaemia and the intermittent use of small doses (5 mg) of the drug intravenously. The side-effects of the drug are also reduced if the sympathetic nervous system is already inhibited by methyldopa or adrenergic blocking agents. Thus, a loading dose of methyldopa (1000 mg) with hydrallazine given by intermittent bolus doses (5 mg, i.v.i.) is an option that is recommended. Monitoring of the fetus is essential during lowering of high blood pressure as fetal heart rate abnormalities may be detected in cases where there is fetal affectation. Although dihydralazine is not the ideal drug, it is easy to administer, relatively cheap, and most obstetricians are familiar with its use.

## OTHER ACUTE-ACTING ANTIHYPERTENSIVES

Labetalol is a combined $\alpha$- and $\beta$-adrenergic which can be given intravenously. It lowers blood pressure smoothly but rapidly, without the tachycardia characteristic of dihydralazine. The dosage regimen recommended by Walker[15] is a slow intravenous injection of 50 mg followed by an infusion 5 mg/ml. The infusion can be initiated at 12 ml/h and titrated to achieve the desired blood pressure control. The agent may also be useful in the presence of unexplained ventricular arrhythmias associated with hypertensive crises of pregnancy as reported by Bhorat et al.[16] There have been no adverse effects on the uteroplacental circulation reported with the use of labetalol.

Nifedipine, a calcium channel blocker, is an effective vasodilator and acts rapidly when given orally. Moretti et al[17] did not report any side-effects on the uteroplacental circulation using Doppler waveform analysis despite reports from animal studies of a decrease in uteroplacental blood flow and fetal hypocalcaemia with the use of nifedipine. Randomised studies have shown that nifedipine is associated with fewer episodes of hypotension and causes less tachycardia when compared to dihydralazine.[18,19] There is concern, however, from case reports that nifedipine, when used in conjunction with magnesium sulphate, may result in marked hypotension because of the compounded effects of the magnesium ion on calcium channel functions.[20] Nifedipine may be used orally sublingually, and its' time of onset of action is rapid; its use as a tablet swallowed but not bitten, results in its action within a period of 10–15 min, while a slow release capsule has a slower onset of action (60 min), but a more prolonged effect. More recently, concern has emerged about the rapid action of nifedipine and its association with hypotension and increased risk of myocardial infarction in non-pregnant patients and in pregnant patients with the combined use of ritodrine in preterm labour.[21] Myocardial infarction and death have been cited as potential adverse effects in non-pregnant patients with hypertension and ischaemic heart disease receiving long-term treatment with the drug.[22,23] Nifedipine capsules are now contra-indicated in pregnancy in some countries.[24]

Considering the increased cardiac output and myocardial oxygen demands attendant with pregnancy, nifedipine may predispose to potential adverse effects even in the absence of coronary artery disease.

Isradipine, a recently introduced potent calcium channel blocker, when compared to dihydralazine, has been found to be effective and safe in a randomised study of 40 patients by Maharaj et al.[25] More studies are required to verify these findings.

Other intravenous agents have also been used in pregnancy. Moodley and Gouws[26] reported that Epoprostenol, a potent intravenous prostaglandin preparation, caused less tachycardia than dihydralazine whilst achieving a similar antihypertensive effect. Roussouw et al[27] reported on a cohort of 20 patients where Ketanserin, a selective serotonin-2-receptor blocker which also inhibits platelet aggregation, was compared to dihydralazine. Ketanserin appears to be safer as no hypotension occurred and high blood pressure was reduced more gradually. A similar study from The Netherlands, found that the anti-hypertensive effects of ketanserin and dihydralazine were comparable, but there were significantly fewer maternal complications associated with ketanserin.[28] Urapidil, a post-synoptic α-1 adrenoreceptor antagonist was compared to dihydralazine in a randomised controlled study involving 26 patients.[29] The results of this study showed that urapidil had a more predictable haemodynamic effect, reduced blood pressure without venous adverse effects, and it additionally caused a reduction in intracerebral blood pressure. It is important to note that the majority of the above studies have been conducted on a small number of patients and ideally these results should be reproduced in studies with statistically acceptable number of patients.

Other agents such as sodium nitroprusside and nitroglycerine may be utilised intravenously. These drugs mandate intra-arterial blood pressure monitoring, together with other critical care monitoring facilities. Sodium nitroprusside is also potentially toxic to the fetus.

## LONG-TERM ORAL ANTIHYPERTENSIVE AGENTS

It is now accepted that antihypertensive agents are of benefit and most institutions utilise their own protocols for the use of antihypertensive drugs. Methyldopa is the preferred long-term antihypertensive agent in pregnancy; its safety has been established by case control studies and no serious fetal side-effects have yet been documented.[30,31] It does cross the placental barrier and accumulates in relatively high concentrations in the amniotic fluid. However, its minor effects, such as transient reduction in neonatal blood pressure for a short period and a slight decrease in the fetal heart rate, are of no clinical importance. Further, children born to mothers who received methyldopa during pregnancy have been followed-up and assessed at the age of 7 years and have been found to be no different from their controls.[32] Long-term safety is thus established.

A stepped care approach is used for long-term antihypertensive therapy in pregnancy. Methyldopa is thus the first step. It is normally used in the form of a loading dose of 500–1000 mg followed by 250–750 mg four times a day. A daily dose of 2 g is usually not exceeded as further effects are not seen with a daily dose above this. Sedation and tiredness are common complaints but postural hypotension is an uncommon problem in pregnancy.

If a second drug is required, then a variety of drugs are recommended by various authors.[2,30,31] Clinical familiarity with use in achieving good blood pressure control is probably what matters. Beta blockers have the advantage of fewer subjective side-effects, but their safety in pregnancy still remains a cause for concern. There have been reports of low birth weight babies with the long term use of β-blockers. Table 2 summarises the commonly used antihypertensive agents.

**Table 2** Commonly used antihypertensive agents in pre-eclampsia

| Class | Drug | Starting dose | Maximum dose (24 h) |
|---|---|---|---|
| Centrally acting | Methyldopa | 250 mg q.i.d. | 4 g |
| α₁ Blockade | Proazosin | 1 mg b.d. | 20 mg |
| Calcium channel blockers | Nifedipine | 10 mg tds/qid | 120 mg |
| α,β–Blockers | Labetalol | 200 mg tds | 2400 mg |

## SEIZURE PROPHYLAXIS

The most significant randomised clinical trial on the subject of anticonvulsants in eclampsia was the Collaborative Eclampsia Trial.[33] This study was designed to assess the effects on recurrent convulsions and on maternal mortality of different anticonvulsants, viz. $MgSO_4$, phenytoin and diazepam in eclampsia. It provided data on 1680 women with eclampsia. There were two comparisons in this study; in the comparison of $MgSO_4$ with diazepam, women allocated $MgSO_4$ had a 52% lower risk of recurrent convulsions (95%: CI 64% to 37%) than those on diazepam. In the phenytoin arm, women allocated $MgSO_4$ had a 67% lower risk of recurrent convulsions (95%: CI 79% to 47%) than those on phenytoin. These reductions in the risk of recurrent convulsions were also reflected in non-significant trends to fewer maternal deaths amongst women allocated $MgSO_4$. The study concluded that there was compelling evidence in favour of $MgSO_4$ rather than phenytoin or diazepam for the treatment of eclampsia.

More recently, a meta-analysis on randomised trials on the use of $MgSO_4$ in pre-eclampsia/eclampsia by Chein et al[34] has shown that in the prevention of further fits in eclampsia, the odds of having recurrent seizures were significantly lower with $MgSO_4$ compared with phenytoin, diazepam and lytic cocktail.

A criticism of many of the clinical randomised trials has been that maternal mortality should be the primary outcome measure, and not the frequency of recurrent convulsions. However, the aim of clinical treatment of women with eclampsia is prevention of further convulsions, in the belief that such management is associated with a reduction in maternal morbidity and mortality. The Collaborative Eclampsia Trial, even with its large number of 1680 patients, lacked the power necessary to demonstrate differences in mortality amongst the different intervention groups.[33] Further trials would be required to show significant reductions in maternal mortality in meta-analysis.

$MgSO_4$ is also used in the management of pre-eclampsia to prevent the first fit and Lucas et al[35] showed that the use of $MgSO_4$ also resulted in significantly lower odds of having seizures, compared with phenytoin. Although this study suggests that these results may be generalised to all women with hypertension in pregnancy as the trial included women with varying severity of pre-eclampsia, ranging from mild hypertension without proteinuria, to severe proteinuric hypertension, the Caesarean section rates were also higher in the women treated with $MgSO_4$. The high Caesarean section rates could be regarded as a potential undesirable effect of magnesium sulphate therapy.

There is ongoing debate about whether prophylactic anticonvulsant therapy is required at all and whether this therapy causes more harm than good. There are no appropriate clinical tests to assess which women are at risk of convulsions and, to date, there is little evidence that benefit outweighs harm. There have also been few published randomised trials comparing anticonvulsants with either no anticonvulsant or placebo.[31–34] The total number of patients included in these studies was 300. In the randomised study by Moodley and Moodley,[36] 228 women with severe pre-eclampsia including women with impending eclampsia were randomised to $MgSO_4$ therapy ($n = 112$), or no anticonvulsant therapy ($n = 116$). All women received antihypertensive therapy. One woman allocated $MgSO_4$, developed eclampsia.

Clearly, randomised trials including large numbers of women are required to evaluate whether anticonvulsants are necessary in pre-eclampsia.

Improved understanding of the mechanism of eclamptic convulsions has also contributed to a more rational choice of anticonvulsant agent. It has been suggested that the underlying pathology may be cerebral oedema secondary to ischaemia,[13] and that magnesium may act as an anticonvulsant by relaxation of cerebral vasospasm,[33] or by blocking some of the neuronal damage associated with cerebral ischaemia.[31] More recently, Naidu et al studied the neuropathophysiology of 65 eclamptics utilising single photon emission, cerebral computerised tomographic scan and transcranial Doppler assessment of the middle cerebral artery.[37] Their findings strongly suggest that the pathophysiological mechanism of eclamptic seizures is primary cerebral vasospasm with resultant ischaemia and cerebral oedema. This strengthens the hypothesis that $MgSO_4$ can be an effective anticonvulsant.

Magnesium sulphate should be the anticonvulsant of choice over diazepam or phenytoin in the treatment of eclampsia or in the most severe forms of pre-eclampsia where its value may outweigh the neonatal risks. This does not mean that obstetricians should not give due attention to early detection of pre-eclampsia by providing appropriate antenatal and timeous delivery of women at risk of developing pre-eclampsia. Furthermore, large randomised clinical trials to evaluate interventions to prevent eclampsia in women with pre-eclampsia, comparing routine anticonvulsant versus none, should be performed. The routine anticonvulsant for this comparison should be $MgSO_4$. The results of a large randomised international trial of 14000 patients comparing $MgSO_4$ to placebo for the treatment of women with pre-eclampsia is awaited, prior to recommendations being made for use of $MgSO_4$ for prophylaxis against convulsions in severe pre-eclampsia.

## COAGULATION DEFECTS

An increase in factor VIII R: Ag and a decrease in antithrombin represent the commonest haematological abnormalities in pre-eclampsia.[38] These tests, however, are relatively inaccessible to clinical monitoring. The platelet count is, therefore, used as the standard clinical test. Serial readings from a baseline early in pregnancy are more valuable than a single reading and platelet counts can be used both for monitoring progression of the disorder, and decision making. Reduction in platelet counts are probably due to increased consumption at a microvascular level where platelets adhere to damaged endothelium.[43] Platelet counts of $100 \times 10^9/l$ are abnormal and should be confirmed by peripheral smear to exclude clumping, a cause of spurious thrombocytopenia and to test for haemolysis. Haemolysis is also examined by plasma concentrations of haptoglobin.[39] In addition, other features of disseminated intravascular coagulation (DIC) should be examined. These include fibrinogen levels, fibrinogen degradation products and prolonged thrombin time. Thus, in patients with persistent low platelet counts (below $100 \times 10^9/l$), a DIC screen should be performed. In addition, patients with counts $< 70 \times 10^9/l$ may have a platelet function defect, particularly if there is clinical evidence of bleeding (viz. haematuria, petechial haemorrhage), and this should also be investigated for by performing a bleeding time or thromboelastography, a test for dynamic function of coagulation factors. It is important to remember that platelet counts may drop further following delivery and only recover by the fourth postpartum day. Katz et al showed that 61 of a cohort of 375 pre-eclamptics had platelet counts of < 100 x 10$^9$/l and 51 of these had risen to > 100 x 10$^9$/l by the fourth postoperative day.[40] If platelet counts do not increase by the fourth post-partum day, such patients should be investigated for thrombotic thrombocytopenia and thrombophilias. It is also important to point out that in severe/or neglected pre-eclamptics/eclamptics, and in those with hypertension and abruptio placentae, platelet transfusions may be necessary if platelet counts are < 50 x 10$^9$/l and there is uncontrollable hypertension, clinical evidence of bleeding and the patient requires a Caesarean section.[41–43]

In the presence of low platelet counts (< 100 x 10$^9$/l), liver dysfunction should be looked for; the HELLP syndrome occurs in 2–12% of pre-eclamptic patients and has an insidious course. Platelet counts in such circumstances should be evaluated frequently.

## ANAESTHESIA ANALGESIA

Continuous epidural analgesia is undoubtedly of benefit for vaginal and operative delivery in pre-eclampsia. The prevention of increases in catecholamine release prevents further elevations in blood pressure values during uterine contractions. It abolishes excessive maternal bearing down during the second stage of labour and it thus allows a controlled delivery. Furthermore, there is some evidence to suggest that it may improve uteroplacental perfusion.[46]

The patient should be fully conscious, have had an adequate cardiac preload and a coagulopathy ought to be excluded prior to insertion of an epidural catheter. A platelet count of above 69,000/mm$^3$ is acceptable.[45] Orlikowski et al reported that a platelet count of 75,000/mm$^3$ should be associated with adequate haemostasis.[41] This was based on a study of 47 pre-eclamptic or eclamptic patients of whom 37% had a platelet count of below 150,000/mm$^3$ and 14% had a platelet count below 100 000/mm$^3$.

The safety of regional anaesthesia in patients on aspirin therapy is uncertain. In the past, bleeding time (BT) was used as a screening test prior to regional anaesthesia. A recent meta-analysis which reviewed 1000 publications, concludes that BT cannot be used to predict haemorrhages.[42] Payne et al compared BT with thrombo-elastography on blood samples taken before and 4 weeks following aspirin therapy (75 mg/day).[43] Although the bleeding times were prolonged, none were greater than 10 min. The thrombo-elastography results showed no changes. They suggest that low dose aspirin does not markedly affect BT and that thrombo-elastogram be performed (prior to epidural analgesia administration) as it gives a view of the entire coagulation system.

If general anaesthesia is indicated, then the following risks should be borne in mind: (i) possible presence of laryngeal oedema which makes intubation difficult and hazardous; (ii) the pressor response to intubation may precipitate an arrhythmia or pulmonary oedema; (iii) risk of aspiration; (iv) the decrease in uteroplacental flow may be hazardous if the fetus is growth retarded; and

(v) neuromuscular blockade – there may be difficulties if the patient has received $MgSO_4$.

The above issues are extremely important and need to be carefully considered in the management of all severe pre-eclamptic patients. It is vital that such patients be evaluated and treated at a tertiary institution or regional centres where the following issues can be included in their management: (i) admission to a high-care unit; (ii) appropriate maternal and fetal evaluation; (iii) appropriate maternal and fetal surveillance; (iv) individual care by a multi-disciplinary team (obstetrician, neonatologist, anaesthetist, nursing staff); and (v) delivery when indicated, viz. uncontrollable hypertension (as defined previously), impending eclampsia, organ failure, viable fetus with (a) resistant decelerations, (b) non-reactive cardiotocograph, (c) absent baseline variability for more than 1 h, (d) oligohydramnios, (e) reverse diastolic blood flow on Doppler velocimetry; gestational age of greater than 34 weeks; and (f) severe growth impairment.

## ECLAMPSIA

Estimates of eclampsia, the occurrence of convulsions associated with signs of pre-eclampsia (hypertension and proteinuria) vary widely from 1 in 100 to 1 in

**Table 3** Symptoms and signs of impending eclampsia

| | |
|---|---|
| 1. | Severe frontal headache |
| 2. | Epigastric pain/tenderness |
| 3. | Nausea/vomiting |
| 4. | Visual blurring |
| 5. | Hyper-reflexia/sustained clonus |

**Table 4** Principles of management of eclampsia

1. Immediate care
   maintain airway
   left lateral position
   oxygen administration
2. Abort convulsions
   diazepam 10 mg i.v.
   or
   clonazepam 1 mg i.v.
3. Seizure prophylaxis
   magnesium sulphate
4. Maintain diastolic blood pressure of 95–105 mmHg
5. Coagulation screen/renal function/platelet count
6. Haemodynamic stabilisation followed by delivery within 6–8 h
7. Postpartum
   24–48 h of intensive care
8. N.B. Ventilatory support for at least 24 hours, if:
   poor arterial blood gases
   unconsciousness/Glasgow Coma Scale < 8
   extreme restlessness
   laryngeal oedema

**Table 5**  MgSO$_4$ regimens used in eclampsia

| Regimen | Loading dose | Maintenance dose |
|---|---|---|
| Pritchard et al[46] | 4 g over 3–5 min i.v. 10 g i.m. | 5 g, 4 hourly i.m. |
| Zuspan[47] | 4 g over 5–10 min i.v. | 1–2 g/h i.v. |
| Sibai[48] | 6 g over 20 min i.v. | 2 g/h i.v. |

i.m., intramuscularly; i.v., intravenously

2000 pregnancies (Table 3).[33] Although uncommon in developed countries, it is still a major cause of maternal morbidity and mortality world-wide and accounts for 5000 maternal deaths/year internationally.[33]

The following factors have been identified as risk factors for maternal morbidity and mortality – late referral to a tertiary hospital, delay in hospitalisation, lack of transport, unbooked status of patients, high parity, a state of unconsciousness and multiple seizures prior to admission.[44]

## MANAGEMENT OF ECLAMPSIA

The principles of management are outlined in Table 4. For the purposes of practical management guidelines, treatment can be divided into that for the eclamptic who has no impairment of consciousness following a seizure, and those who have marked impairment.[44]

### Minimal or no impairment of consciousness

If the patient is convulsing, this should be shortened or aborted with the administration of diazepam 10 mg i.v. or clonazepam 1 mg i.v. MgSO$_4$ is then used to prevent further convulsions as indicated earlier.

MgSO$_4$ may be administered by various regimens (Table 5).[46–48]

If the intramuscular regimen is used, it is important to ensure that before administration of each subsequent maintenance dose: (i) urine output is above 30 ml/h; (ii) patella reflexes are intact; and (iii) respiratory rate is adequate.

The intravenous regimen is advantageous to utilise as the patient does not need to receive repeated intramuscular injections which can be painful and may be associated with a risk of abscess development. The intravenous regimen, however, necessitates close maternal surveillance with availability of appropriate resuscitative facilities. In Durban, South Africa, we currently use a loading dose of 6 mg MgSO$_4$ over 20 min intravenously.[44] This is followed by a MgSO$_4$ infusion at 2 g/h until 24 h post-delivery. Serum magnesium levels are performed in select cases, viz. oliguric patient, development of symptoms and signs of magnesium toxicity, renal failure and recurrent convulsions. Routine serum magnesium levels are not utilised. Chissel et al compared intravenous and intramuscular MgSO$_4$ regimens in pre-eclamptic patients and found that both regimens produced similar serum magnesium levels.[49]

The blood pressure should not be lowered too rapidly as cerebral perfusion may be lowered with exacerbation of cerebral ischaemia. Furthermore, uteroplacental blood flow may also be adversely influenced with resultant fetal jeopardy. The DBP should be gradually lowered to 90–100 mmHg and systolic blood pressure to 140–150 mmHg. Dihydralazine (6.25 mg, i.v.) administered as a bolus over 4–5 min is the drug of choice. A labetalol infusion 120 μg/min is an alternative in the presence of maternal tachycardia. Other rapid-acting agents, viz. diazoxide, sodium nitroprusside and nitroglycerine, are usually preserved for use in the intensive care unit setting, or prior to intubation in theatre.

The eclamptic patient warrants meticulous surveillance, especially the cardiovascular system. The heart rate should be monitored continuously with an ECG monitor as these patients are prone to ventricular arrhythmias. Non-invasive blood pressure monitoring and pulse oximetry should be performed continuously and documented every 15 min. Intra-arterial blood pressure monitoring is recommended in the extremely restless or deeply unconscious patient as blood pressure are often labile. CVP monitoring is vital to correct the contracted intravascular status without causing a circulatory overload. Ringer's lactate is recommended as an intravenous fluid at a rate of 100 ml/h. A Swan Ganz catheter may be indicated in a select group of patients, viz. intractable cardiac failure or oliguria. Insertion of a Swan Ganz catheter is not without complications[50] and, therefore, it should only be used if the appropriate expertise for its use is available.

### Marked impairment of consciousness

This group of patients often has raised intracranial pressure (ICP) and thus it is important to lower blood pressure gradually or the ICP may rise even further. Airway management may necessitate intubation if the patient is extremely restless (due to cerebral oedema), deeply unconscious, has poor arterial blood gases or has extensive laryngeal oedema. In such situations, a Caesarean section should be performed following haemodynamic stabilisation with postoperative ventilation for at least 24 h. The use of steroids and/or diuretics should be considered to reduce cerebral oedema. Dexamethasone (32 g i.v. and 8 g 6 hourly intramuscularly for 24 h) is used in such cases. CAT scanning and MRI are not routine investigations but are performed in specific situations, viz. the presence of focal neurological signs, atypical eclampsia or for research purposes. Transcranial Dopplers and SPECT scans are also being utilised as research tools and are vital for the understanding of the disease process.

## FURTHER MANAGEMENT

Investigations performed should include a haemoglobin level, platelet count, urea, electrolyte status and a coagulation screen. A peripheral smear and liver function test is indicated in the presence of thrombocytopenia (which may present in up to 50% of patients with hypertensive crises of pregnancy). A platelet function test is warranted if platelets are above $50,000/mm^3$, a platelet transfusion is indicated for operative procedures or during the second stage of labour. Urine output should be monitored hourly. Fetal surveillance is necessary in the viable fetus.

## MODE OF DELIVERY

A Caesarean section is recommended in the following situations: (i) all deeply unconscious patients (unless delivery is imminent); (ii) all unco-operative patients due to restlessness; (iii) if vaginal delivery is unlikely to occur within 6–8 h from the onset of the first eclamptic seizure; (iv) there is an obstetric indication for a Caesarean section; or (v) fetal distress.

A general anaesthetic is recommended for Caesarean section unless the patient is fully conscious, co-operative, has had a single seizure, blood pressure is well controlled and blood biochemistry is satisfactory. The anaesthetist should be informed if drugs are used. Relevant issues constitute: (i) the hypertensive response to laryngoscopy, airway suctioning, intubation and extubation; and (ii) the management of laryngeal oedema.

If the patient is delivering vaginally, one should assist the second stage of labour in order to avoid the rise in maternal blood pressure with each uterine contraction. Furthermore, ergometrine is contra-indicated in the third stage. In the post-partum period, the first 24–48 h are especially important as blood pressure may fluctuate and patient is still at risk for developing complications. Major fluid shifts occur during this period. Oliguric patients who have not responded to fluid challenge may benefit from low doses of dopamine (1–5 $\mu$g/kg/min) to improve urine output.[51] Antihypertensives are usually required for 24–48 h and need to be gradually decreased. $MgSO_4$ is administered for 24 h post delivery.

The neonatal assessment is important, especially in the scenario of preterm deliveries, abruptio placenta or a maternal coagulopathy.

## CONTRACEPTION

This is of paramount importance. Steroidal contraception may be prescribed. Puerperal tubal ligations should be avoided because of the attendant risks of thrombo-embolic disease and pulmonary embolism.

## POSTNATAL ASSESSMENT

At the 6th week postnatal assessment, the presence of hypertension or proteinuria necessitates referral to a physician for further investigations. Pregnancy should be advised only if the blood pressure and renal function tests return to normal. It is important to counsel the patient on booking early in future pregnancies. The advantages include possible administration of low dose aspirin and detection of pre-eclampsia as early as possible.

## RECURRENCE

The risk of recurrence varies from 1.9% to 24.9%.[52–54] Daughters of eclamptic patients have a 3% risk of developing eclampsia and a 25% risk of developing pre-eclampsia. It is important to note that, until the precise cause of pre-eclampsia and eclampsia is ascertained, continuing problems of pre-eclampsia/eclampsia can only be improved with public health education, female education, improvement in socio-economic standards, early recognition and evaluation of pre-eclamptic patients and appropriate management of pre-eclampsia.

## KEY POINTS FOR CLINICAL PRACTICE

We make the following recommendations for the management of patients with eclampsia and severe pre-eclampsia:

- 1. All severe pre-eclamptics and eclamptics should be managed in special regional centres with the appropriate expertise.

- 2. Continuous monitoring of blood pressure, pulse rate, ECG and central venous pressure is required as the cardio-vascular system is extremely labile in this condition and can deteriorate in seconds.

- 3. The airway should be maintained and protected. Any patient with a Glasgow Coma Scale of less than 9 should be intubated. Nursing staff at district hospitals and community clinics should be taught how to position an unconscious patient, insert an oral airway and administer oxygen.

- 4. An arterial partial pressure of oxygen of at least 100 mmHg should be maintained. Mechanical ventilation may be necessary.

- 5. Blood pressure should be carefully and slowly lowered, the diastolic pressure should be lowered by not more than 30 mmHg in order to maintain cerebral perfusion.

- 6. Seizures should be prevented or terminated as soon as possible. $MgSO_4$ is the anticonvulsant of choice for this purpose. Efficient transport facilities must be available and personnel at district hospitals and community clinics should be capable of administering anticonvulsants.

- 7. The fetus should be delivered within 6–12 h of admission; Caesarean section is often indicated. General anaesthesia, administered by a skilled anaesthetist, is recommended. Where these facilities are not available, epidural anaesthesia would be adequate, provided a hypotensive episode is prevented with sufficient intravenous pre-loading and coagulopathy is excluded by estimation of crude clotting time, fibrinogen levels and platelet counts.

- 8. An eclampsia team should be organised, since the problems developed by these patients are multifactorial. Personnel (an obstetrician, obstetric anaesthetist and critical care nurse) experienced in the management of these patients need to work together, in order to improve patient outcome

  While prevention of pre-eclampsia/eclampsia must await an under-standing of its aetiology, improvement in antenatal care, together with active management of the disease when it develops, will improve both fetal and maternal prognosis.

### References

1  Maharaj B, Moodley J. Management of hypertension in pregnancy. Cont Med Educ 1991; 12: 1581–1589

2   Davey D A, MacGillivray I. The classification of hypertensive disorders of pregnancy. Am J Obstet Gynecol 1988; 158: 175–215

3   Brown M A, Buddle M L, Farrell T, Davis G, Jones M. Randomised trial of management of hypertensive pregnancies by Korotkoff phase IV or phase V. Lancet 1998; 352: 777–781

4   Calhoun D A, Oparil S. Treatment of hypertensive crises. N Engl J Med 1990; 332: 1177–1183

5   Finnerty A A J. Hypertensive encephalopathies. Am J Med 1972; 52: 672–678

6   Anumba D O C, Robson S C. Management of pre-eclampsia and the HELLP syndrome. Curr Opin Obstet Gynecol 1999; 11: 149–156

7   Odendaal H J, Pattinson R C, Du Toit R. Fetal and neonatal outcome in patients with severe pre-eclampsia before 34 weeks. S Afr Med J 1987; 71: 555–558

8   Sibai B M, Taslima M, Abdella T N et al. Maternal and perinatal outcome of conservative management of severe pre-eclampsia in the mid-trimester. Am J Obstet Gynecol 1985; 152: 32–37

9   Moodley J, Koranteng S A Rout C. Expectant management of early onset of severe pre-eclampsia in Durban, South Africa. S Afr Med J 1993; 83: 584–587

10  Odendaal H J, Pattinson R C, Bam R et al. Aggressive or expectant management for patients with severe pre-eclampsia between 28–34 weeks gestation : a randomised controlled trial. Obstet Gynecol 1990; 76: 1070–1075

11  Sibai B M, Akl S, Fairlie F, Moretti M. A protocol for managing severe pre-eclampsia in the second trimester. Am J Obstet Gynecol 1990; 163: 733–738

12  Helewa M, Heaman M, Robinson M A, Thompson L. Community-based home care programme for the management of pre-eclampsia. Can Med Assoc J 1993; 149: 829–834

13  Richards A M, Moodley J, Bullock M R R, Downing J W. Maternal deaths from neurological complications of hypertensive crises in pregnancy. S Afr Med J 1987; 71: 487–489

14  Vink G, Moodley J, Philpott R H. Effect of dihydralazine on the fetus in the treatment of hypertension in pregnancy. Obstet Gynecol 1980; 55: 519–522

15  Walker J J. Hypertensive drugs in pregnancy. Clin Perinatol 1991; 18: 845–867

16  Bhorat I, Naidoo D P, Moodley J. Continuous electrocardiographic monitoring in hypertensive crises in pregnancy. Am J Obstet Gynecol 1991; 164: 530–533

17  Moretti M M, Fairlie F M, Akl S et al. The effect of nifedipine therapy on fetal and placental Doppler waveforms in pre-eclampsia remote from term. Am J Obstet Gynecol 1990; 163: 1844–1848

18  Seabe S J, Moodley J, Becker P. Nifedipine in acute hypertensive emergencies in pregnancy. S Afr Med J 1989; 76: 248–250

19  Fenakel K, Fenakel E, Apleman Z et al. Nifedipine in the treatment of severe pre-eclampsia. Obstet Gynecol 1991; 77: 331–337

20  Waisman G D, Mayorga L M, Camera M I et al. Magnesium plus nifedipine potentiation of hypotensive effect in pre-eclampsia? Am J Obstet Gynecol 1988; 159: 308–309

21  Psaty B M , Heckbert S R, Koepsell T D et al. The risk of myocardial infarction associated with antihypertensive drug therapies. JAMA 1995; 275: 620–625

22  Buring J E, Glynn R J, Hennekens C H. Calcium channel blockers and myocardial infarction. A hypothesis formulated but not yet tested. JAMA 1995; 274: 654–655

23  Horton R. Spinning the risks and benefits of calcium antagonists. Lancet 1995; 346: 586–587

24  New Zealand Ministry of Health. Managing high blood pressure in pregnancy. Prescriber Update 1994; 7: 2–10

25  Maharaj B, Khedun S M, Moodley J et al. A comparative study of intravenous isradipine and dihydrallazine in the treatment of severe hypertension in pregnancy in Black patients. Hypertens Pregnancy 1997; 16: 1–9

26  Moodley J, Gouws E. A comparative study of the use of epoprostenol and dihydralazine in severe hypertension in pregnancy. Br J Obstet Gynaecol 1992; 99: 727–730

27  Rossouw H J, Howarth G, Odendaal H J. Ketanserin and hydralazine in hypertension in pregnancy – a randomised double blind trial. S Afr Med J 1995; 85: 525–528

28  Bolte A C, van Eyck J, Kanhai H H et al. Ketanserin versus dihydralazine in the management of severe early onset pre-eclampsia. Am J Obstet Gynecol 1999; 180: 371–375

29  Wacker J, Werner P, Walter Sack I, Bastert G. Treatment of hypertension in patients with pre-eclampsia: a prospective parallel group study comparing dihydralazine with urapidil. Nephrol Dialys Transplant 1998; 13: 318–325

30 Redman C W G. Fetal outcome in a trial of antihypertensive treatment in pregnancy. Lancet 1976; ii: 753–756

31 Redman C W G. Treatment of hypertension in pregnancy. Kidney Int 1980; 18: 267–278

32 Cockburn J, Moar V A, Ounstead M, Redman C W G. Final report of study on hypertension during pregnancy. Lancet 1982; i: 647–649

33 Eclampsia Trial Collaborative Group. Which anticonvulsant for women with eclampsia? Evidence from the Collaborative Eclampsia Trial. Lancet 1995; 345: 1455–1463

34 Chein P F W, Khan K S, Arnott N. Magnesium sulphate in the treatment of eclampsia and pre-eclampsia : an overview of the evidence from randomised trials. Br J Obstet Gynaecol 1996; 103: 1085–1091

35 Lucas M J, Leveno K J, Cunningham F G. A comparison of magnesium sulphate with phenytoin for the prevention of eclampsia. N Engl J Med 1994; 333: 201–252

36 Moodley J, Moodley V V. Prophylactic anticonvulsant therapy in hypertensive crises of pregnancy – the need for a large, randomised trial. Hypertens Pregnancy 1994; 13: 245–252

37 Naidu K, Moodley J, Corr P, Hoffmann M. Single photon emission and cerebral computerised tomographic scan and transcranial Doppler sonographic findings in eclampsia. Br J Obstet Gynaecol 1997; 104: 1165–1172

38 Mobbs C, Moodley J, Kenoyer G. Antithrombin III in eclampsia. Clin Exp Hypertens 1985; B4: 105–106

39 Redman C W G. Hypertension in pregnancy. In: Chamberlain G. (ed) Turnbull's Obstetrics. Edinburgh: Churchill Livingstone, 1995; 441–470

40 Katz V L, Thorpe T N, Lozas L, Boues W A. The natural history of thrombocytopenic associated with pre-eclampsia. Am J Obstet Gynecol 1990; 163: 1142–1143

41 Orlikowski C F P, Rocke D A, Murray W B et al. . Thromboelastography changes in pre-eclampsia and eclampsia. Br J Anaesth 1996; 77: 157–161

42 Rodgers R P C, Levin J. A critical reappraisal of bleeding time. Semin Thromb Haemost 1990; 16: 1–20

43 Payne A, Orlikowski C, Moodley J, Rocke D A. Thromboelastography as a measure of coagulation in high risk pregnant patients receiving low dose aspirin. J Obstet Gynaecol 1993; 13: 222–226

44 Moodley J, Daya P. Eclampsia – a continuing problem in the developing world. Int J Gynecol Obstet 1993; 44: 9–14

45 Beilin Y, Zahn J, Camerford M. Safe epidural in 30 parturients with platelet counts between 69 000 and 98 000 mm$^3$. Anesth Analg 1997; 85: 385–388

46 Pritchard J A, Cunningham F G, Pritchard S A. The Parklands Memorial Hospital protocol for treatment of eclampsia: evaluation of 245 cases. Am J Obstet Gynecol 1984; 148: 951–963

47 Zuspan F P. Problems encountered in the treatment of pregnancy-induced hypertension. Am J Obstet Gynecol 1978; 131: 591–596

48 Sibai B M. Magnesium sulphate is the ideal anticonvulsant in pre-eclampsia – eclampsia. Am J Obstet Gynecol 1990; 162: 1141–1145

49 Chissel S, Botha J H, Moodley J, McFadyen L. Intravenous and intramuscular magnesium sulphate regimens in severe pre-eclampsia. S Afr Med J 1994; 84: 607–610

50 Mantel G D, Maikin J D. Low dose dopamine in postpartum pre-eclamptic women with oliguria: a double-blind, placebo controlled, randomised trial. Br J Obstet Gynaecol 1997; 104: 1180–1183

51 Robin E D. Death by pulmonary artery flow directed catheter: time for a moratorium? Chest 1987; 97: 727–731

52 Adelusi B, Ojengbede O A. Reproductive performance after eclampsia. Int J Obstet Gynecol 1986; 24: 183–189

53 Chesley L C, Annitto J E, Cosgrove R A. The familial factor in toxaemia of pregnancy. Obstet Gynecol 1968; 32: 303

54 Sibai B M, Sarinoglu C, Mercer B M. Eclampsia VII. Pregnancy outcome after eclampsia and long-term prognosis. Am J Obstet Gynecol 1992; 166: 1757–1761

# Drug use in pregnancy

This article is about a broad range of drugs which have some psycho-active properties and which are used for non-therapeutic reasons in pregnancy. Some such drug use is probably fundamental in most human societies, but there have been profound global changes in range, type and scale of drug use over the last few decades.

Although drug effects in the brain are inevitably complex, a widely accepted hypothesis is that all the drugs I discuss (with the possible exception of benzodiazepines) appear to have a common final pathway. They all act by increasing dopamine release.[1,2] They do this in different ways. Cocaine blocks dopamine re-uptake by strongly binding to the re-uptake transporter. Opioids mimic the natural transmitters endorphin and encephalin, switching off GABA neurones that tonically inhibit dopamine cell firing. Alcohol similarly acts through GABA, but also blocks glutamate receptors. Nicotine affects dopamine release through a nicotinic acetyl choline pathway. But for all of them, the common end-point where dopamine is released forms part of a circuit known as the brain reward system, consisting of a small group of nerve cells extending from the ventral tegmental area of the midbrain to limbic areas such as the nucleus accumbens, with projections to the pre-frontal cortex.[1,2] This system is involved in natural reward re-inforcement processes which are essential for survival, such as obtaining food and water. All drugs of misuse (and perhaps also video games!) exert their effect by commandeering this existing reward system and massively short circuiting the natural reward environment. This is a very basic process, and explains why drug taking is ubiquitous. The markedly reduced activity in the brain reward circuits on withdrawal also explains dependence. What remains largely unknown is why some individuals become drug dependent while a larger number do not.

**Mr Frank Johnstone** MD FRCOG, Senior Lecturer, Department of Obstetrics and Gynaecology, University of Edinburgh and Consultant, Simpson Memorial Maternity Pavilion, Edinburgh, UK

But, although drug taking has always occurred, there are several new features that make this a pressing and highly significant global concern. Over the past few decades, use has spread to most countries of the world. This is due partly to a general increase in use of psycho-active drugs, improvements in communication and transportation and the globalisation of the world economy. Indeed, tobacco companies have used international trade agreements to open up markets in the developing world, and the same factors facilitating trade in legal goods also facilitate trade in illicit drugs.[3] Illicit drug injection in particular has rapidly increased, and had been reported in 121 countries by 1996. This may be regarded as a 'technologically superior' method of administration because it produces a rapid, strong drug effect and is cost efficient.[3] A further new theme in the developed world is the widespread acceptance and the defining nature of particular drugs in different youth and leisure sub-cultures. Club culture, atmosphere, music, and clothing have all been profoundly influenced by specific drugs. For many complex reasons, the world is, therefore, entering a new, widespread relationship with drugs. The type of drugs will vary, but the relationship is likely to be permanent.

Pregnancy has the potential to be an important event in the natural history of drug misuse. Many women, who do not acknowledge any problem with their drug pattern, may present for the first time to the health care system because of the pregnancy. This presents a window of opportunity for harm minimisation and education. Pregnancy can be a great motivator. Her partner and family may also be influenced to exert a positive effect on the woman herself, to support subsequent childcare and to help her break the cycle of inter-generational morbidity.

As we will see, drug use in pregnancy is already known to be a major public health problem. What remains less clear, but worrying, is the extent of long-term developmental effects on the child. This is a very significant pregnancy issue, and should be the concern of all health care workers involved in maternity care.

## SOME EFFECTS OF DRUGS ON PREGNANCY

Information about drug effects is often difficult to interpret. Effects in animal studies (often with high doses) may be due to maternal toxicity rather than direct effects on the fetus (e.g. drug induced anorexia). There may be selection bias based on obvious chaotic drug use, so that the women studied are quite unrepresentative of population use. The small numbers studied may be inadequate to study infrequent events. Because of editorial and reviewer bias there may be preferential publication of studies which report harmful effects.[4] There is difficulty in ascertaining and measuring drug use, particularly where this is illicit. Many drug users are polydrug users and this makes it difficult to isolate the effect of one drug. And, most importantly, there are major problems in separating the effects of drug use from the other adverse personal, psychological and social circumstances in which drug use is taking place. This is a particular difficulty in relating specific intra-uterine fetal drug exposure to long-term behavioural effects as the child grows up. These issues have been well discussed.[5]

## Opioids

Injecting street heroin is dangerous and in most cohorts of users the mortality is at least 1% each year. The commonest cause of death is respiratory depression due to overdose. The other major medical complications relate largely to non-sterile injecting, resulting in transmission of hepatitis B, and most importantly hepatitis C and HIV.

There is no convincing evidence that opioids cause fetal abnormalities. Large numbers of women have taken these drugs in pregnancy; thus, it seems unlikely that they are major teratogens. They probably have a small inhibiting effect on fetal growth, though this is less than the effects of smoking.[6] In all large studies, there is a modest increase in perinatal mortality due to preterm delivery and late pregnancy stillbirth, but it is uncertain how much of this is a drug effect rather than due to the effect of other variables.[7] Preterm labour does seem to be more common in women injecting drugs rather than taking orally, possibly related to a higher risk of alternation between intoxication and withdrawal with relatively short acting injected drugs.[6] An increase in meconium staining of the liquor is also consistently reported, again perhaps related to episodes of fetal drug withdrawal.

There is a high rate of neonatal abstinence syndrome (NAS), ranging from 50–90% in women taking opiates daily.[8] Some signs are usually seen within the first 24–72 h after birth, though this may be later with methadone. Symptoms may last for weeks or even months in a mild form. Typically, babies feed poorly and have tremor on handling, a shrill cry, sneeze, and may have watery stools. Untreated, they can develop projectile vomiting and electrolyte disturbance, seizures and coma. There is a relationship between maternal dose, serum drug levels and severity of NAS, but this is not a close one.[9,10] However, NAS is less likely to be a serious problem at methadone dosage < 20 mg. Most babies just need support and patience, some need drug treatment and a few need more intensive neonatal care.

There is strong evidence that sudden infant death syndrome is increased in babies born to mothers who take opiates in pregnancy. The largest study, of 1760 cases of sudden infant death syndrome, showed a 7 times increased risk with maternal methadone use and a 5 times increased risk with heroin use. After correction for high-risk variables, the relative risks were 3.6 and 2.3, respectively.[11]

Information on the long-term consequences of *in utero* exposure to opioids is contradictory and inconclusive. The same applies to the long-term effects of neonatal abstinence syndrome, Drug effects, and the consequences of an unstable, impoverished environment, are very difficult to disentangle; but this remains an area of concern.

## Cocaine

As well as its central action, this drug has important peripheral effects on inhibition of re-uptake of noradrenaline in presynaptic nerve terminals. Catecholamines diffuse from the nerve terminals, and the resulting high vascular levels cause vasoconstriction, tachycardia, hypertension and perhaps uterine contractility. This peripheral action provides a plausible theoretical mechanism for adverse pregnancy effects.

There is a huge amount of clinical descriptive evidence that cocaine is associated with pregnancy complications. The mother is at risk from rare but dramatic events such as myocardial infarction, cerebrovascular accident, subarachnoid haemorrhage, hepatic rupture, cardiac arrhythmias as well as fatal injuries. Similarly, placental abruption, fetal cerebral injury, and intrauterine death all seem to have occurred temporally related to cocaine use. However, these are uncommon events and because of their infrequency tend not to emerge as significant associations with cocaine in population data.

The vasoconstrictive properties of cocaine raise the possibility that there might be fetal damage during episodes of fetal ischaemia or subsequent reperfusion. The pattern of defects reported are certainly consistent with this, and similar defects can be produced in animals. If this is the mechanism, then cocaine could affect the fetus at variable periods throughout gestation and not just the first trimester. However, the overall population risk for users does not seem very high, perhaps because only those with high dosage at key gestations are vulnerable.[12,13] A large number of studies in women are consistent in reporting a decrease in birth weight. Animal studies show a dose-related decrease in uterine blood flow, which fits with this. There is also a reduction in fetal size in rhesus monkeys. The consistency of the finding of impaired fetal growth in studies with different approaches suggests that this may be a true effect. Preterm delivery is common and, although it is very difficult to adjust for multiple co-variates, this is probably also a direct drug effect.[12,13] Follow-up studies on children are rather fragmentary and not conclusive. This difficult area, along with discussion of fetal cerebral effects, has recently been reviewed.[13]

## Nicotine

Of the 4000 compounds in tobacco smoke, there is good evidence that nicotine is the key drug of addiction and nicotine, carbon monoxide and cyanide are thought to have the greatest adverse effect on the fetus. Unlike many of the drugs discussed this is legal, but it is important not to confuse legality with safety. World-wide, this is the most harmful drug for pregnancy. Smokers are at increased risk for an alarming number of pregnancy complications and, although most risk increases are relatively modest (around 1.5–2.5), this assumes enormous significance in the light of the numbers of pregnancies involved.[14–16] As always with drugs, the situation is complex because women who smoke in pregnancy have a higher rate than non-smokers of other health risk behaviours, social disadvantage, and emotional disturbance. Nevertheless, the evidence for a specific drug effect is unequivocal.

As a brief summary of what will be well-known to all readers of this chapter, there are well documented increased risks of spontaneous abortion, ectopic pregnancy, placenta praevia, placental abruption, preterm premature rupture of the membranes and preterm delivery. Birth weight is depressed by about 250 g, with an increased risk of significant intra-uterine growth restriction.[17] Intra-uterine death in late pregnancy is more common.[18] Overall, at least in the US, smoking causes an estimated 20–30% of the low birth weight rate and 10% of fetal and infant mortality.[19] Postnatally, maternal milk production is reduced by about 30%. There are strong relationships with sudden infant death syndrome;[20] respiratory disease and hospital admission in the first year of life; and an ongoing effect on respiratory disease in childhood.[21] There are small effects on physical, mental and behavioural development of the child, of uncertain clinical significance. These include poorer reading and language skills, and conduct disorder in boys.

There may be other long-term complications. Potentially carcinogenic tobacco metabolites are present in the first urine of babies whose mothers smoked in pregnancy. The babies of women who smoke were found to have a much higher frequency of a genomic deletion event that is commonly found in leukaemias and lymphomas of early childhood.[22] Studies should examine whether maternal smoking predisposes to cancer in the offspring later in life.

### Benzodiazepines

These are widely available street drugs. They cause dependency and withdrawal, which can, rarely, be serious with seizures.

There are reports showing the same pattern of abnormalities, particularly cleft lip-palate, and suggesting possible restriction of growth and brain development.[23] However, two studies found no evidence of any increase in abnormalities, and there is no conclusive evidence to suggest that therapeutic use is associated with an increased risk of malformations or any specific type of defect.[24] Drug misusers may take huge amounts of drug, and the fetal risks in these pregnancies are uncertain.

Diazepam overdose in 25 pregnancies was not accompanied by obvious fetal problems.[25] Withdrawal may occur in the neonate, typically with irritability and slowness to feed and respond. There may be 'floppy infant syndrome' with poor suck, feeble cry, hypotonia, and sometimes poor temperature control.

### Cannabis

This is the most widely used illicit drug. Cannabis refers to the crude material derived from the plant; marijuana to the mixture of crushed leaves, twigs and seeds; hashish to the resin obtained by pressing and scraping the plant. Although Delta 9-THC is the major psycho-active ingredient, there are 61 chemicals unique to cannabis as well as several hundred chemicals common to other plants.

Most studies have not reported an association between pre-natal marijuana exposure and morphological abnormalities of the baby. Some studies have reported lower birth weight and shorter gestation, but reports are not consistent.[26] Few studies have addressed effects on postnatal development but no consistent abnormalities have been reported.

### Amphetamines

The evidence that amphetamine abuse increases the risk of adverse pregnancy outcome has been well reviewed.[5] There are the usual problems of interpretation, but the clinical reports of increased congenital abnormalities and reduced birth weight are biologically plausible and supported by similar effects being found in animal studies. Data currently available do not allow any accurate estimate of risk.

## Designer drugs

A number of analogues of fentanyl, mescaline, amphetamines and phenyl-cyclidine have been produced. The most widely used drugs at present are amphetamine analogues. 'Ecstasy' (3,4, methylenedioxymethyl amphetamine, MDMA) is one derivative related chemically to both amphetamines and hallucinogens. Complications of use are rare but potentially devastating.

Preliminary reports to a Teratology Monitoring Service suggested there might be an excess rate of fetal anomaly, particularly ventricular septal defect, in 70 pregnancies where the woman had taken ecstasy.[25] Several animal experiments suggest these drugs cause fetotoxicity, prematurity, and growth restriction but results are not consistent.

## Alcohol

This is the only one of these drugs which is proven to be teratogenic. Fetal alcohol syndrome (FAS) has been reviewed in a previous issue of this series. A wide range of other alcohol-related birth defects appear to occur with heavy drinking.[27] These adverse effects have been well documented with very high maternal intakes. Whether lower intakes can also cause mild fetal damage is uncertain, and a safe level of maternal alcohol consumption has not been established. Judging by animal experiments, alcohol may affect fetal brain development at any gestation. Threshold effects on subsequent reading, spelling and arithmetic abilities in children have been reported at low intakes.[28]

## Volatile substances

The mother who continues to abuse solvents is at risk of sudden death, or, if use is prolonged, of causing permanent damage to her central nervous system or other organs. For every ecstasy death, 11 people die of inhaling volatile substances found in domestic consumer products. The commonest substance is cigarette lighter refills (butane) but a wide range of products are used.

Some studies in rats show that intermittent acute high concentrations of solvent cause growth restriction and developmental delay in the pups. In humans there is uncertainty about whether there is a discrete fetal solvent syndrome. Overall, there is enough information to suggest that solvent abuse may be associated with fetal abnormality and growth restriction effects rather similar to FAS.[29]

## OPTIONS FOR DRUG MANAGEMENT

Many women who are not truly dependent on their drug will stop spontaneously as soon as they know they are pregnant. This applies to 15–20% of women who smoke, to many women who use ecstasy or cannabis episodically, and it is also true of some controlled users on opiates. For those women remaining on drugs, management depends on the drug used.

The most widely used drug, and the most significant for its pregnancy effects, is nicotine. It must be understood that nicotine causes dependence, with a recognised withdrawal syndrome, and indeed it is claimed to be the most powerful addictive agent known. It is said that most girls who smoke 3 cigarettes as adolescents will become dependent, with an average duration of dependence of 40 years.[30] Sadly, having been recruited in adolescence, half of all smokers die because of the habit, one-third of them before the age of 65 years.[31] As one review cataloguing the illnesses caused by smoking concluded: '20% of all deaths in developed countries are caused by smoking: an enormous human cost which can be completely avoided'.[32]

Nicotine has minimal psycho-active effect, and the strong need to smoke is largely to relieve withdrawal, the markedly reduced activity in the brain reward circuits. However, the nicotine withdrawal syndrome is not an important cause of clinical morbidity, and cessation can be advised without incurring serious risks for mother or child. In addition, the reduction in birth weight can be prevented by successful cessation of smoking in the first half of pregnancy.[33] A meta-analysis of randomised controlled trials of smoking cessation interventions showed a 50% increase in smoking cessation, and a decrease in low birth weight risk.[34] Indeed, this is one of the few effective interventions in obstetrics proven in randomised controlled trials. Therefore, antenatal care should include advice to stop smoking, with easy access to programmes to support those who choose this. Brief intervention by family doctors is effective. 'Cutting down' is probably not a useful aim. Dependent users will keep their nicotine concentrations constant at a wide range of cigarettes smoked.[17] Achieving changes in smoking behaviour in pregnant women is difficult, and most women may be unable to quit at that particular time in their life.

For most other drugs, much of the skill in management lies in planning realistic aims with each individual pregnant woman. Many women say they would like to stop drugs but, in the particular situation at the time in their life, this may not be possible for them. Trying to persuade the woman to stop drugs may simply alienate her, lead to return to a more chaotic drug use pattern, and result in non-attendance for antenatal care. Therefore, the different options of detoxification, substitution and maintenance and other aspects of damage limitation need to be considered with full understanding of the woman's aspirations and particular social and psychological circumstances. Bury and Bickler have excellently described this assessment and subsequent management.[35]

Injection of heroin is the archetypal drug related behaviour, and the basis of most of what is known about drug dependence. It is important to understand that this is a chronic remitting and relapsing disorder, for many women lasting for years or even decades. The primary aims are engaging the woman in treatment and harm minimisation.

For most women who are dependent and who have a long-standing opiate habit, substitution and maintenance is usually the preferred option. This has the advantage of allowing a more stable life-style, may remove the need for prostitution or criminal behaviour to raise money for street drugs, and it reduces injection with all its dangers. The drug of choice is methadone linctus. This cannot be injected; given in high doses it reduces the craving for heroin; it eliminates opiate withdrawal symptoms for 24–36 h; and because of this long action it offers stability of drug levels. The risk of overdose and potentially death if other drugs are taken, and the likelihood of neonatal abstinence syndrome, must be understood by the woman. Methadone maintenance treatment has been extensively researched, and has been shown to be effective.[36] Substitution should be prescribed as part of a package including social and psychological support.

Acute detoxification in pregnancy is not often appropriate but should be an option. The belief that withdrawal is a risk for the fetus is based on three lines of evidence. These are: (i) case reports where violent intra-uterine movements immediately preceded fetal death; (ii) one study showing high catecholamine levels in amniotic fluid when the mother was withdrawing; and (iii) the adverse effects of naloxone precipitated opiate withdrawal in pregnant ewes. Despite all of this, the risks of withdrawal have probably been exaggerated in the past, and can be minimised by appropriate drug therapy to the mother. Detoxification can be carried out in the mid trimester quite safely and this has a place in overall management.[37]

Slow reduction may be preferred by some women for opiates, and is necessary for benzodiazepines. The size of each reduction depends on the drug and the dose that is being taken and what the drug user thinks she can cope with. The key issues are that reduction should be gradual, stepwise, and tailored to the woman's response. It is not usually appropriate to reduce more often than weekly or fortnightly but, with strong motivation and starting early in the second trimester, it may be possible to achieve dosages which are unlikely to cause significant neonatal abstinence syndrome (for example, a dose of less than 20 mg of methadone).

Methadone plasma levels decrease during pregnancy because of an increased fluid space and a large tissue reservoir. There may also be alterations in the rate of metabolism of the drug by the placenta and fetus. This suggests that, if anything, the pregnant woman may require an increase in methadone in late pregnancy. Similarly, in the postnatal period, a reversal of these effects may lead to increased plasma levels of methadone, with potential toxic effects.[8]

Much of the management of drug misuse is damage limitation rather than cure, and in patients who continue to inject, it is essential to ensure that they have access to clean equipment, by needle exchange.

It is very important for each care agency to be able to offer a full range of options for drug management. It is also essential that a full range of help is available for housing, financial and psychological problems. The immediate priorities of attracting into treatment and retaining in treatment mean that help has to be offered, not only with stabilising drug use but also with stabilising life-style and reducing death rate. These aims acquire particular urgency in pregnancy.

## MATERNITY CARE IN DRUG USERS

This tests the organisation of maternity programmes. Care should be community based, to fit in with her and her family, and if necessary with home visits. The necessary supervision and care of the child has then already been anticipated by care during pregnancy. Care requires a detailed picture of drug habit and background, carrying out appropriate screening, ensuring that appropriate educational messages are conveyed, and making sure that aims are definitely planned and understood.

Another important obligation on community care staff is effective liaison and communication with other agencies. This means firstly resolving the woman's anxieties about other personnel being involved and making sure that she feels she is remaining in control. It also means that the relevant members of the team (and this may include family doctor, drug counsellor, pharmacist, social worker, obstetrician and midwife), are all giving the same messages. Nothing is so guaranteed to reduce confidence as different agencies giving out different messages. For a team to be effective, people should know each other, know how to make contact quickly and easily, and be used to doing so.

If the pregnant woman is defaulting from appointments, this may mean that the antenatal visit was not a priority at that particular time, but it might mean that she does not like the atmosphere provided and that she does not feel the care is geared for her. This may be helped by not giving early appointments, by ensuring that she has correctly noted the appointment time, by showing some flexibility and by treating her with courtesy and consideration.

The opiate using woman should be warned that neonatal abstinence syndrome may occur, that her dose is not a reliable predictor, that it can present after several days and can last for weeks. She needs also to know that NAS is usually easily manageable. The baby needs her support, understanding and patience. The evidence is that if properly looked after, the baby will come to no short-term developmental harm.

Repeated non-sterile injection over years destroys peripheral veins, often leaving track marks (thrombosed, fibrosed veins). Venous access may be very limited, even in women who stopped injecting years before. Usually, a small amount of blood can be obtained peripherally by taking time, asking her advice about likely sites and using the smallest needle or butterfly. Occasionally, external jugular veins have to be used.

Antenatal fetal monitoring may sometimes be necessary. Cardiotocography is commonly non-reactive, particularly in the first few hours after opiates, but baseline variability usually still occurs. Biophysical profile is less affected and will usually be normal even after drug ingestion. But, again, fetal activity may be greatly reduced and often repeat or extended monitoring is required. As a general rule, effects are maximal in the first few hours after drug use, and are worse if a new drug or an excessive dosage has been taken. Drug use reduces fetal activity (and hence fetal heart rate accelerations) but will not usually cause oligohydramnios or fetal heart rate decelerations.

Occasionally, there may be concern about the ability of the woman to look after her child. This happens if previous children are in care, or there is a history of abuse, if she has a chaotic life-style, or is socially isolated with no support network. Case discussions are important at an early stage to involve all interested parties, to forestall emergency meetings and crisis confrontation later. Case discussions ensure that women are getting the help they need and provide a framework for deciding whether a formal case conference is necessary. Many women worry that their baby may be taken away into care purely because they use drugs. This of course should not be true.

Occasionally, there may be incidents involving violence or the threat of violence, most often caused by the partner or visiting friends in hospital. Welsby has accurately captured the disruption caused by some drug users:

'normal patients are often surprised and afraid when confronted with the unpredictable atmosphere of free floating restlessness and aggression in waiting areas'.[38] Women attending for care in hospital, or who have to be admitted to hospital, are entitled to feel that they are in a safe and secure environment, where nothing must be added to their already deep concern about their pregnancy. Sometimes, these incidents are quite unpreventable by staff or the woman herself. But sometimes grievances and niggles are allowed to build without being satisfactorily resolved, to the point where there is confrontation. In order to forestall this, it is important that all staff use positive inter-personal skills, such as empathy, legitimisation, respect, support and partnership in order to create a calm reassuring basis for management. Greenwood has aptly described the appropriate type of attitude as 'flexible rigidity'. There has to be a preparedness to be sensitive to the needs of the individual, and a readiness to be flexible with changing situations but, at the same time, it is essential that the rules and limits of behaviour are clearly understood.[38]

Many women have fears that their needs in labour will not be recognised or met, and that they will experience antagonism during their care. It is very important that the midwife makes a particular effort to be re-assuring and supportive. Careful explanation at all times in their labour is appreciated.

Adequate pain relief can be obtained with opiates although much more frequent injections are likely to be needed. Because of the high fear about pain which many drug users have, epidural anaesthesia may be very useful. Substitution treatment with methadone does not cover pain relief, which is needed in addition (methadone is a relatively poor analgesic).

Naloxone must not be used to reverse opioid induced respiratory depression in the newborn because of the risk of precipitating an acute opiate withdrawal crisis.

After delivery, a chart scoring for neonatal abstinence syndrome is helpful for all concerned. This is, of course, only one aspect of assessment. Withdrawing babies can usually be treated without drug management, with lots of cuddling, small frequent feeds, and patience. Babies may need neonatal unit care to maintain hydration and may need sedation. The logical drug is simply replacement of opiate, and neonatal morphine solution can be used. Chlorpromazine is the most commonly used drug in the UK, but in theory this is not an ideal drug because of the prolonged duration of elimination of metabolites.

Although there are recommendations that women should not breast feed unless they are taking less than 20 mg of methadone daily, this advice does not seem to be based on good evidence.

## CONCLUSIONS

This article is about an attitude to drug use in pregnancy. Drug use is not a marginalised activity, is now embedded in our culture, is a major world concern for pregnancy, and is an issue which will not go away. As well as the short-term effects we know about, much of the future significance will depend on more far reaching effects, such as attention and learning deficits in the offspring.[39]

There are two recent very useful volumes, the first a good source of information about different drugs,[39] the second an excellent practical guide to the management of drug users.[40]

At bottom, management of the pregnant drug user is not intrinsically much different from any other problem in pregnancy. The same general principles apply, the requirements and the issues may just be more obvious. There is a need for good, accurate information, clear communication, mutual respect, support and a partnership of care. So nothing new! Most drug users have the same aspirations for family life as other women and most will cope very well.

## References

1  Koob G. Drug addiction: the yin and yang of hedonic homeostasis. Neuron 1996; 16: 893–896

2  Nutt D J. Addiction: brain mechanisms and their treatment implications. Lancet 1996; 347: 31–36

3  Des Jarlais D C. Systems issues. In: Robertson R. (ed) Management of Drug Users in the Community; A Practical Handbook. London: Arnold, 1998; 39–53

4  Koren G, Shear H, Graham K, Einarson T. Bias against the null hypothesis: the reproductive hazards of cocaine. Lancet 1989: ii; 1440–1442

5  Plessinger M A. Prenatal exposure to amphetamines: risks and adverse outcomes in pregnancy. Obstet Gynecol Clin North Am 1998; 25: 119–138

6  Johnstone F D, Raab G M, Hamilton B A. The effect of human immunodeficiency virus infection and drug use on birth characteristics. Obstet Gynecol 1996; 88: 321–326

7  Johnstone F D. Drug abuse in pregnancy. Contemp Rev Obstet Gynaecol 1990; 2: 96–103

8  Kaltenbach K, Berghella V, Finnegan L. Opioid dependence during pregnancy: effects and management. Obstet Gynecol Clin North Am 1998; 25: 139–151

9  Malpas T J, Darlow B A, Lennox R, Horwood L J. Maternal methadone dosage and neonatal withdrawal. Aust N Z J Obstet Gynaecol 1995; 35: 175–177

10  Doberczak T M, Kandall S R, Friedmann P. Relationships between maternal methadone dosage, maternal-neonatal methadone levels, and neonatal withdrawal. Obstet Gynecol 1993; 81: 936–940

11  Kandall S R, Gaines J, Haabel L, Davidson G, Jessop D. Relationship of maternal substance abuse to subsequent sudden infant death syndrome in offspring. J Pediatr 1993; 123: 120–126

12  Holzman C, Paneth N. Maternal cocaine use during pregnancy and perinatal outcomes. Epidemiol Rev 1994; 16: 315–334

13  Plessinger M A, Woods J R. Cocaine in pregnancy. Obstet Gynecol Clin North Am 1998; 25: 99–118

14  Fredricsson B, Gilljam H. Smoking and reproduction: short and long term effects and benefits of smoking cessation. Acta Obstet Gynecol Scand 1992; 71: 580–592

15  Kendrick J S, Merritt R K. Women and smoking: an update for the 1990s. Am J Obstet Gynecol 1996; 175: 528–535

16  Kramer M S. Determinants of low birth weight: methodological assessment and meta-analysis. Bull World Health Organ 1987; 65: 633–737

17  Ellard G A, Johnstone F D, Prescott R J, Ji-xian W, Jian-hua M. Smoking during pregnancy: the dose dependence of birthweight deficits. Br J Obstet Gynaecol 1996; 103: 806–813

18  Cnattingius S, Haglund B, Meirik O. Cigarette smoking as risk factor for late fetal and early neonatal death. BMJ 1988; 297: 258–261

19  Kleinman J C, Pierre M B, Madans J M, Land G H, Schramm W F. The effects of maternal smoking on fetal and infant mortality. Am J Epidemiol 1998; 127: 274–282

20  MacDorman M F, Cnattingius S, Hoffman H J, Kramer M S, Haglund B. Sudden infant death syndrome and smoking in the United States and Sweden. Am J Epidemiol 1997; 146: 249–257

21  Upton M N, Watt G C M, Smith G D, McConnachie A, Hart C L. Permanent effects of

maternal smoking in offspring's lung function. Lancet 1998; 352: 453

22 Finette B A, O'Neill J P, Vacek P M, Albertini R J. Gene mutations with characteristic deletions in cord blood T lymphocytes associated with passive maternal exposure to tobacco smoke. Nat Med 1998; 4: 1144–1151

23 Laegreid L, Hagberg G, Lundberg A. Neurodevelopment in late infancy after prenatal exposure to benzodiazepines – a prospective study. Neuropediatrics 1992; 23: 60–67

24 Czeizel A. Lack of teratogenicity of benzodiazepine drugs in Hungary. Reprod Toxicol 1988; 1: 183

25 National Teratology Information Service (NTIS). Br J Clin Pharmacol 1998; 45: 184

26 Lee M-J. Marihuana and tobacco use in pregnancy. Obstet Gynecol Clin North Am 1998; 25: 65–83

27 Pietrantoni M, Knuppel R A. Alcohol use in pregnancy. Clin Perinatol 1991; 18: 93–111

28 Konovalov H V, Kovetsky N S, Bobryshev Y Y, Ashwell K W S. Disorders of brain development in the progeny of mothers who used alcohol during pregnancy. Early Hum Dev 1997; 48: 153–166

29 Jones H E, Balster R L. Inhalant abuse in pregnancy. Obstet Gynecol Clin North Am 1998; 25: 65–83

30 Russell M A H. The nicotine addiction trap: a 40-year sentence for four cigarettes. Br J Addiction 1990; 85: 293–300

31 Bartecchi C E, Mackenzie T D, Schrier R W. The human costs of tobacco use (1). N Engl J Med 1994; 330: 907–912

32 Wald N J, Hackshaw A K. Cigarette smoking: an epidemiological overview. Br Med Bull 1996; 52: 3–11

33 Macarthur C, Knox E G. Smoking in pregnancy: effects of stopping at different stages. Br J Obstet Gynaecol 1988; 95: 551–555

34 Dolan-Mullen P, Ramirez G, Groff J Y. A meta-analysis of randomised trials of prenatal smoking cessation interventions. Am J Obstet Gynecol 1994; 171: 1328–1334

35 Bury J, Bickler C. Prescribing for drug users. In: Robertson R (ed) Management of Drug Users in the Community; A Practical Handbook. London: Arnold, 1998; 214–247

36 Ward J, Hall W, Mattick R P. Role of maintenance treatment in opioid dependence. Lancet 1999; 353: 221–226

37 Dashe J S, Jackson G L, Olscher D A, Zane E H, Wendel G D. Opioid detoxification in pregnancy. Obstet Gynecol 1998; 92: 854–858

38 Johnstone F D. Drug addiction and obstetric practice. In: Bewley S, Ward H. (eds) Ethics in Obstetrics & Gynaecology. London: RCOG Press, 1994; 237–249

39 Woods J R (ed) Obstet Gynecol Clin North Am 1998; 25

40 Robertson R. (ed) Management of Drug Users in the Community; A Practical Handbook. London: Arnold, 1998

J. Guy Thorpe-Beeston

# 9

# Immune thrombocytopenia in pregnancy

Platelets are small anucleated corpuscles derived from bone marrow megakaryocytes. In both the pregnant and non-pregnant states, mature platelets circulate for 8–9 days. Platelets act to repair defects in the vascular endothelium and reduce haemorrhage by promoting blood clot formation. When activated, typically by vessel wall trauma, platelets become adherent to themselves and all surfaces including glass. Hence the need to collect blood for platelet counts in bottles containing anticoagulants such as sodium heparin or citrate. Endothelial damage promotes platelet aggregation and degranulation which in turn stimulates the release of prostaglandin and thromboxane $A_2$, amplifying the platelet clumping and vasoconstriction.

## NORMAL PLATELET COUNT IN PREGNANCY

The normal non-pregnant platelet count is 150–400 x $10^9$/l. During pregnancy the platelet count falls progressively, but tends to remain in the normal range.[1-3] The incidence of thrombocytopenia is greatest in the third trimester and this has been attributed to haemodilution and platelet consumption in the placenta. If the platelet count has fallen below 150 x $10^9$/l in the majority of cases there is no accompanying disease process.

The incidence of thrombocytopenia at booking in a study of over 4000 women was found to be 0.4% in contrast to the finding of thrombocytopenia in 7.6% of women at delivery in a study of nearly 7000.[4,5] The causes of thrombocytopenia in pregnancy may be related to increased consumption or destruction or, much less commonly, to a decreased production as may occur in malignant disease (Table 1). In the majority of cases, the platelet count returns to normal 4–6 weeks post partum. Very occasionally – more commonly if there is an associated prolonged bleeding time – the possibility of von Willebrand disease or a qualitative platelet disorder should be considered.[4]

**Mr J. Guy Thorpe-Beeston** MA MD MRCOG, Consultant Obstetrician, Chelsea & Westminster Hospital, 369 Fulham Road, London SW10 9NH, UK

**Table 1** Classification of thrombocytopenia in pregnancy

1. Spurious
2. Gestational
3. Autoimmune:
    Idiopathic
    Drug induced
    HIV
4. Pre-eclampsia and HELLP syndrome
5. Disseminated intravascular coagulation
6. Haemolytic uraemic syndrome
7. Folate deficiency
8. Congenital, e.g. May-Hegglin anomaly, hereditary macrothrombocytopenia
9. Marrow aplasia, malignant infiltration

## SPURIOUS THROMBOCYTOPENIA

Spurious or laboratory-induced thrombocytopenia has become more common since the automation of blood counts and if blood for platelet estimation is collected in EDTA-anticoagulated bottles. It has been estimated to occur in 1–2% of all samples. If thrombocytopenia is suspected, a second blood count using a fresh sample together with blood film examination should be performed. This will exclude laboratory error, sample clotting and EDTA-induced platelet agglutination.[6–8]

## GESTATIONAL THROMBOCYTOPENIA

This condition has also been termed benign or incidental thrombocytopenia. There is no history of autoimmune disease and the other possible causes of thrombocytopenia such as pre-eclampsia have been excluded. Typically, the condition is mild with a platelet count of 120–150 x $10^9$/l, although moderate (50–120 x $10^9$/l), and severe (< 50 x $10^9$/l) thrombocytopenia have been described. Many studies have documented the normal fetal and maternal outcome in such cases. In the largest study involving over 15,000 women, Burrows and Kelton noted the incidence of thrombocytopenia to be 4.8%, having excluded autoimmune disease and pre-eclampsia; there was no neonatal morbidity.[9] In another large study of 730 women, the incidence of thrombocytopenia was 3.6% (range 30–143 x $10^9$/l); again, no neonatal morbidity was noted and none of the 26 infants had a platelet count of less than 100 x $10^9$.[10]

Although there appears to be no significant fetal morbidity, fetal and/or neonatal thrombocytopenia may occur in 4–13% of these cases.[5,11] The mechanism of neonatal thrombocytopenia has not been determined and it has recently been suggested that in nearly 50% of such cases there may be an underlying maternal autoimmune condition.[12] Clearly, the greater the intensity of investigation for possible autoimmune disease the greater the apparent detection rate will be (Table 2). The benefits of thorough investigation in reaching a firm diagnosis and its implications for the current and future pregnancies must be weighed against the expense and whether the knowledge of this information confers benefit on the patient.

Sometimes, it may not be possible to distinguish gestational and autoimmune thrombocytopenia. The diagnosis of gestational thrombocytopenia relies on the

**Table 2**    Investigation of thrombocytopenia

| | |
|---|---|
| 1. | Full blood count on two occasions |
| 2. | Blood film examination |
| 3. | Clotting profile including KCCT, PT, fibrinogen concentration |
| 4. | Platelet autoantibodies |
| 5. | Lupus anticoagulant, anticardiolipin and antinuclear antibodies |
| 6. | Liver and renal function tests |
| 7. | Bone marrow aspiration |

exclusion of the other possible causes and is helped by the knowledge that a platelet count was normal either before, or in the early part of, a pregnancy. If this is the case, then prognosis appears to be extremely good and the platelet counts tend to return to a normal value following delivery. Aggressive medical or obstetric intervention should be avoided.[13] Delivery should attempted vaginally unless there are other obstetric indications for operative delivery. Provided the platelet count is > 80 x 10$^9$/l, most anaesthetists will be happy to offer epidural anaesthesia.[14] If the platelet count is hovering at or below this figure, it may be sensible to discuss other forms of pain relief with mother prior to labour, for example patient controlled analgesia. Postnatally, fetal cord blood should be sampled at the time of delivery and serial maternal counts undertaken to ensure that the maternal count returns to a normal value.

## AUTOIMMUNE THROMBOCYTOPENIA

The incidence of autoimmune thrombocytopenia is estimated to be 1–2 per 1000 pregnancies.[5] In the majority of cases, there are no adverse maternal sequelae and it is rare to see severe bleeding. Autoimmune thrombocytopenic purpura may present with bruising and is seen in 1–2 cases per 10,000 pregnancies.[15] This autoimmune disease is most common in women of childbearing age. The immune destruction of platelets is facilitated by autoantibodies directed against platelet surface antigens. In most cases, the antibody is IgG which may cross the placenta. The placenta also has receptors for the Fc (constant fragment) of the antibody further encouraging the transport of antibodies across the placenta, which may then cause fetal thrombocytopenia. The ability of immunoglobulins to cross the placenta seems to improve with advancing gestation.

Despite the low maternal platelet count and the transmission of antibodies across the placenta, fetal or neonatal intracranial haemorrhage is very rare. In a recent review of 601 neonates born to mothers with autoimmune thrombocytopenia only 6 (1%) had an intracranial haemorrhage.[16] Bussel and colleagues also concluded that the incidence of neonatal intracranial haemorrhage in mothers with autoimmune thrombocytopenia was 1–2%.[17] Overall, therefore, the risk of autoimmune thrombocytopenia being the cause of intracranial haemorrhage is approximately 2 in 100,000 births.[16]

Gestational thrombocytopenia is, therefore, approximately 40–70 times as prevalent and nearly always follows a benign course. In the largest study to date, only one infant was noted to be thrombocytopenic although this infant had trisomy 21 and an abnormal bone marrow.[9]

A recent study has concluded that screening pregnant women for thrombocytopenia has been 'technologically driven and passively accepted'.[18] The authors highlighted the discrepancies that exist between the well-recognised criteria for a successful screening programme and the situation that currently exists for maternal platelet examination. Thus, with an incidence of intracranial haemorrhage of 2 in 100,000 births resulting from autoimmune thrombocytopenia, screening for the condition is unlikely to bring about major improvements in public health. The condition does not have a recognisable or early asymptomatic phase and the natural history is poorly understood. At best the positive predictive value of a low maternal platelet count predicting fetal thrombocytopenia is approximately 1%. Finally, because of the large overlap between gestational and autoimmune thrombocytopenia, the purported interventions to improve fetal outcome, namely cordocentesis and caesarean section, both of which are associated with significant morbidity and rarely mortality, are not justified.[18]

## THE DIAGNOSIS

The diagnosis of autoimmune thrombocytopenia, like gestational thrombo-cytopenia is one of exclusion. Measurement of platelet associated immuno-globulin (PAIgG), unfortunately, is not helpful as these antibodies may be present in over 50% of women with gestational thrombocytopenia. Lescale and colleagues tested the sera of 160 women with presumed gestational thrombo-cytopenia and 90 women with presumed autoimmune thrombocytopenia for the presence of indirect and platelet-associated IgGs, IgMs and complement C3. Although indirect IgG was found in significantly more women with immune thrombocytopenia, platelet-associated IgG was elevated in the majority of women in both groups. The study concluded that it is not possible to distinguish gestational from autoimmune thrombocytopenia on the basis of currently available platelet antibody tests.[19] Currently, the best evidence to support a diagnosis of immune thrombocytopenia is a history of thrombocytopenia that predates the pregnancy.

## MANAGEMENT

The British Society of Haematology has suggested that management decisions should be based on the following factors:

1. *Available treatments to raise the maternal platelet count all carry a risk of significant side effects.*
2. *Haemorrhage due to thrombocytopenia in the mother is very unlikely if the platelet count is > 50 x 10⁹/l at the time of delivery.*
3. *The incidence of fetal thrombocytopenia in presumed maternal autoimmune thrombocytopenia is low.*
4. *The nadir of the platelet count in the affected fetus is 2–5 days post delivery*
5. *The risks of spontaneous fetal haemorrhage in utero and during normal vaginal delivery is low.*[6]

If not already underway, the investigations detailed in Table 2 should be undertaken. Close liaison between the obstetrician, haematologist and, if appro-priate, the neonatologist is necessary. Assuming that the thrombocytopenia is

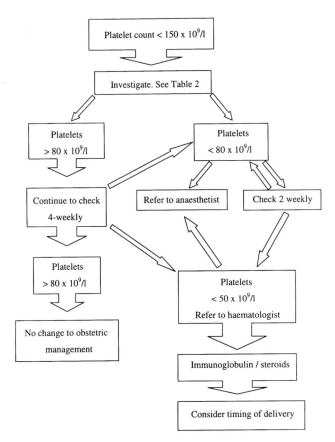

**Fig. 1** Antenatal management of thrombocytopenia.

thought to be autoimmune in nature, no active measures need be taken until the platelet count falls below $50 \times 10^9/l$, as bleeding is very unlikely. However, it would be advisable for the individual to see the anaesthetist to discuss forms of pain relief other than an epidural. If the platelet count falls further, the patient should be referred to the haematologists for a probable bone marrow biopsy (Fig. 1).

Once the platelet count has fallen below $50 \times 10^9/l$, the risk of bleeding at delivery increases; therefore, treatment should be considered although, in practice, the platelet count will often have to be considerably less than this before problems ensue. The earlier in the pregnancy the fall in platelets is apparent, the greater the likelihood of significant complications. The decision to treat will depend principally on the platelet count and the gestation. If a patient should become symptomatic and develop the rare complications of bruising or petechiae, treatment is always indicated.

## MATERNAL TREATMENT

The two principal treatments are the use of corticosteriods or intravenous IgG. If the duration of treatment is likely to be short, then steroids may be used. For example, steroids may be appropriate if one is attempting to elevate the maternal platelet count to a level at term that will allow her to have regional anaesthesia.

Similarly, if a low maintenance dose of steroid proves adequate, this may be an acceptable form of treatment.[20–22] Steroids act both by inhibiting platelet antibody production and increasing platelet production in the bone marrow. However, several potential side-effects may occur which are particularly unwanted in pregnancy, e.g. hypertension, weight gain, gestational diabetes, post partum psychosis and osteoporosis. The risk of fetal complications is minimal as approximately 90% of prednisolone or hydrocortisone are metabolised by the placenta.[23] A starting dose of oral prednisolone (1 mg/kg/day), based on a pre-pregnancy weight, is advised, aiming to reduce the dose to 10 mg daily, provided this is sufficient to maintain the platelet count above 50 x $10^9$/l.[6] Approximately 80% of patients will respond to steroids within 3–6 weeks.[24,25] Clearly, this time lag prior to observing a response may be unacceptable if the pregnancy is approaching term, although it is certainly a cheaper option than intravenous IgG. In contrast, the latter, however, will bring about a maternal platelet response in 4–6 days in 70% of cases.[26]

Intravenous administration of monomeric polyvalent human IgG in doses greater than those produced by the mother prolongs the clearance time of circulating immune complexes (IgG-coated platelets) by binding of the Fc portion on the macrophage in the maternal reticulo-endothelial system. An initial dose of 0.4 g/kg/day for 5 days by intravenous infusion will usually result in a clinically important increase in the maternal platelet count within a week of treatment. The length of effect is variable, but may often be 2–3 weeks or more. Treatment can then be repeated if appropriate.[6] This regimen will usually require the patient's admission to hospital for 5 days. More recently, alternative regimens have been considered using 1 g/kg/day given over 8 h on one day. This uses overall a much lower dose of IgG and may be repeated after 2 days; consequently it is much cheaper. Side-effects are not common although anaphylaxis is always possible and the first dose should always be administered with considerable caution. The risk of infection is of particular concern and hepatitis C transmission has been reported.[27]

The aim of treatment is to elevate the maternal platelet count to > 50 x $10^9$/l prior to delivery. If the count can be increased further, then clearly epidural anaesthesia can safely be used and, provided the pregnancy is sufficiently mature, induction of labour can be considered. The balancing act of maternal well-being and fetal gestation is one with which most obstetricians are familiar, but these dilemmas need to be carefully explained to the patient and the rationale for any decision diligently recorded in the notes. It should also be recognised that, although a useful treatment, this therapy is not a cure.

In rare cases, the maternal platelet count fails to respond to either steroid or IgG therapy. As a last resort, splenectomy has been considered in extreme and symptomatic cases. It has been associated with significant fetal and maternal loss and since the advent of IgG is rarely used.[21,22,28] It does, however, potentially provide a cure or long-term improvement as the spleen is the site of both antibody production and antibody coated platelet destruction. It is best performed in the second trimester. Prior to surgery, all patients should receive appropriate vaccination with pneumocax and oral penicillin for life prophylactically. The platelet count should be elevated with intravenous IgG. Transfused platelets given just prior to surgery only have a very short half-life and are best used if abnormal bleeding occurs.

Historically, other treatments have been used in autoimmune thrombocytopenia, but most are strictly contra-indicated in pregnancy, for example vincristine and cyclophosphamide. The experience of using azothioprine in pregnancy has stemmed from transplant patients and generally the outcome has been favourable.[29] Immune thrombocytopenia is a disorder caused by the destruction antibody coated platelets by the reticulo-endothelial system. Some authors have advocated the use of anti-D because of its comparable efficacy and lower cost. However, its onset of action is not as rapid and anti-D is not widely used for this indication.[30]

## FETAL ASSESSMENT

The falsely-held assumption that maternal autoimmune thrombocytopenia was associated in a significant number of cases with fetal thrombocytopenia and its worse sequelae, namely intracranial haemorrhage, led many authors to advocate an extremely aggressive approach to the investigation of the possible fetal thrombocytopenia. Although the overall incidence of thrombocytopenia in babies born to mothers with maternal autoimmune thrombocytopenia is approximately 11%, the fetal risk of severe problems is extremely small unless there is a pre-existing history of the condition.[31] The initial approach relied on an estimation of the fetal platelet count by obtaining a capillary fetal blood sample using the technique of fetal scalp sampling in early labour. Scott and colleagues defined fetal thrombocytopenia as a platelet count of less than 50 x $10^9$ and used fetal scalp blood samples obtained during labour to decide if abdominal or vaginal delivery was appropriate. In 12 cases, three fetuses were found to have a low platelet count and were delivered by caesarean section. In all cases the outcome was good.[32] This approach, however, has a number of failings. Firstly, false positive results have been described because of sample contamination with maternal blood or liquor.[24,33] Secondly, the technique can only be used once sufficient cervical dilation has occurred during labour to permit fetal scalp sampling. Finally, an abnormal result would lead to an emergency caesarean section, the benefits of which have never been proven.

The next advance, therefore, was to try and assess the fetal platelet count before labour and this has been possible since the advent of cordocentesis.[32,34–36] The results of these studies have confirmed that the fetal platelet count is not associated with any maternal indices of well-being, in particular the maternal platelet count. Secondly, that there is a good relationship between the fetal platelet count at cordocentesis and the subsequent neonatal count. Finally, that cordocentesis is not without risk and may necessitate emergency delivery. Differing definitions have been used to define fetal thrombocytopenia and, although in general a caesarean section was recommended if the platelet count was less than 50 x $10^9$, no benefit was shown in the fetal outcome and no comments were made about possible resulting maternal morbidity. The risk of a procedure-related complication in these studies was 3%. The role of caesarean section in the management of autoimmune thrombocytopenia has been questioned by two recent studies which showed no increase in the risk of fetal intracranial haemorrhage for thrombocytopenic neonates delivered vaginally compared with those delivered abdominally.[9,37] In one study, 4 of 31 neonates with a platelet count of less than 50 x $10^9$ showed no evidence of intracranial haemorrhage even though three had been delivered vaginally.[37] Furthermore, a review of the literature concluded that there was no significant association between the rate of intracranial haemorrhage (estimated to be 3% in infants born with a platelet count of less than $100 \times 10^9$) and the mode of delivery.[37] Assessment of the fetal platelet count does not, at present, appear justified except, perhaps, in pregnancies where there is a history of fetal thrombocytopenia in a previous pregnancy. The use of caesarean section in minimising the risk of fetal intracranial haemorrhage has not been proven.

The most important assessment in the baby should occur in the neonatal period and it is recommended that all neonates should have the platelet count assessed. In those cases of neonatal thrombocytopenia, particularly those who may be symptomatic and have bruising or petechiae, supportive therapy may include a platelet infusion or the use of steroids or immunoglobulins.

## THROMBOCYTOPENIA ASSOCIATED WITH HIV INFECTION

Human immunodeficiency virus positive women may manifest thrombocytopenia similar to women with immune thrombocytopenia, increasing the risk of fetal thrombocytopenia and haemorrhage.[38] In a retrospective study of 890 HIV positive pregnant women in France, 25 (2.8%) were thought to be thrombocytopenic as a result of their infection; 16 (55%) of these women were treated with zidovudine, corticosteroids or intravenous gammaglobulins. Only 1 infant was noted to be thrombocytopenic at birth and sadly went on to develop early-onset acquired immunodeficiency syndrome.[39] Assessment of the fetal platelet count by cordocentesis in such cases may increase the risk of fetal inoculation with maternal HIV and, therefore, should be avoided. Caesarean section with appropriate antiviral drug regimens given immediately prior to delivery is the current recommended mode of delivery for HIV positive women, irrespective of the fetal platelet count.

## ALLOIMMUNE THROMBOCYTOPENIA

Fetal and neonatal thrombocytopenia may result from maternal alloantibodies (IgG) directed against alloantigens located on fetal platelets crossing the placenta and destroying the fetal platelets. The disease process is similar to red cell allo-immunisation, however it may occur in first pregnancies. There is no maternal thrombocytopenia; however, the resulting fetal thrombocytopenia may result in fetal intracranial haemorrhage in 20% of cases.[40] This condition including the complex immunology and treatment has been recently reviewed.[41,42]

### References

1. Tygart S G, McRoyan D K, Spinnato J A, McRoyan C J, Kitay D Z. Longitudinal study of platelet indices during normal pregnancy. Am J Obstet Gynecol 1986; 154: 883–7
2. Sill P R, Lind T, Walker W. Platelet values during normal pregnancy. Br J Obstet Gynaecol 1985; 92: 480–3
3. Burrows R F, Kelton J G. Incidentally detected thrombocytopenia in healthy mothers and their infants. N Engl J Med 1988; 319: 142–5
4. How H Y, Bergmann F, Koshy M, Chediak J, Preperin C, Gall S A. Quantitative and qualitative platelet abnormalities during pregnancy. Am J Obstet Gynecol 1991; 164: 92

5. Burrows R F, Kelton J G. Thrombocytopenia at delivery: a prospective study of 6715 deliveries. Am J Obstet Gynecol 1990; 162: 731–4

6. Letsky E A, Greaves M. Guidelines on the investigation and management of thrombocytopenia in pregnancy and neonatal alloimmune thrombocytopenia. Br J Haematol 1996; 95: 21–6

7. Solanki D L, Blackthorn B C. Spurious thrombocytopenia during pregnancy. Obstet Gynecol 1985; 65: 14S

8. Mayan H, Salomon O, Pauzer R, Farfel Z. EDTA-induced pseudothrombocytopenia. South Med J 1992; 85: 213

9. Burrows R F, Kelton J G. Fetal thrombocytopenia and its relation to maternal thrombocytopenia. N Engl J Med 1993; 329: 1463–6

10. Nagey D A, Alger L S, Edelman B B, Heyman M R, Pupkin M J, Crenshaw Jr C. Reacting appropriately to thrombocytopenia in pregnancy. South Med J 1986; 79: 1385

11. Kaplan C, Daffos F, Forestier F et al. Fetal platelet counts in thrombocytopenic pregnancy. Lancet 1990; 336: 979

12. Ajzenberg N, Dreyfus M, Kaplan C, Yvart J, Weill B, Tchernia G. Pregnancy-associated thrombocytopenia revisited: assessment and follow-up of 50 cases. Blood 1998; 92: 4573–80

13. Aster R H. 'Gestational' thrombocytopenia: a plea for conservative management. N Engl J Med 1990; 323: 264–6

14. Letsky E A. Haemostasis and epidural anaesthesia. Int J Obstet Anesth 1991; 1: 51–4

15. Kessler I, Lancet M, Borenstein R, Berrebi A, Mogilner B M. The obstetrical management of patients with immunologic thrombocytopenic purpura. Int J Gynecol Obstet 1982; 20: 23–8

16. Payne S P, Resnik R, Moore T R, Hedriana H H, Kelly T F. Maternal characteristics and risk of severe neonatal thrombocytopenia and intracranial haemorrhage in pregnancies complicated by autoimmune thrombocytopenia. Am J Obstet Gynecol 1997; 177: 149–55

17. Bussel J B, Druzin M L, Samuels P, Cines D. Thrombocytopenia in pregnancy. Lancet 1991; 337: 251

18. Rouse D J, Owen J, Goldenberg R L. Routine maternal platelet count: an assessment of a technologically driven screening practice. Am J Obstet Gynecol 1998; 179: 573–6

19. Lescale K B, Eddleman K A, Cines D B et al. Antiplatelet antibody testing in thrombocytopenic pregnant women. Am J Obstet Gynecol 1996; 74: 1014–8

20. McMillan R. Chronic idiopathic thrombocytopenic purpura. N Engl J Med 1981; 304: 211–2

21. Martin J N, Morrison J C, Files J C. Autoimmune thrombocytopenic purpura: current concepts and recommended practices. Am J Obstet Gynecol 1984; 150: 86–96

22. Carloss H W, McMillan R, Crosby W H. Management of pregnancy in women with immune thrombocytopenic purpura. JAMA 1980; 244: 2756–8

23. Smith T, Torday J S. Steroid administration in women with autoimmune thrombocytopenia. N Engl J Med 1982; 306: 744–5

24. McCrae K R, Sammuels P, Schreiber A D. Pregnancy-associated thrombocytopenia: pathogenesis and management. Blood 1992; 80: 2697–714

25. Biswas A, Arulkumaran S, Ratnam S S. Disorders of platelets in pregnancy. Obstet Gynecol Survey 1994; 49: 585–94

26. Sullivan C A, Martin J N. Management of the obstetric patient with thrombocytopenia. Clin Obstet Gynecol 1995; 38: 521–34

27. Yap P L, McOmish F, Webster O D B et al. Hepatitis C transmission by intravenous immunoglobulin. J Hepatol 1994; 21: 455–60

28. Bell W R. Hematologic abnormalities in pregnancy. Med Clin North Am 1977; 61: 165–203

29. Letsky E A, Warwick R. Haematological problems. In: James D K, Steer P J, Weiner C P, Gonik B. (eds) High Risk Pregnancy. London: WB Saunders, 1996; 337–72

30. Blanchette V, Carcao M. Intravenous immunoglobulin G and anti-D as therapeutic interventions in immune thrombocytopenia purpura. Transfus Sci 1988; 19: 279–88

31. Samuels P, Bussel J B, Braitman L E et al. Estimation of the risk of thrombocytopenia in the offspring of pregnant women with presumed immune thrombocytopenia. N Engl J Med 1990; 323: 229–35

32. Scott J R, Cruikshank D P, Kochenour N K, Pitkin R M, Warenski J C. Fetal platelet counts in the obstetric management of immunologic thrombocytopenic purpura. Am J Obstet Gynecol 1980; 136: 495–9

33. Moise Jr K J, Patton D E, Cano L E. Misdiagnosis of a normal fetal platelet count after coagulation of intrapartum scalp samples in autoimmune thrombocytopenic purpura. Am J Perinatol 1991; 8: 295–6

34. Daffos F, Forestier F, Kaplan C, Cox W. Prenatal diagnosis and management of bleeding disorders with fetal blood sampling. Am J Obstet Gynecol 1988; 158: 939–46

35. Moise Jr K J, Carpenter R J, Cotton D B, Wasserstrujm N, Kirshon B, Cano L E. Percutaneous umbilical cord sampling in the evaluation of fetal platelet counts in pregnant patients with autoimmune thrombocytopenia purpura. Obstet Gynecol 1988; 72: 346–50

36. Garmel S H, Craigo S D, Morin L M, Crowley J M, D'Alton M E. The role of percutaneous umbilical blood sampling in the management of immune thrombocytopenic purpura. Prenat Diagn 1995; 15: 439–45

37. Cook R L, Miller R C, Katz V L, Cefalo R C. Immune thrombocytopenic purpura in pregnancy: a reappraisal of management. 1991; 78: 578–83

38. Glantz J C, Roberts D J. Pregnancy complicated by thrombocytopenia secondary to human immunodeficiency virus infection. Obstet Gynecol 1994; 83: 825–7

39. Mandelbrot L, Schlienger I, Bongain A et al. Am J Obstet Gynecol 1994; 171: 252–7

40. Bussel J B, Berkowitz R L, McFarland J G, Lynch L, Chitkara U. Antenatal treatment of neonatal alloimmune thrombocytopenia. N Engl J Med 1988; 319: 1374–8

41. Carroll S G, Nicolaides K H. Maternal and fetal thrombocytopenia. In: Studd J. (ed) Progress in Obstetrics and Gynaecology 13. Edinburgh: Churchill Livingstone 1998; 43–54

42. Kelsey H, Rodeck C. Fetal thrombocytopenia. In: Fisk N M, Moise K J. (eds) Fetal Therapy. Cambridge: Cambridge University Press, 1997; 164–83

*Anne Szarewski*

# 10

# What's new in contraception?

The ideal contraceptive would be 100% effective, with no health risks or side effects, independent of intercourse, easily and completely reversible, easily administered and used independently of the medical profession. However, such a method does not yet – and may never – exist. In practice there is, therefore, a trade-off between efficacy and safety. Methods which are very safe, such as barriers or natural family planning, unfortunately are not very effective. Meanwhile, the very effective methods, the hormonal contraceptives and IUDs, raise more concerns about health risks and side-effects.

The last few years have seen a number of new methods come onto the market in the UK, thereby increasing choice and, hopefully, uptake of contraception. In addition, new information has become available about some of the established methods.

## THE COMBINED PILL

Four years have now elapsed since the UK Committee on Safety of Medicines (CSM) issued its statement about the risk of venous thrombo-embolism (VTE) with second and third generation oral contraceptive pills. During those 4 years, the one undisputed fact is that the termination rate in England and Wales rose by at least 8% following the scare.[1]

VTE is rare in young women, with the incidence estimated at being around 5 per 100,000 per year. The risk in pregnancy is higher, at 60 per 100,000 per year. Studies have previously shown that women on low dose, second generation pills have a risk of VTE of approximately 30–40 per 100,000 per year. The new studies suggested that women using pills containing the progestogens, desogestrel and

**Dr Anne Szarewski** MBBS DRCOG PhD MFFP, Senior Clinical Research Fellow in Gynaecological Oncology, Department of Mathematics, Statistics and Epidemiology, Imperial Cancer Research Fund, PO Box 123, Lincoln's Inn Fields, London WC2A 3PX and Senior Clinical Medical Officer, Margaret Pyke Centre for Study and Training in Family Planning and Reproductive Health Care, 73 Charlotte Street, London W1P 1LB, UK

**Table 1** Mortality from various causes (based on ICD coding) by age in women (England & Wales 1992). Annual death rate per million women

| | Age (years) | | | |
|---|---|---|---|---|
| | 15–24 | 25–34 | 35–44 | 15–44 |
| Acute myocardial infarction | 1 | 5 | 33 | 39 |
| Pulmonary embolism | 1 | 1 | 1 | 3 |
| Cerebral infarct | 1 | 2 | 5 | 8 |
| Phlebitis, thrombophlebitis, deep vein thrombosis & embolism | 3 | 2 | 6 | 11 |
| Ovarian cancer | 2 | 8 | 38 | 48 |
| Pregnancy | | | | 60 |
| Home accidents | | | | 40 |
| Road deaths | | | | 80 |

Risk of death in the next year for a female smoker aged 35 years is 1670 per million women. From Statement from the Clinical and Scientific Committee of the Faculty of Family Planning and Reproductive Health Care, 1995.[7]

gestodene, had a risk of VTE of 30 per 100,000 per year (Table 1).[2] In 1995, the CSM advised doctors that, because second generation pills now appeared, in these studies, to have a reduced risk, of 15 per 100,000 per year, desogestrel and gestodene-containing pills should no longer routinely be used as first choice contraceptives.[3]

There has been much debate regarding possible sources of bias (particularly prescriber bias) and confounding in these original studies, especially in view of the fact that later studies, which were better able to control for such factors, generally show no difference between second and third generation pills. However, given that the absolute risk (of both incidence and mortality), whichever figure is taken, is so small, this is essentially a legal, rather than a medical issue.

An appeal against the CSM's guidelines was heard by the Medicines Commission late in 1998. As a result, third generation pills have been re-instated as first-line contraceptives, allowing doctors to prescribe freely once more.[4] There is still a requirement for absolute risks of VTE to be stated separately for second and third generation pills in the data sheets (amended to 15 for second generation and 25 for third generation pills), but this is now for information only. A similar appeal has also been successful in Germany.

Third generation pills have benefits in terms of quality of life,[5] but this aspect is, unfortunately, difficult to quantify. Third generation progestogens, while still giving good cycle control, are less androgenic than second generation products and, therefore, tend to be better for women who have problems with acne, hirsutism, and weight gain.[6,7] These are termed 'minor' side effects, but have been shown to greatly influence compliance.[8] It is noteworthy that a norgestimate-containing pill (which was not evaluated in the three studies of VTE risk) has recently been licensed by the US FDA for the treatment of acne, having been proved effective in a randomised placebo-controlled trial.[9] Further scientific studies of other third generation pills are needed to clarify the anecdotal reports of their beneficial effects.

The risk of breast cancer in oral contraceptive users has been the topic of a number of pill scares in the last 15 years. A recent overview of 90% of the studies so far carried out[10] suggests a small increase in risk (relative risk 1.24) for women who are current users of oral contraceptives. This excess risk declines progressively after cessation of use, disappearing altogether after 10 years. There was no effect of pill dose or of duration of use. Breast cancers diagnosed in pill users were clinically less advanced than those in never-users, and were less likely to have spread beyond the breast. This would suggest that mortality from breast cancer might actually be reduced in pill users.

The lack of both a duration of use and a dose-response effect makes a causal association unlikely. There are two plausible explanations for these results, either or both of which may play a part. Firstly, it is possible that the pill accelerates the growth of tumours which were already present, thus making them clinically obvious earlier. A second possibility is that of surveillance bias; women who take the pill may be more 'breast aware' and are also more likely to be seeing doctors and nurses regularly, allowing the opportunity for advice and examinations. This would explain the earlier diagnosis in pill users compared with never-users, who may be less exposed to medical contact.

Both the Faculty of Family Planning of the Royal College of Obstetricians and Gynaecologists and the Committee of Safety of Medicines have stated that there need be no change in prescribing practice as a result of the breast cancer overview.

Reassuring evidence of the safety of the combined pill comes from the Royal College of General Practitioners' Study, which has recently published data on a 25 year follow-up of its cohort of 46,000 women.[11] Most of the data relate to use of high dose pills, but even these had no overall effect on mortality over the 25 year period (RR 1.0, 95% CI 0.9–1.1). In addition, any effects of the pill ceased within 10 years of stopping the method.

## EMERGENCY CONTRACEPTION

Emergency contraception has been the focus of much discussion in the last few years. The Yuzpe hormonal regimen, consisting of 100 µg ethinyloestradiol plus 500 µg levonorgestrel, repeated 12 h later, is well established.[12] There is increasing pressure for hormonal methods to be made available via nurses[13] and, more controversially, through pharmacies.[14,15] One of the arguments against pharmacy prescription of emergency contraception is that women would use it irresponsibly. A randomised controlled trial has shown that women given a reserve pack of the Yuzpe method (Schering PC4) to keep at home were indeed more likely to use it when an accident occurred.[16] However, they were not more likely to abandon their routine contraceptive method as a result. The control group, who were given information about the method and its availability, were less likely to obtain it and, at the end of the study, had a higher (though not significantly) rate of unintended pregnancies. Such provision would obviously be useful for couples using barrier methods, but one should not forget that women using the pill sometimes forget to restart a packet on time (or miss a number of pills) and would, therefore, also benefit from a reserve packet of the emergency pill.

The debate has been further fuelled by a recent randomised, double-blind trial demonstrating the efficacy of a progestogen-only emergency contraceptive.[17] In this study, 1998 women were randomly assigned either to the Yuzpe regimen or to receive levonorgestrel 750 µg, repeated 12 h later. The failure rates were 3.2% (95% CI 2.2–4.5) and 1.1% (95% CI 0.6–2.0), respectively.

As well as being more effective, the levonorgestrel regimen was associated with significantly fewer side-effects, particularly nausea (23% versus 51%, $P < 0.01$) and vomiting (6% versus 19%, $P < 0.01$).

A more surprising finding was that the efficacy of both methods was significantly greater if they were commenced within 24 h of coitus. This is in contrast to previous findings[18] and merits further investigation. If true, there are important implications for service provision which will make, at the very least, provision of a reserve packet more acceptable, and indeed, highly desirable. Administration of the first dose as early as possible may make the timing of the second dose highly inconvenient (for example in the middle of the night). On-going studies are investigating the necessity of the second dose of hormones, and its timing.

The levonorgestrel regimen has been recently licensed in the UK as Levonelle-2. This consists of two tablets each of 750 µg of levonorgestrel, to be given 12 h apart.

Now that a progestogen-only emergency contraceptive is licensed, the calls for pharmacy-based and nurse prescribing are likely to grow louder and more insistent. The already small risk to health of an oestrogen-containing preparation will be further reduced when only progestogen is used. However, the actual decisions will depend ultimately on the pharmaceutical industry and the regulatory authorities.[15]

Amidst all the arguments about hormonal methods, it should not be forgotten that, at present, the most effective emergency contraceptive is still the insertion of a copper intra-uterine device,[12] and that this also has the greatest flexibility in terms of timing: it can be fitted up to 5 days after the earliest predicted date of ovulation, regardless of how many times unprotected intercourse has occurred.

Looking to the future, mifepristone has great potential for use as an emergency contraceptive. Two recent studies have investigated the use of 600 mg mifepristone as a single dose given within 72 h of unprotected intercourse and in both no pregnancies occurred in the mifepristone group. Nausea and vomiting were less common than with the Yuzpe regimen, but there was a delay in the onset of menstruation, which may limit the acceptability of the method.[12] Surprisingly, a recent WHO study[19] suggests that even this problem may be largely overcome without loss of efficacy if the dose of mifepristone is lowered to as little as 10 mg.

## INJECTABLES

### Injectable progestogens

Of the two available in the UK, depo medroxyprogesterone acetate and norethisterone oenanthate, only the former (Depo Provera or DMPA) is licensed for long-term use and is far more widely used. The efficacy of Depo-Provera given in a dose of 150 mg intramuscularly every 12 weeks is well established. Five large, controlled multicentre studies have been conducted, showing an in-use failure rate of 0.0–0.7 per 100 woman-years.[20]

After many years of neglect, the method is gradually being accepted as an effective, simple and relatively safe choice. Use of DMPA is independent of intercourse and also independent of the user's memory (and thus of continuing motivation), other than remembering the 12 weekly appointments. For many women this is a great advantage. For certain women, DMPA offers the advantage of not requiring storage and not being obvious in use, enabling them to maintain secrecy about their use of contraception. The injection itself is more acceptable since the present 1 ml formulation was introduced – the former 3 ml injection was more uncomfortable.

The probability of achieving amenorrhoea on DMPA is higher than for other progestogen-only methods[20] and may be an advantage to some women, who can understand that it is not dangerous and welcome the freedom which amenorrhoea brings. In addition, certain women will benefit from an improvement in symptoms such as dysmenorrhoea, menorrhagia (and, therefore, anaemia). There have also been anecdotal reports of an improvement in symptoms of premenstrual syndrome.[20]

Like the combined oral contraceptive pill, DMPA offers protection against ectopic pregnancy and is sometimes used in the palliation of symptoms of endometriosis (since it induces amenorrhoea). Also, like the combined pill, it may offer protection against pelvic inflammatory disease, because of the effect of progestogen on cervical mucus.[20] This would make it a better choice than the intra-uterine contraceptive device for young women who are forgetful pill takers and may be at risk of sexually transmitted disease.

There are no oestrogen-related side-effects or health risks associated with this preparation and it does not inhibit lactation. DMPA has no appreciable effects on blood pressure or thrombosis risk.[20,21] In this, it has an advantage over the combined oral contraceptive pill, and provides a simple, effective alternative for women who cannot use the pill for these reasons. Similarly, it has been suggested that women who suffer from focal migraine and are, therefore, advised against use of the combined oral contraceptive pill can still use progestogen-only contraceptives.[22,23] Although the POP is medically safe in these circumstances, in young women it is less effective, and involves strict time keeping, which will be disadvantages for some women.

The method is reversible although there is a median delay in return of fertility of 6 months (not including the duration of the last injection). Disturbances of menstruation can occur which may be marked and unpredictable. With repeated injections, however, women tend to become amenorrhoeic and, indeed, the majority are likely to achieve this within a year. If frequent bleeding is a problem, two approaches (apart from counselling, which is most important) can be tried. The next injection can be given early, by as much as 4 weeks, and this can be done repeatedly. Alternatively, the woman can be given a short course of oestrogen, either as oestradiol (as used in HRT), or simply a packet of the combined pill (if this is not contra-indicated).

Although there has been much publicity about the risk of breast cancer in beagles given enormous doses of DMPA, a large WHO study[24] has shown no overall increase in the risk of breast cancer in women (RR 1.2, 95% CI 0.96–1.52): there was a slightly increased risk within the first 4 years of use; but, since this was greatest after the first injection and diminished rather than increased with duration of use, the observation is more likely to be due to some kind of bias, for example surveillance bias.

The WHO study[20,25] also showed no increase in risk for either cervical or ovarian cancers. In the case of endometrial cancer, there was a 5-fold protective effect (RR 0.2, 95% CI 0.1–0.8).

The issue of whether long-term users of DMPA may be at risk of having reduced bone density due to ovarian suppression was first raised in a small case-control study from New Zealand in 1991.[26] However, the use of volunteers and poor matching of cases and controls for known risk factors for osteoporosis has detracted from this and the same group's recent publication.[27-29] A study of 185 cases, using consecutive attenders (with 91% compliance) from the UK has not confirmed Cundy's findings.[30] In addition, although the majority of DMPA users had low oestradiol levels, this bore no correlation with their bone densities. It is, therefore, doubtful whether oestradiol level measurements are of any value in these women. The results of two prospective studies, currently underway in the US, are eagerly awaited in order that this controversy be laid to rest. In the interim, it should be remembered that DMPA users may, as individuals, be at risk of osteoporosis because of their other characteristics; for example, they are more likely to be heavy smokers. In older users, this may be worth considering; even if synthetic oestrogen is contra-indicated, they can still be given natural oestrogen supplementation as used in HRT.

The greatest obstacle to the use of Depo Provera is undoubtedly adverse public (including health professionals) perception. In addition, it cannot be stressed enough that counselling women about potential side-effects is extremely important. The method is, at least temporarily, irreversible. This means that, in many cases, if a woman develops a side-effect for which she was not prepared, there is little that can be done except wait for the injection to wear off. Not surprisingly, such women are (justly) upset, complain, and may resort to litigation. Appropriate counselling, with the provision and discussion of information leaflets, is essential before the first injection.

### Combined oestrogen–progestogen injectables

Cyclofem, a combination of medroxyprogesterone acetate (25 mg) and oestradiol cypionate (5 mg) in a 0.5 ml dose, is a new injectable contraceptive, which has been successfully used in world-wide trials and may be marketed in the UK in the next couple of years. WHO studies have shown first year failure rates of 0.2 per 100 woman years.[31] An advantage of this preparation is that there is far less menstrual disturbance than with progestogen-only injectables.[20] However, the injections have to given monthly, which is clearly inconvenient for many women. Self injection appears to be a viable option, which is being further investigated.[31]

## IMPLANTS

The levonorgestrel-releasing subdermal implants Norplant and Norplant 2 have been extensively reviewed in this series recently[32] and, therefore, will not be dwelt upon here. These implants have, like injectables, suffered from unwarranted bad publicity and are now relatively neglected in the UK. However, the launch of a new, single rod implant, Implanon, in 1999 should be welcomed.

Many of the problems associated with Norplant were related to the insertion and removal of the six implants. A significant advantage of Implanon is that it consists of a single, semi-rigid rod, measuring 40 mm x 2 mm, which is considerably easier both to insert (taking on average, under 2 min) and remove (3 min).[33] The rod is supplied in a sterile, disposable applicator and insertion does not require a skin incision. Removal, using a 'pop-out' technique, is facilitated by the rigidity of the capsule.

The implant releases between 30–40 µg 3-ketodesogestrel (etonogestrel) per day and lasts for 3 years. This hormone level is designed to achieve complete inhibition of ovulation and so far, in the world-wide phase III clinical trials, there has not been a single pregnancy.[34] It should be noted that inhibition of ovulation is achieved through suppression of luteinising hormone alone; endogenous oestradiol is, therefore, still produced as a result of the action of follicle stimulating hormone.

The incidence of acne appears to be slightly lower than with the levonorgestrel implants.[35] Amenorrhoea is more common in Implanon users than with Norplant (18–25% versus 2–7%, respectively). However, irregular bleeding can be a problem, as with all progestogen-only methods.[36]

## The levonorgestrel-releasing intra-uterine system (Mirena)

The Mirena consists essentially of a Nova T frame, within the stem of which is a steroid reservoir containing 52 mg levonorgestrel, designed to release 20 µg of hormone per 24 h into the uterine cavity. Because of the reservoir, the stem is slightly wider than that of the Nova T, which may necessitate cervical dilatation in nulliparous women. Its efficacy is approximately 0.3 per 100 woman years[37] and it is now licensed for 5 years,[38] though its real duration of action is probably up to 7 years. It should be noted that the Mirena is not licensed for use as an emergency contraceptive.

As with all progestogen-only methods, irregular bleeding can be problem initially, but tends to become very light and infrequent with prolonged use. Indeed, such is the profundity of the endometrial suppression, that the device has been shown to be preferable to hysterectomy for the treatment of menorrhagia in a randomised trial,[39] with other studies showing a reduction in blood loss of 97% after 12 months' use. It is, therefore, a simple, fertility-conserving alternative to both hysterectomy and endometrial resection.[37]

There is no increase in the risk of pelvic infection with this device and ectopic pregnancy is rare (0.02 per 100 woman-years). Despite the very low blood levels of hormone (lower than with any other hormonal method), some women do experience progestogenic side-effects, such as acne.

In the next couple of years, it is hoped that the Mirena will be licensed for the treatment of menorrhagia, and also for use in hormone replacement therapy. Studies have already demonstrated that the device provides endometrial protection in HRT for both peri- and postmenopausal women[37] and smaller devices for use in postmenopausal women are under development. The oestrogen can then be given by whatever route is preferred. This provides continuous combined therapy for women of all ages, with many achieving amenorrhoea and with few progestogenic side-effects. Preliminary data also suggest that the Mirena may be useful in the treatment of endometrial hyperplasia, and this leads on to the possibility that it may also be beneficial in the prevention/treatment of fibroids, and to reduce the endometrial proliferative effects of tamoxifen in women using this therapy. Finally, women who suffer severe premenstrual syndrome (PMS) and are being treated with oestradiol by patches or implants, may be better served by continuous, low dose intra-uterine progestogen rather than oral cyclical therapy.

## Copper intra-uterine devices (IUDs)

The life-span of copper IUDs is becoming longer, with the Copper T380 'slimline' now licensed for 10 years. Randomised trials[40,41] have compared the Copper T380 'slimline' with both the Nova T and the Mirena. The Mirena was the most effective of the three, with a cumulative 5 year pregnancy rate of 0.5 per 100 women, rising to 1.1 at 7 years. The more surprising finding, however, was that the Nova T had a cumulative 5 year pregnancy rate of 5.9 per 100 women. Meanwhile, the cumulative pregnancy rate at 7 years was 1.4 for the Copper T380.

Unfortunately, the T380 has recently been withdrawn for commercial reasons. It is hoped that this will shortly be replaced by the Population Council equivalent, the Copper T 380A. Meanwhile, the Nova T 380, which also contains the same amount of copper, has been introduced. Early studies show the efficacy to be comparable, though slightly lower than the Copper T 380 (pregnancy rates of 1.6 versus 0.4 at 2 years).[45] Currently the Nova T 380 has a 5 year licence.

## The Gynefix

The Gynefix is a novel, frameless IUD, which has been designed to try and overcome the problems of expulsion, heavy bleeding and increased dysmenorrhoea associated with the use of conventional, framed devices (Fig. 1). It consists of six copper cylinders (5 mm x 2.2 mm each) on a monofilament polypropylene thread. The upper and lower cylinders are crimped onto the thread to secure placement. At the upper end of the thread is a knot, which is implanted into the fundal myometrium, acting as an anchor. Specific training is required to fit this device, as the insertion technique is quite different to that for conventional IUDs.

The device is licensed for 5 years and studies to date have shown a failure rate of 0.5 per 100 woman-years. There have been no ectopic pregnancies or cases of pelvic inflammatory disease reported so far, and expulsion rates appear to be less than 1 per 100 woman-years. Although there are limited data available, it appears that bleeding and dysmenorrhoea may be reduced

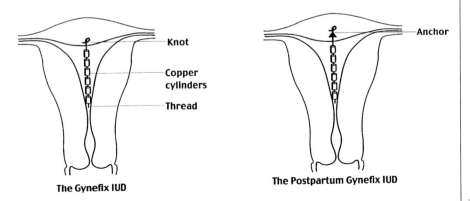

**Fig. 1** Drawing of Gynefix and postpartum Gynefix.

compared with conventional copper IUDs.[42] This may make it preferable for nulliparous women, as well as those who have experienced problems with pain or expulsion with previous IUDs. Postabortal and postpartum versions have also been developed. The postpartum version, Gynefix PP has a slightly thicker polypropylene thread, and an injection moulded, cone shaped 4 mm x 5 mm biodegradable body immediately below the knot. This cone gradually biodegrades over 2–5 weeks and, therefore, moulds to the involuting uterus. The postabortal version, Gynefix PT, has the same thread as the PP, with a slightly bigger anchoring knot compared to the standard model, to enhance the retention force. Studies so far suggest that they are comparable to the standard version in tolerability, efficacy and continuation rates.[42]

### The Persona

Natural family planning enters the age of technology (Fig. 2). This is basically a micro-computer attached to a micro-laboratory. It is based on measurement of levels of luteinising hormone and oestrone-3-glucuronide (E3G) in early morning urine. The woman is required to insert test sticks dipped in her urine: the device then calculates the likely date of ovulation well in advance and allows for sperm survival. She is thus shown 'green light' days, when conception is unlikely and 'red light' days when conception may well occur. With perfect use, failure rates are in the region of 6 per 100 woman-years. However, more typical user failure rates are much higher.[43]

Monitor and Test Stick

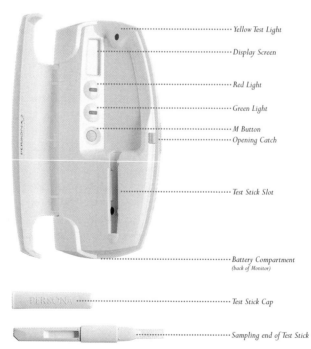

Yellow Test Light

Display Screen

Red Light

Green Light

M Button
Opening Catch

Test Stick Slot

Battery Compartment
(back of Monitor)

Test Stick Cap

Sampling end of Test Stick

**Fig. 2** Persona monitor and test stick reproduced with the permission of Unipath.

The device needs to be programmed for at least 3 months before a couple can rely on it. The woman is required to test her urine on 16 days in the first cycle and on 8 days in subsequent cycles. All this information is stored in the device's computer to produce a unique record for each individual woman.

The manufacturer states that the device is not suitable for women whose cycle lengths fall outside the range 23–35 days. It also cannot be used by women who are breast-feeding, suffer from polycystic ovary syndrome, have menopausal symptoms, or are on hormonal medication (and for 3 months after stopping such medication). A problem which many women do not anticipate is that the use of the emergency pill (of either type) following an 'accident' results in the necessity to reprogramme the device – this means it cannot be relied upon for the next 3 months.

Persona has advantages for couples who wish to use natural family planning, in that it takes away much of the subjectivity of the sympto-thermal method and its greater predictive accuracy results in fewer abstinence days (8 on average, compared to 12). However, the best use failure rate is still high compared to other methods and it should, therefore, be viewed as most suitable for couples spacing, rather than preventing a pregnancy.

## BARRIER METHODS

The arrival of the polyurethane condom is welcome, as it has a number of advantages over latex condoms. It is thinner, odour-free and is suitable for people who are sensitive to latex rubber. In addition, in contrast to latex condoms, it is not corroded by oil-based lubricants.

Meanwhile, the contraceptive sponge has been withdrawn from the UK market, as have the spermicidal gels not based on nonoxynol 9. The latter is a significant drawback, particularly for users of the diaphragm who are allergic to nonoxynol, as there are now no alternatives.

A number of new over-the-counter diaphragm/cervical cap devices (for example the Lea's Shield, Femcap) may come on to the market in the next year or two. However, they appear to be no more effective than the conventional diaphragm.

## FEMALE STERILISATION

Sterilisation is traditionally viewed as the final and most effective form of contraception. However, this may no longer be the case. The US Collaborative Review of Sterilisation[44] followed up over 10,000 sterilised women for nearly 15 years and showed that after 10 years, the cumulative failure rates of some techniques were much higher than expected (Table 2), particularly in women who had been sterilised while young (under 27 years). However, for a UK audience, it should be noted that the Filshie clip was not included in this review. Another worrying finding was that one-third of the pregnancies were ectopic, presenting a significant risk to health. During the last 10 years, extremely effective, reversible methods have become available, and, given the rising divorce rate, sterilisation may no longer be the most sensible, or even the most effective option for many women.

**Table 2** One-year, 5-year and 10-year cumulative probability of pregnancy (per 1000 tubal sterilizations with 95% confidence intervals) by method and age at sterilization. Reproduced from Peterson et al[44] with permission of the *American Journal of Obstetrics and Gynecology.*

| Age | No. | Cumulative probability | | |
| --- | --- | --- | --- | --- |
| | | 1-year | 5-year | 10-year |
| **18–27 years** | | | | |
| Bipolar coagulation | 693 | 3.0 (0.0–7.1) | 26.4 (12.5–40.4) | 54.3 (28.3–80.4) |
| Unipolar coagulation | 280 | 3.7 (0.0–11.1) | 3.7 (0.0–11.1) | 3.7 (0.0–11.1) |
| Silicone rubber band | 994 | 9.5 (3.3–15.7) | 18.2 (8.9–27.5) | 33.2 (10.6–55.9) |
| Spring clip | 694 | 24.1 (12.5–35.8) | 45.3 (28.8–61.8) | 52.1 (31.0–73.3) |
| Interval partial salpingectomy | 120 | 0.0 (0.0–0.0) | 9.7 (0.0–28.6) | 9.7 (0.0–28.6) |
| Post partum salpingectomy | 707 | 1.5 (0.0–4.3) | 7.8 (1.0–14.6) | 11.4 (1.6–21.1) |
| **28–33 years** | | | | |
| Bipolar coagulation | 786 | 2.6 (0.0–6.2) | 18.7 (8.1–29.3) | 21.3 (9.6–33.0) |
| Unipolar coagulation | 549 | 0.0 (0.0–0.0) | 2.0 (0.0–5.8) | 15.6 (0.0–31.4) |
| Silicone rubber band | 1199 | 4.3 (0.5–8.1) | 9.0 (3.4–14.6) | 21.1 (6.4–35.9) |
| Spring clip | 487 | 21.2 (8.2–34.3) | 31.3 (15.1–47.5) | 31.3 (15.1–47.5) |
| Interval partial salpingectomy | 137 | 7.5 (0.0–22.0) | 15.4 (0.0–36.6) | 33.5 (0.0–74.3) |
| Post partum salpingectomy | 625 | 0.0 (0.0–0.0) | 5.6 (0.0–11.9) | 5.6 (0.0–11.9) |
| **34–44 years** | | | | |
| Bipolar coagulation | 788 | 1.3 (0.0–3.8) | 6.3 (0.1–12.5) | 6.3 (0.1–12.5) |
| Unipolar coagulation | 603 | 0.0 (0.0–0.0) | 1.8 (0.0–5.3) | 1.8 (0.0–5.3) |
| Silicone rubber band | 1136 | 4.5 (0.6–8.4) | 4.5 (0.6–8.4) | 4.5 (0.6–8.4) |
| Spring clip | 414 | 5.0 (0.0–11.9) | 10.4 (0.2–20.5) | 18.2 (0.0–36.4) |
| Interval partial salpingectomy | 168 | 12.3 (0.0–29.2) | 18.7 (0.0–39.6) | 18.7 (0.0–39.6) |
| Post partum salpingectomy | 305 | 0.0 (0.0–0.0) | 3.8 (0.0–11.4) | 3.8 (0.0–11.4) |

# THE FUTURE

Within the next year Cerazette, a desogestrel-containing progestogen-only pill (POP) is likely to become available. The dose is 75 µg of desogestrel daily and it has been designed to inhibit ovulation, in contrast to currently available POPs. Early studies suggest that roughly 50% of women bleed infrequently or become amenorrhoeic. It also appears that, because ovulation is inhibited, there is a 12 h pill taking safety margin rather than 3 h. This should make it a much more attractive proposition for many women.

Hormone delivery systems are becoming more varied, with both transdermal patches and vaginal rings under investigation. Apart from solving the perennial problem of forgetfulness in taking pills, hormonal dose is reduced, thereby hopefully reducing the incidence of both side effects and health risks.

The 'male pill' may not be a figment of our imagination for much longer. Various combinations of androgen-only and androgen-progestogen combinations are under investigation. However, an actual pill has been difficult to produce and it is likely that the first versions will be injections or subcutaneous pellets. Although there has been much scepticism about the acceptability of a male pill, there is also a more general feeling that contraceptive responsibility should be shared and many men in stable relationships appear to be keen to take part.

## References

1 Office for National Statistics. Abortion statistics: legal abortions carried out under the 1967 Abortion Act in England and Wales, 1996. Series AB no. 23. London: HMSO
2 Spitzer W O. The 1995 pill scare revisited: anatomy of a non-epidemic. Hum Reprod 1997; 12: 2347–2357
3 Committee on Safety of Medicines. Combined Oral Contraceptives and Thromboembolism. London: CSM, 1995
4 Medicines Control Agency. Combined Oral Contraceptives containing Desogestrel or Gestodene and the Risk of Venous Thromboembolism. Current Problems in Pharmacovigilance 1999; 25
5. CPMP Position Statement 19th April 1996
6. Guillebaud J. Advising women on which pill to take. BMJ 1995; 331: 1111–1112
7 Statement from the Clinical and Scientific Committee of the Faculty of Family Planning and Reproductive Health Care. Risk of venous thromboembolism and the combined oral contraceptive pill. 15th December 1995
8 International Working Group on Enhancing Patient Compliance and Oral Contraceptive Efficacy, Consensus Statement. Br J Fam Plann 1993; 18: 126–129
9 Redmond G P, Olson W H, Lippman J S, Kafrissen M E, Jones T M, Jorizzo J L. Norgestimate and ethinyl estradiol in the treatment of acne vulgaris: a randomized, placebo-controlled trial. Obstet Gynecol 1997; 89: 615–622
10. Collaborative Group on Hormonal Factors in Breast Cancer. Breast cancer and hormonal contraceptives: collaborative reanalysis of individual data of 53,297 women with breast cancer and 100,239 women without breast cancer from 54 epidemiological studies. Lancet 1996; 347: 1713–1727
11 Beral V, Hermon C, Kay C, Hannaford P, Darby S, Reeves G. Mortality associated with oral contraceptive use: 25 year follow up of cohort of 46,000 women from The Royal College of General Practitioners' oral contraception study. BMJ 1999; 318: 96–100
12 Glasier A. Emergency postcoital contraception. N Engl J Med 1997; 337: 1058–1064
13 Kishen M, Presho M. Emergency contraception – a prescription for change. Br J Fam Plann 1996; 22: 22–27

14 Matheson C I, Smith B H, Flett G et al. Over-the-counter emergency contraception: a feasible option. Fam Pract 1998; 15: 38–43

15 Paintin D. Providing hormonal emergency contraception: a lesson from the UK. IPPF Med Bull 1998; 32: 2–3

16 Glasier A, Baird D. The effect of self-administering emergency contraception. N Engl J Med 1998; 339: 1–4

17 WHO Task Force on Postovulatory Methods of Fertility Regulation. Randomised controlled trial of levonorgestrel versus the Yuzpe regimen of combined oral contraceptives for emergency contraception. Lancet 1998; 352: 428–433

18 Trussell J, Ellertson C, Rodriguez G. The Yuzpe regimen of emergency contraception: how long after the morning after? Obstet Gynecol 1996; 88: 150–154

19 WHO Task Force on Postovulatory Methods of Fertility Regulation. Comparison of three single doses of mifepristone as emergency contraception: a randomised trial. Lancet 1999; 353: 697–702

20 Population Reports 1995 New era for injectables. Series K, No. 5

21 WHO Collaborative Study of Cardiovascular Disease and Steroid Hormone Contraception. Cardiovascular disease and use of oral and injectable progestogen-only contraceptives and combined injectable contraceptives. Contraception 1998; 57: 315–324

22 Luscombe H. The relevance of migraine to contraceptive use. Br J Fam Plann 1992, 18: 18–19

23 MacGregor A E, Guillebaud J. Recommendations for clinical practice – combined oral contraceptives, migraine and ischaemic stroke. Br J Fam Plann 1998; 24: 53–61

24 WHO Collaborative Study of Neoplasia and Steroid Contraceptives. Breast cancer and depot-medroxyprogesterone acetate: a multinational study. Lancet 1991; 338: 833–838

25 WHO Collaborative Study of Neoplasia and Steroid Contraceptives. Reports relating to ovarian, endometrial and liver cancers. Int J Cancer 1991; 49: 182–195

26 Cundy T, Evans M, Roberts H, Wattie D, Ames R, Ried I R. Bone density in women receiving depot medroxyprogesterone acetate for contraception. BMJ 1991; 303: 13–16

27 Cundy T, Cornish J, Roberts H et al. Spinal bone density in women using depot medroxyprogesterone contraception. Obstet Gynecol 1998; 92: 569–573

28 Szarewski A, Christopher E, Guillebaud J. Bone density in women receiving depot medroxyprogesterone acetate for contraception [letter]. BMJ 1991 303: 467

29 Szarewski A, Mansour D. Spinal bone density in women receiving depot medroxyprogesterone acetate for contraception. Obstet Gynecol 1999; 93: 629–630

30 Gbolade B, Ellis S, Murby B, Randall S, Kirkman R. Bone density in long term users of depot medroxyprogesterone acetate. Br J Obstet Gynaecol 1998; 105: 790–794

31 Muller N. Self-injection with Cyclofem. IPPF Med Bull 1998; 32: 1–3

32 Mascarenhas L, Newton J. Contraceptive implants. In: Studd J. (ed) Progress in Obstetrics and Gynaecology, vol 12. Edinburgh: Churchill Livingstone, 1996; Ch. 15

33 Mascarenhas L. Insertion and removal of Implanon. Contraception 1998; 58 (Suppl): 79S–85S

34 Croxatto H B, Makarainen L. The pharmacodynamics and efficacy of Implanon, an overview of the data. Contraception 1998; 58 (Suppl): 91S–99S

35 Urbancsek J. An integrated analysis of non-menstrual adverse events with Implanon. Contraception 1998; 58 (Suppl): 109S–115S

36 Affandi B. An integrated analysis of vaginal bleeding patterns in clinical trials of Implanon. Contraception 1998; 58 (Suppl): 99S–109S

37 Hampton N. Intrauterine progestogens. J Br Men Soc 1998; June: 56–61

38 Harrison-Woolrych M, Raine J M. Levonorgestrel intrauterine device can be left in place for five years. BMJ 1998; 317: 149

39 Lahteenmaki P, Haukkamaa M, Puolakka J et al. Open randomised study of use of levonorgestrel releasing intrauterine system as alternative to hysterectomy. BMJ 1998; 316: 1122–1126

40 Sivin I, Stern J, Coutinho E et al. Prolonged intrauterine contraception: a seven year randomized study of the levonorgestrel 20 mcg/day (LNG 20) and the copper T380Ag IUDs. Contraception 1991; 44: 473–480

41 Andersson K, Odlind V, Rybo G. Levonorgestrel-releasing and copper-releasing (Nova T) IUDs during five years of use. Contraception 1994; 49: 56–72

42 Wildermeersch D, Batar I, Webb A et al. GyneFIX. The frameless intrauterine contraceptive implant – an update; for interval, emergency and postabortal contraception. Br J Fam Plann 1999; 24: 149–159

43 Bonnar J, Flynn A, Freundl G, Kirkman R, Royston P, Snowden R. Personal hormone monitoring for contraception. Br J Fam Plann 1999; 24: 128–135

44 Peterson H B, Xia Z, Hughes J M, Wilcox L S, Tylor L R, Trussell J (for the US Collaborative Review of Sterilisation Working Group). The risk of pregnancy after tubal sterilisation: findings from the U.S. Collaborative Review of Sterilisation. Am J Obstet Gynecol 1996; 174: 1161–1170

45 Batar I, Kuukankorpi A, Rauramo I, Siljander M. Two year clinical experience with Nova T 380 – a novel copper-silver IUD. Adv Contracep 1999; 15: 37–48

**11**

*Jon Hyett  Basky Thilaganathan*

# Obstetric management at the limits of neonatal viability

Preterm delivery, defined as delivery before 37 weeks' gestation, occurs in approximately 6–10% of all pregnancies. Obstetric management is focused around measures to prevent spontaneous premature delivery and, if delivery is thought to be inevitable, to optimise neonatal outcome. In pregnancies complicated by pre-eclampsia, utero-placental insufficiency and premature rupture of membranes, the antenatal strategy is to monitor the fetus and mother for the specific problems associated with these conditions. In such pregnancies, elective preterm delivery is usually effected when the fetal and maternal risks of continuing are deemed to outweigh those of preterm birth. Regardless of whether preterm delivery is spontaneous or a consequence of obstetric intervention, it is important that we have a good understanding of the neonatal mortality and morbidity associated with this pregnancy outcome. This is not only needed to balance the relative risks of delivery and continuing the pregnancy, but also to establish the preferred mode of delivery and the level of neonatal care to be offered.

The major determinant of neonatal outcome after preterm delivery is gestational age. The defined margin of neonatal viability may vary considerably between hospitals, but is generally accepted to lie somewhere between 23 and 25 weeks' gestation. Most neonatal intensive care units (NICUs) report survival rates exceeding 80% for neonates delivered at $\geq 28$ weeks' gestation. The long-term outcome of delivery after 27 weeks' gestation is good enough to justify an aggressive approach to fetal and neonatal care. Survival after delivery at 22 weeks' gestation is anecdotal and is frequently associated with profound, long-

**Mr Jon Hyett** MRCOG, Specialist Registrar, Department of Obstetrics and Gynaecology, University College Hospital, London WC1E 6AU, UK

**Dr Basky Thilaganathan** MD MRCOG, Senior Lecturer/Consultant and Director, Fetal Medicine Unit, St George's Hospital, Blackshaw Road, London SW17 0QT, UK,

**Table 1** EPICure mortality data

|  | 22 weeks | 23 weeks | 24 weeks | 25 weeks |
|---|---|---|---|---|
| Number of live births | 146 | 263 | 363 | 398 |
| Admissions to NICU | 15% | 54% | 81% | 90% |
|  | (n = 22) | (n = 142) | (n = 294) | (n = 359) |
| Number of survivors to discharge | 2 | 30 | 97 | 186 |
| Survival (% of live-births) | 1.4% | 11.4% | 26.7% | 46.7% |
| Survival (% of admissions) | 9% | 21% | 33% | 52% |

term disability for the child. Although delivery at the margin of neonatal viability is relatively infrequent, perinatal management of these pregnancies will be mainly determined by the anticipated neonatal outcome.

## PERINATAL MORTALITY ASSOCIATED WITH EXTREMELY PREMATURE DELIVERY

Due to the relatively low number of births at the limit of viability, the risk of neonatal mortality cannot be assessed, with any confidence, by a retrospective audit within an individual unit. Until recently, therefore, we have mainly relied on meta-analysis of multiple small studies to produce working estimates of neonatal mortality after extremely premature delivery. However, the retrospective nature of data collection, and the levels of obstetric and neonatal expertise influence these analyses. More recently, the results of a national, prospective multicentre study of extremely premature delivery (EPICure) have become available.[1] EPICure recorded the mortality and morbidity of 837 neonates admitted to NICU between 22 and 25 weeks' gestation (Table 1).

There is a daily improvement in neonatal survival rate of 1–2% between 23–24 weeks' and 3% between 24–25 weeks' gestation. Survival is also significantly

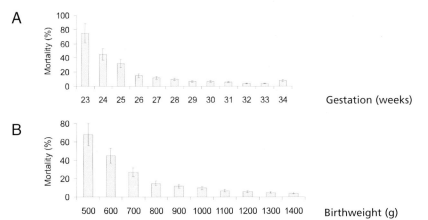

**Fig. 1** Estimated mortality risk by birth weight and gestational age on the basis of singleton infants born in National Institutes of Child Health and Human Development Neonatal Research Network Centers between 1 January 1993 and 31 December 1994. Reproduced with permission of the *American Journal of Obstetrics and Gynecology* from Stevenson et al.[2]

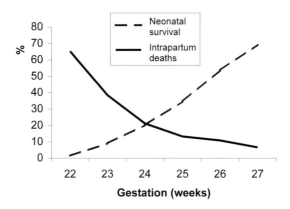

**Fig. 2** Neonatal survival and intrapartum morbidity at the margins of neonatal viability.[3]

associated with increasing birth-weight, female sex and being Afro-Caribbean. With these factors in mind, specific neonatal mortality charts have been established, in an attempt to help clinicians predict survival after preterm delivery (Fig. 1).[2] As fetal weight, sex and ethnicity cannot be altered; these data stress the potential benefit of prolonging gestation by even a few days.

These data also show how the outcome of premature delivery is determined not only by neonatal mortality, but also by the rate of still-birth. Many pregnancies presenting in premature labour with a live fetus at this early gestation will result in still-birth. Most published studies on neonatal outcome ignore the effect of selection before delivery, as they record outcome after live birth or admission to NICU. This so called 'hidden mortality' is due to the decision on the part of the parents and medical staff not to actively intervene in the course of labour (Fig. 2).[3] It is, therefore, evident that obstetric decisions critically influence outcome of extremely premature delivery. Similarly, units that actively intervene at these gestations to effect a live-birth are likely to have increased rates of neonatal mortality and morbidity.

## NEONATAL MORBIDITY IN SURVIVORS OF EXTREMELY PREMATURE DELIVERY

The fact that neurodevelopmental and other disabilities are associated with extremely premature delivery is not in dispute. The definition and diagnosis of disability, timing of the onset of disability and limited numbers of survivors available for study, hinder evaluation of the effects of extremely premature delivery on subsequent handicap. Disabilities include cerebral palsy, blindness, epilepsy and chronic oxygen dependency, as well as learning and attention deficits. These effects are often underestimated by the obstetrician as they are usually only detected with long-term paediatric follow-up.

Whilst the rate of cerebral palsy over the last two decades has remained constant in neonates delivered at term, it has increased 25–30-fold in neonates weighing < 1500 g (Fig. 3).[4] The EPICure study recorded the incidence of specific disabilities at 1-year follow-up in surviving infants (Table 2). Collectively, 11% of infants delivered at 23–25 weeks were reported to be free of any impairment,

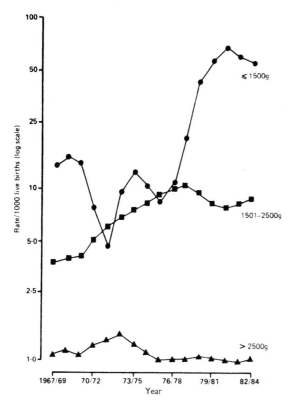

**Fig. 3** Birth-weight specific trends in cerebral palsy. Reproduced with permission of the *Archives of Disease in Childhood* from Pharoah et al.[4]

whilst 29% had major disabilities as defined as abnormal neurology, developmental delay or need for home oxygen.[5] Although the probability of survival in the EPICure cohort depends on gestational age, there were no significant gestation-specific differences in morbidity in survivors.

## AETIOLOGY OF PREMATURE DELIVERY

A recent study in Western Australia reported that 54% of very preterm deliveries (< 33 weeks' gestation) were associated with preterm pre-labour rupture of the

**Table 2** EPICure 1-year morbidity data

|  | 23 weeks | 24 weeks | 25 weeks |
|---|---|---|---|
| Number of infants | 33 | 90 | 177 |
| Abnormal neurology | 6% | 14% | 13% |
| Suspect neurology | 27% | 11% | 11% |
| Severe visual impairment | 12% | 4% | 3% |
| Major neurological problem | 15% | 18% | 18% |
| Developmental delay | 21% | 18% | 16% |
| Home oxygen | 24% | 13% | 7% |
| Cough and wheeze | 33% | 29% | 33% |
| Feeding problems | 27% | 27% | 21% |

membranes or idiopathic preterm labour, 18% with antepartum haemorrhage and 21% with pre-eclampsia.[6] These deliveries, therefore, fall into two groups: (i) pregnancies where labour occurs spontaneously, often with no obvious underlying cause; and (ii) those where pregnancies are interrupted for reasons of maternal or fetal health. The emphasis of management, therefore, differs widely, and these two groups are dealt with separately below.

## SPONTANEOUS PRETERM DELIVERY

Spontaneous premature labour often occurs quickly, frequently presenting out-of-hours and allowing less preparation for the arrival of the premature neonate. Clinical management and further research, therefore, needs to be directed towards the identification of high-risk pregnancies and the development of strategies to prevent and protect against preterm labour. Maternal and fetal evaluation after admission are also important to maximise the chances of normal survival after birth.

### Fetal pulmonary maturation

There is convincing evidence that administration of corticosteroids to mothers prior to premature delivery reduces the incidence of neonatal respiratory distress syndrome, intraventricular haemorrhage and infant mortality. However, a recent meta-analysis of randomised studies did not show a significant benefit at gestations of less than 28 weeks.[7] The most likely reason for the latter finding is the very small number of neonates studied. Indeed, the data from the EPICure trial show that the neonatal survival is significantly associated with use of antenatal steroids, but not with postnatal surfactant therapy.[1] A policy of prophylactic corticosteroid administration to mothers at risk of extremely premature delivery is supported. The value of weekly repeated corticosteroid administration against increased risk of premature delivery has not been scientifically evaluated. The use of repeated corticosteroid administration should be avoided until both the efficacy and safety of the policy is determined.

### Tocolysis

Although there are a number of different agents currently in use, β-adrenergic agonists, such as ritodrine, are the most commonly used tocolytic world-wide. The multifactorial aetiology of preterm labour makes it unlikely that we will find a single drug capable of arresting its course. Ritodrine significantly reduces the number of women that deliver within 24–48 h of commencing administration.[8] The rationale for usage has been that fetal pulmonary maturation can be safely induced in this time period. However, ritodrine use has not been shown to significantly improve perinatal mortality nor have a beneficial effect on birth-weight or prolongation of the pregnancy.

Tocolysis may be most useful in delaying delivery whilst corticosteroids administered upon admission take effect. An immediate concern with the use of such drugs is the considerable adverse maternal effects that could potentially occur. Preliminary results from studies on nitric oxide donors such as glyceryl trinitrate (GTN) suggest that they have a similar efficacy to ritodrine, but with fewer serious adverse maternal effects.[9] That GTN is equally efficacious and a safer drug than ritodrine, remains to be confirmed by larger randomised studies.

## Antibiotics

The policy of routine use of antibiotics for preterm labour and preterm pre-labour rupture of membranes (PPROM) is questionable. Randomised studies have shown little maternal or fetal benefit in the case of preterm labour, whilst in PPROM a reduction in the number of deliveries within one week is not associated with any reduction in perinatal mortality.[10] These findings are not surprising for a number of reasons. Firstly, the diagnosis of premature labour is difficult, as the normal criteria of more frequent and painful contractions with progressive effacement and dilatation of the cervix are often not predictive of imminent delivery. Consequently, the precise diagnostic criteria vary between studies, making direct comparison difficult. Secondly, as treatment is instigated before a pathogen is isolated, blind prophylaxis is used with different drugs being used various studies. Thirdly, dosages are tailored to achieving therapeutic maternal serum levels, although the focus of infection is presumably at the chorio-amniotic interface where drug levels are unknown. Finally, most studies have examined pregnancy outcome before 32 or 37 weeks of pregnancy, rather than examining the effect management around the margins of neonatal viability. It remains to be determined whether the UK ORACLE study is able to produce gestation specific data on the benefits and hazards of antibiotic use.

## Emergency cervical cerclage

Women presenting with painless cervical dilatation, regardless of a previous history of cervical incompetence, are often considered as candidates for emergency cervical cerclage. The low prevalence of this condition and the unexpected nature of its presentation have meant that there is a paucity of scientific information. Most studies are retrospective or observational in nature and invariably have only a few patients. Nevertheless, the data of these studies suggest that there may be significant prolongation of the pregnancy, but considerable infective maternal morbidity.[11] Emergency cervical cerclage should be considered in cases presenting with symptoms and signs suggestive of cervical incompetence.

# PREVENTION OF PRETERM DELIVERY

Various groups have proposed strategies for labelling pregnancies at high risk on the basis of social and environmental factors and the history of both past and present pregnancies. The strongest risk factor is a history of previous preterm birth, making risk assessment less effective for women in their first pregnancy. Even the best forms of assessment are of poor predictive value, placing as many as 15% of women in a high risk group whilst identifying just 40% of pregnancies which deliver before 37 weeks.[6] Numerous other methods of screening have also been suggested, reflecting the various mechanisms purported to cause preterm delivery.

## Genital tract infection

The relationship between lower genital tract infection and preterm labour is well established. Bacterial vaginosis, which describes complex changes in vaginal flora characterised by a predominance of anaerobic organisms, has consistently been found in a high proportion of women with preterm labour.[12] Consequently, it has been suggested that women should be screened and treated for bacterial vaginosis and preliminary reports in a high-risk population showed a significant reduction in the risk of preterm birth.[13] A similar screening and treatment programme in low-risk women did not, however, show a significant reduction in the risk of spontaneous preterm delivery.[14]

## Cervico-vaginal fetal fibronectin assay

Increased levels of fetal fibronectin in cervico-vaginal secretions have also been used as a marker for preterm delivery.[15] This glycoprotein is a component of the extracellular matrix in fetal membranes and its appearance in cervico-vaginal secretions after 20 weeks' gestation may indicate disruption of the interface between the fetal membranes and the uterine wall. Various groups have proposed that increased levels of fetal fibronectin may, therefore, be used either as a screening test to identify pregnancies at high-risk of preterm delivery. Furthermore, fetal fibronectin may have a useful role to play in the diagnosis of preterm labour. In a prospective study of 763 patients attending with threatened preterm labour, a positive fetal fibronectin test was associated with a 26-fold increase in the risk of delivery within the next 7 days.[16]

## Cervical incompetence

Cervical incompetence, defined clinically following repeated painless mid-trimester miscarriage or early preterm birth, is another important, although relatively uncommon cause of preterm birth. There is limited evidence to suggest that the insertion of a cervical suture early in pregnancy is effective in reducing the incidence of preterm delivery.[17]

A recent screening study, of 2,567 low-risk singleton pregnancies showed that the relative risk of preterm delivery increased as the cervical length at 23 weeks decreased.[18] The cervical length was ≤ 15 mm in only 1.7% of the population and this group contained 86% of deliveries ≤ 28 weeks' and 58% of deliveries ≤ 32 weeks' gestation. A sub-analysis of 43 pregnancies with a cervical length ≤ 15 mm suggests that insertion of a Shirodkar suture at this relatively late stage may reduce the future risk of premature delivery 10-fold.[19] These data suggest that measuring cervical length may be a useful method of predicting preterm labour. Furthermore, a short cervix may be indicative of an element of cervical incompetence and insertion of a cervical suture may be helpful in delaying preterm birth.

## Home uterine activity monitoring

Having established a high-risk group, some authors advocate regular monitoring of uterine activity, which can even be done at home with results transferred to the hospital by modem. Patients with a high level of uterine activity can then be treated with bed rest, tocolytics or even antibiotics. There is, however, no evidence that this successfully prevents preterm delivery or improves perinatal outcome.

## IATROGENIC PRETERM DELIVERY

Iatrogenic delivery generally takes place after a period of heightened surveillance, allowing preparation for elective delivery of a premature infant in a unit where senior neonatal support will be readily available. Taking severe pre-eclampsia as an example, aggressive management involves early delivery and is, therefore, associated with a high rate of perinatal mortality and morbidity. Expectant management risks fetal death or asphyxia *in utero* as well as increased neonatal morbidity. A recent study has, however, shown a significantly lower neonatal morbidity with no associated increase in maternal morbidity in pregnancies managed expectantly.[20] Transferring patients to units with high level neonatal facilities, but then managing them conservatively may, therefore, gain most benefit. Collecting patients in this manner concentrates experience and allows expectant management to be pursued more vigorously.

### Uterine artery Doppler screening

The aim of early identification of pregnancies at risk of pre-eclampsia and intra-uterine growth retardation is to increase antenatal surveillance for these particular pregnancy complications. The ultimate aim is to reduce maternal and fetal morbidity through the institution of therapies that have shown promise in disease palliation and/or prevention. Unfortunately, the majority of studies of high-risk women using aspirin or calcium supplementation have been disappointing. The most likely reason for this failure is that a large proportion of normal pregnancies was included in these studies, diluting any possible beneficial effects. Uterine artery Doppler screening is an effective screening tool at 24–26 weeks, but this may be too late for treatment. Unfortunately, in earlier pregnancy, the specificity and positive predictive value of uterine artery Doppler is poorer. It appears that a combination of maternal serum biochemical analysis and uterine artery Doppler may provide effective screening at an early enough stage of pregnancy for the potential benefits of therapy to be realised.[21]

## MULTIPLE PREGNANCY

Epidemiological studies show that multiple pregnancies have a significantly increased risk of preterm delivery. A study of 33,873 women who delivered between 1982–1986 showed that whilst preterm birth affected 9.6% of singleton pregnancies, it affected 54% of multiple gestations.[22] Whilst only 2.6% of all neonates born were twins, they represented 12.2% of all preterm infants and were born at significantly earlier gestations. The mortality of twins born before 28 weeks of gestation was 1.6 times higher than that of singleton pregnancies, but survivors did not have a higher rate of major handicap.

Simple measures, such as a policy of encouraging mothers of twins to finish work early (by 28 weeks of gestation), reducing their level of activity and

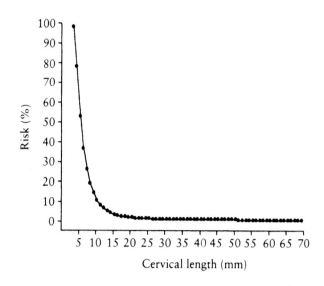

**Fig. 4** Risk of spontaneous delivery at ≤ 32 weeks according to cervical length at 23 weeks of gestation. Reproduced with permission of *Ultrasound in Obstetrics and Gynecology* from Heath et al.[19]

education about preterm birth have been shown to significantly decrease its incidence, particularly before 34 weeks of gestation. The importance of reducing activity is reinforced by recent findings of transvaginal ultrasound, which show that, at later gestations, the cervix shortens by up to 30% upon standing.[23] A prospective randomised study of twin pregnancies showed that the addition of home uterine monitoring to patient education about preterm labour led to higher numbers of women seeking early medical advice, allowing suppression of labour and improving pregnancy outcome.[24] Fetal fibronectin appears to be as sensitive a marker for preterm labour in multiple pregnancies as it is in high-risk studies of singleton pregnancies, but there is no data concerning the effectiveness of subsequent intervention. Assessment of cervical length by transvaginal ultrasound is better than digital examination for predicting birth before 34 weeks of gestation, but is not as sensitive a test as it is with singleton pregnancies.[25]

More recently, it has been shown that chorionicity is an important determinant of pregnancy outcome. Chorionicity can be accurately determined by transabdominal ultrasound at 10–14 weeks of pregnancy[26]. Monochorionic twins are all monozygotic and are associated with a higher incidence of mortality and morbidity than dichorionic twin pregnancies.[27] Fetal loss before 24 weeks of gestation is 6 times higher in monochorionic twins whilst the risk of perinatal mortality, delivery before 32 weeks and low birth-weight doubles (Fig. 4). Twin–twin transfusion syndrome appears to be one of the main aetiological factors increasing the morbidity and mortality of monochorionic twins. This condition is caused by in imbalance of placental perfusion and results in severe growth restriction in the donor twin and high output cardiac failure in the recipient. The increased cardiac output of the recipient results in polyhydramnios, which leads to premature delivery of two infants that are already compromised. If chorionicity is determined early in

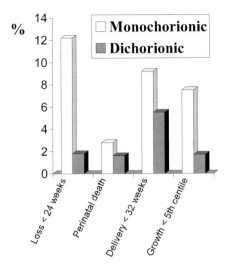

**Fig. 5** The hidden mortality and morbidity of monochorionic twins.[27]

pregnancy, surveillance for monochorionic pregnancies can be increased and acute second trimester twin–twin transfusion is more likely to be recognised. Although further treatment of this condition continues to be the subject of much debate, pregnancy outcome may be improved (Fig. 5).[28]

## MODE OF DELIVERY

The optimal mode of delivery at extremely premature gestations is not known. Randomised studies and meta-analyses have too few patients to make any firm conclusions. The merits, therefore, of an elective Caesarean section policy over an expectant approach, remain to be established. Furthermore, there is considerable maternal mortality and morbidity associated with operative delivery at this gestation. The dangers of tocolytics, anaesthetics, classical Caesarean section and maternal sepsis secondary to chorioamnionitis should not be ignored when decisions about extremely premature delivery are made.

## NEONATAL CARE

The care of pregnancies at risk of preterm delivery before 28 weeks should take place in a hospital with appropriate experience. The rarity of such deliveries and the financial implications of such health care delivery, make it necessary that this level of perinatal care is only available in certain units. The level of experience is extremely influential in dictating outcome. In a national survey of extremely premature deliveries in Sweden, the perinatal mortality rate was 30% in tertiary centres and 46% in level IIa units with full perinatal services.[29]

The outcome of infants born at extremely premature gestations, who have required full cardiopulmonary resuscitation at delivery, is so poor that it is doubtful whether it should be routinely attempted.[30] Reports so far have shown that there are few survivors after the use of vasopressor drugs in the first week of life after extremely premature delivery. Any such survivors inevitably stand an extremely high risk of subsequent severe handicap. Careful consideration should, therefore, be given before advocating a routine policy of aggressive cardiopulmonary resuscitation at this gestation.[31]

## DECIDING ON PERINATAL MANAGEMENT

### Medical role

Once extremely premature delivery is thought to be inevitable, the gestational age and conditions predisposing to the delivery should be assessed. The data presented in this review allow obstetricians and neonatologists to crudely evaluate the likelihood of neonatal survival and probability of long-term handicap. It would appear appropriate from the available evidence to discourage active treatment at a 22 week delivery and to encourage parents expecting delivery of a 26 week fetus to take up intensive neonatal care.

The management at 23–25 weeks, however, presents far more difficulties. Although, intensive care cannot be denied to these neonates, an approach that considers the risks from an obstetric, neonatal and parental perspective is advocated. Set guidelines, however, are inappropriate, as they do not allow flexibility for unexpected outcomes such as a 23 week neonate born with good vital signs, or a 25 week neonate requiring full cardiopulmonary support. Policies for management must also be emergent to allow for developments in the late neonatal period, such as germinal layer or intraventricular haemorrhage, parenchymal cysts and hydrocephalus.

Due to the time involved in collating and reporting this information, current practice is based on the evidence of the early 1990s, before the development and widespread use of technologies such as artificial surfactant, nitric oxide, extra-corporeal membrane oxygenation and oscillatory ventilation. It is, therefore, important that we keep sight of the changing limit of viability associated with advances in neonatology. As survival at earlier gestations improves, our per-ception of the limit of viability must change.[32] It is also difficult to produce a concise definition of 'viability', as this must address ethical and legal, as well as medical issues.[32,33] It would, therefore, seem sensible to ensure that data are also recorded at the margin of viability, including births at 22 weeks and less than 500 g.

### Parental decisions

Parents have established preconceptions about the value and prognosis of extremely premature delivery. As the latter is a relatively rare event, it is unlikely that many will have relatives or friends who have been through a similar pregnancy. Often the media presents the only consistent, widely available and believable source of information. This is naturally biased towards 'miracle' births, is anecdotal in nature and rarely spells out the details of negative outcome. Sadly, little is done to contradict the popular belief that extremely premature delivery is associated with good outcome, until the parents are facing the prospect of delivery. Doctors are equally culpable of unintentional misinformation: NICUs often have boards full of pictures showing smiling faces of survivors, but rarely remind us that just as many neonates did not survive.

The obstetrician and neonatologist should provide accurate information about maternal risks and neonatal outcome, so that parents may develop realistic expectations. Parents' decision making is complicated by a numerous factors such as previous experiences, prior expectations, perceived risks and even religious and cultural beliefs. Providing information alone is unhelpful, without ensuring that parents comprehend the full extent of the potential problems associated with extremely premature delivery. The information communicated at this highly emotionally charged time is critical in influencing the parents' final decisions. This must be managed in a sensitive manner, so as not to damage the trust that is implicit to the patient–doctor relationship. The parents will disregard any information provided no matter how well intentioned, if they do not trust their carers. Often, it is the latter situation that leads to difficult ethical dilemmas, such as parents requesting full cardio-pulmonary resuscitation in a 22 week neonate, or withdrawal of care in an 800 g, 25 week female neonate that has already received steroids antenatally.

## CONCLUSIONS

The management of pregnancy at risk of extremely premature delivery is complicated by our inability to accurately predict the neonatal outcome. Therefore, access to intensive care cannot be denied to these neonates, but rather we should advocate a consultative approach to care in these situations. The key to effective management is provision of accurate information to the parents and ascertaining that their expectations are realistic for the outcome of the pregnancy. Based on available information, the obstetrician, neonatologist and parents should be encouraged to plan an individual course of management for the mother and neonate. These plans should be emergent, to allow clinicians to be flexible about unexpected or unpredictable clinical situations.

### References

1  Costeloe K for the EPICure Study Group. EPICure: Survival and morbidity of extremely preterm infants at discharge from hospital. (Program Issue, Annual Meeting of the American Pediatric Society and Society for Pediatric Research). Pediatr Res 1998; 43: Abstract 1230

2  Stevenson D K, Wright L L, Lemons J A et al. Very low birth weight outcomes of the National Institutes of Child Health and Human Development Neonatal Research Network; January 1993 to December 1994. Am J Obstet Gynecol 1998; 179: 1632–1639

3  Tin W, Wariyar U, Hey E. Changing prognosis for babies of less than 28 weeks' gestation in the North of England between 1983 and 1994. Northern Neonatal Network. BMJ 1997; 314: 107–111

4  Pharoah P O D, Cooke T, Cooke R W I, Rosenbloom L. Birthweight specific trends in cerebral palsy. Arch Dis Child 1990; 65: 602–606

5  Marlow N for the EPICure Study Group. EPICure: Health status of survivors of extreme prematurity at one year. (Program Issue, Annual Meeting of the American Pediatric Society and Society for Pediatric Research). Pediatr Res 1998; 43: Abstract 1288

6  Lockwood C J. The diagnosis of preterm labor and the prediction of preterm delivery. Clin Obstet Gynecol 1995; 38: 675–687

7  Crowley P. Corticosteroids prior to preterm delivery. In: Enkin M W, Keirse M J N C, Renfrew M J, Neilson J P. (eds) Pregnancy and Childbirth Module of the Cochrane Database of Systematic Reviews. Updated quarterly, London: BMJ Publishing

8  Preterm Labor Investigators Group. Treatment of preterm labour with the beta-adrenergic agonist ritodrine. N Engl J Med 1992; 327: 308–312

9  Black R S, Lees C C, Thompson C et al. Fetal and maternal cardiovascular effects of transdermal glyceryl trinitrate versus intravenous ritodrine in acute tocolysis. Obstet Obstet Gynecol 1999; 94: 572–576

10  Crowley P. Antibiotics in preterm labour with intact membranes. In: Enkin M W, Keirse M J N C, Renfrew M J, Neilson J P. (eds) Pregnancy and Childbirth Module of the Cochrane Database of Systematic Reviews. Updated quarterly, London: BMJ Publishing

11  Olatunbosun O A, al Nuaim L, Turnell R W. Emergency cerclage compared with bed rest for advanced cervical dilatation in pregnancy. Int Surg 1995; 80: 170–174

12  Hillier S L, Nugent R P, Eschenbach D A et al. Association between bacterial vaginosis and preterm delivery of a low-birth-weight infant. N Engl J Med 1995; 333: 1737–1742

13  Hauth J C, Goldenberg R L, Andrews W W, DuBard M B, Copper R L. Reduced incidence of preterm delivery with metronidazole and erythromycin in women with bacterial vaginosis. N Engl J Med 1995; 333: 1732–1736

14  McDonald H M, O'Loughlin J A, Vigneswaran R et al. Impact of metronidazole therapy on preterm birth in women with bacterial vaginosis flora (*Gardnerella vaginalis*): a randomised, placebo controlled trial. Br J Obstet Gynaecol 1997; 104: 1391–1397

15  Jones G, Poston L. The diagnostic accuracy of cervico-vaginal fetal fibronectin in predicting preterm delivery: an overview. Br J Obstet Gynaecol 1998; 105: 244

16  Peaceman A M, Andrews W W, Thorp J M et al. Fetal fibronectin as a predictor of preterm birth in patients with symptoms: a multicentre study. Am J Obstet Gynecol 1997; 177: 13–18

17  Anonymous. Final report of the Medical Research Council/Royal College of Obstetricians and Gynaecologists multicentre randomised trial of cervical cerclage. MRC/RCOG Working Party on Cervical Cerclage. Br J Obstet Gynaecol 1993; 100: 516–523

18  Heath V C F, Southall T R, Souka A P, Elisseou A, Nicolaides K H. Cervical length at 23 weeks of gestation: prediction of spontaneous preterm delivery. Ultrasound Obstet Gynecol 1998; 12: 312–317

19  Heath V C F, Souka A P, Erasmus I, Gibb D M F, Nicolaides K H. Cervical length at 23 weeks of gestation: the value of Shirodkar suture for the short cervix. Ultrasound Obstet Gynecol 1998; 12: 318–322

20  Sibai B M, Mercer B M, Schiff E, Friedman S A. Aggressive versus expectant management of severe pre-eclampsia at 28–32 weeks' gestation: randomized controlled trial. Am J Obstet Gynecol 1994; 171: 818–822

21  Konchak P S, Bernstein I M, Capeless M D. Uterine artery Doppler velocimetry in the detection of adverse obstetric outcomes in women with unexplained elevated maternal serum $\alpha$-fetoprotein levels. Am J Obstet Gynecol 1995; 173: 1115–1119

22  Gardner M O, Goldenberg R L, Cliver S P, Tucker J M, Nelson K G, Copper R L. The origin and outcome of preterm twin pregnancies. Obstet Gynecol 1995; 85: 553–557

23  Arabin B, Aardenburg R, van Eyck J. Maternal position and ultrasonic cervical assessment in multiple pregnancy. Preliminary observations. J Reprod Med 1997; 42: 719–724

24  Dyson D C, Crites Y M, Ray D A, Armstrong M A. Prevention of preterm birth in high-risk patients: the role of education and provider contact versus home uterine monitoring. Am J Obstet Gynecol 1991; 164: 756–762

25  Crane J M, Van den Hof M, Armson B A, Liston R. Transvaginal ultrasound in the prediction of preterm delivery: singleton and twin gestations. Obstet Gynecol 1997; 90: 357–363

26  Sepulveda W, Sebire N J, Hughes K, Odibo A, Nicolaides K H. The lambda sign at 10–14 weeks of gestation as a predictor of chorionicity in twin pregnancies. Ultrasound Obstet Gynecol 1996; 7: 421–423

27  Sebire N J, Snijders R J, Hughes K, Sepulveda W, Nicolaides K H. The hidden mortality of monochorionic twin pregnancies. Br J Obstet Gynaecol 1997; 104: 1203–1207

28  Ville Y, Hecher K, Gagnon A, Sebire N, Hyett J, Nicolaides K. Endoscopic laser coagulation in the management of severe twin-to-twin transfusion syndrome. Br J Obstet Gynaecol 1998; 105: 446–453

29  Finnstrom O, Olausson P O, Sedin G et al. The Swedish national prospective study on extremely low birthweight infants. Incidence, mortality, morbidity and survival in relation to level of care. Acta Paediatr 1997; 87: 503–511

30  Sims D G, Heal C A, Bartle S M. Use of adrenaline and atropine in neonatal resuscitation. Arch Dis Child 1994; 70: F3–F9
31  O'Shea T M, Kothadia J M, Roberts D D, Dillard R G. Perinatal events and the risk of intraparenchymal echodensity in very-low-birthweight neonates. Paediatr Perinat Epidemiol 1998; 12: 408–412
32  Dunn P M, Stirrat G M. Capable of being born alive? Lancet 1984; i: 553–535
33  Morrison J J, Rennie J M. Changing the definition of perinatal mortality. Lancet 1995; 346: 1038

*Nahid Siraj  Richard Johanson*

# The second stage of labour

In this chapter, we aim to review the literature on the management of the second stage of labour, including reference to relatively common management issues as well as more specialised 'complications' of labour.

The second stage of labour is diagnosed when the fetal head is visible at the introitus or when there are other signs of full dilatation, such as perineal stretching, blood stained discharge or anal dilatation. Vaginal examination can be performed earlier if the mother experiences an urge to bear down or if there are changes in the fetal heart rate suggesting increased compression (e.g. early decelerations). Ideally, the second stage should progress smoothly, with a delivery of a live baby without any intervention, but it has been termed the most 'dangerous journey a human ever undertakes'. In some labours, 'watchful waiting' is all that is required but in others a variety of 'interventions' may be necessary to avoid fetal or maternal distress.

The Confidential Enquiry into Stillbirths and Deaths in Infancy[1] and a number of medico-legal overviews[2] reinforce the dangers of the second stage of labour. Ignoring abnormal CTGs or attempting instrumental delivery inappropriately in the second stage of labour are the most common causes of medical negligence. The second stage of labour remains a controversial area and, as yet, there are no College guidelines for management. Primary clinical research has covered many aspects of the second stage, and systematic reviews of the current evidence can be found in the Cochrane Library. We have attempted to refer to 'best evidence' wherever possible, but recognise the contributions to individualised decision making that past experience and patient's expectations make.

**Ms Nahid Siraj** MBBS MRCOG, Staff Grade, Obstetrics and Gynaecology Directorate, North Staffordshire Hospital, Newcastle Road, Stoke on Trent ST4 6QG, UK (for correspondence)

**Mr Richard Johanson** BSc MA MD MRCOG, Consultant Obstetrician and Gynaecologist, Obstetrics and Gynaecology Directorate, North Staffordshire Hospital, Newcastle Road, Stoke on Trent ST4

# DURATION OF THE LABOUR

The second stage of labour itself has two phases. The first phase starts with full dilatation and ends when the bearing down efforts start. The second phase is termed 'expulsive'. In most situations, the first phase will be unrecognised, as frequent routine vaginal examinations are no longer undertaken.

The current view appears to be that there should not be any arbitrary limit on the duration of the second stage of labour, providing that maternal and fetal condition remain satisfactory. Terminating the second stage of labour electively, simply on the basis of duration, will increase the incidence of unnecessary instrumental deliveries and caesarean sections.

During the expulsive phase of the second stage, there is a gradual lowering of the umbilical vein and artery pH, with progressive respiratory acidosis and lactic acidemia. Although uncommon, undetected intrapartum asphyxia at this stage may lead to hypoxic ischaemic encephalopathy in the neonate. Adverse maternal outcomes associated with a prolonged second stage include postpartum haemorrhage, puerperal fever, low backache and pelvic floor denervation.[3]

A retrospective review of perinatal morbidity/mortality performed on 6,041 nulliparous women who had reached the second stage of labour with a live singleton, cephalic fetus with a birth-weight of more than 2.5 kg[4] showed that a second stage which lasted more than 3 h was seen in 11% of nulliparous women and of more than 5 h in 2.7%. Despite these prolonged labours, no perinatal deaths unrelated to anomalies occurred and there was no significant relationship between the second stage duration and a low 5 min Apgar score, neonatal seizures or admission to the Neonatal Intensive Care Unit.[4] On the basis of an audit of over 25,000 deliveries in the North West Thames Region, Paterson concluded that it is reasonable to expect multiparous women without epidurals to be delivered within 1 h of onset of the second stage. The duration allowed in multiparous women with epidurals or in nulliparous women (either with or without an epidural) will depend on the rate of the progress.[5] When considering a second stage that is 'prolonged', it is important that factors influencing the duration should be checked, such as parity, use of epidural, fetal position, strength of contractions, fetal size and 'perineal resistance'. Generally, a conservative approach will allow a spontaneous delivery or safer instrumental delivery at a lower station.[4]

## PUSHING

Over the years, the second stage of labour has been thought of as being hazardous to both maternal and fetal well-being. It is not surprising, therefore, that procedures have been developed for shortening the second stage of labour. Common questions asked are when should pushing start, how long should pushing last and how best should a mother push?

Pushing in the expulsive phase of the labour can either be directed or spontaneous (where the patient will follow her own instinct).[6] Traditionally, the Valsalva manoeuvre has been used for directed pushing. At the beginning of each contraction, the woman takes a deep breath, holds it and then pushes against a closed glottis. During this procedure, there is an increase in blood pressure which is followed by hypotension. The fluctuations seen in blood

**Table 1** Forced bearing down in second stage of labour

| | |
|---|---|
| Reduced | Length of labour |
| Increased | Abnormal fetal heart pattern |
| | Low cord pH |
| | Low Agpar score |

pressure during this manoeuvre may result in burst capillaries in the woman's eyes and face.[7] Changes in maternal blood pressure and respiration could also negatively influence utero-placental blood flow and significantly decrease fetal cerebral oxygenation.[8] These effects could be particularly detrimental if the fetus has already been compromised, or if the duration of directed maternal pushing is prolonged.

With 'spontaneous pushing', the woman follows her own instinct. This is frequently characterised by 5–6 pushes during each contraction, with each push lasting an average of 5 s.[9] Most spontaneous bearing down efforts are accompanied by the release of air, with several breaths being taken between each effort. Spontaneous pushing also helps with the gradual distension of the perineum and encourages even distribution of pressure by the presenting part, which may result in fewer tears.[10]

When the fetal head reaches the pelvic floor, it causes perineal stretching, stimulating Ferguson's reflex, which leads to further bearing down efforts. However, the mother can also sense the urge to push when the fetal head is pressing on the rectum or the sacral plexus, if the baby is big or in an 'occipito-posterior' position. The need to bear down does not necessarily correlate with full dilatation of the cervix; therefore, a vaginal examination should be carried out to check dilatation and fetal station. If the head is low, and the woman has an urge to push, she should be encouraged to continue, even if there is still a 'rim' of cervix left. On the other hand, if the cervix is fully dilated but the presenting part remains high, it is thought that the premature urge to push should be discouraged because this will result in maternal exhaustion with a very low chance of spontaneous vaginal delivery (Table 1).

## POSITION

Throughout time, and across all cultures, women have tended to deliver in an upright or all-fours position. French obstetricians, Paré in particular, favoured delivery on a bed and since then delivery in the recumbent position has become standard practice in most supervised deliveries. The different positions (upright, sitting, squatting, kneeling) adopted by women during the second stage of labour have been examined in numerous observational studies. Advantages and disadvantages of the different positions have been discussed (Table 2 and Fig. 1).

**Table 2** Dorsal position – possible disadvantages

| |
|---|
| Compression of the inferior vena cava and aorta |
| Narrower birth canal |
| Loss of gravity |
| Loss of pelvic mobility |
| Inefficient uterine contractions |

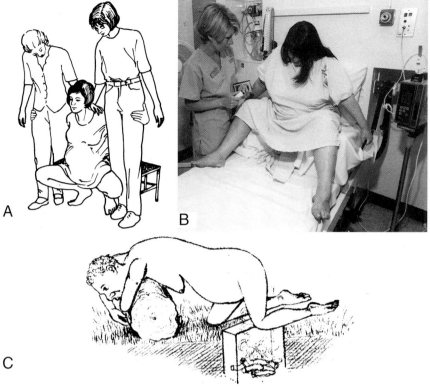

**Fig. 1** Different positions adopted by women during the second stage of labour: (A) squatting; (B) sitting; and (C) 'all fours'

The supine position, because of caval compression will affect utero-placental blood flow and may cause maternal fainting or fetal distress. Therefore, left lateral or semi-recumbent positions are advised to prevent caval compression. However, these positions may be hard to maintain throughout labour and do not increase the crucial pelvic dimensions. The upright position of kneeling has been strongly recommended,[11] as it increases the subpubic space, allowing a more anterior passage of the presenting part and putting less pressure on the perineum. Squatting has been advocated to prevent caval compression, increase the diameter of the pelvic outlet and facilitate maternal expulsive effort. As Western women find maintenance of a squatting position difficult, alternatives have been tried. Birthing chairs have been tried in many countries but controlled trials have shown them to be associated with more postpartum haemorrhage and with increased third degree tears.[12] These complications have both been thought to be due to a lack of perineal support. Subsequently a 'birth cushion' has also been introduced, which does give perineal support.[13] This reduces the direct pressure on the perineum by supporting the buttocks and the thighs. It facilitates better co-ordinated and more effective pushing efforts, and is associated with a lower rate of operative delivery and shortened second stage. In another randomised controlled trial,[14] a squatting stool (which allows the mother to sit down in between contractions but to squat whilst pushing) showed no increase in the incidence of postpartum haemorrhage, third degree tears or vulval haematomas in the upright group and again the incidence of episiotomies was lower. A pooled analysis of randomised trials comparing upright versus supine positions for the second stage of labour showed that women who adopted the upright posture, experienced less pain, perineal trauma and fewer episiotomies. Indeed, the overall normal vaginal delivery rate was slightly higher in the upright group.[14]

Changing position during the second stage of labour has been shown to improve the strength of uterine contractions, reducing the incidence of fetal heart rate abnormalities and, therefore, also reducing the risk of instrumental delivery.[15] Care-givers should help and encourage labouring women to change positions during labour rather than simply keeping to the semirecumbent position on the bed. However, as in other areas, maternal choice is important. Evidence-based information leaflets on position for delivery are available from the Midwives Information and Resource Service (MIDIRS).[16]

During antenatal classes, women should have the opportunity to discuss the different positions for labour and for delivery. It may also be useful for women to know that maternal position in the latter part of pregnancy can affect fetal position. If the fetus is lying in an occipito-posterior or occipito-lateral position, it may lead to a prolonged and painful labour and difficult delivery. A single trial has shown promising short term effects of using 'hand and knees' posture during late pregnancy when the fetus is in this position. However, no large studies have yet been undertaken to prove its true effectiveness.[15]

## EPISIOTOMY

Episiotomy was first described by Auld in the 18th Century. By the early 1970s, it had become a widely accepted obstetric intervention performed by midwives and obstetricians throughout the world. As the practice has steadily increased, the use of episiotomy has been rightfully questioned. This is an operative procedure which is associated with increased blood loss and increased haematoma, infection and abscess formation, leading to increased early and late morbidity. Over the years, suggested maternal benefits of episiotomy have been a reduction in the incidence of 3rd and 4th degree perineal tears, the preservation of perineal muscle function and a reduction in fetal asphyxia, cranial trauma and cerebral haemorrhage. A recent Cochrane Systematic Review[17] has examined the practice of liberal versus restricted use of episiotomy. This meta-analysis of five randomised controlled trials involved 4650 women having a vaginal birth. Restricted use of episiotomy, when compared with liberal episiotomy use, was found to be associated with a reduced risk of posterior perineal trauma. There was, however, an increased risk of anterior vaginal and labial trauma. No differences in pain, dyspareunia or urinary incontinence were found. There were no differences seen between the restricted and liberal groups in terms of postpartum perineal pain, or in urinary and pelvic floor symptoms.[18] In a subgroup where perineometry and electromyograms were undertaken, no differences were seen. On the other hand, there is no evidence that routine episiotomy prevents intra-cranial haemorrhage or intrapartum asphyxia. In a review which included observational studies and longer term follow-up, Renfrew and co-workers were certain that use of episiotomy should be restricted to essential indications.[19]

In terms of achieving a 'normal delivery with an intact perineum', changing positions during labour may be of value. Other factors include a reduction in the

**Table 3**  How to avoid long-term morbidity

| |
|---|
| Intact perineum |
| Restricted versus liberal episiotomy |

use of epidurals,[20] physiological pushing during the second stage of labour (which is associated with less fetal distress than directed pushing) and perineal trauma is less with the use of Ventouse rather than forceps.[21] Judicious use of episiotomy remains advisable when there is a 'rigid' perineum causing increased tissue resistance and a delay in the spontaneous vaginal delivery, or if there is fetal distress (marked by a prolonged fetal bradycardia or late decelerations during the 'perineal phase' of the second stage of labour), when delivery does not seem to be imminent (Table 3).

## USE OF EPIDURAL ANALGESIA

Epidural analgesia is undoubtedly an effective form of pain relief. It does carry risks, however, some of which are related to its mode of action. The pain of the second stage of labour is transmitted by the second, third and fourth sacral spinal segments. A complete blockage of this pathway will relax the pelvic floor muscles, which may delay the rotation of the fetal head and, by diminishing the bearing down reflex, decrease the efficiency of maternal pushing effort, prolonging the second stage and increasing the need for oxytocin administration and instrumental delivery.[22] Epidural analgesia may also be linked to an increase in uterine infection.[23]

However, despite early suggestions to the contrary,[20] epidural analgesia does not appear to be associated with an increase in caesarean section for failure to progress.[24] Delayed pushing during the second stage of labour can increase the rate of spontaneous vaginal delivery[22] and reduce the rate of instrumental deliveries.[25] It is also possible for an epidural to be sited for the first time during the second stage of labour. For example, this might be when the cervix is fully dilated but the presenting part remains high with associated maternal distress, or if there are premature bearing down efforts due to the malposition of the fetus. In this situation, the epidural should abolish the premature urge to push and may allow spontaneous descent of the fetal head.[20]

## USE OF SYNTOCINON

Although the cervix is fully dilated, the head may fail to descend in the second stage due to inefficient uterine contractions (particularly in the primigravid patient). The main objection raised in respect of using oxytocin in the second stage of labour is the risk of cephalopelvic disproportion and uterine rupture.[26] O'Driscoll and co-workers,[27] in a study of 1000 consecutive cases, showed an incidence of cephalopelvic disproportion of 1% and no cases of uterine rupture in primigravid patients. Use of oxytocin in the second stage of labour will facilitate normal delivery and reduce the need for rotation or forceps delivery.[28] Care should be taken in using oxytocin in the second stage of labour in multiparous women, and in those with a previous caesarean section.

## FETAL DISTRESS DURING THE SECOND STAGE OF LABOUR

In the second stage of labour, the CTG will frequently show deceleratory changes which may be physiological. Early decelerations occur in 16.2% of traces during the last 30 min of labour.[28] These result from head compression and have been shown to be associated with a normal fetal acid/base status.[29] Isolated episodes of fetal bradycardia or fetal tachycardia occurring in otherwise normal fetal heart rate patterns are probably not worrying on their own; but, if associated with decreased variability or decelerations, then it is important to expedite delivery or to perform a fetal blood sample (if the patient is in the early phase of the second stage of labour). The incidence of variable decelerations during the second stage of labour is almost 50%.[28] Cord compression is considered to be an important cause and persistent or worsening variable decelerations will require delivery. Late decelerations occur in only 4.4% of cases during the last 30 min of the labour.[28] Persistent late decelerations in the second stage of labour are an indication for delivery of the fetus. Despite these recommendations, only a third of worrying CTGs will be associated with acidosis.[30] In many cases, fetal blood sampling in the second stage of labour is justifiable, as it may avoid unnecessary instrumental delivery or caesarean section.

## OCCIPITO POSTERIOR POSITION

The occipito posterior position has been found to be associated with a number of factors, including an anthropoid pelvis, inefficient uterine contractions, the use of epidural and an anterior placenta. When the head engages, the occiput is usually lateral but will rotate anteriorly during labour in four cases out of five. In those where the occiput is posterior, the sagittal suture will most commonly be in the right oblique diameter. If flexion increases during labour, the occiput will become the leading part, rotating anteriorly when it reaches the pelvic floor. In describing this rotation, much emphasis has traditionally been placed on different pelvic types.[31] However, the importance of pelvic tone is now becoming more widely recognised. High dose epidural blocks are associated with an increased risk of occipito posterior position and the need for rotational forceps. It is recognised that such mechanical problems may be overcome by efficient uterine action.[27,32] When deflexion persists, or increases, the bregma will be the part which reaches the pelvic floor first, by which it will be rotated forwards, causing a persistent occipito posterior position. In some patients with a persistent occipito posterior fetus, the presenting part descends further without rotation and is spontaneously born 'face to pubis'. Persistent occipito posterior occurs in approximately 4.5% of deliveries.[33]

Gardberg and Tuppurainen[34] analysed labours complicated by persistent occipito posterior position in a retrospective review of 3648 deliveries. The average duration of both first and second stages of labour were significantly increased in the occipito posterior deliveries. The frequency of operative interventions; vacuum extraction, forceps and caesarean section were all increased. Dystocia was the main cause given for caesarean delivery. Pearl and co-workers[35] found a high incidence of severe perineal laceration and episiotomy in their occipito posterior position group and also an increased incidence of Erb's palsy and facial nerve palsy following forceps delivery in this group. Sultan and

**Pre-requisites for delivery with the Ventouse**
1. Full dilatation of the cervix and full engagement of the head
2. Co-operation of the patient
3. Good contractions should be present

**Basic rules for delivery with the Ventouse**
1. The delivery should be completed within 15 min of application
2. The head, not just the scalp, should descend with each pull
3. The cup should be re-applied no more than twice (and after one detachment an experienced operator should be summoned)
4. If failure with the Ventouse occurs despite good traction do not try the forceps as well

co-workers[36] found that the occipito posterior position at delivery significantly increased the risk of third degree obstetric anal sphincter tears. High cervical spinal cord injury in neonates has been reviewed from two tertiary care centre hospitals in Canada and the common feature in all cases was a forceps delivery with a rotation from an occipito posterior presentation.[37]

If the fetal head is low in the pelvic cavity, then the baby can be delivered in the direct OP position; however, if the occipito posterior position is diagnosed in the early phase of the second stage of labour, then the head should be allowed to descend and rotate if needed with syntocinon. Epidural analgesia can be offered as it will stop the premature urge to push, and also provide an effective form of analgesia if instrumental delivery is needed. If a baby in an occipito posterior position requires delivery when the head is still in the mid-cavity, then clinical judgement should be used before attempting a trial of vacuum or forceps. There is no place for forceful instrumental delivery.

## INSTRUMENTAL DELIVERY

The major hazard of instrumental delivery, with either the Ventouse or forceps is injury to mother and/or baby. Fetal injury more often than not is associated with failure to deliver and multiple instrumentation. To minimise the chances of any maternal or fetal damage, the basic rules for delivery with the Ventouse should be followed (Table 4).

### Causes and management of failure to deliver with the Ventouse

It has been suggested that failure rates of less than 1% should be achieved with well-maintained apparatus and correct technique (Table 5).[38,39] However, in routine practice, Johanson and co-workers[40] achieved a vaginal delivery with the first instrument used in 86% of cases. Each of the following factors contributed to the failures:

1. *Failure to use the correct cup type. Failures with the silicone rubber cup group will be common if it is used inappropriately when there is deflexion of the head, excess caput, a big baby or a prolonged second stage of labour.*
2. *Inadequate initial assessment of the case: (i) the head being too high – a classic mistake is to assume that because caput can be felt below the ischial spines the*

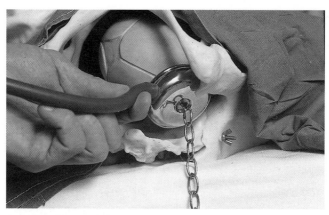

**Fig. 4**   Inserting the 'posterior' Ventouse cup

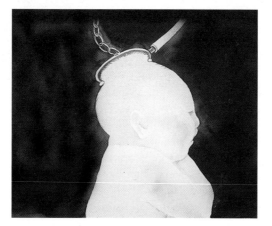

**Fig. 5**   Correct application of 'posterior' Ventouse cup

*head must be engaged; or (ii) mis-diagnosis of the position and attitude of the head – attention to simple detail will minimise the occurrence of this problem.*

3. *Either too anterior or lateral placements will increase the failure rate.[41] If the cup placement is found to be incorrect, it may be appropriate to begin again with correct placement; mid-line over the occiput.*

4. *Failures due to traction in the wrong direction. These may be amenable simply to a change in angle of traction.*

5. *Excessive caput. Rarely even with the metal cups adequate traction is not possible because of excessive caput. Careful consideration in these cases must be given to delivery by Caesarean section unless the head is well down, in which case forceps can be used.*

6. *Poor maternal effort. There is no doubt that maternal effort can contribute substantially to the success of the delivery. Adequate encouragement and instruction should be given to the mother.*

7. *The incidence of (true failure) is low and usually secondary to outlet contraction.*

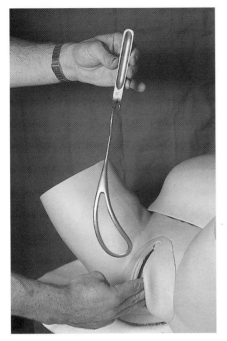

**Fig. 6** Application of forceps blade

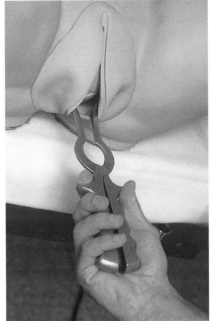

**Fig. 7** Correct pull with forceps

## Pre-requisites for delivery with forceps

1. *It is essential that the head is fully engaged on abdominal palpation. This is particularly important with a face presentation.*

2. *It is generally advised that catheterisation and an episiotomy are required for forceps delivery.*

3. *It is essential that the position of the head is carefully noted. If occipito-transverse or occipito-posterior complications are more likely.*

4. *It is essential that the operator checks the forceps pair that he/she has been given. It may be useful to check the maximum diameter between the two blades as well (a pair that is not true will have maximum diameter as little as 7 or 7.5 cm. The maximum diameter should be at least 9 cm).*

5. *The blades must lock easily. Do not force them to close.*

6. *The first pull is downwards and then upwards. If the head does not descend, consider whether the station is higher than first thought or whether the position is occipito posterior.*

**Table 5** Avoiding instrumental delivery

Many thousands of deliveries could be avoided each year
Companionship/fetal blood sampling/better management of epidurals/more leniency in terms of defining prolongation of labour

## TWIN DELIVERY

Many authors recommend using an epidural for twin labours and delivery. If the accommodation of twins is anything other than vertex–vertex, this can be justified in terms of analgesia for possible intrauterine manipulations required in the 2nd stage for delivery of the second twin. Alternatively, having an anaesthetist present and ready to administer anaesthesia if complications arise is a satisfactory alternative.

Although this combination of vertex–vertex is considered low-risk and will most frequently be delivered by a midwife, an obstetrician should be present as complications with delivery of the second twin can occur. Delivery of the first twin is undertaken in the usual manner and, thereafter, the majority of second twins would have been delivered within 15 min.[42]

After the delivery of the first twin, abdominal palpation should be performed to assess the lie of the second twin. It is helpful to use ultrasound for confirmation, which is also useful for checking the fetal heart rate. If the lie is longitudinal with a cephalic presentation, one should wait until the head is descending then perform amniotomy with a contraction. If contractions do not ensue within 5–10 min after delivery of the first twin, then an oxytocin infusion should be started. If an assisted delivery becomes necessary, then the vacuum extractor has a number of advantages. It may be applied at a higher station than the forceps and causes less vaginal or perineal trauma. If the cervix is no longer fully dilated, using a 4 cm cup may be easier.

If the second twin is non-vertex (which occurs in about 40% of twins), vaginal delivery is considered safe. Rabinovici and co-workers[43] carried out a randomised study of vaginal and caesarean deliveries where the second twin's presentation was non-vertex. Although the study only included 60 twins, the results showed no difference in 5 min Apgar scores, or in any other indices of neonatal morbidity between the two groups. There are numerous other reports on the safety of vaginal delivery for non-vertex second twin. Laros[44] had no fetal losses in either group of second twins, with 74 being delivered by caesarean and 76 being delivered vaginally. Chervenak and co-workers[45] examined a series of 93 vertex/breech and 46 transverse twin combinations. Amongst the babies that delivered vaginally weighing more than 1500 g, there were no cases of neonatal death or intra ventricular haemorrhage. Fishman and co-workers[46] reviewed 390 vaginally-delivered second twins and reported no significant differences in neonatal outcome between vaginal breech and vaginal vertex.

If the second twin is a breech, the membranes can be ruptured once the breech is fixed in the birth canal. A total breech extraction should be performed if fetal distress occurs or if a footling breech is encountered. Complications are less likely if the membranes are not ruptured until the feet are held by the operator. Where the fetus is transverse, external cephalic version can be successful in over 70% of cases.[47] The fetal heart rate should be closely monitored and ultrasound can be helpful to demonstrate the final position of the baby. If external cephalic version is unsuccessful, given that the operator is experienced, an internal podalic version can be undertaken.

The technique used for internal podalic version has been described by Rabinovici and co-workers.[48] A fetal foot is identified by recognising a heel through intact membranes. The foot is grasped and pulled gently and continuously lower into the birth canal. The membranes are ruptured as late as possible. This procedure is easiest when the transverse lie is with the back superior or posterior. If the back is inferior or if the limbs are not immediately palpable, ultrasound may help to show the operator where they would be found. This will minimise the unwanted experience of bringing down a fetal hand in the mistaken belief that it is a foot.

Many clinicians choose caesarean section when the first twin presents as a breech, because of concern about 'interlocking'. However, this complication is extremely rare. Cohen and co-workers[49] reported 'interlocking' occurring only once in 817 twin pregnancies. Oettinger and co-workers[50] compared the outcome of breech presenting twins over two time periods where the caesarean section rate increased from 21% to almost 95%, and found no change in neonatal morbidity or mortality. They did, however, find an increase in maternal morbidity in association with a caesarean section delivery.

## BREECH DELIVERY

As in cephalic presenting births, a vaginal breech delivery is more likely to be successful if both mother is not 'too small' and the baby not 'too big'.[51,52] The presentation should be either frank (hips flexed, knees extended) or complete (hips flexed, knees flexed but feet not below the fetal buttocks). The literature shows a significantly increased mortality/morbidity in footling breech, due principally to an increased incidence of cord prolapse, and entrapment of the after coming head by an incompletely dilated cervix.[52] There should be no evidence of feto-pelvic disproportion, with a pelvis clinically thought to be adequate and an estimated fetal weight of <4000 g (ultrasound or clinical measurement).[52] In some smaller women, it may be appropriate to exclude a vaginal breech option where the estimated fetal weight is < 4000 g. Although X-ray pelvimetry has figured prominently in protocols for planned vaginal birth, none of these studies was able to confirm the value of this examination in selecting those women who were more likely to succeed in a trial of labour or to have any effect on perinatal outcome.[52] There should be no evidence of hyperextension of the fetal head and fetal abnormalities should have been searched for.[52,53] In the Canadian consensus on breech management at term, it was felt that that trial of labour should only be precluded with medical/obstetric complications which are likely to be associated with mechanical difficulties at delivery.[52] Examples would be medical conditions where the mother was not allowed to push or where the pelvis was known to be contracted. Ophir and co-workers[54] offered 66% of patients with a previous caesarean section a trial of labour of whom 79% delivered their breech infants vaginally.

In the Canadian consensus of breech management at term,[52] further guidelines on intrapartum management have been drawn up. Careful monitoring of fetal well-being and progress of labour are emphasised without being absolute. For example, there is no evidence that epidural analgesia is essential, indeed it does not offer any unique advantage for term breech pregnancy and may be associated with prolongation of the 2nd stage.[55] In selected cases, induction or augmentation may be justified.[52] Fetal blood sampling from the buttocks provides an accurate assessment of the acid/base status (when the fetal heart rate trace is suspect).[56] It has been suggested that all operators should be given training to be able to undertake a symphysiotomy should the head be entrapped.[57,58]

Although much emphasis is placed on adequate case selection prior to labour, a recent survey of outcome of the undiagnosed breech in labour managed by experienced medical staff showed that safe vaginal delivery can be achieved.[59]

## PROLAPSED CORD

Traditionally, management of umbilical cord prolapse has included the knee-chest or Trendelenburg positioning and manual elevation of the presenting part of the fetus above the pelvic inlet to relieve cord compression. However, an important advance in the management of umbilical cord prolapse has been the development of 'bladder filling'. Bladder filling was first proposed by Vago in 1970[60] as a method of relieving pressure on the umbilical cord. Bladder filling raises the presenting part of the fetus off the compressed cord for an extended period of time, thereby eliminating the need for an examiner's fingers to displace the presenting part.[60–62] A number 16 Foley catheter with a 5 ml balloon is placed into the urinary bladder. The bladder is filled via the catheter with about 500 ml normal saline by a standard infusion set. The quantity of saline needed is determined by the removal of cord compression, which will usually occur when the distended bladder appears above the pubis.[60] The balloon is then inflated, the catheter is clamped, and the drainage tubing and urine bag are attached and secured. This procedure has a further advantage in that the full bladder may decrease or inhibit uterine contractions. The bladder is emptied by unclamping the catheter before opening the peritoneal cavity for caesarean delivery.

## SHOULDER DYSTOCIA[63]

The need for rehearsals of simple routines for management of shoulder dystocia has been emphasised in the most recent Confidential Enquiry into Stillbirths and Deaths in Infancy (CESDI) report.[1] A well-tried sequence of steps is as follows:

1. *Call for help.* This includes calling the most experienced obstetrician available, a paediatrician and an anaesthetist.

2. *Episiotomy.* Although it has been suggested that episiotomy does not affect the outcome of shoulder dystocia,[64] there is strong evidence to suggest that the incidence of vaginal lacerations with shoulder dystocia is high and, therefore, doing an episiotomy to reduce the chance of having severe lacerations is recommended. The main reason for recommending doing an episiotomy is to allow the operator more space to use the hollow of the sacrum to deliver the posterior shoulder.

3. *McRobert's manoeuvre.* Both thighs are sharply flexed against the abdomen. This position serves to straighten the sacrum relative to the lumbar vertebrae and causes cephalic rotation of the pelvis to occur which helps

free the impacted shoulder.[65] Lurie and co-workers[66] reviewed 76 cases of shoulder dystocia and found that McRobert's manoeuvre was sufficient to achieve delivery of the impacted shoulder in 67 cases (88%).

4. *Moderate traction and suprapubic pressure.* Suprapubic pressure is applied to displace to reduce the bisacromial diameter and push the anterior shoulder underneath the symphysis pubis.[66] It is important to know where the fetal back lies so that pressure is applied in the right direction. At this stage only moderate downward traction is applied, strong traction as well as fundal pressure should be avoided. Baskett and co-workers[67] stated that increased traction on the head was associated with the greatest degree of neonatal trauma. Gross and co-workers[68] warned against fundal pressure.

5. *Deliver posterior arm and shoulder.* The hand of the operator should be passed up to the fetal axilla and the posterior shoulder should be hooked down (there is always more room in the hollow of the sacrum). Traction on the posterior axilla usually enables the operator to bring the posterior arm within reach. If the cubital fossa is within reach, backward pressure on it will result in disengagement of the arm which can then be brought down, by getting hold of the hand and sweeping it across the chest.[66] This process is similar to the Pinard method of bringing down a leg in breech presentation. This procedure is usually successful. Once the posterior shoulder is down the anterior shoulder is easily disimpacted.

## FACE PRESENTATION

Face presentation commonly prolongs the second stage of labour due to the poor line of thrust between the body and the head of the fetus. Descent is usually followed by internal rotation, with the chin passing anteriorly. It must be remembered that the biparietal diameter is usually approximately 7 cm behind the advancing face, so that even when the face is distending the vulva, the biparietal diameter has only just entered the pelvis. Descent is thus always less advanced than vaginal examination would suggest, even when one allows for the gross oedema which is usually present. The value of abdominal examination in such cases cannot be over stressed.

Anterior rotation having occurred, the neck comes to lie behind the symphysis pubis and the head is born by flexion, causing considerable posterior perineal distension by the occiput in the process. An episiotomy is often necessary to avoid extensive tearing. The shoulders and body are born in the usual way. With a mentoanterior position in labour no interference is necessary whilst satisfactory progress continues. With satisfactory uterine action, spontaneous delivery or easy 'lift out' (forceps only) delivery will ensue in 80% or more cases.

Even with mentoposterior positions, anterior rotation will occur in the second stage in 45–65% of cases, so that persistent mentoposterior position or mentotransverse arrest is encountered in only 10% of face presentations. In cases of persistent mentoposterior position, the neck is too short to span the 12 cm of the anterior aspect of the sacrum. Delivery is usually impossible unless, as can happen with a very small fetus or one which is macerated, the shoulders can enter the pelvis at the same time as the head. A persistent mentoposterior presenting fetus will usually be delivered by caesarean[69] to reduce fetal and maternal morbidity.[70]

## KEY POINTS FOR CLINICAL PRACTICE

- There should not be any arbitrary upper limit for the duration of the second stage of labour

- More attention should be paid during the expulsive phase of the second stage of labour

- Physiological pushing should be encouraged

- Women should be encouraged to adopt different positions to facilitate the delivery of the fetus

- Routine and liberal use of episiotomies cannot be justified

- Oxytocinon can be used in the second stage of labour, if necessary

- Use of epidural is associated with prolonged second stage of labour and increased incidence of instrumental delivery

- If instrumental delivery will not be simple, fetal blood sampling should be carried out for fetal heart rate abnormality in the second stage of labour

- Careful use of both Ventouse and forceps will minimise fetal and maternal injuries

- Vaginal delivery of twins should be considered a safe option

- If labour proceeds without complications, a vaginal breech should remain a possibility

- Prolapsed cord can be managed safely with 'bladder filling'

- Shoulder dystocia routines should be regularly rehearsed

- Face presentation – metoanterior is suitable for forceps delivery

## ACKNOWLEDGEMENTS

We thank Claire Rigby, Clinical Effectiveness Co-ordinator for her assistance and Miss Hema for her helpful comments.

### References

1 Confidential Enquiry into Stillbirths and Deaths in Infancy. London. Maternal and Child Health Research Consortium. 1997
2 Ennis M, Vincent C A. Obstetric accidents: a review of 64 cases. BMJ 1990; 300: 1365–1367
3 Watson V. The duration of the second stage of labour. Modern Midwife 1994; 21–22
4 Menticoglou S M, Manning F, Harman C. Perinatal outcome in relation to second stage duration. Am J Obstet Gynecol 1995; 173: 906–912
5 Paterson C M. The characteristics of the second stage of labour in 25,069 singleton deliveries in the North West Thames health region. Br J Obstet Gynaecol 1992; 9: 377–380

6   Nikodem V C. Sustained (valsalva) vs exhalatory bearing down in 2nd stage of labour [revised 03 October 1993] In: Enkin M W, Keirse M J N C, Renfrew M J, Neilson J P, Crowther C (eds) Pregnancy and Childbirth Module. In: The Cochrane Pregnancy and Childbirth Database [database on disk and CDROM]. The Cochrane Collaboration; Issue 2, Oxford: Update Software; 1995

7   Burns K. The second stage of labour. A battle against tradition. Midwives Chronicle and Nursing Notes 1992; 92–96

8   Aldrich CJ. The effect of maternal pushing on fetal cerebral oxygenataion and blood volume during the second stage of labour. Br J Obstet Gynaecol 1995; 102: 448–453

9   Barnett M, Humerick S. Infant outcome in relation to second stage labour pushing method. Birth 1982; 9: 221–229

10  Way S. To push or not to push? Professional Care of Mother and Child 1991; 53

11  Gardosi J, Sylvester S, B-Lynch C. Alternative positions in the second stage of labor: a randomised controlled trial. Br J Obstet Gynaecol 1989; 96: 1290–1296

12  Nikodem V C  Keirse M J N C , Renfrew M J et al. (eds) Upright vs recumbent position during second stage of labour (Cochrane Review). In: The Cochrane Library; 1997. Oxford, Update Software

13  Gardosi J, Hutson N, Lynch C. Randomised, controlled trial of squatting in the second stage of labour. Lancet 1989; ii: 74–77

14  De Jong P R, Johanson R B, Baxen P, Adrians V D, Van der Westhuisen S, Jones P W. Randomised trial comparing the upright and supine positions for the second stage of labour. Br J Obstet Gynaecol 1997; 104: 567–571

15  Hofmeyr G J. Hands/knees posture in pregnancy for malposition of presenting part [revised 04 October 1993]. In: Enkin M W, Renfrew M J, Neilson J P, Crowther C (eds) Pregnancy and Childbirth Module. In: The Cochrane Pregnancy and Childbirth [database on disk and CDROM]. The Cochrane Collaboration; Issue 2, Oxford: Update Software; 1995

16  MIDIRS. Positions in Labour and Delivery, vol 5, 1st edn. Bristol: MIDIRS and the NHS Centre for Reviews and Dissemination, 1995

17  Carroli G, Belizan J, Stamp G. Episiotomy policies in vaginal births (Cochrane Review). In: The Cochrane Library; Issue 3, 1998. Oxford: Update Software

18  Klein M C, Gauthier R J, Jorgensen S H et al. Does episiotomy prevent perineal trauma and pelvic floor relaxation? online Obstetrical and Gynecological Survey. Online J Curr Clin Trials 1992; July 1 (Doc No 10): 238-239

19  Renfrew M J, Hannah W, Albers L. Practices that minimize trauma to the genital tract in childbirth: a systematic review of the literature. Birth 1998; 25: 143—60

20  Howell CJ. Epidural vs non-epidural analgesia in labour (Cochrane Review). In: The Cochrane Library, Issue 3, 1998. Oxford: Update Software

21  Johanson R B, Menon V. Vacuum extraction vs forceps delivery (Cochrane Review). In: The Cochrane Library, Issue 3, 1998. Oxford: Update Software

22  Maresh M, Choong K H, Beard R W. Delayed pushing with lumbar epidural analgesia in labour. Br J Obstet Gynaecol 1983; 90: 623–627

23  Ramin S, Gambling D R, Lucas M J, Sharma S K, Sidawi J E, Leveno K J. Randomised trial of epidural versus intravenous analgesia during labour. Obstet Gynecol 1995; 86: 783–789

24  Halpern S H, Leighton B L, Ohlsson A, Barrett J F R, Rice A. Effect of epidural vs parenteral opioid analgesia on the progress of labor. JAMA 1998; 280: 2105–2110

25  Vause S, Congdon H M, Thornton J. Immediate and delayed pushing in the second stage of labour for nulliparous women with epidural analgesia. A randomised controlled trial. Br J Obstet Gynaecol 1998; 105: 186–188

26  Kirwan P. Oxytocin and the second stage of labour. Ir J Med Sci 1983; 152(5): 201–202

27  O'Driscoll K, Jackson R J A, Gallagher J T. Active management of labour and cephalopelvic disproportion. J Obstet Gynaecol Br Commonwealth 1970; 77: 385–389

28  Kreb H B. Intrapartum fetal heart rate monitoring. Am J Obstet 1979; 133: 762–780

29  Beard R W, Filshie G M. The significance of the changes in the continuous fetal heart rate in the first stage of labour. J Obstet Gynaecol Br Commonwealth 1971; 78: 865–883

30  Larry C, Gilstrap L C I, Johne M D, Hauth M D. Second stage fetal heart rate abnormalities and type of neonatal acidemia. Obstet Gynecol 1987; 70(2): 191-195

31  Richtie J W K, Charles R. Malpositions of the occiput and malpresentations. In: Whitfield

N. (ed) Dewhurst's Textbook of Obstetrics and Gynaecology for Postgraduates, 5th edn. Oxford: Blackwell, 1994; 346–367

32  O'Driscoll K, Meagher D. Active management of labour. In: Progress of Labour, Second Stage. Eastbourne: W B Saunders; 1980; 7: 47–50

33  Gimovsky M, Hennigan C. Abnormal fetal presentations. Curr Opin Obstet Gynecol 1995; 7: 482–485

34  Gardberg M, Tuppurainen M. Persistent occiput posterior presentation – a clinical problem. Acta Obstet Gynecol Scand 1994; 73: 45–47

35  Pearl M L, Roberts J M, Laros R K et al. Vaginal delivery from the persistent occiput posterior position. Influence on maternal and neonatal morbidity. J Reprod Med 1993; 38: 955–961

36  Sultan A H, Kamm M A, Hudson C N, Bartram C I. Third degree obstetric anal sphincter tears: risk factors and outcome of primary repair. BMJ 1994; 308: 887–891

37  Menticoglou S M, Perlman M, Manning F A. High cervical spinal cord injury in neonates delivered with forceps: report of 15 cases. Obstet Gynecol 1995; 86: 589–594

38  Bird G C. Gothenburg N. (eds) Vacuum Extractor Manual. Gothenburg; 1982

39  Bird G C. The use of the vacuum extractor. Clin Obstet Gynecol 1982; 9: 641–661

40  Johanson R B, Rice C, Doyle M et al. A randomised prospective study comparing the new vacuum extractor policy with forceps delivery. Br J Obstet Gynaecol 1993; 100: 524–530

41  Vacca A. The place of the vacuum extractor in modern obstetric practice. Fetal Med Rev 1990; 2: 103–122

42  Rayburn W F, Lavin J P J, Miodovnik M, Varner M W. Multiple gestation: time interval between delivery of the first and second twins. Obstet Gynecol 1984; 63: 502

43  Rabinovici J, Barkai G, Reichman B et al. Randomised management of the second nonvertex twin: vaginal delivery or caesarean section. Am J Obstet Gynecol 1987; 156: 52

44  Laros R K, Dattel B J. Management of twin pregnancy: the vaginal route is still safe. Am J Obstet Gynecol 1988; 158: 1330

45  Chervenak F A, Johnson R E, Berkowitz R L et al. Is routine caesarean section necessary for vertex-breech and vertex-transverse twin gestations? Am J Obstet Gynecol 1984; 148: 1

46  Fishman A, Grubb D K, Kovacs B W. Vaginal delivery of the nonvertex second twin. Am J Obstet Gynecol 1993; 168: 861

47  Chervenak F A, Johnson R E, Berkowitz R L, Hobbins J C. Intrapartum external version of the second twin. Obstet Gynecol 1983; 62: 160

48  Rabinovici J, Barkai G, Richman B, Serr D M, Mashiach S. Internal podalic version with unruptured membranes for the second twin in transverse lie. Obstet Gynecol 1988; 71: 4280–4300

49  Cohen M, Kohl S G, Roisenthal A H. Fetal interlocking complicating twin gestation. Am J Obstet Gynecol 1965; 91: 407

50  Oettinger M, Ophir E, Markowitz J et al. Is caesarean section necessary for delivery of a breech first twin? Gynecol Obstet Invest 1993; 35: 38

51  FIGO. Recommendations of the FIGO Committee on perinatal health on guidelines for the management of breech delivery. Eur J Obstet Gynecol Reprod Biol 1995; 58: 89–92

52  Hannah W J, and Workshop Participants. The Canadian consensus on breech management at term. J SOGC 1994; 16: 1839–1858

53  Rojansky N, Tanos V, Weinstein D. Sonographic evaluation of fetal head extension and maternal pelvis in cases of breech presentation. Acta Obstet Gynecol Scand 1994; 73: 607–611

54  Ophir E, Oettinger M, Yagoda A, Markovits Y, Rojansky N, Schapiro H. Breech presentation after cesarean section: always a section? Am J Obstet Gynecol 1989; 161: 25–28

55  Chadha Y C, Mahmood T A, Dick M J, Smith N C, Campbell D M. Breech delivery and epidural analgesia. Br J Obstet Gynaecol 1992; 99: 96–100

56  Brady K, Duff P, Read J A, Harlass F E. Reliability of fetal buttock sampling in assessing the acid-base balance of the breech fetus. Obstet Gynecol 1989; 74: 886–888

57  Menticoglou S M. Symphysiotomy for the trapped aftercoming parts of the breech: a review of the literature and a plea for its use. Aust N Z J Obstet Gynecol 1990; 30: 1–9

58  Spencer J O A. Symphysiotomy for vaginal breech delivery. Br J Obstet Gynaecol 1987; 94: 716–718

59  Nwosu E C, Walkinshaw S, Chia P, Manasse N, Atlay R D. Undiagnosed breech. Br J

Obstet Gynaecol 1993; 100: 531–535

60 Hankin, Clark et al. Operative Obstetrics; Diagnosis and management of uterine inversion. 1995; 273–281

61 Caspi E, Lotan Y, Schreyer P. Prolapse of the cord: Reduction of perinatal mortality by bladder insilation and cesarean section. Isr J Med Sci 1983; 19: 541–545

62 Chetty R M, Moodley J. Umbilical cord prolapse. S Afr Med J 1980; 57: 128–129

63 Louca O, Johanson RB. Shoulder dystocia. In: O'Brien P M S. (eds) The Yearbook of Obstetrics & Gynaecology. London: RCOG Press, 1998; 6: 73–84

64 Nocon J, McKenzie A, Thomas L, Hansell R. Shoulder dystocia: an analysis of risks and obstetric manoeuvres. Am J Obstet Gynecol 1993; 168: 1732–1737

65 Hernandez C, Wendel G. Shoulder dystocia. Clin Obstet Gynecol 1990; 33: 3

66 Lurie S, Ben-Arie A, Hagay Z. The ABC of shoulder dystocia management. Asia-Oceania J Obstet Gynecol 1994; 20: 195–197

67 Baskett T F, Allen A C. Perinatal implications of shoulder dystocia. Obstet Gynecol 1995; 81: 14–17

68 Gross T, Sokol R, Williams T, Thompson K. Shoulder dystocia. A fetal physician risk. Am J Obstet Gynecol 1987; 156: 1408–1418

69 Daw E. Management of the hyperextended fetal head. Am J Obstet Gynecol 1976; 124: 113–115

70 Cruikshank D P, Cruikshank J E. Face and brow presentation: a review. Clin Obstet Gynecol 1981; 24: 333–351

*Michelle Laybourn  Anthony M. Mander*

# The role of computerised antenatal fetal heart rate analysis in obstetric practice

The oldest method of assessing the fetal heart rate is auscultation. The first association between audible abnormality of the fetal heart and risk to the fetus was suggested by Evory Kennedy in 1833.[1] Kennedy was also the first to point out that the fetal heart rate is affected by uterine contractions. When Jacques Kergaradec[1] (1787–1877) studied auscultation, the only application of the knowledge was to confirm that the fetus was alive. However, he made the perceptive observation which foresaw the potential for antenatal fetal heart monitoring 'will it not be possible to judge the state of health or disease of the fetus from the variations that occur in the beat of the fetal heart'.

The work of Hon[1] on detailed analysis of the fetal heart rate in labour demonstrated that the use of modern instrumentation methods aided the elucidation of clinical fetal distress. Hon's efforts were aimed to find a reliable means of accurately demonstrating reversible fetal distress. The antenatal cardiotocography (antenatal CTG) came about as a result of experience gained from electronic fetal heart monitoring in labour.

The antenatal CTG has been in use for several decades. The problem exists – are the parameters in labour the same as those used in a non-stressed fetus in the antenatal period? Druzin said of the antenatal electronic CTG 'the ability to predict the *healthy fetus* is its strength, the inability to distinguish the *sick fetus* is its weakness'.[2] Antenatal CTG developed into using stress tests.

## Contraction stress test

The idea of the contraction stress test was to mimic labour using Oxytocinon and, therefore, aid interpretation by using intrapartum parameters during

**Dr Michelle Laybourn** MB ChB, House Officer General Surgery, Tameside General Hospital, Fountain Street, Ashton under Lyne OL6 9RW, UK

**Mr A.M. Mander** FRCOG, Consultant Obstetrician/Gynaecologist, The Royal Oldham Hospital, Rochdale Road, Oldham OL1 2JH, UK (for correspondence)

contractions. The antenatal stress test is no longer widely used, other than in the US. The contraction test is expensive, very time consuming and inconvenient to the mother.

## Non-stress test

The non-stress test shows reaction to fetal heart to normal events such as Braxton Hicks contractions or fetal movement. Studies confirm that fetal well-being is predictable by the normal reactive non-stress test.

The interpretation of non stress antenatal CTG tracings is extremely difficult. Interpretation of the traces is subjective and inconsistent between observers, not only on the same occasion, but also between the same observer on different occasions.[3-6] Scoring systems offered advantages, but by the 1970s it was realised that this would be an ideal task for a computer,[7] as it will apply a given set of rules stringently.

The problem is that both the antenatal non-stress test and contraction stress tests have a high incidence of negative predictive value, i.e. they have good predicting fetal well-being when normal but because they have high false positive results further investigation is necessary to confirm abnormal findings.

These other methods of investigating and assessing fetal well-being include:

## Biophysical profile

A biophysical profile provides more information about the fetal condition; it looks at liquor volume, movement, tone, fetal heart rate and fetal breathing. The test has its limitations. It is time consuming and expensive to do. In practical terms, only liquor volume and fetal heart rate are now often used, though many other modifications have been suggested to the original bio-physical profile.

## Doppler blood flow studies

Doppler blood flow, a useful investigation, can only be done on a limited number of women as it is time consuming requiring highly specialist equipment and very skilled operators. Consequently, the dilemma exists as to how to identify the patients at risk requiring this limited facility. Randomised controlled trials show that Doppler studies are not a useful screening tool for the fetus at risk, but useful for fetal assessment and for monitoring the severity of the situation where growth restriction is diagnosed.

The problems of interpretation of antenatal CTGs are difficult to standardise. Therefore, an objective numerical analysis for measuring fetal heart rate patterns was developed by Redman and Dawes.[8-11]

Dawes was the first to appreciate that, without objective numerical measurements, the interpretation of human fetal heart rate patterns could never be exact. He recognised that to analyse the large volume of data, computerised methods are necessary. Dawes was quick to capitalise on new computer technology to develop a system that is now used as a clinical tool and was also honoured by a British Design Award in 1990 for the elegance of its presentation and methods.[12] The first generation machine was known as System 8000.

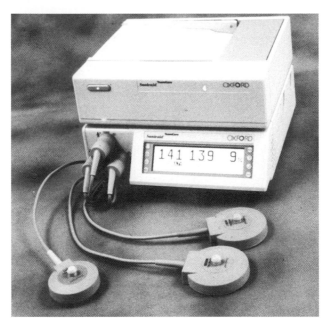

**Fig. 1** The System 8002.

This system Dawes and his team in Oxford developed was a method of computerised analysis for ultrasound derived fetal heart rate. It concluded that the most useful measures of fetal heart rate analysis are variations and accelerations.[13] The system consisted of a cardiotocograph and computer, and was also capable of analysing data obtained remotely with a similar monitor then transmitted via modem.

## COMPUTERISED ANTENATAL FETAL HEART RATE ANALYSIS

System 8002 (Fig. 1) [9–11] is a method of numerical analysis of the antenatal fetal heart rate as an aid to the management of 'high risk' women from 26 weeks onwards.[3,14,15] The sensors are attached to the abdomen in the same way as for a non-computerised CTG, and the woman is asked to record any fetal movements she feels using a hand held button. Data are initially analysed after 10 min recording; the first step being to fit a baseline which is then adjusted according to further data. Analysis of variation is now calibrated according to the gestational age of the fetus as high variation is higher in a more mature fetus, whereas low variation tends to be lower.

### Parameters analysed

1. *High and low variation*      The record is considered to be abnormal if there is no episode of high variation.

2. *Long term variation*      This is the average of the differences between minimum and maximum pulse intervals in each minute.

| 3. *Accelerations* | Although these are not considered to be a good enough predictor of normality they are included in the analysis as they are the traditional feature identified visually. |
| 4. *Decelerations* | These are counted and those of 50 lost beats or more are listed individually on the report. |
| 5. *Basal heart rate* | |
| 6. *Fetal movements* | These are recorded by the mother. |
| 7. *Contractions* | A contraction is recorded if the external uterine pressure rises more than 16% for 30 s or more. |
| 8. *Signal loss* | If this exceeds a threshold value a warning is issued for the midwife to adjust the position of the transducer. |

## Dawes Redman criteria

These have been derived from the analysis of over 48,000 records and provide rules for determining whether a record is normal or if the patient requires further clinical review and investigation, i.e. a definite answer as to whether a record is normal or not.[14]

1. *There must be an episode of high variation (sign of normality) that is above the 1st centile for gestational age.*

2. *There should be no large decelerations, or any deceleration (regardless of size) at the end of the record.*

3. *The basal heart rate should be between 116–160 beats per minute.*

4. *There should be no evidence of sinusoidal heart rhythm.*

5. *The short term variation is 3 ms or greater.*

6. *There should be no error at the end of the record.*

At the end of a recording, a printout gives a summary of data and states whether the criteria were met or not (Fig. 2).

Greater emphasis is now placed on the measurement of short-term rather than long-term variation.[15] Each minute is divided into 16 epochs (3.75 s each) and the mean pulse interval for each epoch is found. The difference between adjacent epochs is then averaged. A mean value for all the minutes is displayed at the end of the record. This has been shown to be independent of basal heart rate in the absence of periods of low variation and to correlate with metabolic acidosis and intra-uterine death.

**Table 1** Short term variation and metabolic acidaemia[17,18]

| STV (ms) | % Likelihood of metabolic acidaemia or intra-uterine death |
|---|---|
| > 4 | 0 |
| 3.5–4.0 | 8 |
| 3.0–3.5 | 29 |
| 2.5–3.0 | 33 |
| < 2.5 | 72 |

Reprint   for
Date of recording   18-Feb-00
Record Number        A 467

Reference No.
Time of recording   12:56
Gestation 38 weeks   4 days

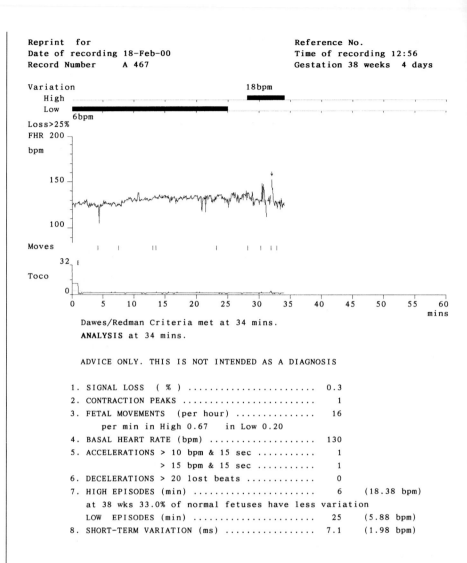

**Fig. 2** Typical print out from System 8002 summarising data.

Long-term variation (LTV) is susceptible to slow sinusoidal rhythms which may be misinterpreted as episodes of high variation. It also depends on the proportion of episodes of low and high variation and the basal heart rate which may vary in any FHR record.[3] Short-term variation (STV) is a more useful measurement, as it has been shown to correlate directly with the development of metabolic acidaemia and ultimately fetal death (Table 1).[16]

A rough approximation of LTV can be obtained by multiplying STV by 5.5, although direct assessment of STV is now recommended.

The Dawes System 8002 also provides other advantages over visual analysis; these include better quality records, better use of time spent recording and adjustment for changing fetal behavioural states (Table 2).

**Table 2** Fetal heart antenatal monitoring

|  | Pinard auscultation | Doppler auscultation | Doppler fetal monitor visual monitor | System 8002[9-11] computerised Doppler analysis |
|---|---|---|---|---|
| **From** | 24 weeks | 12 weeks | 26 weeks | 26 weeks |
| **Record** | Audible only to observer | Audible to observer and patient | Very tracing . operator dependant Paper tracing only stored | Non operator dependant. Data can be stored electronically enabling detailed study later |
| **Interpre-tation** | Subject to listener variability. Difficult in obese patient or noisy environment | Easy audible interpretation of heart rate. Irregularities difficult to interpret | 'Visual' interpretation difficult.[3-6] Large inter- and intra-observer error. Lot of training needed | Scoring system removes possibility of observer error. Good detailed information. Very little training needed |
| **Time** | 1 min | 1 min | 30–60 min with unspecified end point | Quick, time saving, reliable. 12 min if Dawes Redman criteria met[14] |
| **Equipment costs** | £2 | £150 | £5,000–£10,000. Expensive in staff and time. Rain forests of paper | £5,000 |
| **Prediction of fetal well-being** |  |  |  |  |
| Healthy fetus[2] | Fair | Fair | Good | Good |
| Sick fetus[3] | Poor | Poor | Poor | Good [17,18] |

## HOW TO USE COMPUTERISED ANTENATAL FETAL HEART RATE ANALYSIS IN CLINICAL PRACTICE

The Royal Oldham Hospital had used computerised antenatal CTGs for about 10 years, and usage increased with the opening of an Antenatal Day Unit. As we found little information in the literature regarding its role in antenatal care and management, we undertook a study[19] with the following aims:

1. *To obtain demographic information about women referred for computerised antenatal fetal monitoring.*

2. *To investigate the mechanism of referral and clinical indications for computerised monitoring.*

3. *To determine if and how monitoring influences the subsequent management and outcome of pregnancy.*

In our study, data were obtained by retrospective analysis of the case notes of 118 women who were delivered over 6 weeks during Autumn 1997. This included gestational age, referral mechanism, reason for monitoring, time taken to meet the Dawes Redman criteria and short-term variation. Gestational age at delivery was recorded, as were mode of delivery and method of induction of labour (if one was used). The gender and birth weight of the infant were noted as were its Apgar scores at 1 and 5 min after birth.

The principal measure of outcome was defined as fetal growth, measured using a customised growth chart.[20–22] Each chart takes account of the body mass index, parity and ethnic group of the mother, thereby producing an individual chart for the projected growth of the fetus. Customised charts eliminate the inaccuracy of charts based on large population studies which have not been updated in line with changes in population demographics. (This is particularly important in Oldham, where 20% of the obstetric population is of Asian origin; hence the use of customised growth chart is of paramount importance.) Approximate weights can be obtained by ultrasound measurement of the circumference of the fetal abdomen, and these can then be plotted on the chart and compared to the centile lines as the pregnancy progresses.

The birth-weight and the gestational age at birth were plotted on the customised growth chart. Statistical analysis was performed using SPSS software.

## Demographic information about women referred for computerised antenatal fetal monitoring

There was no significant difference in the demographic data between women who were monitored and those who were not – it would seem that there is no particular 'at risk' group based on demographic parameters.

## Mechanisms of referral and clinical indications for computerised monitoring

Most women who had abdominal pain or decreased fetal movements were self-referrals and it is interesting that the two most common clinical indications for computerised antenatal CTG were the result of maternal perception (see Tables 3 & 4).

Far fewer women were referred by their GP than any other mechanism. This is possibly because pregnant women generally see the community midwife rather than the GP. There was a high proportion of self referrals. Women are informed about the antenatal day unit when they attend the booking clinic and there is also information in their hand-held notes. It is also likely that women may have attended the day unit in a previous pregnancy or heard about the service from other sources, e.g. the community midwife. Some consultants also give out information about the day unit with kick count charts for recording fetal

**Table 3** Mechanism of referral for computerised antenatal fetal monitoring

| | | |
|---|---|---|
| Antenatal clinic | 56 | 47% |
| Self referral (M) | 47 | 40% |
| Community midwife | 11 | 9% |

M indicates maternal rather than medical perception.

**Table 4** Clinical indication for computerised antenatal fetal heart rate analysis

| | | |
|---|---|---|
| Reduced fetal movements (M) | 37 | 31% |
| Abdominal pain (M) | 24 | 20% |
| Hypertension | 19 | 16% |
| IUGR | 10 | 8% |
| Other | 11 | 9% |
| Postmature | 8 | 7% |
| APH | 6 | 5% |
| Diabetes | 3 | 3% |

*Note*: the first two indications (51%) are maternal (M) rather than medical perceptions.

movements in the third trimester of pregnancy, which may account for the large number of self-referrals due to decreased fetal movements.

All the women who were monitored could be defined as high risk. Abdominal pain and decreased fetal movements are subjective perceptions, so it is not surprising that most were self-referrals, compared to objective measurements, such as fetal growth, which led to clinic or midwife referrals.

During the initial review of case notes, it was found that several women in whom monitoring would have been appropriate (e.g. intra-uterine growth retardation and poor obstetric history) had not been referred. The reasons for this are not clear, the lack of antenatal protocols for the use of the System 8002 might have contributed.

### Data obtained by computerised antenatal fetal heart rate analysis
The time taken to meet the Dawes Redman criteria was 10 min in 46 (39%) cases. The maximum time taken was 60 min and the mean was 17 min. In 17 cases, the criteria were not met during the first monitoring, and it was repeated. In 8 cases, the monitoring was stopped before the criteria had been met.

The short-term variation ranged from 4.5 ms to 16.8 ms with a mean of 8.9 ms. There was no significant difference in these values between ethnic groups or between male and female infants. This confirms that there is no difference in variation between sexes. The findings of Oguer and Steer confirm that gender does not affect fetal heart rate.[23]

### Differences with subsequent referrals for computerised antenatal fetal heart rate analysis
A subsequent referral was more likely to be made by the woman herself than a first referral (34/74, 46% compared to 47/118, 40%). No substantial

differences in indication for referral or mode of delivery were found in women referred more than once. Differences were found in the action taken following a subsequent episode of monitoring.

### Correlation between variables

Spearman correlation coefficients were calculated for various combinations of variables. Time taken to reach the Dawes Redman criteria was found to correlate with short term variation (rs = −0.6146), i.e. the higher the short-term variation, the shorter the time taken. Time taken was not found to correlate with body mass index or with gestational age at monitoring.

Monitoring was stopped in 8 cases before the criteria were met. It is not clear why this was, though it seems unlikely that this was at the request of the mother, as 40% were self-referrals. It is possible that some traces were seen by a doctor or midwife and thought to be satisfactory, on the criteria of a non stress test and were thus discontinued. If this is the case, it rather defeats the point of using the computerised system.

Most women who referred themselves because of decreased fetal movements were monitored once and were not re-referred after discharge back to routine care, indicating that the use of System 8002 is an effective method of reassurance.

It is reassuring that the monitoring was repeated if the criteria were not met, this was due to the absence of a high episode in all 17 cases. It is possible that this was related to the behavioural state of the fetus at the time of monitoring.

The fact that women were more likely to be admitted after a second or third referral for monitoring may indicate a lower threshold for admission, even if the data from the monitor were within normal limits.

There are no guidelines issued about the frequency of repeat computerised monitoring. Women who were monitored many times generally achieved consistent readings for short-term variation. Daily or alternate day monitoring may offer an alternative to admission.

## How monitoring influences the subsequent management and outcome of pregnancy

### Subsequent management of women referred for computerised antenatal fetal monitoring

Discharge back to routine antenatal care was the most common action taken after monitoring (50, 42%). The monitoring was quite often repeated the next day if a poor tracing was obtained or the criteria not met. Significant abnormalities in the results of monitoring triggered clinical intervention of 15 women admitted; five women had delivery expedited as a result of computerised monitoring, including two who had immediate induction of labour and one who had an emergency Caesarean section. The remaining 10 were admitted and subsequently allowed home before delivery.

### Outcome of pregnancy following computerised antenatal fetal monitoring

**Mode of delivery.** Most women (85, 72%) were delivered vaginally and 12 (10%) underwent delivery by Ventouse. Labour was induced in 49 women

(41.5%). Twelve women (10%) had elective Caesarean sections, for a variety of reasons. Nine women (8%) had emergency Caesarean sections, one for cephalo-pelvic disproportion following trial of labour, and the others for fetal distress and failure to progress in the second stage of labour (Table 5).

A higher proportion of women had labour induced in the study group than over the previous year and a binomial test found this to be highly significant ($P < 0.0005$).

There was no other significant difference in mode of delivery. From this one can infer that computerised monitoring is revealing cases where delivery should be expedited.

There was a significantly higher rate of induction of labour among women who had been monitored using the computerised system, than that for all women in 1996. Monitored mothers in whom labour was induced were more likely to have an instrumental delivery, indicating that there is possibly a lower threshold for intervention in women who have previously been considered 'high risk'.

No significant differences were found regarding gender of infant, Apgar scores or gestational age at delivery.

**Outcome.** Significantly more infants had weights below the 10th centile on their customised growth chart ($P = 0.009$) and significantly fewer had weights above the 90th centile ($P = 0.05$); that is, babies of women who had been monitored were more often small for gestational age.

A significantly larger number of infants had weights below the 10th centile than would be expected ($P = 0.009$), and fewer had weights above the 90th centile ($P = 0.05$). This may be because the customised growth charts are not adjusted for gender of infant. It is more likely to have occurred because intra-uterine growth retardation is one of the indications for monitoring, and is often associated with several of the other indications.

Retrospective analysis of all singleton pregnancies in our hospital[21] in 1995 revealed that more infants with a birth-weight < 10th centile by customised charts alone had been born by emergency Caesarean section (23.5% versus 2.6%), that more had had Apgar scores less than 7 at 1 min (29.4% versus 8.7%) and that these infants had a higher rate of admission to special care (23.5% versus 0.8%) than those defined small by population charts alone, despite similar induction rates (29.0% versus 24.0%) and similar birth-weights (3062 g versus 2892 g).

We have not attempted to investigate the attitudes and opinions of staff and patients with regard to computerised antenatal fetal monitoring though this clearly is an important area for further study.

**Table 5** Mode of delivery compared to those of all deliveries in 1996

|  | Monitoring<br>n = 118 | All (1996)<br>n = 3137 |
| --- | --- | --- |
| Induced | 42% | 27% |
| Normal | 72% | 74% |
| Ventouse | 10% | 8% |
| Forceps | 0 | 2% |
| Emergency Caesarean | 8% | 7% |
| Elective Caesarean | 10% | 8% |

# PROTOCOL FOR THE FUTURE USE OF COMPUTERISED ANTENATAL FETAL HEART RATE ANALYSIS

Mothers with viable pregnancies (24 weeks) are given information regarding fetal movements and maternally perceived symptoms such as uterine pain and bleeding and how to fill in a kick count chart. The mothers are told to attend the Antenatal Day Unit if problems occur. On referral, examination and assessment is made with the System 8002 monitoring (see Fig. 3). Pregnancies with risk factors or signs and symptoms suggestive of risk are referred for assessment and fetal monitoring on the System 8002.[17,18] (In the presence of an abnormal System 8002 result in a premature fetus, giving corticosteroids should be considered in case early delivery is indicated.)

Ultrasound scan for assessment of fetal growth is arranged if none was performed in the previous 2 weeks

Normal growth on customised growth chart with adequate liquor volume is very reassuring and mothers are discharged with the advice to keep kick count charts. However, fetal growth restriction (< 10th centile on customised chart) and/or oligohydramnios (amniotic fluid index < 5 cm ) are indications for Doppler blood flow waveform studies of the umbilical artery.

A normal Doppler blood flow study is usually repeated after 1 week and a growth scan after 2 weeks. Mothers with normal fetal growth and normal Doppler but oligohydramnios, have System 8002 monitoring daily.

An abnormal Doppler blood flow result with fetal growth restriction is an indication for admission for closer twice daily System 8002 monitoring and

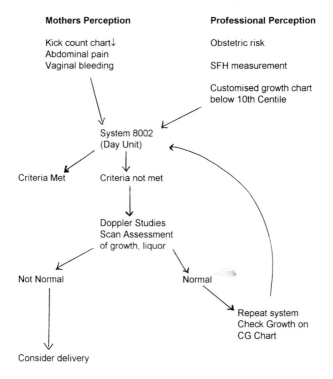

**Fig. 3** Protocol for the use of computerised antenatal fetal heart rate analysis in obstetrics.

**Table 6**  Antenatal risk factors

Poor obstetric history
Maternal conditions – cardiac disease, diabetes
Suspect maternal drug abuse
Suspect fetal anomaly
Vaginal bleeding (M)
Uterine pain (M)
Multiple pregnancy
Intra-uterine growth retardation (restriction)
Antepartum haemorrhage
Hypertension or pre-eclampsia
Abnormal symphysis fundal height measurement
Oligohydramnios
Previous questionable FHR tracing
Decreased fetal movements (M)
Abnormal umbilical Doppler waveform

M = maternal perception and symptoms which need investigation.

Doppler is repeated on alternate days. Grossly abnormal Doppler (i.e. absent end diastolic flow or reversed diastolic flow) indicates the need for emergency delivery irrespective of gestational age.

With regard to midwifery and obstetric staff, current classifications of a high risk fetus give a complacent view of our abilities to pick out the at-risk fetus.[21] We recommend that the classification of the high risk fetus antenatally be carefully analysed as suggested in Table 6. The kick count chart should be utilised as above. Symphysis fundal height measurements should be charted by the attendants in primary and secondary care with appropriate referral. There is little justification for not using customised growth charts in clinical practice.

If obstetricians persist in using obsolete and inaccurate methods of predicting the at-risk fetus, it is not surprising that our midwifery colleagues and the informed lay public find much of our practice pseudo-scientific and even suspect, leading to lack of credibility.

## WHY IS THE USAGE OF THE SYSTEM SO PATCHY?

Computerised antenatal fetal heart rate analysis is quick, cheap and provides very good information. Why is it not used more widely in the UK where the system originated? Geographically its uptake is sporadic.

To our knowledge, over 23 maternity units throughout the UK use the system. Uptake is greater in other countries, Italy and Norway have the highest system 'population' to the national birth rate, followed by Finland. In Germany, numbers are increasing rapidly perhaps because of a large multicentre trial taking place there. The highest number in use is in Poland. In all, over 51 countries use the Dawes system which is marketed world wide with the exception of the US.

Furthermore, it is puzzling that there is so little data on the use of computerised antenatal fetal heart analysis in clinical practice; is it due perhaps to lack of awareness of the system? A 'Luddite' reluctance by health professionals to accept computer interpretation of clinical data? The absence of clearly defined risk factors in antenatal care?

Computerised antenatal fetal heart analysis has many advantages – it is non-operator dependent, time saving and reliable and, since data can be stored electronically, it enables detailed research and audit to be undertaken and thus provides a good basis for evidence-based medicine. It should, therefore, be more widely used in obstetric practice.

## CONCLUSIONS

We recommend the establishment of proper protocols for the use of antenatal computerised fetal heart analysis; fundamental to this is the establishment of appropriate risk criteria for patients, medical and midwifery staff.

We strongly feel there is a need to update guidelines and protocols for antenatal care to improve the identification of the baby at risk. These should utilise maternal perceptions, the use of symphysis fundal height measurements and appropriate flow management protocols for the use of the System 8002 in clinical practice to identify the very high risk fetus and lead to more detailed assessment.

There is undoubtedly a need to produce appropriate audit criteria to assess the efficacy of such clinical protocols and guidelines.

Finally, computerised antenatal fetal heart rate analysis provides an objective assessment of fetal well-being and importantly is especially effective in reassuring mothers who have referred themselves to hospital. It should be more widely used in obstetric practice.

---

**KEY POINTS FOR CLINICAL PRACTICE**

- Computerised antenatal fetal heart analysis has many advantages – it is non-operator dependent, time saving and reliable and, since data can be stored electronically, it enables detailed research and audit to be undertaken and thus provides a good basis for evidence-based medicine.

- Computerised antenatal fetal heart rate analysis provides an objective assessment of fetal well-being and importantly is especially effective in reassuring mothers who have referred themselves to hospital.

---

ACKNOWLEDGEMENTS

The authors gratefully acknowledge the assistance of the Departments of Obstetrics and Clinical Audit at The Royal Oldham Hospital, the Statistics Support Unit of Manchester Medical School, Jackie Miller for her help in the production of this paper and our colleague Mr Aziz for his help and advice.

*References*

1  Baskett T F. Eponyms and Names in Obstetrics and Gynaecology. London: RCOG Press, 1996; 98–99, 107–108

2 Druzin M. Antepartum Fetal Assessment. Boston: Blackwell, 1992
3 Flynn A M, Kelley J, Matthews K. Predictive value of, and observer variability in several ways of reporting antepartum cardiotocograms. Br J Obstet Gynaecol 1982; 89: 434–440
4 Trimbos J B, Keirse M J N C. Observer variability in assessment of antepartum cardiotocograms. Br J Obstet Gynaecol 1978; 85: 900–906
5 Cheng L C, Gibb D M F, Ajayi R A, Soothill P W. A comparison between computerised (mean range) and clinical visual cardiotocographic assessment. Br J Obstet Gynaecol 1992; 99: 817–820
6 Dawes G S, Redman C W G. Correspondence. Br J Obstet Gynaecol 1993; 100: 701–705
7 Sokol R J, Chik L (eds) Perinatal Computing – An Overview. Acta Obstet Gynaecol Scand Suppl 1982; 109: 7–82
8 Dawes G S, Lobb M, Moulden M, Redman C W G, Wheeler T. Antenatal cardiotocogram quality and interpretation using computers. Br J Obstet Gynaecol 1992; 99: 791–797
9 Catanzarite V A, Jelovsek F R. Computer applications in obstetrics. Am J Obstet Gynecol 1987; 156: 1047–1053
10 Street P, Dawes G S, Moulden M, Redman C W G. Short term variation in abnormal antenatal fetal heart rate records. Am J Obstet Gynecol 1991; 165: 515–523
11 Mantel R, van Geijn H P, Ververs I A P, Copray F J A. Automated analysis of near term ante-partum FHR in relation to behavioural states: the Sonicaid system 8000. Am J Obstet Gynecol 1991; 165: 57–65
12 Obituary. The Times; Monday 20 May 1996; p 19
13 Spencer J A D. In: Studd J (Ed). Fetal heart rate variability. Progress in Obstetrics and Gynaecology. Edinburgh: Churchill Livingstone, 1989; 7: 103–121
14 Dawes G S, Moulden M, Redman C W G. System 8000: computerised antenatal FHR analysis. J Perinat Med 1991; 19: 47–51
15 Sonicaid System 8002 Technical Specification. Oxford: Oxford Instruments UK Ltd
16 Ribbert L S M, Snijders R J M. Nikolaides K H, Visser G H A. Relation of fetal blood gases and data from computer-assisted analysis of fetal heart rate patterns in small for gestation fetuses. Br J Obstet Gynaecol 1991; 98: 820–823
17 Street P, Dawes G S, Moulden M, Redman C W G. Short term variation in abnormal antenatal fetal heart rate records. Am J Obstet Gynecol 1991; 165: 515–523
18 Personal communication, Prof. C W G Redman, 4th March 1999
19 Laybourn M, Mander A M. Computerised antenatal electronic fetal monitoring in obstetric practice (oral presentation). Abstracts of the 13th Congress of European Association of Gynaecologists and Obstetricians (EAGO), Jerusalem, May 1998; 95
20 Henson G, Dawes G S, Redman C W G. Characterization of the reduced heart rate variation in growth retarded fetuses. Br J Obstet Gynaecol 1984; 91: 751–755
21 Leeson S, Aziz N. Customised fetal growth assessment. Br J Obstet Gynaecol 1997; 104: 648–651
22 Gardosi J, Chang A, Kalyan B, Sahota D, Symonds E M. Customised antenatal growth charts. Lancet 1992; 349: 283–287
23 Ogueh O, Steer P. Gender does not affect fetal heart rate variation. Br J Obstet Gynaecol 1998; 105, 1312-1314

*Sara Paterson-Brown*

# Elective caesarean section – a woman's right to choose?

Traditionally, caesarean sections (CS) have been reserved for those situations where labour or vaginal delivery have been considered dangerous to either mother or baby and high rates of CS are met with knee-jerk reactions of disapproval. There is no evidence to support any specific target rate, however, and the recent drive in America to reduce the CS rate to 15% by the year 2000 has been criticised[1] as causing increased maternal and fetal damage. Aiming at reducing CS rates generally may, therefore, do some individuals a disservice: what matters most is that those women and babies who need CS get it, while those who do not are saved unnecessary surgery.

Although CS is becoming increasingly safe and evidence is mounting regarding risks of labour and vaginal delivery, there is no doubt that the evidence, as it stands, remains grossly incomplete. Despite this, the balance of acceptability between abdominal and vaginal delivery is changing. Whether maternal choice should be added to this equation when deciding how to deliver a woman is the subject of this review.

## ETHICS OF CHOICE

The doctor–patient relationship is complex and private, requiring mutual respect and trust. The doctor is there to advise, and act in accordance with accepted medical practice within the constraints, if any, set by the patient. The patient's right to refuse or limit treatment is well tested and universally acknowledged, but the opposite right to request certain interventions, while perfectly acceptable in many situations, seems to have caused significant controversy when relating to caesarean sections.[2–6]

**Miss Sara Paterson-Brown** FRCS MRCOG MA, Consultant in Obstetrics and Gynaecology, Queen Charlotte's and Chelsea Hospital, Goldhawk Road, London W6 0XG, UK

## Examples of choice in obstetrics and gynaecology

The unfavourable response to patient autonomy in pregnancy is surprising, as there are many situations in the field of obstetrics and gynaecology where women's opinions and preferences are very much respected. Infertility is a minefield of ethical dilemmas, but patients assert positive rights of request for fertility treatment with its attendant risks even when they already have live children. They assert positive rights when requesting definitive treatment for unpleasant, but not dangerous, conditions: such as menorrhagia or urinary incontinence and even sterilisation to save themselves the daily inconveniences of contraception. How can we discredit 'positive right' in the context of patient choice for caesarean sections when we live with it in so many other professional situations?

## Current guidance on choice

The recommendations from *Changing Childbirth*[7] that women should have a pivotal role in their obstetric care reflected public and professional opinion in the UK. The expectation, however, was that this would encourage an increase in natural childbirth and home deliveries. Some of the choices made are contrary to those expected, being towards more, rather than less, medicalisation and intervention, but that does not mean that we should be questioning the initial premise.

In the UK, clinical governance is going to become a part of everyday life, and the booklet brought out by the General Medical Council on good medical practice[8] guides us to patient choice quite deliberately: 'patients want to be sure that their doctors...respect their views and wishes when treating them', and 'medical and clinical teams must have a positive attitude to patients and listen to their wishes and needs'.

These recommendations are not guiding doctors into a role of simply 'doing what the patient wants', but they are clear in their suggestion that we should be involving women in decisions concerning their care. Such involvement must be accompanied by information, counselling and then advice, all of which may be time consuming, but is difficult to criticise on any other grounds. Few patients will not follow the doctor's advice if it is given willingly and impartially, and doctors should not feel threatened by this development, but embrace the opportunity for dialogue, helping the woman to become involved in decision-making.

If we are to conclude that women should not be allowed to choose an elective CS, then we must be satisfied that the risks of the CS are so much worse than those of labour that we can exclude patient preference from the equation.

## BALANCE OF THE RISKS

It is interesting to reflect on an obstetric situation where there is patient and/or obstetrician anxiety: a woman with an uncomplicated pregnancy of a well-grown singleton fetus at term who has had a previous obstetric catastrophe of a non-recurring cause, or previous numerous first trimester miscarriages, or prolonged infertility treatment. A perfectly common and acceptable course of action in these scenarios is for her to be delivered by elective CS at term. If we believe this is truly the safest way to deliver these 'precious' pregnancies, why do we not afford all mothers and babies similar concern?

In any decision to deliver by elective CS, something must have tipped the balance of risks, or of the acceptance of those risks, away from labour and vaginal delivery. Trying to be precise about what these often subtle factors are can be frustratingly difficult, but there is no doubt that in obstetric situations which are not completely normal, including previous CS, breech presentation and problems in labour, maternal involvement and choice are playing an increasingly important part.[9–13] Is the medical balance of risks in these situations so delicately poised that maternal choice **can** be accepted as legitimate while the balance of risks in an uncomplicated pregnancy are so overwhelmingly in favour of labour and vaginal delivery that it should have no influence on decision making?

To take this argument further, we must explore the risks to infant and mother of elective CS versus labour (labour as opposed to vaginal delivery or normal delivery must be used as the comparator, as no woman entering labour can be guaranteed a particular type of delivery).

## FETAL RISKS

### Risks of awaiting spontaneous labour

Unexpected antepartum stillbirth, although tragic, is not uncommon and increases 8-fold from 0.7 per 1000 on-going pregnancies at 37 weeks to 5.8 per 1000 ongoing pregnancies at $\geq 43$ weeks (Fig. 1).[14] If the risk of death increases as gestation advances from 37 weeks, what other lesser damage is occurring silently? We believe that less than 10% of cases of cerebral palsy are attributable to intrapartum insult and most are accounted for by antenatal events – we do not know what proportion of these occur at term. If subtle changes are effecting death, it is not unreasonable to suppose that lesser insults could effect damage at this time. This problem requires much more attention and research, but at present is a significant factor to remember when balancing

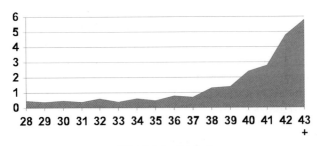

**Summed mortality at each gestation per 1000 ongoing pregnancies**

Weeks gestation

**Fig. 1** Risks of awaiting labour expressed as summed mortality at each gestation per 1000 ongoing pregnancies. (Adapted from Hilder et al.[14])

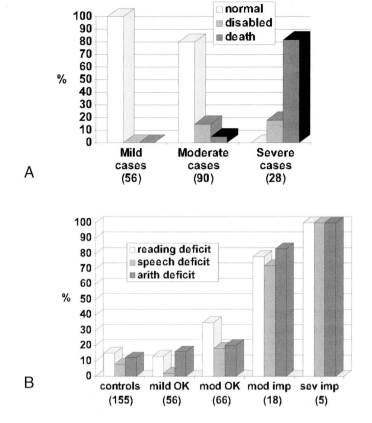

**Fig. 2** Eight year follow-up of 174 babies suffering birth asphyxial neonatal encephalopathy. (**A**) Crude outcomes relative to mild, moderate or severe neonatal encephalopathy. (**B**) fine outcomes relative to severity of encephalopathy and the crude outcome assessment (e.g. ''mod OK' are those cases of moderate encephalopathy with normal crude outcome assessment, and 'mod imp' are those with obvious crude outcome problems). Adapted from Robertson et al.[17]

elective delivery at 39 weeks against waiting indefinitely for spontaneous labour to ensue.

## Risks of labour

Of all babies born over 1500 g in the UK, 1 in 1561 will die due to intrapartum events.[15] Over half of these deaths are deemed avoidable,[15] which still leaves the risk of fetal death in labour at 1 in 3000 with exemplary care. The trouble is, with the best will in the world, mistakes do happen, and in no case is such a mistake deliberate, or indeed even recognised in most cases until after the event under the tyranny of hindsight. With shortages in midwifery staffing in the UK which has reached a critical level, combined with decreasing experience of junior doctors, this situation may deteriorate further.

Neonatal encephalopathy occurs at a rate of about 1 in 260 term babies of which approximately 15% are directly attributable to intrapartum events, i.e. 1 in 1750 labours.[16] However ghastly the short-term stresses of having a baby admitted to the neonatal intensive care unit must be, the long-term consequences of neonatal encephalopathy are most relevant in this context. Robertson et al[17] investigated crude and fine outcomes of 174 babies who had suffered asphyxial neonatal encephalopathy at 8 years of age and found significant mortality and morbidity (Fig. 2). Ingemarson et al[18] conducted a 4-year follow-up on 102 babies born with an umbilical cord gas pH of less than 7.05 and compared them with 100 controls and found significant speech deficits in those infants who had been acidaemic at birth (19 of 102 compared to 8 of 100, respectively, $P = 0.03$).

## Risks of vaginal delivery

During vaginal delivery, the baby may sustain birth trauma in different ways and the problem is that, by definition, such damage is unexpected. Even when considering shoulder dystocia, most cases occur in babies not deemed to be macrosomic before (or even after) delivery. Instrumentation may be needed with risks of laceration or nerve palsies from the use of forceps, or of cephalo-haematoma or retinal haemorrhages from ventouse extraction. Quantifying these complications is complex, as it depends on the obstetric population and the intrapartum care provided, but is not insignificant.

## Risks of elective CS

The natural birthing process stresses and squeezes the infant during its descent through the birth canal, and this helps it adapt to extra-uterine life. Electively delivering a baby abdominally pre-empts spontaneous labour reflective of fetal maturity and also deprives it of this physiological (if sometimes dangerous) stress: hence, such babies may be disadvantaged. There is good evidence[19] demonstrating that, in the immediate postnatal period, respiratory function is more likely to be compromised in infants delivered by elective CS (Table 1). In practical terms, this risk can be minimised by delaying elective delivery until 39 completed weeks gestation, where the combined risk of transient tachypnoea and respiratory distress syndrome occurs in 1.8% of infants.[19]

**Table 1**  Respiratory morbidity associated with elective CS

| Gestation (weeks) | Total number elective CS | Total number | Rate per TTN + RDS | Odds ratio 1000 CS |
|---|---|---|---|---|
| 37 | 366 | 27 | 73.8 [49.1–106.1] | 14.3 [8.9–23.1] |
| 38 | 1063 | 45 | 42.3 [31.1–56.2] | 8.2 [5.5–12.3] |
| 39 | 505 | 9 | 17.8 [8.0–33.5] | 3.5 [1.7–7.1] |
| 40 | 243 | 1 | 4.1 [0.1–22.8] | 0.8 [0.1–5.8] |
| 41 | 164 | 1 | 6.1 [0.2–33.5] | 1.2 [0.2–8.6] |

Adapted from Morrison et al,[19] [95% confidence intervals].

There is a complete lack of evidence concerning bonding and breast feeding in mother–baby pairs where the CS was requested in the absence of pathology. All work available refers to medically indicated CS with their attendant confounding variables including unplanned procedures, general anaesthesia, sick women, babies requiring special care, etc., and, by definition, it is inappropriate to compare these with successful vaginal delivery mother–baby pairs. This is an area which requires further research; no conclusions can be drawn on current evidence.

### Long-term fetal effects from different modes of delivery

Recent work has demonstrated that rats born by CS under general anaesthesia have a heightened response to stress, and the implications drawn from this are that increased sensitivity of dopamine pathways could increase the risk of schizophrenia in humans born by CS.[20,21] On the other hand, evidence from Sweden has demonstrated a link between adverse events during labour or delivery and subsequent suicide by violent means as an adult.[22] Clearly, further work needs to be done in this area.

## MATERNAL RISKS

The problem with looking at the evidence available on maternal outcomes relative to mode of delivery is the heavy bias against CS derived purely from the populations of women studied. All CS, whether elective or emergency, prelabour or intrapartum, are usually grouped together, and have been performed for clinical reasons including maternal disease, rather than for maternal choice in otherwise healthy individuals. It is, therefore, hardly surprising that mortality, morbidity and satisfaction are worse in the CS groups.

### Maternal mortality

With the reservations described above, evidence available from South Africa is that those women who require a CS are more likely to die than those women who achieve a successful vaginal delivery.[23] The ratio of risk corrected for the reasons for the CS are approximately 5:1 CS versus vaginal delivery, and 1.5:1 for emergency intrapartum versus elective CS. This is obviously a hugely important area, and yet the confidential enquiry into maternal deaths in the UK, which had previously devoted a chapter to CS deaths, has dropped it from its most recent report.[24] Instead, the deaths are dealt with in the relevant chapters of the conditions resulting in death suggesting that CS is not considered the most important feature of these deaths. This is supported by the observation that there has yet to be a death reported in the UK of a previously fit woman who has undergone an elective CS under epidural anaesthetic with thromboprophylaxis and antibiotic cover.

One of the problems in the UK is that we do not have accurate figures on the number of CS being carried out each year, let alone why they are being done, and this makes estimates of deaths attributable to CS impossible. This problem is being addressed by the Maternity Hospital Episode Statistics system, but is not yet solved.[25]

In Massachusetts, a study looking at 2,803,596 live-births[26] from 1954–1985 found that, although the CS rate quadrupled, the maternal mortality rate remained constant. The maternal death rate directly attributable to these clinically indicated CS was 5.8 per 100,000 CS deliveries, while the total death rate in women delivered vaginally was 10.8 per 100,000 vaginal deliveries. This puts death rates more into perspective, but, with such low death rates in those countries not only able to provide safe conditions for CS but also able to audit them, it will take some time before this risk is fully appreciated in those few otherwise fit women who have a CS purely for maternal choice.

## Maternal morbidity

The most meaningful comparisons of morbidity need to be between those women having an elective CS and those undergoing labour. No such studies have been done in fit healthy women with no medical indication for CS but comparisons of elective CS versus trial of labour in specific obstetric situations have been performed. The results of many these trials are conflicting, but the most recent and largest studies demonstrate that elective CS appears safer than trial of scar[27] or trial of breech delivery.[28]

Given the dearth of information on comparative risks of CS and labour, we must investigate the risks of CS and vaginal delivery separately.

### Short-term risks relative to mode of delivery
Short-term morbidity after elective caesarean section has been quantified by Obwegeser et al[29] as 2% urinary infections, 1% wound infection and 12% maternal anaemia in a group of 108 women undergoing elective caesarean section for breech presentation. More recently,[28] elective CS and vaginal delivery both had maternal morbidity rates of less than 2% while in those having emergency CS, rates approached 3%.

It is commonly believed that the general recovery after CS is slower than after vaginal delivery, but recent evidence from Scotland shows that instrumental vaginal delivery causes significantly more maternal morbidity than either CS or normal vaginal delivery and that the recovery of women delivered by the latter two methods is comparable.[30] A very important message from this is that vaginal delivery at almost all costs is not necessarily appropriate, whatever our CS targets are.

The more we use regional analgesics for pain relief in labour the higher the instrumental vaginal delivery rate will be,[31] and the real problem we have is that our social habits make this increasingly likely: how can we expect women to tolerate the severe pains of labour when our normal everyday habits are to avoid pain whenever possible, and to do everything with as little effort as possible? We have local anaesthetics for dentistry (the drilling of which lasts a matter of minutes), we take analgesics available over the counter for headaches and some of us can not even elevate from the semirecumbent to switch off the television. The shortage in midwifery staffing does little to help and discouraging the use of pethidine in order to promote breast-feeding may further exacerbated the situation.

### Future obstetric performance after CS
The implications for future childbearing are the most relevant long-term consequences of CS. Unfortunately, the evidence we have on this follows on

**Table 2**  Risk of placenta praevia and placenta accreta after caesarean section

| Number previous CS | Incidence of placenta praevia | Of those with placenta praevia incidence of placenta accreta | Overall risk of placenta accreta |
|---|---|---|---|
| 0 | 0.26 | 5% | 0.01% |
| 1 | 0.65 | 24% | 0.16% |
| 2 | 1.8 | 47% | 0.85% |
| 3 | 3 | 40% | 1.2% |
| 4 | 10 | 67% | 6.7% |

Adapted from Clark et al.[32]

from CS which were clinically indicated in a variety of complicated circumstances and, therefore, give us the worst possible case scenarios. This area needs much more research, especially focused on those CS done electively in fit women who had antibiotic prophylaxis. The fact remains that, in the follow-up studies available, there are significant risks associated with future fertility.

The incidence of placenta praevia and placenta accreta increase almost linearly after each previous CS (see Table 2),[32] and placental abruption is increased by 2–4-fold.[33] As the risk of these complications increases the more children a women has, her future reproductive intention is very relevant to any individual woman's caesarean threshold.

### Psychological sequelae

Although all women entering labour face the risks of emergency CS, instrumental vaginal delivery and perineal trauma, the majority will achieve a normal vaginal delivery giving them an enormous sense of achievement and fulfilment. Whatever the outcome, however, the pain experienced – which can be combined with overwhelming fear and a feeling of loss of control – can have profound effects on the woman both short and long-term. The recovery after labour depends on individual circumstances, but post-traumatic stress disorder is being increasingly recognised. This can have tremendous implications for the woman's future and especially on sexual relations and childbearing.[34] The evidence available to suggest CS is traumatic does not relate to those done for choice where we have no evidence either way.

### Long-term problems from vaginal delivery

The anal sphincter is ruptured in 35% of women with their first vaginal delivery.[35] Only a few of these are diagnosed clinically and, of those recognised and repaired, 85% will still have a defect at follow-up, with 50% being symptomatic.[36] One of the problems with anal incontinence is the embarrassment women feel and, therefore, this condition is very under-reported.[37] In a recent study in the UK, 24% of 54 multiparae were faecally incontinent and 60% had defective anal sphincters.[38] Urinary incontinence occurs in up to a third of women after vaginal delivery[39] and a recent study from Oregon investigating 150,000 women demonstrated an 11% life-time risk of requiring surgery for either urinary incontinence or prolapse.[40]

## SENSIBLE STRATEGIES TO MINIMISE RISK

Currently, the evidence is incomplete and much more work needs to be done on investigating the complications of labour, vaginal delivery and CS, but there is no doubt that the way ahead must focus on minimising risk whatever way the woman needs to be delivered.

### Caesarean section

Thromboprophylaxis, antibiotics, regional blockade and early mobilisation should already be standard practice, but we need to work more on surgical techniques to establish the optimum uterine closure, to reduce the likelihood of future placentation complications.

### Labour

Despite the fact that active management of labour has yet to be proved effective in any randomised trial, there can be no doubt of the value of intensive one-to-one care of women appropriately prepared antenatally. How valuable early amniotomy is will remain debatable, but the process of accurate diagnosis of labour is something that few units can boast of or audit. Any approach to labour which demands a thinking, critical review of women as they prepare for, present and labour can only be advantageous. Let us not forget that 45% of the intrapartum deaths investigated by CESDI had suboptimal antepartum care.[15]

## GROUNDS FOR REFUSAL

When faced with a woman requesting an elective CS because she cannot accept the risks of labour as given impartially, while accepting the known and theoretical risks of CS, how should one respond? The evidence is inconclusive and, therefore, in such situations the patient's opinions and values should matter. On what grounds could we refuse?

### Unnatural

As doctors we must do no harm, yet this does not mean doing nothing, and it remains that the pregnant woman needs to be delivered either vaginally or abdominally. CS is a surgical procedure and, as such, could be considered 'unnatural' – indeed you could argue that medicine is unnatural – but is it? Evolution, which is based on natural selection, includes the development of the brain and the intelligence to adapt to the trials of life. Hence, the human has a large brain with which to think and a narrow pelvis with which to move. Natural selection is taking us towards more difficult childbirth which we are intelligent enough to overcome.[41]

### Financial

The Audit Commission report in the UK costed CS at £780 more than vaginal delivery.[42] These CS included emergency and elective procedures which were medically indicated and, therefore, once again we have the problem of not being able to compare like with like. More recently, MacKenzie has costed CS as £24 more than IOL in nulliparous women and £174 more in multiparae.[43] Furthermore, this cost is only one of many that should be taken into the equation when considering elective CS against labour. The long-term health costs of future deliveries, future pelvic floor dysfunction and future corrective surgery are unaccounted for, as are the overwhelming medical negligence costs of brain damaged babies.

### Not feasible logistically

We must also consider whether it would be possible to satisfy the demands for elective CS in fit healthy women. On first impressions, one may think that performing CS for choice would increase the work-load significantly, but the demand is likely to be very small, as discussed below, and the logistics of staffing an acute unit with a variable work-load is much more complex and inefficient than staffing a theatre list. Midwives are in very short supply in the UK, which is sadly something that is unlikely to improve in the short-term and, therefore, planned delivery and maximising health care assistant roles in the postnatal period could be seen as more efficient, cost effective and also potentially achievable.

## THE LIKELY DEMAND

Given the above limited evidence on the risks of elective CS in a fit healthy woman, compared to the much more readily available evidence of the shortcomings of labour, it is hardly surprising that some women are beginning to opt for elective CS. Obstetricians are clearly exposed to the worst of the obstetric scenarios and, therefore, it is perhaps not surprising that, when London obstetricians were questioned about their preferences in the hypothetical situation of being at term with an uncomplicated singleton cephalic fetus, a not insignificant minority (17%) would opt for CS for themselves or their partner.[44] The noteworthy feature of the Al-Mufti study is not so much the overall CS preference rate but the female to male differences: 31% of females as opposed to 8% of males would choose an elective abdominal delivery in a completely uncomplicated pregnancy of a singleton cephalic fetus at term. This difference in choice between men and women cannot be because of professional exposure on the labour ward. What then? Is it that women are more likely to describe their embarrassing symptoms to the female gynaecologists or are the latter just more sympathetic to them?

We know that in Italy, where obstetricians are obliged to do what their patients request, 4% of women choose CS. We do not have comparable figures from the UK, but there is no doubt that maternal request has a big impact on CS for less than completely normal circumstances. Jackson and Irvine[10] demonstrated that 38% of all elective CS done in a district general hospital in the UK were for maternal request in the absence of any contra-indication to vaginal delivery, mostly in women with previous CS scars, and we know from Australia and the US[9,27] that 50% of women with a previous CS will request another one.

It is perhaps not so surprising that women are becoming intolerant of risk when one thinks how 'expectant' we have all become. Our lives are more safe and controlled now than ever before: perinatal, infant and maternal mortality are at an all time low in the developed world, and we can plan our families and have prenatal diagnosis to reduce the likelihood of abnormality. It is, therefore, understandable that some people will request a medicalised, controlled and safe method of delivering their baby.

## CURRENT OPINION

In the UK, the opinion stated in a *British Medical Journal* editorial in 1987[45] suggested that it was medically negligent to perform a CS for maternal request alone. This is now being challenged. Editorials in the two leading UK journals published the same week in March 1997,[46,47] after the Audit Commission report[42] stated that:

> those who favoured technology over nature were comfortably in the majority...cost and effectiveness issues need to be considered alongside woman's views. If the two conflict obstetricians should support the woman not the auditor.[46]

and that:

> The trend for use of caesarean section, coupled with greater emphasis on individual autonomy has clearly progressed too far for a return to paternalistic directions to women on how they should give birth. Instead the emphasis should be on comparisons of the implications of vaginal versus CS delivery. The uptake of CS in women made aware of such information will clearly be more appropriate than any current 'desirable' targets.[47]

### Informing women

The most crucial area to address in this whole debate is the fact that women must be appropriately informed. Consumer groups aim to educate generally but do not address personal characteristics, while professionals address these individual features but are in danger of being influenced by anecdotal experience and bias. We are all aware of the impression that a woman's decision is largely dependent on the doctor involved in the counselling. It is often felt that junior doctors who are training amidst already high CS rates are not adequately experience to perform this role; but, if we agree that senior trainees or consultant must be involved, it is then illogical for these women to be supervised in their delivery by the junior doctor. There is no easy answer to this problem other than to support the recent drive for more consultant input into intrapartum care.

### Technicians

One professional worry is that obstetricians are in danger of becoming technicians[4] and shedding responsibility for their actions by 'blaming' patient choice. This shedding of responsibility is unacceptable in any case where a woman decides to opt for a course that her doctor believes inappropriate. Whether this be a refusal of treatment or a request for inappropriate intervention, the doctor has a duty to try to advise and persuade further. In most cases, consensus will be reached; this issue of maternal choice only arises after all such information and advice has been offered. In such a situation, any woman challenging a firm medical opinion must have a very good reason for doing so (she is after all in a relatively weak position when faced with an experienced, informed and confident professional) and this should be explored. With the evidence so incomplete, we cannot judge her acceptance of some risks in preference to others as wrong just because they differ from ours.

### Message to the public

Another major area of concern in this debate relates to its misinterpretation: **if we agree (and many do not) that CS should be done for maternal request in specific cases, it does not mean that the profession is suggesting that CS is good and labour and vaginal delivery are bad.** This is a false conclusion which is not supported by the available evidence. The fact is that we have inadequate evidence, and further research is needed to establish how to minimise the risks as well as to investigate the longer term outcomes of either approach in different clinical situations. Neither does it mean that CS should be seen as an easy option during intrapartum care, with lower threshold to resorting to this method of delivery. Emergency CS in labour is the worst of all worlds and should be avoided by appropriate antenatal planning and rigorous intrapartum care.

## CONCLUSIONS

The increasing dialogue between all groups of patients and doctors across the specialties should not be seen as a threat to professional opinion and judgement. It should be a stimulus to the profession to help them communicate with their patients and increase patient satisfaction with the services we provide. However, if we are to converse and involve patients in this way, we cannot then discard their opinions and preferences as irrelevant to the decision making process if they happen to differ from our own. The risks of CS and labour are real but different, and if fully explained to the woman, she should be allowed to accept one set of risks over the other – after all she is the person who has to live with the consequences. An elective CS in a fit healthy woman is neither unsafe nor bad practice if she truly understands the risks involved and is adamant that she cannot accept the risks of labour or vaginal delivery.

### References

1 Sachs B P, Kobelin C, Castro M A, Frigoletto F. The risks of lowering the caesarean delivery rate. N Engl J Med 1999; 340: 54–57
2 Paterson-Brown S, Fisk N M. Caesarean section: every woman's right to choose? Curr Opin Obstet Gynecol 1997; 9: 351–355
3 Paterson-Brown S, Amu O. Should doctors perform an elective caesarean section on request? BMJ 1998; 317: 462–465
4 De Zulueta P, Norman B, Crowhurst J A et al. Elective caesarean section on request [letter]. BMJ 1999; 318: 120–122
5 Stirrat G M. The place of caesarean section. Contemp Rev Obstet Gynaecol 1998; 10: 177–183

6  Gilbert S. Doctors report rise in elective caesareans. New York Times 1998; Vol CXLVIII no 51, 288

7  Expert Maternity Group. Changing Childbirth. London: HMSO, 1993

8  General Medical Council. Maintaining good medical practice. London: GMC, 1998

9  Lau T K, Wong S H, Li C Y. A study of patients' acceptance towards vaginal birth after caesarean section. Aust N Z J Obstet Gynaecol 1996; 36: 155–158

10  Jackson N V, Irvine L M. The influence of maternal request on the elective caesarean section rate. J Obstet Gynaecol 1998; 18: 115–119

11  Mould T A J, Chong S, Spencer J A D, Gallivan S. Women's involvement with the decision preceding their caesarean section and their degree of satisfaction. Br J Obstet Gynaecol 1996; 103: 1074–1077

12  Lescale K B, Inglis S R, Eddleman K A, Peeper E Q, Chervenak F A, McCullough L B. Conflicts between physicians and patients in non-elective cesarean delivery: incidence and the adequacy of informed consent. Am J Perinatol 1996; 13: 171–176

13  Graham W J, Hundley V, McCheyne A L, Hall M H, Gurney E, Milne J. An investigation of women's involvement in the decision to deliver by caesarean section. Br J Obstet Gynaecol 1999; 106: 213–220

14  Hilder L, Costeloe K, Thilaganathan B. Prolonged pregnancy: evaluating gestation specific risks of fetal and infant mortality. Br J Obstet Gynaecol 1998; 105: 169–173

15  Maternal and Child Health Research Consortium. Confidential Enquiry into Stillbirths and Deaths in Infancy, 4th Annual Report. (1997) London: Maternal and Child Health Research Consortium (Chiltern Court, 188 Baker Street, London NW1 5SD, UK), 1997

16  Adamson S J, Louisa M A, Badawi N, Burton P R, Pemberton P J, Stanley F. Predictors of neonatal encephalopathy in full term infants. BMJ 1995; 311: 598–602

17  Robertson C M, Finer N N, Grace M G A. School performance of survivors of neonatal encephalopathy associated with birth asphyxia at term. J Pediatr 1989; 114: 753–760

18  Ingemarsson I, Herbst A, Thorngren-Jerneck K. Long-term outcome after umbilical artery acidaemia at term birth: influence of gender and duration of fetal heart-rate abnormalities. Br J Obstet Gynaecol 1997; 104: 1123–1127

19  Morrison J J, Rennie J M, Milton P J. Neonatal respiratory morbidity and mode of delivery at term: influence of timing of elective caesarean section. Br J Obstet Gynaecol 1995; 102: 101–106

20  El-Khodor B F, Boksa P. Birth insult increases amphetamine-induced behavioural responses in the adult rat. Neuroscience 1998; 87: 893–904

21  Vaillancourt C, Boksa P. Caesarean section birth with general anaesthesia increases dopamine-mediated behaviour in the adult rat. Neuroreport 1998; 9: 2953–2959

22  Jacobson B, Bygdeman N. Obstetric care and proneness of offspring to suicide as adults: case control study. BMJ 1998; 317: 1346–1349

23  Lilford R J, Van Coeverden deGroot H A, Moore P J, Bingham P. The relative risks of caesarean section (intrapartum and elective) and vaginal delivery: a detailed analysis to exclude the effects of medical disorders and other acute preexisting physiological disturbances. Br J Obstet Gynaecol 1990; 97: 883–892

24  Anon. Report on Confidential Enquiries into Maternal Deaths in the UK 1994-6. London: HMSO, 1998

25  Macfarlane A. At last – maternity statistics for England. BMJ 1998; 316: 566–567

26  Sachs B P, Yeh J, Acker D, Driscoll S, Brown D A J, Jewett J-F. Cesarean section-related mortality in Massachusetts, 1954–85. Obstet Gynecol 1988; 71: 385–388

27  McMahon M J, Luther E R, Bowes W A, Olshan A F. Comparison of a trial of labour with an elective second cesarean section. N Engl J Med 1996, 335: 689–695

28  Roman J, Bakos O, Cnattingius S. Pregnancy outcomes by mode of delivery among term breech births: Swedish experience 1987–1993. Obstet Gynecol 1998; 92: 945–950

29  Obwegeser R, Ulm M, Simon M, Ploeckinger B, Gruber W. Breech infants: vaginal or cesarean delivery? Acta Obstet Gynecol Scand 1996, 75: 912–916

30  Glazener C M A, Abdalla M, Stroud P, Naji S, Templeton A, Russell I T. Postnatal maternal morbidity: extent, causes, prevention and treatment. Br J Obstet Gynaecol 1995; 102: 282–287

31  Howell C J. Epidural vs non-epidural analgesia in labour (Cochrane Review) In: Oxford: The Cochrane Library, issue 3, update, 1998

32  Clark S L, Koonings P P, Phelan J P. Placenta previa/accreta and prior cesarean section. Obstet Gynecol 1985; 66: 89–92

33  Hemminki E, Merilainen J. Long-term effects of cesarean sections: ectopic pregnancies and placental problems. Am J Obstet Gynecol 1996, 174: 1569–1574

34  Jolly J, Walker J, Bhabra K. Subsequent obstetric performance related to primary mode of delivery. Br J Obstet Gynaecol 1999; 106: 227–232

35  Sultan A H, Kamm M A, Hudson C N, Thomas J M, Bartram C I. Sphincter disruption during vaginal deliveries. N Engl J Med 1993; 329: 1905–1911

36  Sultan A H, Kamm M A, Hudson C N, Bartram C I. Third degree obstetric anal sphincter tears: risk factors and outcome of primary repair. BMJ 1994; 308: 887–891

37  MacArthur C, Bick D E, Keighley M R B. Faecal incontinence after childbirth. Br J Obstet Gynaecol 1997; 104: 46–50

38  Frudinger A, Halligan S, Bartram C I, Spencer J A D, Kamm M A Changes in anal anatomy following vaginal delivery revealed by anal endosonography. Br J Obstet Gynaecol 1999; 106: 223–227

39  Wilson P D, Herbison R M, Herbison G P. Obstetric practice and the prevalence of urinary incontinence three months after delivery. Br J Obstet Gynaecol 1996; 103: 154–161

40  Olsen A L, Smith V J, Bergstrom J O, Colling J C, Clark A L. Epidemiology of surgically managed pelvic organ prolapse and urinary incontinence. Obstet Gynecol 1997; 89: 501–506

41  Steer P. Caesarean section: an evolving procedure? Br J Obstet Gynaecol 1998; 105: 1052–1055

42  Audit Commission. First Class Delivery: Improving Maternity Services in England and Wales. Abingdon: Audit Commission Publications, 1997

43  MacKenzie I Z. Should women who elect to have caesarean sections pay for them? BMJ 1999; 318: 1070

44  Al-Mufti R, McCarthy A, Fisk N M. Survey of obstetricians' personal preference and discretionary practice. Eur J Obstet Gynecol Reprod Biol 1997; 73: 1–4

45  Hall M. When a woman asks for a caesarean section. BMJ 1987; 294: 201–202

46  Drife J. Maternity services: the Audit Commission reports. BMJ 1997; 314: 844

47  Anon. What is the right number of caesarean sections? Lancet 1997; 349: 815

*Gautam Khastgir John Studd*

# Oestrogen and osteoporosis

Osteoporosis is a disease of major public health importance which affects over one-third of all postmenopausal women causing severe pain, disability and even mortality.[1,2] It has been referred as the 'silent epidemic' because it is usually clinically apparent only when fractures occur by which time the disease is well-established and perhaps irreversible. The problem is common in the Western world but there are also reports of a high prevalence in the Asian population.[3] In the UK, there are over 200,000 osteoporotic fractures each year and the cost to the National Health Service is estimated to be £940 million.[4] With the increase in ageing population, it has been estimated that the number of osteoporotic fractures would double over the next 50 years.[4] Hence, there is a need for an effective osteoporosis management strategies, as recognised by the Department of Health Advisory Group on Osteoporosis.[5] This has been supported by a recent publication of 'evidence-based' clinical guidelines for the prevention and treatment of osteoporosis.[4]

The association of osteoporosis and oestrogen deficiency has been known for over 50 years, since Fuller Albright noted that 40 of his 42 osteoporotic patients were postmenopausal women.[6] In recent years, the causal relationship between the menopause and osteoporosis has been confirmed due to oestrogen deficiency induced accelerated bone loss.[7] Hence, oestrogen replacement therapy (ERT) is the logical and appropriate first-line intervention to consider for the prevention and treatment of osteoporosis. In postmenopausal women, ERT not only arrests bone loss,[8-15] but also improves bone mineral density (BMD)[17-22]

**Dr Gautam Khastgir** MD FRCS MRCOG, Subspecialty Senior Registrar in Reproductive Medicine and Honorary Lecturer in Obstetrics and Gynaecology, Department of Obstetrics and Gynaecology, Imperial College School of Medicine, Chelsea & Westminster Hospital, 369 Fulham Road, London SW10 9NH, UK (Present address for correspondence: F E 8 Salt Lake Sector III, Calcutta 700 091, India)

**Mr John Studd** DSc MD FRCOG, Consultant Gynaecologist, Dept of Obstetrics & Gynaecology, Imperial College School of Medicine, Chelsea & Westminster Hospital, 369 Fulham Rd, London SW10 9NH, UK

leading to a reduced risk of osteoporotic fracture.[23-29] These findings have been consistently shown in both clinical[8-22] and epidemiological studies.[23-29]

Many publications have confirmed the role of oestrogen in maintaining skeletal homeostasis both in human and in various animal models.[8-22,30-47] The use of cell culture models and molecular biology techniques have increased our understanding of the basis of oestrogen action on bone cells. The initiation of large controlled trials has confirmed the anti-osteoporotic action of oestrogen in postmenopausal women. Traditionally, ERT has been employed in the prevention of early postmenopausal bone loss,[8-11,18] but its use has been extended to the treatment of established osteoporosis.[16,17,19,21,22,30-32] The aim of this review is to give a summary of the oestrogenic action on bone and the current status of oestrogen replacement as a therapeutic option for the prevention and treatment of postmenopausal osteoporosis.

## MECHANISM OF BONE LOSS AFTER THE MENOPAUSE

The effect of oestrogen deficiency on bone is best understood by considering the structural organization of the skeleton, which is comprised of discrete microscopic units described as basic multicellular units (BMUs).[33] These units consist of a group of bone resorbing cells (osteoclasts) and a group of bone forming cell (osteoblasts) with their respective precursors. They mediate all skeletal activities such as growth and fracture repair, but their main function is to 'remodel' the skeleton. Bone remodelling is a replacement mechanism whereby the BMUs remove microscopic parts of the skeleton at discrete loci by osteoclasts and replace them with new bone formed by osteoblasts.[33] In health there are several million active remodelling sites in the skeleton, but these occupy a minority of the bone surface (15–20%).

Oestrogen deficiency accelerates the rate of bone turn-over with a rapid activation of new bone remodelling units.[34,35] Thus, at any one time, a progressively greater surface of bone will be occupied by remodelling events. Since remodelling implies a net deficit of bone until resorption cavities are

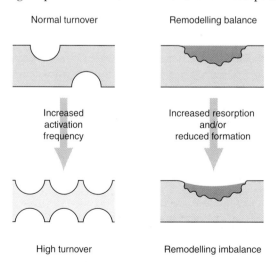

**Fig. 1** Postmenopausal bone loss due to oestrogen deficiency induced changes in bone turnover and remodelling balance.

completely filled, the skeletal volume missing at one time increases (Fig. 1).[36] Because of the prolonged turn-over time of the skeleton, it may take several years to reach a new steady state where the skeletal mass is no longer decreasing. This accounts, in part, for the accelerated bone losses that occur in the early years after the menopause.[37]

In addition, an imbalance between the amount of bone removed and that subsequently incorporated into each remodelling site forms the basis of both age related and menopause related bone loss (Fig. 1).[38] The quantum concept of bone remodelling has suggested that bone loss is either due to deep resorption cavities by osteoclasts or incomplete refilling of normal resorption cavities by osteoblasts.[39] Thus, skeletal mass decreases incrementally with each remodelling event and with accelerated bone turnover after menopause, the rate of bone loss is amplified leading to trabecular thinning.[35,37,40,41] It has been estimated that about two-thirds of the bone loss in old women can be ascribed to the menopause, and about one-third to ageing.[42]

Bone loss associated with oestrogen deficiency and advancing age is accompanied by a breakdown of micro-architecture, which decreases the mechanical competence out of proportion to the amount of bone loss.[40,43-45] As a result of successive deep resorption at a particular site, there is complete perforation and fragmentation of some trabeculae leading to loss of connectivity.[43,46] This could result from increased osteoclast activity caused by so-called 'killer osteoclasts', or to normal osteoclastic resorption defect occurring in relatively thin plates at an increased frequency after the menopause.[35] As a result of trabecular breakdown, there is no bone structure on which new bone formation can occur. In elderly patients with osteoporosis, there is also a decrease in new bone formation, presumably reflecting the inability of osteoblasts to repair adequately.[47,48]

The surface of cancellous bone is much greater than that of cortical bone, despite cancellous bone occupying a minority of the total skeletal mass. Because of such high surface to volume ratio of cancellous bone, osteoporosis commonly affects the cancellous site earlier and more floridly than the cortical site.[7,42] Hence, osteoporotic fractures occur most commonly in the vertebral bodies, proximal femur and distal forearm as these sites have predominantly cancellous bone. The proportion of cancellous to cortical bone may also explain, in part, the occurrence of vertebral crush fracture and Colles' fracture of distal forearm early in the natural history of osteoporosis, whereas hip fractures are a later event.

In the immediate postmenopausal period, bone loss accelerates when as much as 5% or more of trabecular bone and 1.5% of cortical bone are lost annually. This superimposes on age-related bone loss, which has been estimated to be at a rate of 1% per year. The accelerated phase of bone loss slows after 2–4 years in cancellous bone and 5–7 years in cortical bone but the age-related bone loss continues into old age so that by the age of 80 years, bone mass declines to half of its peak value.[42] It has been estimated that women lose 35% of the cortical bone and 50% of cancellous bone in their lifetime.[42,49,50] As a result of postmenopausal bone loss, the life-time risks of sustaining a fracture in a 50-year-old white women has been estimated to be 32% at the vertebra, 16% at the hip and 16% at the wrist.[51] The incidence of postmenopausal fracture increases with age.[52-54] After the age of 60 years, a quarter of all white women have a vertebral crush fracture,[55] which over the age of 70 years affects as many as one out of two women.[52] Similarly, the incidence of hip fracture rises exponentially beyond the age of 50 years.[26]

# EFFECTS OF OESTROGEN ON THE SKELETON

Oestrogen has been shown to regulate different aspects of the bone remodelling process and its effects are now known both at the tissue and cellular levels. The organization of bone into BMUs with a sequential action of osteoclasts and osteoblasts makes it impossible to generalise the findings of cell culture in relation to actual tissue changes. However, bone histomorphometry allows detailed studies of the dynamics of bone remodelling and the activities of individual bone cells.

## Oestrogenic action on bone turn-over

The main action of oestrogen at the tissue level is a reduction of the rate of bone turn-over by limiting osteoclasts to create new erosion cavities.[56] Furthermore, oestrogen suppresses excessive bone resorption and, thereby, corrects the imbalance at each remodelling site.[56–58] However, filling-in of the existing erosion cavities continues so that skeletal mass may increase for some time until a new steady state is achieved. This results in relatively small increments in skeletal mass after a year or so, which should not be interpreted as an anabolic response.

The conventional dose of ERT is considered to be ineffective in replacing the bone loss that has already occurred and in reversing the micro-architectural damage of patients with established osteoporosis.[59] A higher dose of ERT has shown to stimulate bone formation in animal models.[60] Such anabolic effect has recently been evident on human skeleton after long-term higher dose ERT using subcutaneous implants. In women with established osteoporosis, there was a rise in cancellous bone volume, mean wall thickness, trabecular thickness, trabecular number and trabecular connectivity after 6 years of implant therapy.[61] These histological changes occur with about 15–30% increase in BMD at the hip and lumbar spine. Neither the age nor the interval since menopause at the beginning of treatment influenced the histomorphometric variables, which indicates that bone loss is largely reversible with appropriate ERT at any time after the menopause.

## Oestrogenic action of bone cells

The precise mechanisms of oestrogen actions on bone cells are not fully understood, but there is evidence suggesting that it exerts a direct effect as well as indirectly alters local humoral mediators. Oestrogen receptors (ERs) have been identified in osteoblasts[62,63] and, to a lesser extent, in osteocytes and osteoclasts.[64,65] The widespread presence of ERs allows for multiple options in terms of how oestrogens might affect bone and also for the possibility of multifaceted effects. However, these receptors are found in relatively low concentrations when compared with other oestrogen cell targets which implies that additional indirect mechanisms may play an important role in bone conservation.

Oestrogen is a potent inhibitor of osteoclast differentiation and activity, and is also considered as a powerful inducer of apoptosis. It has shown to have direct effects on osteoclasts.[65] However, suppression of bone resorption activity of osteoclasts in cell culture has been found to be dependent on the presence of osteoblasts. This suggests that oestrogen possibly exert its effect on osteoclast indirectly by stimulating osteoblasts to produce factors that are capable of controlling osteoclast cell differentiation and function.[66] These interactions are mediated through a multitude of cytokines and growth factors on which oestrogen has a profound effect. Oestrogen inhibits a number of osteoclast-stimulating mediators, such as interleukin-1 (IL-1), interleukin-6 (IL-6), tumour necrosis factor (TNFα) and stimulates osteoclast-inhibiting mediators, transforming growth factor-β (TGF-β).[67-72] However, in a recent study no difference in marrow plasma levels of IL-1α, IL-1β, and IL-6 were seen in postmenopausal women, irrespective of ERT use.[73] Oestrogen may also protect bone by lowering local prostaglandin concentrations and by reducing the responsiveness of bones to the resorbing effect of parathyroid hormone (PTH).[74]

Oestrogen acts directly on osteoblasts in stimulating bone formation with an increase in type I procollagen.[75,76] It also stimulates osteoblasts to release TGF-β, which mediates bone formation. In addition, oestrogen increases insulin-like growth factor 1 (IGF-1) mRNA levels and reduces parathyroid hormone (PTH) stimulated adenylate cyclase activity, which may also contribute to oestrogen's bone-conserving action.[77] However, the effect of oestrogen on osteoblasts in cell culture is still equivocal with some studies not supporting stimulation of cell proliferation and increased collagen synthesis.[78] These discrepancies may reflect differences in the cell culture method, the osteoblast cell model employed, or a variation in the number of oestrogen receptors. The diversity of response may also indicate that the effects are limited to a subpopulation of bone cells.

## ROLE OF ERT IMMEDIATELY AFTER THE MENOPAUSE

### Effects on bone mineral density

A large number of prospective studies have unequivocally demonstrated that ERT arrests early postmenopausal bone loss.[8-12] Some of these studies have also shown an increase in bone mineral density (BMD) of 2–10% within 12–36 months of ERT.[13-22] The most pronounced increase is seen in vertebral bodies due to maximum cancellous bone, an intermediate rise in proximal femur with a combination of cancellous and cortical bones, while the areas of mainly cortical bone, such as forearm, display only preservation of bone mass. Women with large body frame and lower BMD respond better than slender women and those with higher BMD.[79] The best responders were also furthest past menopause which indicates that the longer the time of oestrogen deprivation the greater the capacity of bone to respond to ERT (Fig. 2A).[20]

There is a definable minimum effective oestrogen (E)/oestradiol ($E_2$) dose for prevention of bone loss in a majority of women (oral $E_2$ valerate/micronised 17β-$E_2$ 2 mg daily; oral conjugated E 0.625 mg daily; transdermal 17β-$E_2$ 50 μg daily; percutaneous gel 17β-$E_2$ 1.5 mg daily; subcutaneous implant 17β-$E_2$ 25–50 mg every 6 months).[80,81] However, some individuals continue to lose bone despite taking the recommended bone-sparing dose of ERT.[15,20] In such women there may be a better response if the ERT dose is increased. This is supported by the fact that the minimum bone sparing circulatory oestradiol level is 300 pmol/l,[22] which may not be achieved with the minimum dose of ERT by the oral and transdermal routes in all women. It is, therefore, recommended that the

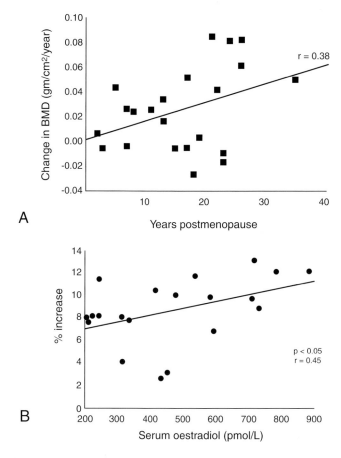

**Fig. 2** Bone mineral density changes with oestrogen replacement therapy according to (**A**) duration since menopause and (**B**) the serum oestradiol levels. Adapted from (A) Lindsay and Tohme[16] and (B) Studd et al[17] with permission.

response to HRT is monitored by BMD scans every 2–3 years to give the appropriate bone-sparing dose. One study has shown no additional effect of higher than the bone-sparing dose of ERT but the dose range was not very wide.[80] Others have reported a progressive dose-related response with ERT[22,82,83] and this is supported by the finding that there is a positive correlation between the percentage increase in BMD and the circulatory oestradiol level (Fig. 2B).[17,20–22]

In general, the oral and transdermal routes of ERT are equally effective in conserving bone loss.[15,20] However, subcutaneous implants produce a higher circulatory oestradiol level and, therefore, result in a greater increase in BMD (8–12%) within 1 year.[17,20,21] This indicates that a reduction in bone remodelling space (4–6%) does not fully account for oestrogen's action on the skeleton.[41,56,57] The potential of subcutaneous ERT to increase BMD has been shown even after many postmenopausal years of oral ERT.[84]

When HRT is initiated at the onset of the menopause, the expected bone loss is prevented for the duration of therapy up to 15 years.[12] However, a cross-sectional study after long-term ERT of similar duration has shown that BMD

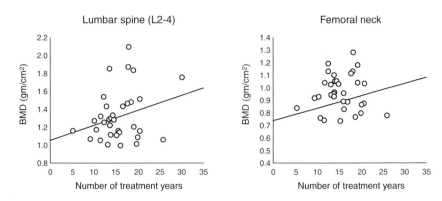

**Fig. 3** Bone mineral density levels according to the duration of oestrogen replacement therapy. Adapted from Naessen and Persson[87] with permission.

at the spine was actually 54.2% greater than non-treated controls.[11] There is also a recent prospective evidence of a continuous increase in bone mass of postmenopausal women treated with oestrogen for 8 years making the spinal BMD 14.8% higher than controls. Bone mass in the forearm was preserved, but was 14.5% higher than in untreated women, who showed a continuous fall during the study period.[85] Such a degree and timing of bone changes indicate a possible anabolic effect, rather than filling in of remodelling space, which is usually completed within 2 years.[41,56,57]

The increase in BMD was even higher (20–25%) with long-term oestradiol implant therapy for 5–30 years.[86,87] Serum levels of oestradiol correlates with BMD at all measurement sites.[87] Interestingly, even with the higher circulatory level of oestrogen, there is a continued dose response and the greatest increase is seen in women with lowest BMD.[22] The rise in BMD has been shown to continue as long as the high dose ERT is being administered (Fig. 3),[86,87] and this results in a very high BMD (> 2–3 standard deviations above the age-matched mean) after 15 years of oestradiol implant therapy.[88] There was no influence of age on BMD, contrasting with non-users who showed an inverse relationship between age and BMD.[86,87] These findings suggest that the anabolic effect of ERT is more likely in those with low BMD and it is also dose and duration dependent.

## Effects on fracture incidence

It has been suggested that, with the use of HRT, an increase in BMD by 10% would decrease the risk of fragility fracture by 50% in the female population.[89–91]. However, the reduction in fracture risk by ERT actually exceeds that expected based on BMD alone.[91,92] This indicates that ERT might also improve bone quality or trabecular architecture, which has an independent contribution on osteoporotic fracture risk.[40,45]

A number of epidemiological studies have confirmed that postmenopausal ERT is associated with a reduction in the fracture risk. Many of these retrospective case-control and cohort studies have shown a compound reduction in relative risk of hip and spinal fracture between 0.5 and 0.75 after ERT (Fig. 4A).[11,23–26] Similarly, in another retrospective cohort study, the relative risk of

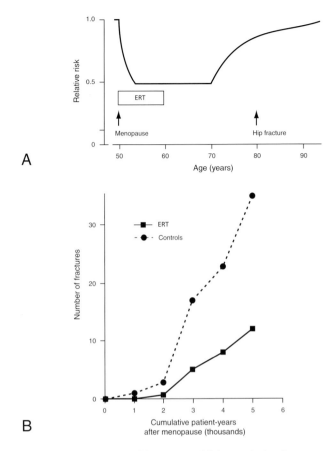

A

B

**Fig. 4:** (**A**) Relative risks of fracture and (**B**) cumulative fracture rates with long term oestrogen replacement therapy (ERT). Adapted from (A) Ettinger et al[11] and (B) Kanis[91] with permission.

distal forearm fracture was 0.3 in women exposed to ERT.[93] In these observational studies, an effect of sampling cannot be excluded as healthier individuals may have sought and taken HRT. However, one randomised controlled prospective study also confirmed a significant reduction in relative risk of vertebral fracture by greater than 0.5 after one year of ERT in post-menopausal women.[19]

Postmenopausal women need to use ERT for at least 5 years before the fracture protective effect is observed.[24] The mean duration of ERT in most studies was far below (3–5 years) the time considered necessary to achieve significant effects on the skeleton (10 years or more). However, even after a long-term ERT (average of 14 years), the incidence of osteoporosis fracture was about 50% lower than control (Fig. 4B).[11] The results were similar for women under and over 75 years of age. In users starting HRT within 5 years of menopause, the relative risk was 0.29 for hip fracture, 0.29 for wrist fracture and 0.50 for vertebral fracture.[28] After an average of 17 years of ERT, an age adjusted relative risk was 0.29 for hip fracture, 0.57 for vertebral fracture and 0.55 for wrist fracture.[29]

## ROLE OF ERT IN OLDER POSTMENOPAUSAL WOMEN

Elderly patients and their doctors often believe that it is too late for ERT but it can actually reduce the rate of bone loss[16,19,21,30–32] and the incidence of fracture at that age.[19] Several prospective studies have evaluated the potential benefit of later initiation of ERT. These short-term studies clearly and consistently show that women who started ERT after the age of 60 years had a substantial increase in BMD leading to significantly greater protection against bone loss compared with never users of same age.[30–32,56,94] With oral or transdermal route of ERT, the BMD increase in the initial 2 years has been reported to be 10–12% at the lumbar spine and 5% at the proximal femur.[16,19,30,56] However, with percutaneous route of ERT the BMD changes were quicker and greater showing an increase of 12.6% at the lumbar spine and 5.2% at the hip after 1 year.[21]

Interestingly, women older than 60 years experienced a greater incremental increase in BMD with ERT compered to younger subjects.[79] The most pronounced increase in BMD was noted in those women furthest from the menopause and consequently with the lowest initial BMD.[16,20–22] The authors concluded that postmenopausal women would benefit from the introduction of ERT at least up to 35 years after the menopause.[16] Hence, contrary to the popular belief, menopausal age appears to be positively, rather than inversely, correlated with the effect of ERT on BMD. The increase in BMD was shown even in older women with established osteoporosis.[16,19] Therefore, ERT can be considered for prevention as well as treatment of established osteoporosis in older women who have been postmenopausal for many years.[16,19,21,30–32] There is no truth in the view that women many years postmenopausal are too old or too osteoporotic for ERT.

## EFFECT OF STOPPING OESTROGEN THERAPY

On withdrawal of ERT, there is an initial bone loss equivalent to the rate in untreated postmenopausal women.[10] Several earlier studies have shown a rapid loss of BMD, which is referred as 'catch-up loss', in the first 1–2 years after cessation of ERT.[31,95] The rate of bone loss was not related to the duration of ERT and was similar to the rate of bone loss in untreated women during the first 2 years of menopause.[95] However, when ERT was stopped after age 65 years, the bone loss was more rapid than in those women of similar age who had never taken ERT.[31] A prospective study has reported that, for up to 7 years, bone loss occurs no more rapidly after stopping treatment than in untreated women and whether catch-up bone loss occurs thereafter is uncertain.[96]

Women who start ERT at the menopause and then stop after some years may lose all bone benefits by age 75 years. In the Framingham study, the bone density was preserved in women less than 75 years who had taken oestrogen for 7 years or more, but little residual effect on bone density in women who were 75 years or older.[27] Similarly, in the Rancho Bernardo study, the BMD of the past early users, who had taken ERT for an average of 10 years and had discontinued it 17 years previously, were similar to those of never users (Fig. 5).[97] In women who have stopped ERT, bone mineral density has been shown to be inversely associated with the number of years since discontinuation of therapy.[97,98] Hence, the option of improving bone mass with ERT has the

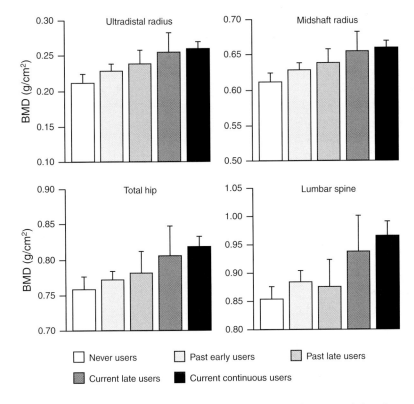

**Fig. 5** Bone mineral density results according to the time of onset and duration use of oestrogen replacement therapy. Adapted from Schneider et al[97] with permission.

additional benefit of extending the period of protection against osteoporosis after stopping the therapy.

Studies on fracture risk suggest that the protective effect is related to the duration of use and benefit appears to diminish rapidly after cessation of ERT.[99] It has been shown that there is a reduced effect on fracture rates in older women who have used ERT in the past (Fig. 4A).[24,100,101] In the study of osteoporotic fractures, no decrease in risk for hip, wrist or non-spinal fractures was noted in past oestrogen users (mean duration 4.8 years).[28] Similarly, in a population of women 65 years and older, only current users of oestrogen had a reduced risk of non-spinal fractures.[28] However, a potential confounding factor in these retrospective epidemiological studies in elderly women is that those with low bone density tend to die sooner.

## IDEAL TIME TO START OESTROGEN

The logical time for starting ERT is at the menopause, which clearly signals an oestrogen deficiency state. This has been the standard recommendation for osteoporosis prevention, as rapid bone loss occurs immediately after the menopause. It was thought that ERT taken for the first 10 years after the menopause would delay bone loss sufficiently to reduce the risk of osteoporotic fractures in old age. Moreover, ERT initiated at older age was not expected to be effective as the 'window of opportunity' would be past and bone loss in these older women was thought to be due to age, not oestrogen deficiency.[102,103] Recent studies have challenged these assumptions. There are several arguments for starting ERT later rather than at the age of menopause.

In order to obtain maximum protection from osteoporosis, women should start ERT at the menopause and continue lifelong.[31,97] This view is supported by the findings of the highest BMD in ever users of ERT over the age of 65 years and continued protection from bone loss as long as ERT was used (Fig. 5).[97] However, it is unlikely that ERT would be continued indefinitely and, if discontinued 5–10 years after the menopause, there is no long-term osteoporosis prevention benefit in old age.[27,28,30,31] It has been estimated that 10 years of ERT following the menopause would defer the risk of fracture by 10 years (Fig. 4A). This is confirmed by the findings that, about 10 years after stopping ERT, the bone density and fracture risks were similar in women who had used and who had not (Fig. 5).[97] Thus ERT would have a progressively decreasing impact on fractures after the age of 70 years, when most fractures occur (Fig. 4A).[104]

Moreover, ERT commenced after the age of 60 years may be as effective in preserving bone if started at the time of menopause and continued into late life (Fig. 5).[97] These findings are compatible with the estimated BMD model of women who did and did not use ERT as described by Ettinger and Gardy (Fig. 6).[105] They predicted that the difference in BMD at the age of 85 between women who use ERT continuously starting at the menopause or at 65 years, to be only between 2–6%. The risk reduction in osteoporotic fracture is most marked in the former group of women (0.73), although women who initiate therapy at the age of 65 years have almost as much protection with risk reduction between 0.57–0.69. However, 5 years treatment of ERT has a transient effect of osteoporotic fracture, irrespective of the age at which treatment is given and targeting intervention at the age of 60–70 years may actually prevent more hip fractures than targeting intervention at the time of the menopause.[104]

Delaying ERT facilitates the identification of women at high risk because BMD at age 60 years is a better predictor of future fracture risk than is

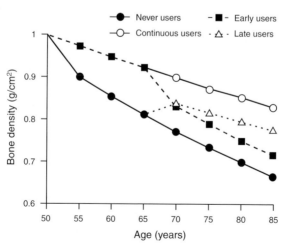

**Fig. 6** Bone mineral density changes with early and late onset as well as short and long-term use of oestrogen replacement therapy after menopause. Adapted from Ettinger and Grady[105] with permission.

perimenopausal BMD. It has been argued that most cost-effective intervention is to reduce or arrest bone loss when early osteoporosis is diagnosed (secondary prevention) than to treat a large group at a younger age (primary prevention), when it is uncertain, who will eventually develop the condition.[27] Such a strategy also reduces the duration of ERT and presumably the risk of breast cancer while still protecting bone.[97] The current opinion suggests that giving ERT for periods of up to 10 years would yield significant benefit with minimised risk of osteoporosis. Longer duration of ERT use should further increase benefit but may increase the risk of breast cancer.

These considerations suggest that targeting ERT at the time of the menopause have less than optimal effects on osteoporotic fractures throughout the lifetime of women. Indeed, it may be preferable to target intervention specifically for osteoporosis at a time later in the natural history of the disorder. This view is supported by the reasonable assumption that treatments are unlikely to be taken for life, and given that most hip fractures occur in the elderly. Thus, there is a growing support for the use of ERT to treat established osteoporosis in older women. However, delaying treatment is not recommended for women who have a premature menopause, menopausal symptoms or osteoporosis. It is an option for recently menopausal women who are asymptomatic, at no particular risk for fracture and can safely wait for 10 years before starting ERT.

## CONCLUSIONS

Postmenopausal osteoporosis is caused by oestrogen deficiency, which increases the rate of bone turnover, along with an excessive resorption and inadequate formation at each remodelling site. The outcome of such remodelling imbalance is an accelerated loss of bone mass leading to progressive thinning and disruption of trabecular architecture that result in a disproportionate loss of bone strength. ERT has been long-proven to be effective in preventing postmenopausal bone loss, but recent studies have also shown that it increases bone mineral density, which continues as long as the therapy is given. This is valid even in elderly women with established osteoporosis who respond better, as the lower the bone mass before therapy the greater is the response. Oestrogen not only decreases the rate of bone turnover and, thereby, reduces the number of resorption cavities, but also corrects the imbalance at each remodelling site, resulting in improved filling of such cavities. Moreover, there is current evidence of an increase in bone formation, particularly with a high dose and long-term ERT. These effects on bone cells are both direct through oestrogen receptors and indirect by the local mediators of bone turnover.

The beneficial effects of ERT in reducing osteoporotic fracture risks are now well-established. Most studies indicate that fracture rates are halved with current or recent past use of ERT. The minimum duration of ERT use to prevent fracture has yet to be firmly established, although some studies suggest that 5 years may be adequate. The minimum circulatory oestradiol level of 300 pmol/l, which is needed for reversal of bone loss, may not be achieved with a low dose oral ERT, particularly conjugated oestrogens. Cessation of ERT results in resumption of usual postmenopausal bone loss and thus the effect of 10 years of ERT is almost completely lost 10 years after stopping the therapy. Hence, current use of ERT is associated with a lower risk of fracture than past use. Since most women are unlikely to take ERT life long, in the absence of menopausal symptoms and any high risk for osteoporosis or heart disease, it is logical to start HRT after the age 60 years at the time when those at risk can be better identified. This view is supported by the finding that, women who take ERT for 10 years, starting late after age 60 years, have similar bone protection to those who are continuing since menopause. Moreover this regimen of osteoporosis prevention gives the option of limiting ERT to 10 years and avoids the increased risk of breast cancer.

## References

1 Melton L J, Chrischilles E A, Cooper C, Lane A W, Riggs B L. How many women have osteoporosis? J Bone Miner Res 1992; 7: 1005–1010

2 Cooper C. Epidemiology and definition of osteoporosis. In: Compston J E. (ed) Osteoporosis: New Perspective on Causes, Prevention and Treatment. London: Royal College of Physicians of London, 1996; 1–10

3 Cooper C, Campion G, Melton III L J. Hip fractures in the elderly: a world wide projection. Osteoporos Int 1992; 2: 285–289

4 The Guideline Development Group. Osteoporosis: Clinical Guidelines for Prevention and Treatment. London: Royal College of Physicians of London, 1999

5 Advisory Group on Osteoporosis. Report to the DoH. Barlow D H (ed). London: Department of Health, 1994

6 Albright F, Smith P H, Richardson A M. Postmenopausal osteoporosis: its clinical features. JAMA 1941; 116: 2465–2474

7 Nilas L, Christiansen C. The pathophysiology of peri- and postmenopausal bone loss. Br J Obstet Gynaecol 1989; 96: 580–587

8 Lindsay R, Hart D M, Aitken J M, MacDonald E B, Anderson J B, Clarke A C. Long term prevention of postmenopausal osteoporosis by oestrogen: evidence of increased bone mass after delayed onset of oestrogen treatment. Lancet 1976; i: 1038–1041

9 Nachtigall L E, Nachtigall R H, Nachtigall R D et al. Estrogen replacement therapy I: a 10 year prospective study in the relationship to osteoporosis. Obstet Gynecol 1979; 53: 277–281

10 Christiansen C, Christiansen M S, McNair P, Hagen C, Stocklund K, Transbol I B. Prevention of early postmenopausal bone loss: controlled 2-year study in 315 normal females. Eur J Clin Invest 1980; 10: 273–279

11 Ettinger B, Genant H K, Cann C E. Long-term estrogen replacement therapy prevents bone loss and fractures. Ann Intern Med 1985; 102: 319–324

12 Al-Azzawi F, Hart D M, Lindsay R. Long term effect of oestrogen replacement therapy on bone mass as measured by dual photon absorptiometry. BMJ 1987; 294: 1261–1262

13 Riis B J, Thomsen K, Strom V, Christiansen C. The effect of percutaneous estradiol and natural progesterone on postmenopausal bone loss. Am J Obstet Gynecol 1987; 156: 61–65

14 Munk-Jensen N, Nielsen S P, Obel E B, Eriksen P B. Reversal of postmenopausal vertebral bone loss by oestrogen and progestogen: a double blind placebo controlled study. BMJ 1988; 296: 1150–1152

15 Stevenson J C, Cust M P, Ganger K F, Hillard T C, Lees B, Whitehead M I. Effects of transdermal versus oral hormone replacement therapy on bone density in spine and proximal femur in postmenopausal women. Lancet 1990; 335: 265–269

16 Lindsay R, Tohme J F. Estrogen treatment with established postmenopausal osteoporosis. Obstet Gynecol 1990; 76: 290

17 Studd J W W, Savvas M, Watson N, Fogelman I, Cooper D. The relationship between plasma oestradiol and increased bone density in postmenopausal women after treatment with subcutaneous hormone implants. Am J Obstet Gynecol 1990; 163: 1474–1479

18 Prince R L, Smith M, Dick I M et al. Prevention of postmenopausal osteoporosis – a comparative study of exercise, calcium supplementation , and hormone replacement therapy. N Engl J Med 1991; 325: 1189–1195

19 Lufkin E G, Wahner H W, O'Fallon W M et al. Treatment of postmenopausal osteoporosis with transdermal estrogens. Ann Intern Med 1992; 117: 1–9

20 Hillard T C, Whitcroft S J, Marsh M S, Ellerington M C, Lees B, Whitehead M I. Long-term effects of transdermal and oral hormone replacement therapy on postmenopausal bone loss. Osteoporos Int 1994; 4: 341–348

21 Holland E F N, Leather A T, Studd J W W. Increase in bone mass of older postmenopausal women with low mineral bone density after one year of percutaneous oestradiol implants. Br J Obstet Gynaecol 1995; 102: 238–242

22 Studd J W W, Holland E F N, Leather A T, Smith R N J. The dose response of percutaneous oestradiol implants on the skeletons of postmenopausal women. Br J Obstet Gynaecol 1994; 101: 787–791

23 Hutchison T A, Polansky S M, Feinstein A R. Postmenopausal oestrogens protect against fractures of hip and distal radius. Lancet 1979; ii: 705–709

24 Weiss N S, Ure C L, Ballard J H et al. Decreased risk of fractures of the hip and lower forearm with postmenopausal use of estrogen. N Engl J Med 1980: 303: 1195-1198

25 Paganini-Hill A, Ross R K, Gerkins V R et al. Menopausal estrogen therapy and hip fractures. Ann Intern Med 1982; 95: 28–31

26 Kiel D P, Felson D T, Anderson J J et al. Hip fracture and the use of estrogen in postmenopausal women – the Framingham Study. N Engl J Med 1987; 317: 1169–1174

27 Felson D T, Zhang Y, Hannan M T, Kiel D P, Wilson P W F, Anderson J J. The effect of postmenopausal oestrogen therapy on bone density in elderly women. N Engl J Med 1993; 329: 2–9

28 Cauley J A, Seeley D G, Ensrud K et al. Estrogen replacement therapy and fractures in older women. Ann Intern Med 1995; 122: 9–16

29 Maxim P, Ettinger B, Spitalny G M. Fracture protection provided by long-term estrogen therapy. Osteoporos Int 1995; 5: 23–29

30 Christiansen C, Riis B J. 17β-Estradiol and continuous norethisterone: a unique treatment for established osteoporosis in elderly women. J Clin Endocrinol Metab 1990; 71: 836–841

31 Quigley M E T, Martin P L, Burnier A M, Brooks P. Estrogen therapy arrests bone loss in elderly postmenopausal women. Am J Obstet Gynecol 1987; 156: 1516–1523

32 Marx C W, Dailey III G E, Cheney C, Vint II V C, Muchmore D B. Do estrogens improve bone mineral density in osteoporotic women over age 65? J Bone Miner Res 1992; 7: 1275–1279

33 Frost H M. Dynamics of bone remodelling. In: Frost H M (ed), Bone Biodynamics. Boston: Little & Brown, 1964; 315–333

34 Wronski T J, Walsh C C, Ignaszewski L A. Histological evidence for osteopenia and increased bone turnover in ovariectomised rats. Bone 1986; 7: 119–123

35 Parfitt A M. Bone remodelling and bone loss: understanding the pathophysiology of osteoporosis. Clin Obstet Gynaecol 1987; 30: 789–811

36 Kanis J A. The restoration of skeletal mass: a theoretical overview. Am J Med 1991; 91: 29–36

37 Dempster D W, Lindsay R. Pathogenesis of osteoporosis. Lancet 1993; 341: 797–805

38 Eriksen E F. Normal and pathological remodelling of human trabecular bone: three-dimensional reconstruction of the remodelling sequence in normal and in metabolic bone disease. Endocr Rev 1986; 7: 379–408

39 Parfitt A M. The cellular basis of bone remodelling: the quantum concept reexamined in light of recent advances in the cell biology of bone. Calcif Tissue Int 1984; 36 (Suppl.): S37–S45

40 Prafitt A M. Trabecular bone architecture in the pathogenesis and prevention of fracture. Am Med J 1987; 82: 68–72

41 Heaney R P. The bone remodelling transient: implications for the interpretation of clinical studies of bone mass changes. J Bone Miner Res 1994; 9: 1515–1523

42 Riggs B L, Wahner H W, Dunn W L et al. Differential changes in bone mineral density of the appendicular and axial skeleton with ageing: relationship to spinal osteoporosis. J Clin Invest 1981; 67: 328–335

43 Parfitt A M, Mathews C H E, Villaneuva A R, Kleerekoper M, Frame B, Rao D S. Relationship between surface, volume and thickness of illiac trabecular bone on ageing and in osteoporosis: implications for microanatomic and cellular mechanism of bone loss. J Clin Invest 1983; 72: 1396–1409

44 Parfitt A M. Age-related structural changes in trabecular and cortical bone: cellular mechanism and biochemical consequences. a) Differences between rapid and slow bone loss. b) Localised bone gain. Calcif Tissue Int 1984; 36: S123–S128

45 Compston J E. Connectivity of cancellous bone: assessment and mechanical implications.

Bone 1994; 15: 463–466

46 Kleerekoper M, Villanueva A R, Stanciu J, Rao DS, Parfitt A M. The role of three dimensional trabecular microstructure in the pathogenesis of vertebral compression fracture. Calcif Tissue Int 1985; 37: 594–597

47 Darby A J, Meunier P L. Mean wall thickness and formation periods of trabecular bone packets in idiopathic osteoporosis. Calcif Tissue Int 1981; 33: 199–204

48 Kelly P J, Pocock N A, Sambrook P N, Eisman J A. Age and menopause-related changes in indices of bone turnover. J Clin Endocrinol Metab 1989; 69: 1160–1165

49 Smith D M, Khairi M R A, Johnston Jr C C. The loss of bone mineral with aging and its relationship to risk of fracture. J Clin Invest 1975; 56: 311–318

50 Mazess R B. On aging bone loss. Clin Orthop 1982; 165: 239–252

51 Cummings S R, Black D M, Rubin S M. Lifetime risks of hip, Colles', or vertebral fracture and coronary heart disease among white postmenopausal women. Arch Intern Med 1989; 149: 2445–2448

52 Jensen G F, Christiansen C, Boesen J, Hegedus V, Transbol I. Epidemiology of postmenopausal spinal and long bone fractures: a unifying approach to postmenopausal osteoporosis. Clin Orthop Rel Res 1982; 166: 75–81

53 Evans J G, Prudham D, Wandless I. A prospective study of fractured proximal femur: incidence and outcome. Public Health 1979; 93: 235–241

54 Riggs B L, Melton L J. Involutional osteoporosis. N Engl J Med 1986; 314: 1676–1686

55 Stevenson J C, Whitehead M I. Postmenopausal osteoporosis. BMJ 1982; 285; 585–588

56 Steiniche T, Hasling C, Charles P, Eriksen E F, Mosekilde L, Melsen F. A randomised study on the effects of estrogen/gestagen or high dose oral calcium on trabecular bone remodelling in postmenopausal osteoporosis. Bone 1989; 10: 313–320

57 Parfitt A M. Bone remodelling: relationship to the amount and structure of bone, and pathogenesis and prevention of fractures. In: Riggs B L, Melton L J. (eds) Osteoporosis: Etiology, Diagnosis, and Management. New York: Raven, 1988; 45–93

58 Turner R T, Evans G L, Wakley G K. Mechanism of action of oestrogen on cancellous bone balance in tibia of ovariectomized growing rats: inhibition of indices of formation and resorption. J Bone Miner Res 1993; 8: 359–366

59 Rosen C J, Kessenich C R. The pathophysiology and treatment of postmenopausal osteoporosis. An evidence based approach to oestrogen replacement therapy. Endocr Met Clin North Am 1997; 26: 295–311

60 Chow J W M, Lean J M, Chambers T J. 17β-oestradiol stimulates cancellous bone formation in female rats. Endocrinology 1992; 130: 3025–3032

61 Khastgir G, Studd J W W, Holland N, Alaghband-Zadeh J, Fox S, Chow J. Histomorphometric evidence of an anabolic effect of oestrogen on bone in older postmenopausal women. Br J Obstet Gynaecol 1998; 105 (Suppl. 17): 6

62 Eriksen E F, Colvard D S, Berg N J et al. Evidence of estrogen receptors in human osteoblast-like cell. Science 1988; 241: 84–86

63 Komm B S, Terpening C M, Benz D J et al. Estrogenic binding, receptor mRNA, and biologic response in osteoblast like osteosarcoma cells. Science 1988; 241: 81–84

64 Pensler J M, Radosevich J A, Higbee R et al. Osteoclasts isolated from membranous bone in children exhibit nuclear estrogen and progesterone receptors. J Bone Miner Res 1990; 5: 797–802

65 Oursler M J, Osdoby P, Pyfferoen J et al. Avian osteoclasts as estrogen target cells. Proc Natl Acad Sci USA 1991; 88: 6613–6617

66 Rodan G A, Martin T J. Role of osteoblasts in hormonal control of bone resorption – a hypothesis. Calcif Tissue Int 1981; 33: 344–351

67 Polan M L, Daniele A, Kuo A. Gonadal steroids modulate human monocyte interleukin-1 (IL-1) activity. Fertil Steril 1988; 49: 964–968

68 Girasole G, Jilka R L. Passeri G et al. 17 β-estradiol inhibits interleukin-6 production by bone marrow-derived stromal cells and osteoblasts in vivo: a potential mechanism for the antiosteoporotic effect of estrogen. J Clin Invest 1992; 89: 883–891

69 Ralston S H, Russell R G G, Gowen M. Estrogen inhibits release of tumour necrosis factor from peripheral blood mononuclear cell in postmenopausal women. J Bone Miner Res 1990; 5: 983–988

70 Jilka R L, Hangoc G, Griasole G et al. Increased osteoclast development after estrogen loss: mediation by interleukin-6. Science 1992; 257: 88–91

71 Kimble R B, Vannice J L, Blowdow D C et al. Interleukin-1 receptor antagonist decreases bone loss and bone resorption in ovariectomised rats. J Clin Invest 1994; 93: 1957–1967

72 Kitazawa R, Kimble R B, Vannice J L et al. Interleukin-1 receptor antagonist and tumour necrosis factor binding protein decrease osteoclast formation and bone resorption in ovariectomised mice. J Clin Invest 1994; 2: 397–406

73 Kassem M, Khosla S, Spelsberg T C et al. Cytokine production in the bone marrow microenvironment: failure to demonstrate estrogen regulation in early postmenopausal women. J Clin Endocrinol Metab 1996; 81: 513–518

74 Pilbeam C C, Klein-Nulend J, Raisz L G. Inhibition by 17β-estradiol of PTH stimulated resorption and prostaglandin production in cultured neonatal mouse calveriae. Biochem Biophys Res Commun 1989; 163: 1319–1324

75 Ernst M, Schmid C, Foresch E R. Enhanced osteoblast proliferation and collagen gene expression by oestradiol. Proc Natl Acad Sci USA 1988; 85: 2307–2310

76 Gray T K, Flynn T C, Gray K M et al. 17β-estradiol acts directly on the clonal osteoblastic cell line UMR 106. Proc Natl Acad Sci USA 1988; 85: 6267–6271

77 Ernst M, Heath J K, Rodan G A. Estradiol effects on proliferation, messenger ribonucleic acid for collagen and insulin-like growth factor-1, and parathyroid hormone-simulated adenylate cyclase activity in osteoblastic cell from calvariae and long bone. Endocrinology 1989; 125: 825–833

78 Keeting P E, Scott R E, Colvard D S et al. Lack of a direct effect of estrogen on proliferation and differentiation of normal human osteoblast-like cells. J Bone Miner Res 1994; 9: 983–991

79 Armamento-Villareal R, Civitelli R. Estrogen action on the bone mass of postmenopausal women is dependent on body mass and initial bone density. J Clin Endocrinol Metab 1995; 80: 776–782

80 Lindsay R, Hart D M. The minimum effective dose of oestrogen for the prevention of postmenopausal bone loss. Obstet Gynecol 1984; 63: 759–773

81 Bouillon B, Burckhardt P, Christiansen C et al. Consensus development conference: prophylaxis and treatment of osteoporosis. Am J Med 1991; 90: 107–110

82 Christiansen C, Christiansen M S, Larsen N E, Transbol I B. Pathophysiological mechanisms of oestrogen effect on bone metabolism. Dose-response relationships in early postmenopausal women. J Clin Endocrinol Met 1982; 55: 1124–1130

83 Ettinger B, Genant H K, Steiger D, Madwig P. Low-dosage micronised 17-β oestradiol prevents bone loss in postmenopausal women. Am J Obstet Gynecol 1992; 166: 479–488

84 Savvas M, Studd J W W, Norman S, Leather A T, Garnett T J. Increased bone mass after one year of percutaneous oestradiol and testosterone implants in post-menopausal women who have previously received long-term oral oestrogen. Br J Obstet Gynaecol 1992; 99: 757–760

85 Eiken P, Pors Nielsen S, Kolthoff N. Effects on bone mass after eight years of hormone replacement therapy. Br J Obstet Gynaecol 1997; 104: 702–707

86 Garnett T, Studd J W W, Watson N, Savvas M. A cross-sectional study of the effects of long-term percutaneous hormone replacement therapy on bone density. Obstet Gynecol 1991; 78: 1002–1007

87 Naessen T, Persson I. Maintained bone density at advanced ages after long term treatment with low dose oestradiol implants. Br J Obstet Gynaecol 1993; 100: 454–459

88 Wahab M, Ballard P, Purdie D W, Cooper A, Willson J C. The effect of long term oestradiol implantation on bone mineral density in postmenopausal women who have undergone hysterectomy and bilateral oophorectomy. Br J Obstet Gynaecol 1997; 104: 728–731

89 Riggs B L, Melton L J. The prevention and treatment of osteoporosis. N Engl J Med 1992; 327: 620–627

90 Dennison E, Cooper C. The epidemiology of osteoporosis. Br J Clin Pract 1996; 50: 33–36

91 Kanis J A. Treatment of osteoporosis in elderly women. Am J Med 1995; 98 (Suppl. 2A): 60–66

92 Barrett-Connor E. Hormone replacement therapy. BMJ 1998; 317: 457–461

93 Spector T D, Brennan B, Harris P A et al. Do current regimens of hormone replacement therapy protect against subsequent fractures? Osteoporos Int 1992; 2: 219–224

94 Kohrt W M, Birge S J. Differential effects of estrogen treatment on bone mineral density of the spine, hip, wrist and total body in late postmenopausal women. Osteoporos Int 1995; 5: 150–155

95  Christiansen C, Christiansen M S, Transbol I. Bone mass in postmenopausal women after withdrawal of oestrogen/gestagen replacement therapy. Lancet 1981; i: 459–461

96  Stevenson J C, Kanis J A, Christiansen C. Bone-density measurement. Lancet 1992; 339: 370–371

97  Schneider D L, Barrett-Connor E L, Morton D J. Timing of postmenopausal estrogen for optimal bone mineral density. The Rancho Bernardo Study. JAMA 1997; 277: 543–547

98  Orwoll E S, Bauer D C, Vogt T M, Fox K M. Axial bone mass in older women. Ann Intern Med 1996; 124; 187–196

99  Michaelsson K, Baron J A, Farahmand B Y et al. For the Swedish Hip Fracture Study Group. Hormone replacement therapy and risk of hip fracture: population based case-controlled study. BMJ 1998; 316: 1858–1863

100  Naessen T, Persson I, Adami H O, Bergstrom R, Bergkvist L. Hormone replacement therapy the risk for first hip fracture: a prospective population based cohort study. Ann Intern Med 1990; 113: 95–103

101  Kanis J A, Johnell O, Gullberg B et al. Evidence for the efficacy of bone active drugs in the prevention of hip fracture. BMJ 1992; 305: 1124–1128

102  Riggs B L, Wahner H W, Seeman E et al. Changes in bone mineral density of the proximal femur and spine with aging: differences between postmenopausal and osteoporotic syndromes. J Clin Invest 1982; 70: 716–723

103  Richelson L S, Wahner H W, Melton L J, Riggs B L. Relative contribution of aging and estrogen deficiency to postmenopausal bone loss. N Engl J Med 1984; 311: 1273–1275

104  Johnell O, Stenbeck M, Rosen M et al. Therapeutic strategies in the prevention of hip fractures with drugs affecting bone metabolism. Bone 1993; 14 (Suppl. 1): S85–S87

105  Ettinger B, Grady D. Maximizing the benefit of estrogen therapy for prevention of osteoporosis. Menopause 1994; 1: 19–24

*Ranee Thakar   Isaac Manyonda*

# Hysterectomy for benign disease – total versus subtotal

Approximately 590,000 hysterectomies are performed every year in the US,[1] and 72,821 were performed in the UK in 1994–1995.[2] This renders hysterectomy the commonest major gynaecological operation, and the vast majority of procedures are performed for benign disease. The operation disrupts the intimate anatomical relationship between the uterus, bowel, bladder and vagina, and inevitably the local nerve supply. It is, therefore, conceivable that hysterectomy may alter the function of these organs, such change being either detrimental or beneficial. The procedure may be total, when both the body of the uterus and the cervix are removed, or subtotal, when the cervix is conserved. In the UK, subtotal hysterectomy is an unpopular procedure, accounting for only 1.47% of the hysterectomies in 1994–1995.[2] This is apparently largely due to a perceived risk of cervical stump carcinoma. However, there are a number of compelling reasons why the British gynaecologist might review his/her views: the incidence of cervical cancer is falling due to more effective screening; in the present climate of medical litigation, the increased risk of ureteric and bladder damage associated with total, but minimised by subtotal, hysterectomy might persuade some to consider whether the former operation is always necessary; and, finally, the conflicting reports from Scandinavia in the early and late 1980s, where the issue was whether one or other operation conferred benefit in terms of urinary, bowel and sexual function, have brought the whole controversy into the public domain, with the popular press reporting polarised views, and women increasingly demanding one or other operation. This chapter reviews current literature on this topic.

**Dr Ranee Thakar** MBBS MRCOG, Subspecialty Trainee in Urogynaecology, Department of Obstetrics and Gynaecology, St George's Hospital, Blackshaw Road, London SW17 0QT, UK (for correspondence)

**Mr Isaac Manyonda** BSc PhD MRCOG, Consultant Gynaecologist, Department of Obstetrics and Gynaecology, St George's Hospital, Blackshaw Road, London SW17 0QT, UK

## EVOLUTION OF HYSTERECTOMY

Charles Clay performed the first recorded hysterectomy in 1843. The patient unfortunately died in the immediate postoperative period. Undaunted, Clay performed another hysterectomy the following year. This was a subtotal hysterectomy and the patient lived for 15 days, dying only because of the carelessness of porters who dropped her on the floor while the nurses where changing the bed linen.[3] Subsequent hysterectomies were all subtotal until 1929, when Richardson performed a hysterectomy which included removal of the cervix.[4] From then on surgeons took heart and increasingly became bold, and total hysterectomies became more common. When the 1940s heralded antibiotics, blood transfusion, modern anaesthesia and improved surgical techniques, total hysterectomy took off as the preferred procedure over subtotal hysterectomy. With the recognition that cancer occasionally developed in the cervical stump, performing subtotal hysterectomy became such an anathema that authors apologised for including a description of the operation in manuals of operative gynaecology, condemning it to the repertoire of the inexperienced surgeon.[5] To this day, most British gynaecologists have little time for this operation: only 1.47% of the 72,821 hysterectomies performed in 1994–1995 were subtotal.[1] A recent postal survey conducted by the authors confirmed the unpopularity of subtotal.[6] However, a series of publications from Finland in the early 1980s indicated that subtotal hysterectomy may have benefits over total hysterectomy.[7-9] Unfortunately, subsequent studies from the same institute could not corroborate the earlier findings, while critics of the latter studies point out that these studies were not comparable to the earlier studies. This has created a controversy at a time when there is emphasis on the practice of evidence-based medicine, and when the popular press and consumers are forcing the debate into the public domain.

## ANATOMICAL CONSIDERATIONS

A change in urinary, bowel or sexual function following hysterectomy may be due to either altered spatial anatomical relationships and/or disruption of the innervation of these structures. The bladder, uterus and rectum are all attached to the pelvic side walls by the endopelvic fascia which, although continuous, has distinct thickening or ligaments. The cardinal and the uterosacral ligaments hold the cervix firmly in place, while the rest of the uterus is free and mobile. Thus the cervix serves as the anchor of support for the entire organ. The pelvic plexus, which is of paramount importance in the co-ordinated contractions of the smooth muscle of the bladder and bowel, is formed by the junction of the pelvic parasympathetic and sympathetic nerves. This plexus is intimately related to the bladder, cervix and vagina and the nerve supply of the pelvic organs is derived from it.[10] It is, therefore, conceivable that damage to this autonomic innervation during pelvic surgery may result in functional disorders of the pelvic viscera and, indeed, it has been suggested that constipation following hysterectomy may be caused by autonomic denervation of the hindgut.[11] Similarly, sympathetic damage produces loss of proximal urethral pressure and parasympathetic damage may cause detrusor areflexia.[12]

During the operation of total hysterectomy, the pelvic plexus may be at risk in four areas. Firstly, the main branches of the plexus passing beneath the uterine arteries may be damaged during the division of the cardinal ligaments.[13] Secondly, the major part of the vesical innervation, which enters the bladder base before spreading throughout the detrusor muscle, may be damaged during blunt dissection of the bladder from the uterus and cervix. Thirdly the extensive dissection of the paravaginal tissue may disrupt the pelvic neurons passing from the lateral aspect of the vagina.[14] Finally, the removal of the cervix will result in loss of a large segment of the plexus which is intimately related to it. The remaining portion of the plexus may be inadequate to deal with afferent impulses from the rectum and the bladder, possibly leading to bladder and rectal dysfunction.[15]

However, hysterectomy may include the removal of structures that are a source of symptoms including endometriomas, myomas, pelvic adhesions and adenomyosis; thus, their removal may remove or minimise these symptoms. It is not inconceivable that excision of these may be more significant than the anatomical distortions and interruptions of the nerve supply referred to above.

## BLADDER FUNCTION FOLLOWING HYSTERECTOMY

Hysterectomy involves dissection of the bladder from the uterus, the process being more extensive for a total than a subtotal hysterectomy. Bladder innervation may, therefore, be altered, but studies have yielded conflicting results. In a retrospective questionnaire, Milson and co-workers[16] found a significant increase in urinary incontinence in women who had previously undergone hysterectomy compared to women who had not (20.8% versus 16.4%). However, retrospective data comparing hysterectomised to non-hysterectomised women are unreliable, since a degree of vesico-urethral dysfunction may be present prior to surgery.[9,16,17] Pary and colleagues,[14] therefore, carried out a prospective study with both subjective and objective assessments of urinary function and found subjective symptoms in 58.3% of women prior to hysterectomy, although urodynamic dysfunction was found in only 38.9%. Postoperatively, they found an increase in urinary symptoms (75%), new urodynamic abnormalities (an additional 30%) and pelvic neuropathy as evidenced by sacral reflex latencies. By contrast, Langer and co-workers[18] evaluated 16 asymptomatic premenopausal women and performed cystometry and uroflowmetry pre-operatively, and again at 4 weeks and 4 months post-hysterectomy, and found no difference in symptoms or urodynamic results. While some have found no more urinary symptoms after hysterectomy than after dilatation and curettage,[19] others compared urinary symptoms after TCRE and similarly found no difference.[20] Another study has even reported a statistically significant decrease in stress incontinence, frequency and nocturia 12 months after total abdominal hysterectomy.[21] It has been hypothesised that decreased urinary stress incontinence following hysterectomy may be due to elevation of the bladder neck by fixation of the vaginal vault to the uterosacral ligaments.[19] Apparent urodynamic or neurological changes post-hysterectomy may not necessarily cause symptoms. Prior and associates[22] found an increase in vesical sensitivity after hysterectomy irrespective of whether it was by vaginal or abdominal approach, and this persisted for at least 6 months, but was not always associated with urinary symptoms. While there is little data on the effect of vaginal as opposed to abdominal hysterectomy, it has been reported that urgency more often followed a vaginal procedure.[23]

The real current debate, however, is whether subtotal hysterectomy confers any benefits over total hysterectomy. In a series of publications from 1983, Kilkku[7–9] extolled the virtues of subtotal hysterectomy with respect to urinary and sexual function, such that in Finland, where Kilkku carried out his studies, 53% of abdominal hysterectomies from 1981 to 1986 were subtotal. Kilkku interviewed 105 patients before total abdominal hysterectomy with bilateral salpingo-oophorectomy (TAH/BSO), and again at 6 weeks, 6 months and 1 year postoperatively. He also interviewed 107 women who underwent subtotal hysterectomy with bilateral salpingo-oophorectomy (STAH/BSO). He found statistically significant differences in urinary symptoms between the two operations. In the total hysterectomy group, 28.6% of the patients reported pre-operative incomplete bladder emptying, which fell to 22.1% post-surgery. In contrast, 35.5% of the STAH/BSO reported incomplete bladder emptying prior to surgery and, by 1 year, the figure had fallen to only 10.3%. Similar trends were found for urinary incontinence and frequency. The authors, therefore, concluded that subtotal hysterectomy was more advantageous.[9] However, subsequent studies by Virtanen and co-workers[21] from the same institute did not concur with Kilkku's findings and by 1991 the rate of subtotal hysterectomy had dropped to 13%.[24] That said, the two studies are not comparable, as Kilkku compared total and subtotal hysterectomy while the study conducted by Virtanen was a longitudinal assessment of total hysterectomy only.

Other workers have also studied the effects of total (TAH) versus subtotal hysterectomy (SAH) on bladder function. Kjuanso et al[25] evaluated urethral closure function pre-operatively and postoperatively in 31 non-randomised patients who underwent SAH ($n = 13$) and TAH ($n = 18$). They found no operation-induced changes in urethral relaxation and functional length, closure pressure or resistance to stress associated with either operation. Lalos and Bjerle[26] performed a randomised comparison of 22 patients, equally divided between total and subtotal hysterectomy. They found no differences in either urodynamic evaluation or in subjective symptoms such as frequency and incontinence. The numbers in these studies were so small that the findings were not statistically significant. It is thus evident that there is insufficient data to allow a valid opinion on the effect of total versus subtotal hysterectomy on urinary function.

To date, there have not been any studies of the effect of vaginal hysterectomy on urinary function. This might be a difficult evaluation, as this operation is frequently chosen when uterovaginal prolapse (e.g. cysto-urethrocele which can cause urinary symptoms) is present. As more and more hysterectomies are carried out by the vaginal route in the absence of prolapse, an evaluation may become possible.

## EFFECT OF HYSTERECTOMY ON BOWEL FUNCTION

The picture is no clearer with regard to bowel function with some reports suggesting an increased incidence of constipation[27] and irritable bowel syndrome[28] following hysterectomy. Taylor et al[29] conducted a case-control study through detailed questionnaires in which post-hysterectomy women and controls were compared, and showed that women with previous hysterectomy were more likely to report infrequent defecation and firmer stool consistency. This study can be criticised, as they excluded women who had extensive bowel operations and those with irritable bowel syndrome in the matched controls but the same exclusions were not applied to the hysterectomy group. Conversely, Prior et al[22] observed that, after hysterectomy, constipation was more likely to disappear than develop. They also found no change in that whole gut transit times in 26 women before and 6 months after hysterectomy.

A retrospective study of 593 women who had hysterectomy (abdominal, vaginal, radical and subtotal) against a control group of 100 women who had laparoscopic cholecystectomy found increased rate of bowel dysfunction in the hysterectomy group. Data obtained through a postal questionnaire indicated that, before hysterectomy, 216 patients (41%) were found to have abnormal defecation patterns whereas 315 (59%) reported having a fully normal defecation pattern. In women who had normal bowel function, 31% reported severe deterioration in bowel function whereas 11% showed moderate changes after hysterectomy. Severe straining was noted in 29% and incomplete and/or digital evacuation in 26% and 16%, respectively. No significant difference in incidence of bowel symptoms was noted in the different types of hysterectomy. When compared to the control group, a significantly lower incidence of bowel dysfunction (9%) was noted in the laparoscopic cholecystectomy group ($P <0.001$). It was also observed that, in patients with changes in bowel function, changes in bladder function were observed more frequently ($P <0.001$) than in the group with no deterioration of bowel function after hysterectomy. Interpretation in retrospective studies, such as this, must be done with caution as there is a reliance on the recall of bowel function going back as long as 5 years.[30]

Numerous attempts have been made to study rectal physiology after hysterectomy using manometry (Table 1). Smith et al[11] and Roe et al[31] studied anal and rectal physiology of women reporting post-hysterectomy constipation. Smith et al[11] studied 14 women with intractable constipation following hysterectomy (12 abdominal and 2 vaginal) and compared them to an asymptomatic group of matched control subjects. Manometry showed no difference in sphincter function and on proctometrogram rectal compliance and volumes appeared to be significantly increased in the post-hysterectomy group, some of these patients demonstrating severe defects in rectal perception to distension. A significant proximal-to-distal motility gradient was demonstrable in the basal state of the control group but not in the post-hysterectomy group. Following stimulation with Prostigmin, the proximal-to-distal motility gradient was further attenuated in the control group. In the post-hysterectomy group, a lesser increase in motility was observed. Furthermore, there was a paradoxical reversal in motility following stimulation in this group, i.e. there was now a significant distal to proximal motility gradient. When Carbacol was administered, a hypersensitive reaction of the colon was noted in the hysterectomised women which is typical of autonomic denervation. The response to Prostigmin would be expected in an organ with incomplete damage to innervation. The observations in this present study suggest that constipation in this special group of patients may occur as a result of incidental injury to the autonomic parasympathetic innervation of the left colon and the rectum. This conclusion is further substantiated by

**Table 1** Anorectal function after simple hysterectomy

| Author | Type of study | Type of hysterectomy | No of patients | Ano-rectal physiology in hysterectomy patients |
|--------|---------------|----------------------|----------------|------------------------------------------------|
| Roe et al 1988[31] | Retrospective | Not mentioned | 14 Hyst, 22 controls, 16 STC | No difference in anal canal pressures, rectosigmoid motility, ano-rectal inhibitory reflex or rectal sensitivity |
| Smith et al 1990[11] | Retrospective | AH (12), VH (2) | 14 Hyst, 14 controls | No difference in anal canal pressures or pudendal nerve motor terminal latency. Reduced rectal sensitivity and increased compliance. Reduced motility |
| Barnes et al 1991[50] | Prospective (pre and 1 week). Comparative | RH (15) | 15 Hyst, 3 controls | No difference in anal canal pressures. Increased distention needed to trigger relaxation. Reduced sensitivity. Controls normal |
| Prior et al 1992[22] | Prospective (pre & 6 weeks) | VH (18), TH (8) | 26 | No difference in anal canal pressures, rectal compliance, ano-rectal inhibitory reflex or motility. Rectal sensitivity increased at 6 weeks |
| Goffeng et al 1997[32] | Prospective (pre, 3 & 11–18 months). Comparative | SH (32), TH (10) | 42 | No difference in anal canal pressures, rectal sensation or whole gut transit |
| Kelly et al 1998[51] | Prospective (pre & 16 weeks) | AH (16), 14 (VH) | 30 | Significantly reduced anal canal squeeze pressure more in multiparous women. No difference in ano-rectal inhibitory reflex, rectal sensation or pudendal nerve latencies |

SH, subtotal hysterectomy; TH, total hysterectomy; VG, vaginal hysterectomy; AH, abdominal hysterectomy; RH, radical hysterectomy.

abnormalities of bladder function noted in the same patients. However, the number of patients involved in this study are small.

In contrast to this study, when Roe et al[31] studied 31 women with slow transit constipation, i.e. intractable constipation that has proved to be resistant to the usual therapeutic measures, they found that 14 (45%) developed severe symptoms following a hysterectomy, usually within the first year of the operation. The rest had symptoms arising *de novo*. When compared to controls, there was no difference in the rectosigmoid motility, rectal compliance or maximal tolerable volume in the hysterectomy group.

Goffeng et al[32] conducted a longitudinal study, pre-operatively and at 3 and 11–18 months after hysterectomy. Detailed interviews enquiring about bowel function were performed along with rectal manometry and whole gut transit time. Anorectal physiology was normal after hysterectomy and no adverse bowel symptoms were noted except for a significant improvement in abdominal pain. There was no difference between total hysterectomy and subtotal hysterectomy.

A prospective study designed to determine the incidence of symptoms suggestive of irritable bowel syndrome arising after hysterectomy and the effect of surgery on pre-existing gastrointestinal symptoms found less marked changes. In women with IBS before hysterectomy, 60% improved after surgery, 20% were worse and new problems with constipation arose in 5%. He concluded that hysterectomy had little, if any, effect on the *de novo* development of irritable bowel syndrome.[33]

A higher incidence of enteroceles (40%) and of perineal descent (25%) have been noticed on defecography after hysterectomy. This could be due to a generalised weakness of the pelvic floor, lending itself to excessive perineal descent and the development of a rectal and vaginal wall prolapse. Both vaginal and abdominal hysterectomies are responsible for weakening of the uterosacral and cardinal ligaments originally attached to the cervix, exposing the anterior rectal and vaginal wall to abdominal pressure.[34]

## HYSTERECTOMY AND FEMALE SEXUALITY

In recent years, research has focused on the possibility that anatomical changes induced by hysterectomy might affect sexuality. Disturbance of the innervation of the cervix and the upper vagina after total hysterectomy could interfere with lubrication and orgasm. The so-called internal orgasm is essentially a cervical orgasm, caused by stimulation of nerve endings in the uterovaginal plexus, which intimately surround the cervix and attach to the upper vagina. Since much of the sensory and autonomic information from the pelvic organs, including the uterus, is channelled through the uterovaginal plexus, it is understandable that loss of a major portion of the uterovaginal plexus through excision of the cervix might have an adverse effect on sexual arousal and orgasm in women who previously experienced internal orgasm. Women who achieve orgasm through clitoral stimulation might not be affected. In those women who had experienced both types of orgasm or in whom sexual response is blended, a decrease in sexual response following hysterectomy might be noted.[15] The other factors contributing to sexual problems could be a reduction in cervical mucous contributing to the vaginal dryness and vaginal shortening.[35]

However, the above are merely theoretical considerations. In reality, the issue of whether hysterectomy affects sexual function is infinitely more complex, since both physical and psychological factors have varying and unquantifiable influences on human sexuality. Women increasingly enquire as to whether hysterectomy is likely to affect their sexual function and, although there is no clear answer, most doctors, and information leaflets, tend to assure women that sexuality is unchanged, and may even improve. Depending on a variety of factors such as cultural beliefs and education, women's views on the role of the uterus may well influence how they will react to hysterectomy. Historically, the uterus has been regarded as the regulator and controller of important physiological functions, a sexual organ, a source of energy and vitality, and a maintainer of youth and attractiveness.[36] Little wonder, therefore, that removal of such an organ might be expected to alter women's perception of self, especially with regard to femininity, attractiveness, sexual desire and ability to respond sexually.[37] However, research has not provided clear-cut answers. It has proven difficult to design protocols that adequately address the potential contribution of both psychological factors and anatomical changes. Psychological studies suggest that post-hysterectomy sexual function is influenced by a wide range of patient characteristics. For example, poor knowledge of reproductive anatomy, pre-hysterectomy negative expectation of sexual recovery following surgery, pre-operative psychiatric morbidity and unsatisfactory pre-operative sexual relations are all associated with poor outcome.[38,39] Pre-hysterectomy factors that are associated with positive post-surgery sexuality include frequency of coitus, frequency of desire, and orgasmic response.[40] In other words, those women who retained an overall desire for sexual activity, and were presumably hampered by negative physical symptoms, might be expected to experience an improvement in their sexual function following hysterectomy.

Interest in the influence of anatomical changes was brought into sharp focus by the series of reports from Scandinavia, already referred to above.[7–9] In the same two groups of women in whom they studied urinary function, Kilkku and his associates compared coital frequency, dyspareunia, libido and frequency of orgasm before surgery and at 6 weeks, 6 months, 1 year and 3 years post-surgery. Both groups showed an equal, but slight reduction in coital frequency, dyspareunia decreased in both groups but statistically more in the STAH group; the frequency of orgasm was significantly reduced in the TAH group but not in the STAH group. Such findings lend credence to Master's observation that 'many women will certainly describe cervical sexual pressure as a trigger mechanism for coital responsivity'.[41] Such women may be handicapped sexually when such a trigger mechanism is removed surgically. More recent reports from the same institute where Kilkku carried out his work, suggest that the negative effect of total hysterectomy on sexual function is not as great as originally perceived.[21] Thus the issue remains unresolved.

## CONCLUDING REMARKS

Whether or not hysterectomy has detrimental effects on urinary, bowel or sexual function, it will continue to be the appropriate treatment for some women. Therefore, the fundamental debate should be whether the operation can be performed in a manner that minimises undesirable effects. To this end, a debate is currently gathering momentum among British gynaecologists as to whether subtotal hysterectomy confers any benefits over total hysterectomy. Subtotal hysterectomy is undoubtedly the safer operation, whatever the skill of the surgeon; there is less bleeding and mobilisation of the bladder, and potentially less disruption of autonomic nervous pathways. Nathorst-Boos and co-workers found a lower morbidity rate with subtotal compared to total hysterectomy and reported that wound infections, haematomas and urinary tract infections may be less common.[42] Vault granulations do not occur with subtotal hysterectomy while they complicate 21% of total hysterectomies.[43] However, in general, the British gynaecologist has a negative view to subtotal hysterectomy. Leaving the cervix behind is often regarded as reflecting surgical inexperience, and advocates of total hysterectomy also argue that cancer may subsequently develop in the cervical stump – subsequent surgery is then rendered difficult while radiotherapy is compromised by the absence of the uterus. However, even in the UK, screening for cancer of the cervix by regular smears has begun to pay dividends, and perspectives on the risk of cancer developing in the stump in patients carefully selected for subtotal hysterectomy are changing. The risk is currently quoted at less than 0.3%.[44] It is, therefore, questionable whether the British gynaecologist should persist in removing a healthy cervix. With the popular press showing a growing interest, it is only a matter of time before women start demanding one or other operation. However, it is imperative that a definitive investigation be undertaken to establish whether removing or retaining the cervix confers any benefits, so that gynaecologists may base any change in surgical practice on scientific evidence rather than fashion. We are currently undertaking a multicentre prospective randomised study comparing the effect of total versus subtotal hysterectomy on urinary, bowel and sexual function, employing both subjective and objective tools including urodynamics and rectal physiological outcomes.

Whichever procedure turns out to be advantageous, the obvious next challenge will be to establish the optimal route of performing the operation. There is a growing momentum to perform hysterectomy by the vaginal route, but the reality in current UK practice is that only 19% of hysterectomies are vaginal.[1] This is despite the fact that it is well established that vaginal hysterectomy is associated with much lower morbidity rate (24.5%) compared to abdominal hysterectomy (42.8%).[45] Minimal access surgery may have additional advantages: there is reduction in wound infections, postoperative pain, time spent in hospital and postoperative convalescence.[46,47] Whether the reduced tissue handling has beneficial effects on bladder, bowel or sexual function is unknown. Donnez and Nisolle have suggested that the technique of laparoscopic assisted subtotal hysterectomy (LASH) may reduce the risk of ureteric, bladder and urethral injury associated with laparoscopic total hysterectomy, while reducing the operating time. Should subtotal hysterectomy turn out to be advantageous over total hysterectomy, then the optimal procedure may well turn out to be a LASH.[48,49]

### References

1 Pokras R, Hufnagel V G. Hysterectomy in the United States, 1965–84. Vital health statistics. Series 13. No 92. Washington DC: Govt Printing Office, 1987; (DHHS publication no. (PHS) 88–1753)

2   Hospital Episode Statistics 1994–1995. London: Department of Health
3   Sutton S. Hysterectomy: a historical perspective. Baillière's Clin Obstet Gynaecol 1997; 11: 1–22
4   Richardson E H. A simplified technique for abdominal panhysterectomy. Surg Gynaecol Obstet 1929; 48: 248–251
5   Howkins J, Stalworthy J. Bonney's Gynaecological Surgery. London: Baillière Tindall, 1974; 282
6   Thakar R, Manyonda I, Robinson G, Clarkson P, Stanton S. Total versus subtotal hysterectomy: a survey of current views and practice amongst British gynaecologists. J Obstet Gynaecol 1998; 18: 267–269
7   Kilkku P, Gronoos M, Hirovnen T, Rauramo L. Supravaginal uterine amputations vs hysterectomy: effects on libido and orgasm. Acta Obstet Gynecol Scand 1983; 62: 147–152
8   Kilkku P. Supravaginal uterine amputation vs hysterectomy: effects on coital frequency and dyspareunia. Acta Obstet Gynecol Scand 1983; 62: 141–145
9.  Kilkku P. Supravaginal uterine amputation vs hysterectomy with reference to bladder symptoms and incontinence. Acta Obstet Gynecol Scand 1985; 64: 375–379
10  Warick R, Williams P L. (eds) Gray's Anatomy, 31st edn. Edinburgh: Longmans, 1980; 1203–1204
11  Smith A N, Varma J S, Binnie N R, Papachrysostomou M. Disordered colorectal motility in intractable constipation following hysterectomy. Br J Surg 1990; 77: 1362–1366
12  Benson J T. Neurophysiology of the female pelvic floor. Curr Opin Obstet Gynecol 1994; 6: 320–323
13  Smith P H, Ballantyne B. The neuroanatomical basis of denervation of the urinary ladder following major pelvic surgery. Br J Surg 1968; 55: 929–933
14  Parys B T, Haylen B, Hutton J L, Parsons K F. The effect of simple hysterectomy on vesicourethral function. Br J Urol 1989; 64: 594–599
15  Hasson H M. Cervical removal at hysterectomy for benign disease. J Reprod Med 1993; 38: 781–790
16  Milsom I, Ekelund P, Molander U, Arvidsson L, Arskoug B. The influence of age, parity, oral contraception, hysterectomy and menopause on the prevalence of urinary incontinence in women. J Urol 1993; 149: 1459–1462
17  Jecquier A M. Urinary symptoms and total hysterectomy. Br J Urol 1976; 48: 437–441
18  Langer R, Neuman M, Ron-el R et al. The effect of total abdominal hysterectomy on bladder function in asymptomatic women. Obstet Gynecol 1989; 74: 205–207
19  Griffith-Jones M D, Jarvis G J, McNamara H M. Adverse urinary symptoms after total abdominal hysterectomy – fact or fiction? Br J Urol 1991; 67: 295–297
20  Bhattacharya S, Mollison J, Pinion S et al. A comparison of bladder and ovarian function two years following hysterectomy or endometrial ablation. Br J Obstet Gynaecol 1996; 103: 898–903
21  Virtanen H S, Makinen J I, Tenho T, Kiiholma P, Hirvonen T. Effects of abdominal hysterectomy on urinary and sexual symptoms. Br J Urol 1993; 72: 868–872
22  Prior A, Stanley K, Smith A R B, Read N W. Effect of hysterectomy on anorectal and urethrovesical physiology. Gut 1992; 33: 264–267
23  Vervest H A, duJong M K, Vervest J S et al. Micturition symptoms and urinary incontinence after nonradical hysterectomy. Acta Obstet Gynecol Scand 1988; 67: 141–146
24  Virtanen H S, Makinen J I, Kiilholma P J A. Conserving the cervix at hysterectomy. Br J Obstet Gynaecol 1995; 102: 587
25  Kujansuu E, Teisala K, Punnonen R. Urethral closure function after total and subtotal hysterectomy measured by urethrocystometry. Gynecol Obstet Invest 1989; 27: 105–106
26  Lalos O, Bjerle P. Bladder wall mechanics and micturition before and after subtotal and total hysterectomy. Eur J Obstet Gynecol Reprod Biol 1986; 21: 143–150
27  Preston D M, Lennard-Jones J E. Severe chronic constipation of young women: idiopathic slow transit constipation. Gut 1989; 27: 41–48
28  Hogston P. Irritable bowel syndrome as a cause of chronic pain in women attending a gynaecological clinic. BMJ 1987; 294: 934–935
29  Taylor T, Smith A N. Effect of hysterectomy on bowel function. BMJ 1989; 299: 300–302
30  van Dam J H, Gosselink M J, Drogendijk A C, Hop W C, Schouten W R. Changes in bowel function after 9.5 ptwithout previous hysterectomy. Dig Dis Sci 1988; 33: 1159–1163
32  Goffeng A R, Andersch B, Antov S, Berndtsson I, Oresland T, Hulten L. Does simple hysterectomy alter bowel function? Ann Chir Gynaecol 1997; 86: 298–303

33 Prior A, Stanley K, Smith A R B, Read N W. Relation between hysterectomy and irritable bowel syndrome: a prospective study. Gut 1992; 33: 814–817

34 Karasick S, Spettell C M. The role of parity and hysterectomy on the development of pelvic floor abnormalities revealed by defecography. AJR 1997; 169: 1555–1558

35 Jewett J F. Vaginal length and incidence of dyspareunia following total abdominal hysterectomy. Am J Obstet Gynecol 1952; 63: 400–407

36 Sloan D. The emotional and psychosexual aspects of hysterectomy. Am J Obstet Gynecol 1978; 131: 598–605

37 Polivy J. Psychological reactions to hysterectomy: a critical review. Am J Obstet Gynecol 1974; 118: 417–426

38 Dennerstein L, Wood C, Burrows G D. Sexual responses following hysterectomy and oophorectomy. Obstet Gynecol 1977; 49: 92–96

39 Helström L, Sorborm D, Bäckström T. Influence of partner relationship in sexuality after subtotal hysterectomy. Acta Obstet Gynecol Scand 1995; 74: 42–46

40 Helström L, Lundberg P O, Sörborm D, Bäckström T. Sexuality after hysterectomy: factor analysis of women's sexual lives before and after subtotal hysterectomy. Obstet Gynecol 1995; 74: 142–146

41 Masters W H, Johnson V. Human Sexual Response. Boston: Little, Brown, 1966; 117

42 Nathorst-Boos J, Fuchs T, von Schoultz B. Consumers attitude to hysterectomy: the experience of 678 women. Acta Obstet Gynecol Scand 1992; 71; 230–234

43 Manyonda I T, Welsh C R, McWhinney N A, Ross C D. The influence of suture materials on vaginal vault granulations after abdominal hysterectomy. Br J Obstet Gynaecol 1990; 97: 608–612

44 Storm H H, Clemmenson I H, Manders T, Brinton L A. Supravaginal uterine amputation in Denmark 1978–1988 and risk of cancer. Gynecol Oncol 1992; 45: 198–201

45 Dicker R C, Greenspan J R, Strauss L T et al. Complications of abdominal and vaginal hysterectomy amongst women of reproductive age in the United States: the collaborative review of sterilisation. Am J Obstet Gynecol 1982; 144: 841–848

46 Phipps J H, John M, Nayak S. Comparison of laparoscopically assisted vaginal hysterectomy and bilateral salpingo-oophorectomy with conventional abdominal hysterectomy. Br J Obstet Gynaecol 1993; 100: 698–700

47 Raju K S, Auld B J. A randomised prospective study of laparoscopic vaginal hysterectomy versus abdominal hysterectomy with bilateral salpingo-oophorectomy. Br J Obstet Gynaecol 1994; 101: 1068–1071

48 Donnez J, Nisolle M. Laparoscopic supracervical (subtotal) hysterectomy (LASH). J Gynecol Surg 1993; 9: 91–99

49 Donnez J, Smets M, Polet R, Basil S, Nisolle M. Laparoscopic supracervical (subtotal) hysterectomy. Zentralbl Gynakol 1995; 117: 629–632

50 Barnes W, Waggoner S, Delgado G, Maher K, Potkul R, Benjamin S. Manometric characterization of rectal dysfunction following radical hysterectomy. Gynecol Oncol 1991; 42(2): 116–119

51 Kelly JL, O'Riordain, Jones E, Alawi E, O'Riordain MG, Kirwan WO. The effect of hysterectomy on ano-rectal physiology. In J Colorect Dis 1998; 13: 116-118

*Nuala Woodman   Michael D. Read*

# Oophorectomy at hysterectomy

Hysterectomy is one of the most commonly performed operations in the UK and the rate appears to be increasing. Currently, some 100,000 hysterectomies are performed annually (compared with 6 times this number in the US). The average age is in the early forties with an increasing number being performed in the thirties. There are estimated to be around two and a half million women in the UK who have undergone a pre-menopausal hysterectomy, of whom there are more than 250,000 who have also have bilateral oophorectomy and this number is increasing annually. Between 20–25% of women in the UK have had a hysterectomy by the time they reach their mid-fifties.

The dilemma over whether to remove or conserve ovaries at the time of hysterectomy has been debated, with varying degrees of passion, for over 100 years.[1] Studies suggesting that function in conserved ovaries is compromised following hysterectomy have supported the prophylactic oophorectomy lobby. On the other hand, proponents of conserving ovaries point to the problems of long-term compliance with oestrogen replacement therapy to prevent significant health risks which could otherwise arise.

A key theme running through all aspects of the debate is the absolute necessity for appropriate communication with the patient, in terms she can understand, so that she can make a decision in full appreciation of the implications whether she decides to have her ovaries removed or conserved.

## ARGUMENTS IN FAVOUR OF OOPHORECTOMY

Whilst the majority of cases of oophorectomy are undertaken for prophylactic purposes, there are a number of pre-existing conditions where it is believed oophorectomy can be therapeutic.

**Mr Michael D. Reid** MD FRCSEd FRCOG, Consultant Obstetrician and Gynaecologist, Women's Health Directorate, Gloucestershire Royal Hospital, Great Western Street, Gloucester GL1 3NN, UK

**Nuala Woodman** MSc, Research Assistant, Women's Health Directorate, Gloucestershire Royal Hospital, Great Western Street, Gloucester GL1 3NN, UK

## Therapeutic indications

### The presence of unilateral benign ovarian disease

Where a woman is known to have unilateral ovarian disease at the time of hysterectomy, there is an increased risk of subsequent benign disease occurring in the other ovary. The incidence of benign ovarian disease in women who have one ovary conserved compared with those who have both conserved is more than doubled.[2] There is a strong argument, therefore, to recommend bilateral oophorectomy for these women.

### Chronic pelvic pain

Chronic pelvic pain is well recognised as a feature of the residual ovary syndrome. The treatment of such pain can be difficult and surgery is often required, although this can be technically difficult with increased risk of damage to the ureters. Women with a pre-existing pelvic pain are most likely to benefit from oophorectomy at the time of hysterectomy.[3]

### Endometriosis

For women with chronic endometriosis, which does not respond satisfactorily to medical suppression therapy or laser ablation (including uterine nerve ablation), hysterectomy and bilateral oophorectomy have commonly been offered. It has been found that the oestrogen replacement therapy, which is necessary for both short-term symptoms and preventing long-term disease, does not cause stimulation of any residual (or newly developing) endometriotic tissue in the majority of women.

In cases where hysterectomy has been performed for menstrual problems and there has been evidence of endometriosis, the decision whether to conserve ovaries often depends on the appearance of the ovaries. However, in cases where the ovaries were apparently normal and were conserved, further surgery for pelvic pain became necessary in up to 47% of cases.[4]

However, the role of hysterectomy and bilateral oophorectomy in this situation has been challenged in both the US and UK suggesting that a more suitable approach is to concentrate on removing endometriotic deposits and associated scar tissue. Reich[5] advocates conserving the uterus in the presence of extensive obliteration of the cul de sac and suggests that oophorectomy is not usually necessary at the time of hysterectomy for endometriosis. In the presence of ovarian disease, he suggests that unilateral oophorectomy is appropriate as, in his series, re-operation was only necessary in 5% of cases, in marked contrast to the findings of Montgomery.[4]

### Pre-menstrual syndrome

As pre-menstrual symptoms occur in around 80% of women, it could be regarded as a 'normal' event. However, some women are severely affected by pre-menstrual syndrome (PMS) and, on occasions, this can be very distressing and severely disabling. Although there are over a dozen 'treatments' promoted for pre-menstrual syndrome, all helping some sufferers but none helping all, there is only one 'cure' for true PMS and that is ovarian failure. The underlying cause of PMS is still unknown. Whilst it is not a simple hormonal imbalance, it is related to the cyclical hormone release from the ovaries associated with ovulation.[6,7] Following hysterectomy alone, pre-menstrual symptoms persist, but not after hysterectomy and bilateral oophorectomy.[8–10] Furthermore, the subsequent oestrogen replacement therapy does not cause a return of symptoms whereas combined oestrogen/progestogen therapy often does.

Bilateral oophorectomy should never be offered lightly to a pre-menopausal woman and, as PMS sufferers are usually in the 35–40 year age group, it is essential that all possible is done to make sure that she has true PMS, that the proposed approach is likely to relieve her symptoms, and that she understands the need for long-term oestrogen replacement therapy together with the risks of non-compliance.

GnRH agonists have been used to treat PMS symptoms with more reliable results when using the injectable preparations[11] compared with the nasal preparations.[12] Both physical and physiological symptoms of PMS improve significantly with this treatment. In order to determine whether the 'PMS' will be 'cured' by hysterectomy, bilateral oophorectomy and oestrogen replacement, a 2–3 month trial of ovarian suppression using a GnRH agonist with add back oestrogen after the first month can be extremely useful in predicting the chances of therapeutic success.[13] This test of ovulation suppression is similar to that used in patents with chronic pelvic pain described by Carey and Slack.[14] In cases of true PMS, the patient (and her family) report that she is a 'new woman' and for these women the operation can significantly improve their quality of life. However, if the symptoms are not improved during this trial period, the woman would not benefit from surgery and she should not be offered the bilateral oophorectomy.

A far greater number of women will be offered, or request, oophorectomy for prophylaxis against the possible future occurrence of problems.

## Prophylactic indications

### Residual ovary syndrome

Following hysterectomy with conservation of ovaries, 3–10% of women will present with pelvic symptoms,[15,16] most commonly cyclical unilateral pain.[17,18]

This condition is more common in women under 35 years at the time of hysterectomy. There are characteristic changes in the ovaries the cause of which may be related to dense adhesions in the ovarian capsule preventing normal cyclical volume changes and subsequent pain. A history of previous pelvic surgery is found in up to 10% of cases and endometriotic cysts in up to 10% of cases. Many women have a history of pain which pre-dates the hysterectomy.

A very interesting, but very rare, variant is the ovarian remnant syndrome in women following hysterectomy with bilateral oophorectomy (usually in the presence of pelvic adhesions and a technically difficult procedure). These women experience symptoms similar to residual ovary syndrome and are found to have normal pre-menopausal FSH levels. It is believed that these women have some residual ovarian tissue following an incomplete excision at the time of the original operation.[19]

Complete removal of the ovaries is technically more difficult at the time of vaginal hysterectomy.[20] It is possible that more cases of ovarian remnant syndrome will emerge following the increase in the proportion of hysterectomies performed vaginally in pre-menopausal women over recent years.

### Benign cyst formation

There is no evidence to suggest that hysterectomy reduces the incidence of benign cyst formation in conserved ovaries although statistics are few. The tendency to bilateral tumour occurrence, either simultaneously or during long-term follow-up,[21] suggests that it would be reasonable to consider oophorectomy where there is a history of surgery for benign cysts whether that was a cystectomy or unilateral oophorectomy.

### Cancer of the ovary

By far the most common reason put forward for prophylactic oophorectomy is to prevent subsequent malignancy in conserved ovaries.

Ovarian cancer is a cause of death for 2% of women in the UK accounting for about 4,000 deaths per year. The problem is not limited to this country, as cancer of the ovary is the leading cause of death from gynaecological cancers in the US (the fifth leading cause of all cancer deaths) and the sixth leading cause of cancer deaths in Singapore.[22,23] It remains difficult to detect in its early stages with no satisfactory screening method. As a result, the overall 5-year survival rate remains around 20–25%. It is against this background that prophylactic oophorectomy is actively promoted as oophorectomy essentially obviates the risk.

Hysterectomy alone reduces the risk of subsequent development of carcinoma of the ovary by 50% over the following 20 years.[24] There is no difference in the prognosis between cancers arising in residual ovaries and cancers arising in non-hysterectomised women. The life-time risk of developing carcinoma of the ovary is up to 2%, increasing significantly in women with a family history (7% for those with two affected relatives). Where there is an established hereditary predisposition, the life-time risk may be as high as 50%.[25]

It is difficult to predict the risk of developing cancer in a residual ovary.[26] However, information is available about the number of women developing cancer who have had previous pelvic surgery and could have had a concomitant prophylactic oophorectomy. Various studies put this figure at 7–18%.[27–31]

## Other considerations

The debate as to whether hysterectomy compromises ovarian function stretches back more than 60 years with the first report of an increase in ovarian failure in young women after hysterectomy being published in 1932.[32] The report of Siddle et al[33] was a turning point in the debate suggesting that ovarian failure occurred up to 4 years earlier in a group of 90 women after hysterectomy compared with a non-hysterectomised control group. However, the authors invited caution in interpretation of their findings, as the diagnosis of ovarian failure was made on clinical grounds and the study population was recruited from a menopause clinic; the women may not, therefore, be representative. These cautions have not always been observed in subsequent publications referring back to this paper. The poor correlation between symptoms and endocrine status in hysterectomised women has been highlighted by Quinn et al.[34]

Indirect support for an increased incidence of premature ovarian failure following hysterectomy comes from a number of studies on bone density.[35–37]

Cardiovascular studies have also suggested a link between hysterectomy and premature ovarian failure.[38,39] Simple hysterectomy is also associated with more severe vasomotor and other menopausal complaints than in women undergoing a natural menopause.[40] There has been considerable debate about the psychological sequelae of hysterectomy for over 100 years. Recent studies suggest that many of the apparent psychologically detrimental effects described after hysterectomy are related to pre-existing dysfunction.

It can be difficult to determine when ovarian failure occurs following hysterectomy. Relying on clinical symptoms is very unreliable[34] and it is more appropriate to rely on estimation of FSH levels and possibly serum oestradiol levels, but for this, there is a significant resource implication.

Some authorities advocate routine oestrogen replacement in all women following hysterectomy even with conservation of ovaries.[41] Support for this approach includes evidence for a gradual reduction in ovarian activity from the age of 40 years with decreasing fertility, falling plasma oestrogen levels, and decline in vertebral bone density.[1] Although the mean age of the menopause in this country is around 51 years, many women experience 'menopausal' symptoms for years before this and these symptoms are alleviated by oestrogen replacement therapy.[42]

If pre-menopausal hysterectomy is associated with a significant risk of premature ovarian failure, this would strengthen the argument in favour of offering prophylactic oophorectomy with subsequent oestrogen replacement. However, the majority of information currently available about any sequelae following hysterectomy is based on cross sectional studies. There is no prospective longitudinal data.

In the Gloucestershire Royal Hospital, we are currently undertaking a study of over 1,000 women who have had hysterectomy for benign disease performed under the age of 47 years; 531 of these women had a simple hysterectomy with conservation of ovaries and a further 521 having hysterectomy and bilateral oophorectomy. Women who have had conservation of ovaries are being followed up yearly with serum FSH assays for 5 years. In longitudinal studies, there can be no short-cuts and the final results will, of necessity, not be available for some time yet; but interim results at the end of year 4 do show some interesting trends. Table 1 shows the numbers of patients by year and route of operation. Table 2 shows the number of confirmed ovarian failures and the time after operation at which this occurred in yearly intervals. Table 3 shows the confirmed ovarian failure group as a percentage of each cohort. The percentage figure shown in the end column is a cumulative total, thus by the

**Table 1** Number of patients by year and route of operation

| Type of operation | 1994 | 1995 | 1996 | 1997 |
|---|---|---|---|---|
| Abdominal | 83 | 58 | 28 | 35 |
| Abdominal + USO | 31 | 42 | 22 | 19 |
| Vaginal | 39 | 59 | 51 | 59 |
| Vaginal + USO | 2 | 0 | 0 | 3 |
| Total | 155 | 159 | 101 | 116 |

USO, unilateral-salpingo oophorectomy.

**Table 2**  Number of confirmed ovarian failures occurring at yearly intervals after the operation

| Year of operation | Year 1 | Year 2 | Year 3 | Year 4 |
|---|---|---|---|---|
| 1994 | 6 | 2 | 3 | 3 |
| 1995 | 3 | 4 | 2 | |
| 1996 | 3 | 0 | | |
| 1997 | 7 | | | |
| All | 19 | 6 | 5 | 3 |

**Table 3**  Confirmed ovarian failures as a percentage of each cohort

| | Confirmed failures | Size of cohort | Percentage |
|---|---|---|---|
| Year 1 | 19 | 491 | 3.9 |
| Year 2 | 18 | 361 | 5.0 |
| Year 3 | 20 | 259 | 7.7 |
| Year 4 | 14 | 121 | 11.6 |

The year 1 cohort includes information from the 1994–1997 groups.
The year 2 cohort includes information from the 1994–1996 groups.
The year 3 cohort includes information from the 1994–1995 groups.
The year 4 cohort includes information from the 1994 group only.
The percentage figures are cumulative.

end of year 4, a total of 11.6% of women who had had hysterectomy had suffered a confirmed ovarian failure. Sixteen women subsequently had their ovaries removed for pain or cyst formation. Our preliminary data, therefore, do not support Siddle's findings. An interesting finding requiring further clarification is the apparent disproportionate increase in premature ovarian failure occurring in women with a previous sterilisation and also in women having vaginal hysterectomy rather than abdominal hysterectomy.

## When should prophylactic oophorectomy be offered?

In the absence of any indications for 'therapeutic' oophorectomy, current thinking in the UK is to discuss oophorectomy in women over the age of 40 years and to recommend it in women over the age of 45 years. Certainly, the majority of gynaecologists would recommend removal of ovaries at the time of abdominal hysterectomy after the menopause.[26] However, it is interesting that the numbers of bilateral oophorectomies at the time of hysterectomy falls after the age of 60 years.[43] This is related to the increasing number of hysterectomies performed vaginally, presumably in association with prolapse in older women. Although proponents find no difficulty with vaginal oophorectomy, with success rates in excess of 90%,[44] others, perhaps more representative of 'middle-of-the-road' gynaecologists, report success rates of less than 70%.[20] It can be difficult to remove the ovaries using the vaginal approach and there may be an increased risk of the ovarian remnant syndrome. It is, however, rather illogical to say on the one hand that one would recommend removal of the ovaries 'automatically' at the time of an abdominal hysterectomy in a post-menopausal woman, yet not to perform it in cases of vaginal hysterectomy in women at increasing risk of ovarian cancer for which we are offering prophylaxis! The increasing use of laparoscopic techniques offers the opportunity to remove the ovaries much more simply at the time of a vaginal hysterectomy both in pre- and post-menopausal women and, therefore, there is no need to restrict the prophylactic oophorectomy to women having abdominal procedures.

The annual statistical reports from the RCOG suggest an increasing trend towards vaginal hysterectomy over the past 10 years. The planned route of the hysterectomy may, in turn, have a bearing on the discussions about the role of prophylactic oophorectomy. It would be very interesting to be able to follow the trends in the UK looking at the number of prophylactic oophorectomies performed in relation to the route of hysterectomy both over the last 10 years and, prospectively, over the next 10 years. For the majority of district general hospitals, the facilitation of bilateral oophorectomy at the time of vaginal hysterectomy is probably the single greatest indication for developing and extending laparoscopic surgical techniques.

## ARGUMENTS FOR CONSERVATION OF OVARIES

There is evidence that retained ovaries work normally after hysterectomy.[17,45,46] Bilateral oophorectomy is a major undertaking in every sense except surgically and the ease with which the ovaries can be removed may bias the decision.

The simplistic view, that the ovaries have no further hormonal function after the menopause, has been shown to be incorrect.[47] Androgens and oestrogens are produced in significant quantities and histological evidence of steroidogenesis is present in post-menopausal ovarian stroma.[48] So there may be an endocrine role for the post-menopausal ovary both directly and via peripheral conversion of androgens.

### Health problems

Following bilateral oophorectomy, the oestrogen lack may cause severe and potentially serious short and long-term health problems.

#### Cardiovascular
Coronary heart disease is the most common serious health problem affecting post-menopausal women. Pre-menopausal oophorectomy is a significant risk factor. Mortality from cerebrovascular causes is predominantly a male problem below the age of 55 years, but overall is greater in females. Oestrogen lack leads to adverse changes in lipid,[49] carbohydrate and insulin metabolism[50] and coagulation and fibrinolytic mechanisms.[51]

#### Osteoporosis
Following ovarian failure, there is a demonstrable bone loss in vertebrae and femoral neck of up to 3% per year in the first 5 years,[52] which is not naturally replaced. However Ravn et al[53] found no association between hysterectomy and decreased bone mineral density.

#### Risk of carcinoma of the breast
The debate regarding the role of hormone replacement and occurrence of carcinoma of the breast continues. Meta-analyses of published studies suggest

a risk of 25–30% above controls when HRT has been used in excess of 15 years.[54] However, these studies were performed on women reaching an actual menopause and there is no significant information on women who have pre-menopausal oophorectomy and subsequent oestrogen replacement. There does not appear to be any increased risk of carcinoma of the breast before the age of 50 years and it may be that, if there is an increased risk with oestrogen therapy, this may be related to the life-time exposure to oestrogens whether this is natural or synthetic, rather than simply to synthetic oestrogens alone. Beyond the age of 50 years, the risks appear to be the same as for non-hysterectomised women. Certainly, there has been no report of increased mortality in women developing breast cancer who are receiving HRT and it may be that the closer surveillance is resulting in very early detection of tumours thus leading to a decrease in the mortality.

## Compliance with long-term oestrogen replacement

Despite the explosion in HRT regimens and modes of delivery in recent years, a number of women have medical contra-indications to hormone replacement therapy and less tangible problems occur in women on hormone replacement. Although the majority of side effects related to hormone replacement therapy are reported in women with an intact uterus receiving combined oestrogen/progestogen therapy, there are a significant number of women on oestrogen replacement alone who complain of side effects, especially breast tenderness and enlargement and weight gain. Some continue to experience 'menopausal' symptoms despite increasing doses of oestrogen and measured oestrogen levels in the normal range. The occurrence of tachyphylaxis is well recognised in women receiving implants.

Even if one accepts the argument that, on balance, prophylactic oophorectomy is appropriate in a particular case, this advice assumes though the long-term compliance with oestrogen replacement. Following hysterectomy and bilateral oophorectomy in a pre-menopausal woman where there is no adequate oestrogen replacement, there may be a reduction in life expectancy of up to 1.4 years.[55]

Experience in non-hysterectomised post-menopausal women suggests a mean compliance with HRT of less than 1 year. Most studies on compliance are based on cyclical combined therapy with monthly withdrawal bleeds and it was felt that this continuing 'menstruation' was a significant reason for discontinuing therapy. Compliance may well be improved with the advent of long cycle and 'no bleed' preparations. However, Spector[56] found a mean duration of only 28 months in women following hysterectomy and bilateral oophorectomy. If this were to be an accurate reflection of the situation, we may well be doing more harm than good in respect of long-term health problems.

In the 521 women who have had hysterectomy and bilateral oophorectomy in our longitudinal study, we have found a 96.5% compliance at 1 year and over 84% compliance at the end of 4 years (see Table 4).

Overall, approximately 35.5% of women stay with the original hormone replacement regimen they started after hysterectomy, although the percentage varies according to the type of hormone replacement, being the greatest with oral preparations. Some 64.5% of women, however, have found it necessary to try different types, brands or doses of hormone replacement to find a regimen

**Table 4** Compliance with HRT therapy at yearly intervals

|  | Size of cohort | Percentage taking HRT |
|---|---|---|
| Initial | 521 | 99.6 |
| After 1 year | 508 | 96.5 |
| After 2 years | 350 | 94.3 |
| After 3 years | 228 | 90.8 |
| After 4 years | 102 | 84.3 |

which suits them. Of this 64.5%, 37.4% have changed their HRT once, 14.3% twice and a further 7 (7%) changing it three times. We have found two patients who have changed their hormone replacement 6 times to find a regimen which suits them.

If the ovaries are to be removed, it is essential that the woman understands that oestrogen replacement needs to be continued at least up to the age of 50 years to avoid any increased risks of osteoporosis and cardiovascular problems. The most important aspect in the discussion about whether to remove the ovaries is the woman's perspective and this depends on the quality of the information given to her.

Each woman considering hysterectomy will have her own individual pattern of symptoms and response to them. The gynaecologist must elicit her initial position, exploring her wishes, expectations and fears regarding surgery. Having established the symptoms, it is appropriate to consider if bilateral oophorectomy would be beneficial, discussing the pros and cons and backing this up with written information for the woman to take home to consider at leisure and discuss with her family. This information should be clearly written in 'plain English' avoiding jargon and unnecessary technical terminology. There is rarely any haste to make a decision and the women can be allowed plenty of time to consider the situation, discussing it further with family, her general practitioner, or getting information from other sources. She should also have the opportunity for further discussion with the gynaecological team and this is an invaluable aspect of the pre-admission clinic allowing opportunity to discuss any points with the medical staff and also the nursing staff in the clinic. It is impossible to overestimate the confusion and potential unhappiness for these women caused by inadequate communication.[57]

### References

1 Studd J. Prophylactic oophorectomy. Br J Obstet Gynaecol 1989; 96: 506–509
2 Plöckinger B, Kölbl H. Development of ovarian pathology after hysterectomy without oophorectomy. J Am Coll Surg 1994; 178: 581–585
3 Beard R W, Kennedy R G, Gangar K F et al. Bilateral oophorectomy and hysterectomy in the treatment of intractable pelvic pain associated with pelvic congestion. Br J Obstet Gynaecol 1991; 98: 988–992
4 Montgomery J C, Studd J W W. Oestradiol and testosterone implants after hysterectomy for endometriosis. Contrib Gynecol Obstet 1987; 16: 241–246
5 Reich H. Laparoscopic surgery For advanced endometriosis. In: The Yearbook of Obstetrics and Gynaecology, vol 6. London: RCOG Press, 1998; 377–393
6 Schmidt B J, Nieman M A, Danaceau M A et al. Differential behavioural effects of gonadal steroids in women with and those without pre-menstrual syndrome. N Engl J Med 1998; 338: 209–216

7  Halbreich U, Rojanskyn N, Palter S. Elimination of ovulation and menstrual cyclicity (with Danazol) improves dysphoric pre-menstrual syndromes. Fertil Steril 1991; 56: 1066–1069

8  Backstrom T, Boyle H, Baird D T. Persistence of symptoms of pre-menstrual tension in hysterectomised women. Br J Obstet Gynaecol 1981; 88: 530–536

9  Casper R F, Hearn M T. The effects of hysterectomy and bilateral oophorectomy in women with severe pre-menstrual syndrome. Am J Obstet Gynecol 1990; 162: 105–109

10  Casson P, Hahn P M, van Vugt D A et al. Lasting response to ovariectomy in severe, intractable pre-menstrual syndrome. Am J Obstet Gynecol 1990; 162: 99–105

11  Muse K N, Cetel N S, Futterman L A et al. The pre-menstrual syndrome: effects of medical ovariectomy. N Engl J Med 1984; 311: 1345–1349

12  Bancroft J, Boyle H, Warner P et al. The use of an LH/RH agonist, Buserelin, in the long term management of pre-menstrual syndromes. Clin Endocrinol 1987; 27: 171–182

13  Mortola J F, Girton L, Fischer U. Successful treatment of pre-menstrual syndrome by combined use of gonadatropin releasing hormone agonist and estrogen/progesten. J Clin Endocrinol Metab 1991; 72: 252

14  Carey M P, Slack M C. GnRH analogue in assessing chronic pelvic pain in women with residual ovaries. Br J Obstet Gynaecol 1996; 103: 150–153

15  Montgomery J B. Discussion on the paper by Randall and Paloucek on the frequency of oophorectomy at the time of hysterectomy. Am J Obstet Gynecol 1968; 100: 724–725

16  Christ J E, Lotze E C. The residual ovary syndrome. Obstet Gynecol 1975; 46: 551–555

17  Grogan R H. Re-appraisal of residual ovaries. Am J Obstet Gynecol 1967; 97: 124–129

18  Siddall-Allum J, Rae T, Rogers V et al. Chronic pelvic pain caused by residual ovaries and ovarian remnants. Br J Obstet Gynaecol 1994; 101: 979–985

19  Siddall-Allum J. The ovarian remnant syndrome. J R Soc Med 1994; 87: 375–376

20  Capen S, Irwin H, Magrin J et al. Vaginal removal of the ovaries in association with vaginal hysterectomy. J Reprod Med 1983; 28: 589–593

21  Randall C L, Hall D W, Armenia C S. Pathology in the preserved ovary after unilateral oophorectomy. Am J Obstet Gynecol 1962; 84: 1233–1240

22  Fong Y-F, Lim F-K, Arulkumaran S. Prophylactic oophorectomy: a continuing controversy. Obstet Gynecol Survey 1998; 53: 493–499

23  Li T C, Saravelos H. Oophorectomy at the same time as hysterectomy. Br J Obstet Gynaecol 1994; 101: 949–936

24  Irwin K L, Weiss N S, Lee N C et al. Tubal sterilisation, hysterectomy and the subsequent occurrence of epithelial ovarian cancer. Am J Epidemiol 1991; 134: 362–369

25  Kerlikowske K, Brown J S, Grady G D. Should women with familial ovarian cancer undergo prophylactic oophorectomy? Obstet Gynecol 1992; 80: 700–707

26  Jacobs I, Oram D H. Prophylactic oophorectomy. Br J Hosp Med 1987; 38: 440–449

27  Bloom M L. Certain observations in a study of 141 cases of primary adenocarcinoma of the ovary. S Afr Med J 1962; 36: 714–716

28  Gibbs E K. Suggested prophylaxis for ovarian cancer. Am J Obstet Gynecol 1971; 111: 756–765

29  Bightler S, Bolke G, Estape P E et al. Ovarian cancer in women with prior hysterectomy. A fourteen year experience at the University of Miami. Obstet Gynecol 1991; 78: 681–684

30  Averette H E, Hoskins V, Nguyen H N et al. National survey of ovarian carcinoma. A patient care evaluation study of the American College of Surgeons. Cancer 1993; 71: 1629–1638

31  Schwarz P E. The role of prophylactic oophorectomy in the avoidance of ovarian cancer. Int J Gynecol Obstet 1992; 39: 175–184

32  Sessums V J, Murphy D P. Hysterectomy and the artificial menopause. Surg Gynaecol Obstet 1932; 55: 286–289

33  Siddle N, Sarrel P, Whitehead M. The effect of hysterectomy on the age at ovarian failure: identification of a sub-group of women with premature loss of ovarian function and literature review. Fertil Steril 1987; 47: 94–100

34  Quinn A J, Kingdom J C P, Murray G D. Relation between hysterectomy and subsequent ovarian function in a district hospital population. J Obstet Gynaecol 1993; 14: 103–107

35  Hreshchyshyn M, Hopkins A, Zyulstra S, Anbar M. The effects of natural menopause, hysterectomy and oophorectomy on lumbar spine and femoral neck densities. J Obstet Gynaecol 1988; 72: 631–638

36  Watson N R, Stuge A W W, Garnet T et al. Bone loss after hysterectomy with ovarian conservation. Obstet Gynecol 1995; 86: 72–77

37  Purdie D W, Steel. (Unpublished data.) In: Studd J W W, Edwards L (eds) Hysterectomy and HRT. London: RCOG Press, 1997; 93

38  Centerwall B S. Pre-menopausal hysterectomy and cardiovascular disease. Am J Obstet Gynecol 1981; 139: 58–61

39  Ritterband A B, Jaffe I A, Densen P M et al. Gonadal functions and the development of coronary heart disease. Circulation 1963; 27: 237–251

40  Oldenhaave A, Lazlo J B, Jaszmann M D et al. Hysterectomised women with ovarian conservation report more severe climacteric symptoms than do normal climacteric women of similar age. Am J Obstet Gynecol 1993; 168: 765–771

41  Edwards L. Patient view on osteoporosis. In: Drife J O, Studd J W W (eds) Proceedings of the 22nd Study Group of the Royal College of Obstetricians and Gynaecologists. London: Springer, 1990; 149–161

42  Jordan J A. Prophylactic oophorectomy at hysterectomy. In: Studd J W W, Edwards L (eds) Hysterectomy and HRT. London: RCOG Press, 1997; 60

43  Parazzini F, Negri E, La Vecchia C et al. Hysterectomy, oophorectomy and subsequent ovarian risk. Obstet Gynecol 1993; 81: 363–366

44  Scheth S S. The place of oophorectomy at vaginal hysterectomy. Br J Obstet Gynaecol 1991; 98: 662–666

45  Metcalfe M G, Braiden V, Livsey J H. Retention of normal ovarian function after hysterectomy. J Endocrinol 1992; 135: 597–602

46  Garcia L R, Cutler W B. Preservation of the ovary: a re-evaluation. Fertil Steril 1984; 42: 510

47  Lucisano A, Russo N, Acampora M G et al. Ovarian and peripheral androgen and oestrogen levels in post-menopausal women: correlations with ovarian histology. Maturitas 1986; 57–65

48  Gronroos M, Klemi P, Saimi T et al. Ovarian production of oestrogens in the post-menopausal ovary. Int J Gynecol Obstet 1980; 18: 93–98

49  Stevenson J C, Crook D, Godsland I F. Influence of age and menopause on serum lipids and lipoproteins in healthy women. Atherosclerosis 1993; 98: 83–90

50  Walton C, Godsland I F, Proudler A J et al. The effects of the menopause on insulin sensitivity, secretion and elimination in non-obese healthy women. Eur J Clin Invest 1993; 23: 466-470

51  Mead T W. Oestrogens and thrombosis in HRT and osteoporosis. In: Drife J O, Studd J W W (eds) Proceedings of the 22nd Study Group of the Royal College of Obstetricians and Gynaecologists. London: Springer, 1990; 223–233

52  Riggs B L, Melton L J. Medical progress: involution of osteoporosis. N Engl J Med 1986; 314: 1676–1686

53  Ravn P, Linda C, Nilas L. Lack of influence of simple menopausal hysterectomy on bone mass and bone metabolism. Am J Obstet Gynecol 1995; 172: 891–895

54  Sands R, Boshoff C, Jones A, Studd J W W. Current opinion: hormone replacement therapy after diagnosis of breast cancer. Menopause 1995; 2: 73–80

55  Speroff T, Dawson M W, Speroff L et al. A risk benefit analysis of elective bilateral oophorectomy: effect of changes in compliance with oestrogen therapy on outcome. Am J Obstet Gynecol 1991; 164: 165–174

56  Spector T D. Use of oestrogen replacement therapy in high risk groups in the United Kingdom. BMJ 1989; 299: 1434

57  Edwards L. The woman's perspective of hysterectomy. In: Studd J W W, Edwards L (eds) Hysterectomy and HRT. London: RCOG Press, 1997; 133

Kevin G. Cooper

# Endometrial ablation

Endometrial destruction as treatment for menorrhagia had been attempted using various blind techniques in the 1950s and 1960s, with limited success. With advances in endoscopic equipment in the 1970s, and borrowing from resection techniques used by urologists, therapeutic hysteroscopic surgery became possible. Electro-resection of the endometrium was described by Neuwirth and Amin in 1976[1] for the removal of submucous fibroids. De Cherney and Polan performed myomectomies using an unmodified urological resectoscope in 1983[2] and, later, successful resection of the endometrium in a series of 21 women in 1987.[3] The first UK results were presented by Magos in 1989[4] who called the procedure transcervical resection of the endometrium (TCRE). In the early 1980s, Goldrath pioneered an alternative effective method of hysteroscopic endometrial ablation using a laser fibre under direct vision.[5] Davis reported his series of laser ablations in the UK in 1989.[6] Following encouraging observational series reports,[7,8] a number of randomised controlled trials were undertaken to evaluate these procedures in the 1990s. These compared transcervical resection of the endometrium and/or laser ablation with hysterectomy,[9-13] and one has compared the two endometrial procedures.[14] A summary of the results of these trials are shown in Table 1. There has been no published data comparing rollerball ablation with these procedures in the context of a randomised trial, although observational series suggest equivalent results.[15-17] These trials along with descriptions of hysteroscopic surgical equipment and techniques have been well covered in previous editions of this series (volumes 9, 10 & 12), and readers are referred to these chapters for complete details.

Dysfunctional uterine bleeding exerts a significant burden on society. A large proportion of women presenting for treatment of excessive menstruation have monthly blood loss within the normal range, but still request help. It is

**Dr Kevin G. Cooper** MSc MD MRCOG, Consultant Gynaecologist, Aberdeen Royal Infirmary, Foresterhill, Aberdeen AB25 2ZB, UK

Table 1 Summary of randomised controlled trials evaluating hysteroscopic endometrial surgery in the surgical management of heavy menstrual loss

| Study | Comparison of patients (TCRE + other) | Number time | Follow-up time (min) | Procedure | Complications | Satisfaction (%) | Hypomenorrhoea (amenorrhoea) % |
|---|---|---|---|---|---|---|---|
| 1 Gannon et al[9], 1991 | Abdominal hysterectomy | 51 (26 + 25) | 9–16 months | 30 – TCRE, 50 – TAH | 0% TCRE 46% TAH | 84% TCRE | 80% TCRE (64% amen.) |
| 2a Dwyer et al[10], 1993 | Abdominal hysterectomy | 196 (97+ 99) | 4 months | 35 – TCRE, 45 – TAH | 4% TCRE 47% TAH | (a) 85% TCRE, (a) 94% TAH | 89% TCRE (13% amen.) |
| 2b Sculpher et al[35], 1996 | | | 2 years | | | (b) 77% TCRE, (b) 96% TAH | 70% TCRE, (13% amen) |
| 3a Pinion et al[11], 1994 | Hysterectomy | 204 (105 + 99) | 12 months | 45- ablation, 61 - hyst | 1% ablation 5% hyst. | (a) 78% ablation (a) 89% hyst | 76% ablation (22% amen.) |
| 3b Aberdeen Endometrial Trials Group[31], 1999 | | | Minimum of 4 years | | | (b) 80% ablation (b) 89% hyst | 97% ablation (45% amen.) |
| 4 O'Connor et al[12], 1997 | Hysterectomy | 172 (116 + 56) | Up to 4 years | 32 – TCRE 66 – hyst | 13% TCRE 45% TAH | 85% TCRE 96% hyst | 21% amen. at 21 months |
| 5 Crosignani et al[13], 1997 | Vaginal hysterectomy | 85 (41 + 44) | 2 years | 13 – ablation 71 - hyst | 0% ablation 2% hyst | 87% ablation 95% hyst | 64% ablation (22% amen.) |
| 6 Bhattacharya et al[14], 1997 | Endometrial laser ablation | 372 (188 + 184) | 2 years | 21 – TCRE 30 – laser | 10% TCRE 14% laser | 91% TCRE 90% laser | 86% TCRE ( %) 85% laser ( %) |

**Table 2**  Hospital statistics for the surgical management of menorrhagia in England

| | Year ending | | | | |
| | 1990 | 1991 | 1992 | 1993 | 1994 |
|---|---|---|---|---|---|
| Hysterectomy | 73,280 | 70,675 | 71,630 | 73,169 | 73,517 |
| Endometrial ablation | 1699 | 4224 | 7878 | 9982 | 9945 |
| Total | 74,979 | 74,899 | 79,508 | 83,151 | 83,462 |

Source: *Hospital Episode Statistics Volume 1: Finished Consultant Episodes by diagnosis, operation and speciality.*

known that women complaining of heavy menstrual loss suffer a significant reduction in health related quality of life.[18-20] Women complaining of heavy menstrual loss, 'menorrhagia', make up 5% of all general practice patients, accounting for over £7 million in prescription charges[21] and up to 12% of new referrals to gynaecology clinics in the UK.[22] There is considerable uncertainty about how best to treat these women once referred to a gynaecologist which is reflected by the variations in hysterectomy rates both nationally and internationally. Within 5 years of referral, up to 60% of women will have had a hysterectomy,[23] and by the age of 55 years, 20% of women in the UK will have had a hysterectomy.[24]

The operative statistics quoted in the above paragraph were gathered before the widespread use of endometrial destructive surgery and these high rates of hysterectomy could be significantly reduced. Endometrial ablative techniques were initially expected to reduce the benign hysterectomy rate, but may not have had the desired effect and instead lead to an overall increase operative interventions (Table 2).[25,26] National operative data (Table 2), are however misleading as they represent all hysterectomies for menorrhagia and do not identify those that were suitable for ablation. Local data, from areas with good uptake of proven endometrial surgical techniques, are more appropriate for inspection and can demonstrate a reduction in benign hysterectomies for menorrhagia (Table 3).[27] National data may be further confused by a preference towards hysterectomy amongst senior gynaecologists as the surgical procedure for menorrhagia,[28] which will skew audit results by reducing uptake of endometrial surgery in eligible women. Finally, the availability of

**Table 3**  Hospital statistics for the surgical management of menorrhagia in Aberdeen

| | 1990 | 1991 | 1992 | 1993 | 1994 | 1995 | 1996 | 1997 |
|---|---|---|---|---|---|---|---|---|
| Benign hysterectomy – any route | 605 | 680 | 620 | 622 | 537 | 560 | 456 | 480 |
| Endometrial destructive surgery | 44 | 116 | 118 | 164 | 290 | 364 | 315 | 307 |
| Total | 649 | 796 | 738 | 786 | 827 | 924 | 771 | 787 |

Source: Information management and technology. Patient administration system. Aberdeen Royal Hospitals NHS Trust, 1998.

these less invasive techniques have almost certainly attracted women for surgical treatment who would not previously have considered a hysterectomy, again increasing the numbers. The possibility that the threshold for surgical treatment has also lowered cannot be discounted. This may result from a combination of increased patient awareness of treatment options and availability, dissatisfaction with medical treatment, and diminishing menstrual tolerance.

## INDICATIONS FOR ENDOMETRIAL DESTRUCTION

What is the place of endometrial destructive surgery in the management of women complaining of heavy menstrual loss? Initially its role was envisaged as an alternative or replacement for hysterectomies undertaken for dysfunctional uterine bleeding. Recommendations were also made that its use should be reserved for women in whom medical treatment had failed. Whilst these are laudable suggestions, are they correct? The present evidence will be examined and then a revised role in the menstrual treatment armamentarium suggested. The second generation ablative techniques will then be considered.

### Endometrial destruction or hysterectomy?

Hysteroscopic endometrial destructive techniques have been shown to be effective with lower morbidity rates and quicker recovery times when compared with hysterectomy in five randomised controlled trials,[9–13] whilst their safety is confirmed by two national audits.[29,30] This degree of evaluation rarely occurs on the introduction of a new surgical procedure into everyday clinical practice. Despite this commendable, continuing evidence-based approach allied to the convincing results, these operations have not had the anticipated effect on hysterectomy rates. From 1991 to 1993, the number of NHS departments providing one of these procedures rose from 56% to 83%.[30] However, in the same timescale, the hysterectomy rate in England remained at above 70,000 (Table 2), despite the fact that almost 50% are undertaken for dysfunctional uterine bleeding,[24] and are, therefore, suitable for endometrial surgery. If the failure of these procedures to make the expected impact occurred through a lack of convincing long-term data, then we can now be reassured. Long-term results are now available from two randomised trials which corroborate the earlier trial results[12,31] and observational data,[32] clearly demonstrating that hysteroscopic surgery is an acceptable alternative to hysterectomy. Satisfaction rates remain high at 80% or more in the long-term. Re-operation rates seem to plateau at 3 years varying from 22% to 38%. The previous significant economic advantages of the hysteroscopic techniques[33,34] are slightly less at this stage, but still evident.[31,35]

Those who regard the re-operation rates as high must remember that these were recruits randomised from cohorts of women who would have had a hysterectomy and hence amenorrhoea. Initial counselling for the ablative techniques may have given unreasonably high expectations for amenorrhoea based on previous observational data (50–60%), whereas realistic rates were somewhat lower (20–40%). An expectation or desire for amenorrhoea has been shown to lead to higher re-operation rates, despite lighter periods being

**Table 4** Indications and recommended counselling for women considering hysteroscopic endometrial surgery as an alternative to hysterectomy

| Indications | Outcomes |
| --- | --- |
| Heavy menstrual loss | Satisfaction rates around 80% |
| Not expecting amenorrhoea | Lighter periods most likely |
| Endometrial atypia excluded | Amenorrhoea in about a third, but cannot predict in whom |
| Uterus less than 12 weeks' size | Significant improvement in quality of life |
| No pelvic infection | True dysmenorrhoea is significantly improved for most women |
| Completed family | Likely reduction in pre-menstrual symptoms |
| Fit for surgical procedure | Risk of hysterectomy between 10–25% after 3–4 years |
| Would undergo hysterectomy if necessary | |

achieved.[36] If appropriate counselling is given with realistic details regarding outcome (Table 4), then these re-operation rates might be reduced. The other possible reasons for increasing numbers of ablative procedures undertaken in the face of static hysterectomy rates were previously mentioned, but undoubtedly include women who would not have undergone a hysterectomy, but are willing to consider endometrial surgery.

## Ablation or medical treatment?

Although hysteroscopic endometrial surgery compared well with, and has many advantages over, hysterectomy, it cannot guarantee amenorrhoea. To find its therapeutic niche the next logical comparison was with standard first line gynaecological management for heavy menstrual loss, medical treatment, which similarly aims to lighten periods. It is logical to conclude that high hysterectomy rates are in part a reflection of the long-term failure of medical therapy. A pragmatic randomised controlled trial comparing transcervical resection of the endometrium with medical treatment was undertaken in women first referred to a gynaecologist with heavy menstrual loss who were not referred for surgery.[20] Women randomised to medical treatment were not subsequently randomised to individual medical treatments, but received a medication chosen by her consultant that had not previously been tried by her general practitioner. No treatments shown to be ineffective in reducing menstrual blood loss in randomised controlled trials were prescribed. The levonorgestrel intra-uterine system was not a medical option in the trial as it was not licensed for the treatment of menorrhagia. It may represent a significant breakthrough in non-surgical management of this condition and further trial results are awaited.

At 4 months, women allocated to transcervical resection were highly significantly more likely to be totally or generally satisfied, to find the treatment acceptable, and would be willing to have the treatment again. The mean number of heavy days, menstrual and pain scores were significantly reduced by medical treatment, but these improvements were modest in comparison with transcervical resection. Haemoglobin levels were significantly increased only following transcervical resection. Quality of life scores were improved in both arms, although only transcervical resection returned them to normal values. Outcome was better following hysteroscopic surgery irrespective of whether or not a woman had previously received treatment from her general practitioner or the type of trial medical management prescribed.

Two year follow-up of the study cohorts consolidated the short-term results.[37] Women allocated medical treatment were highly significantly less likely to be totally or generally satisfied, to find their management acceptable, or to recommend their allocated treatment. In the medical cohort, 59% of women had undergone TCRE, hysterectomy or both, whereas 17% in the TCRE cohort had undergone further surgery; 14% of the medical and 10% of the transcervical resection of the endometrium arm had undergone hysterectomy at two years. These rates are low when compared to previous randomised trials, although these women were not expecting amenorrhoea at recruitment.

A policy of hysteroscopic surgery as primary gynaecological treatment for dysfunctional uterine bleeding is, therefore, effective and safe and does not result in an increase in hysterectomies. The present recommendations stating that hysteroscopic endometrial surgery should be offered once medical treatment has failed cannot be upheld by these findings. An effective endometrial ablative technique should, therefore, be one of a selection of treatments offered by a gynaecologist to all women who have completed their family, with a diagnosis of dysfunctional uterine bleeding, irrespective of what treatment, if any, she received in primary care.

## TREATMENT PREFERENCE

About a third of women referred for treatment of their heavy menstrual loss will have strong preferences with regards to their treatment.[36,38] These treatment preferences are equally divided between medical and surgical options, and identification is important as they have different expectations and outcomes.[36] Women with a strong preference for medical treatment are generally less severely affected by their periods, are more likely to continue with medication or no treatment, and have a high chance of avoiding surgery.[37] Women with a strong surgical preference should be asked whether amenorrhoea is their expected or desired outcome, as these women have higher rates of dissatisfaction and subsequent hysterectomy, this should be discussed as an option from the outset. The final treatment choice should be made by the woman after a full discussion of the advantages and disadvantages of the various treatment options available to her.

## NEW ABLATIVE TECHNIQUES

A reluctance to learn a new surgical technique, with a recognised learning curve, may contribute to the piecemeal uptake of hysteroscopic surgery by gynaecologists in the UK. Through recognition of this problem, a number of 'blind' endometrial ablative procedures, utilising various energy sources have been developed. These ablative techniques which claim to be effective, quick to learn and simple to use include, the uterine thermal balloon,[39,40] cryo-ablation,[41] photodynamic therapy[42] and microwave ablation,[43,44] amongst an ever growing list.

Much of this technological expansion has been driven by medical equipment manufacturers, although some are modifications of innovative older ideas. All report high levels of success, but few have been rigorously evaluated from the point of view of efficacy or safety in the context of well constructed randomised trials. This is indeed unfortunate given the strict scientific policing which accompanied the introduction and ongoing assessment of transcervical resection of the endometrium and laser ablation. These new procedures should be accepted into general use only once they have been satisfactorily compared to one of the proven hysteroscopic techniques. There is no place for the commonly undertaken prospective multicentre observational studies, which are subject to major bias. Apart from eliminating bias, equalising known and unknown prognostic variables, and forming the basis for statistical analyses, random-isation also protects half of the recruits from any unforeseen problems that might arise directly as a result of the new procedure in the short or long-term.

Two of these blind ablative techniques have been evaluated in randomised controlled trials, microwave endometrial ablation (MEA) and the uterine thermal balloon and will be discussed further. Microwave technology will also be explained. Other new ablative procedures, which should only be under-taken within strict trial protocols until their safety and efficacy is proven, are not discussed further.

## Microwave endometrial ablation

Microwave ablation should not to be confused with radio frequency endometrial ablation (RaFEA),[45] which was misnamed 'microwave' by some sources. Microwaves are electromagnetic waves with a wavelength of 0.3–30 cm and frequency, 300–300,000 MHz (between radiowaves and infrared radiation). A 9.2 GHz microwave frequency was determined to be the most effective at producing the 5 mm depth of necrosis necessary to completely destroy the basal layer of the endometrium. A microwave generator, or magnetron, supplies microwave energy to a hand held applicator, as seen in Figure 1. The applicator is an 8 mm diameter, 15 cm circular metal pipe with a dielectric filled waveguide to propagate microwave energy at 9.2 GHz into the uterine cavity. The dielectric extends beyond the tip of the pipe to form the radiating tip. With power levels of 30 W, energies of 1.5–9.3 kJ result and a hemispherical field pattern emanates from the dielectric tip, which, if placed in egg white, causes a symmetrical ball of coagulum of constant thickness. Extensive testing on animal tissue, excised perfused uteri and pre-hysterectomy in vivo specimens have been undertaken and a depth of necrosis of 5–6 mm can be consistently achieved.

Uterine tissue has a very high water content, so the microwave field amplitude is reduced by about 90% approximately 3 mm from the surface of the applicator tip. Beyond this zone of intense microwave heating, further tissue destruction occurs by thermal conduction from the heated region. The total depth of necrosis depends upon the power level used and the length of time it is applied. The pattern of heating at the tip is hemispherical and monitoring the temperature of the adjacent tissue allows control over the depth of necrosis. A thermocouple on the applicator tip measures the temperature on the endometrial surface. There is a second thermocouple in the base of the applicator as a control and to show the temperature gradient. The temperature at the tip is displayed graphically allowing the surgeon to monitor the process of heating and hence treatment. The system computer screen provides the surgeon with a proven temperature band of 70–80°C. An alarm is activated if the temperature exceeds 85°C and automatically shuts off power at 90°C. Another safety feature is that potential perforation can be determined quickly by a failure to establish a temperature gradient if the machine is activated. No earthing is required and there is no energy transmission at the pre-set power levels beyond 6 mm from the applicator tip.

The procedure can be performed under general or local anaesthesia.[46] The cervix is dilated to 8 mm and the length of the cavity measured. The probe is

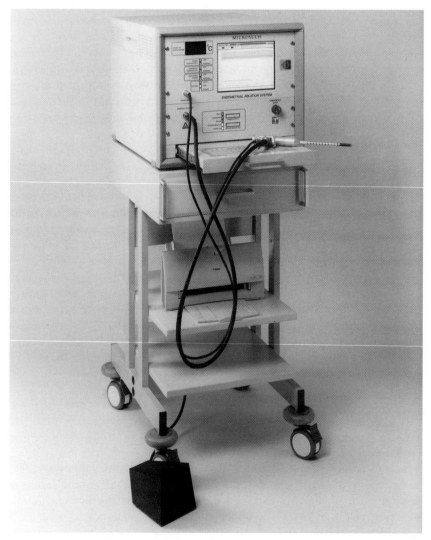

**Fig. 1** Microwave generator and treatment probe.

inserted until the tip reaches the fundus, ensuring that the length inserted is the same as that previously measured. The microwave generator is then activated by depressing the footswitch. Once the temperature reaches 70–80°C, the probe is moved laterally into the cornual region. The temperature reading will transiently fall; then, once the operating temperature is attained again, the probe is moved to the opposite cornua and the process repeated. The probe is then gradually withdrawn whilst maintaining the temperature in the 70–80°C range. The technique effectively 'paints' the uterine cavity with a broad brush of destructive microwave energy.[43] The treatment phase should be stopped once a coloured area appears on the probe shaft. This is set 3 cm from the tip and ensures that the endocervical canal is not treated, which could result in stenosis with subsequent haematometria or pain. The treatment time varies with cavity length, but is usually between 2–3 min.

The first clinical assessment of this ingenious device was undertaken in Bath and the initial results were very encouraging, showing active treatment times of less than 3 min and high satisfaction rates.[43] The first randomised trial comparing microwave endometrial ablation (MEA), with transcervical resection of the endometrium has been completed in Aberdeen and short-term results have been presented.[44] The entry criteria accepted any consenting women wishing endometrial destructive surgery, who had completed their family, had a uterus of 10 weeks' size or less without endometrial atypia. Operations were performed under general anaesthetic 5 weeks following endometrial preparation with goseralin. Microwave ablation was a significantly faster technique than TCRE, the mean total operating time being less than 12 min. Postoperative stay was less following MEA, though not significantly so, whereas analgesia requirements were low and equivalent for both techniques(< 30%). Troublesome bleeding occurred in 5 cases of transcervical resection of the endometrium and no microwave cases. Satisfaction with, and acceptability of, treatment rates are high and equivalent. Health related quality of life was highly significantly improved following microwave ablation.

Analysis of longer term results at one year uphold the 4 month findings, with differences in outcome between the procedures becoming less obvious.[55] Follow-up is to be repeated again at 2 and 4 years. A successful pilot study has now been completed demonstrating the acceptability of MEA performed under local anaesthesia. A prospective randomised trial, funded by the Scottish Office, comparing MEA under local and general anaesthetic commenced in the summer of 1999.

## Uterine thermal balloon

This system utilises a 16 cm long, 5 mm diameter catheter with a heating element contained in a latex balloon on the treatment end (Fig. 2). This apparatus is connected to a control unit which can monitor display and adjust pre-set intra-uterine balloon pressure, temperature and duration of treatment. The deflated balloon and 5 mm catheter are introduced transcervically into the uterine cavity and once in place, 5% dextrose solution is used to inflate the balloon. A minimum pressure of 150 mmHg must be achieved for the device to activate and the system will automatically shut-off if pre-set low and high pressure

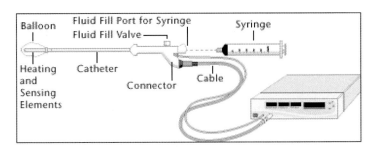

**Fig. 2** The uterine thermal balloon.

limits are reached. Once the balloon pressure stabilises at between 160–180 mmHg, the fluid is then heated to approximately 87°C and treatment is undertaken at this temperature for 8 min. The balloon is then deflated and removed from the cavity.

One randomised trial has been undertaken assessing the uterine thermal balloon to date.[40] As this took place in the US, it was compared with rollerball ablation, the preferred method of hysteroscopic surgery there. Despite convincing evidence of the effectiveness of rollerball ablation, published results are not available from a randomised controlled trial. The methodological structure of this trial was otherwise quite robust with appropriate randomisation. The power calculation was based on a 20% difference in effectiveness, a sizeable difference if attempting to demonstrate similar efficacy and may result in dismissal of important differences between the techniques. Women with submucous fibroids were excluded which necessitated pre-procedure assessment of the endometrial cavity. True menorrhagia was an entry criteria and was determined by pictorial chart assessment of menstrual blood loss.[47] Pre-treatment endometrial preparation with drug therapy was not undertaken which is financially advantageous and would also prevent the known gonadotrophin releasing hormone analogue associated increase in cervical resistance.[48] Instead, 3 min of 5 mm suction curettage was completed to prepare the cavity immediately prior to treatment.

Outcome measures included operative details, pictorial menstrual charts and assessment of satisfaction and pre-menstrual symptoms. A recognised quality of life questionnaire was not utilised. Operative data demonstrated that the thermal balloon was significantly quicker than rollerball ablation and no intra-operative complications occurred. Impressively, 47% of women undergoing balloon therapy were treated under local anaesthesia. Results after 1 year are very encouraging with high and equivalent satisfaction rates of over 80% in both groups. Similarly menstrual scores were highly significantly reduced by both techniques, with a trend of improving scores throughout the year. Amenorrhoea rates were significantly higher following rollerball ablation, 27% compared to 15%, but this should not be regarded as a principal outcome measure. Dysmenorrhoea rates were also decreased in around 70% of women for both techniques. Similarly, premenstrual symptoms were significantly reduced for both, which is a recognised and consistent finding following endometrial destructive procedures.[10,11,20,49]

Important considerations which reduce the generalisibilty of the results are the pre-recruitment identification of women with true menorrhagia which is not normal practice in the UK. Women with heavier menstrual loss, as identified in this study, are known to report higher satisfaction rates and a larger reduction in menstrual loss following ablative treatment.[50] Also, only women with normal cavities were included despite the fact that 15–20% of women with heavy menstrual loss undergoing ablation will have a cavity distorted by a fibroid.[11,44] A multi-centre prospective series evaluating the thermal balloon in 300 women has been published which presents generally similar and supportive results for this technique.[39] It should be re-iterated that there is no place for these uncontrolled series' reports in the assessment of new techniques beyond the initial pilot study stage, and the practice should not be supported.

Whilst the results of both these randomised trials are encouraging, and may herald the mass introduction of these simple-to-use techniques, we must be cautious. Firstly, these results are not generalisible to all blind ablative techniques which must be separately evaluated in there own right. Secondly, if these techniques are undertaken by clinicians with no hysteroscopic experience, problems may arise if there is equipment failure or an intra-operative complication which could be resolved through hysteroscopic surgery. Determination of the endometrial cavity, its characteristics, confirmation of its correct length and re-assurance of its integrity can only be ensured by hysteroscopy, and is routinely undertaken prior to microwave ablation in our department. SERNIPS (the safety and efficacy register for newly introduced procedures) recommends confirmation of correct siting for blind ablative devices with ultrasound, which may be re-assuring, but cannot exclude placement in a false passage. Finally, no pathological specimen is obtained with any ablative technique; therefore, dependence on pre-treatment endometrial biopsy results to exclude atypia or carcinoma is required. The pipelle sampler, the most commonly used endometrial biopsy instrument, samples under 10% of the endometrium and has been shown to miss cases of endometrial cancer when tested on known cases of the disease.[51] Of greater concern, cases of endometrial cancer have been picked up in resection strips from women undergoing transcervical resection of the endometrium who had negative pre-treatment biopsies and hysteroscopy (also one case in Aberdeen).[52,53] The re-assurance of known long-term results and a histological representation of the whole cavity from the resection strips maintains TCRE as our preferred method of treatment if the women desires or requires general anaesthesia.

Where these ablative techniques have an undoubted advantage is in their potential to be widely undertaken using local anaesthetic. Short procedure times, minimising cervical dilatation, in conjunction with little peri-operative instrument manipulation, all contribute to the likely success of ablative procedures under local anaesthetic. A high proportion of women, 47% of thermo-ablative balloon procedures had their procedure under local anaesthetic in the aforementioned randomised trial, and some of these were in the office setting. For women with a preference, these techniques can undoubtedly be successfully completed under local anaesthetic. Whether women without a preference for local anaesthesia can be re-assured that the procedure would be acceptable to them will be clearer once the Aberdeen randomised trial comparing local and general anaesthetic for endometrial ablation is completed.

## CONCLUSIONS

Hysteroscopic surgical techniques have undergone more rigorous assessment in randomised trials than almost any other surgical procedure and can be considered a validated technique.[54] Long-term results are now available in comparative trials with hysterectomy and reassure us of the safety and efficacy of these techniques. Table 3 confirms that the benign hysterectomy rate for menstrual disorders has been reduced from over 600 to less than 500 a year in Aberdeen since the introduction of endometrial surgery. Unfortunately, uptake seems to be incomplete in the UK. Those who did not embrace these procedures, because of a healthy scepticism and need to examine the long-term trial results, should now be re-assured. If the surgical skills and training involved were factors in their hesitancy, then it is time to learn.

Endometrial destruction is also an effective and acceptable first-line treatment for women attending the gynaecologist with heavy menstrual loss. It should not be withheld from suitable women in an effort to pursue medical therapy. Endometrial destructive techniques have the ability to return health related quality of life to normative levels, which, along with the prevention of anaemia, remains the ultimate treatment goal. Whilst these endometrial techniques undergo refinement to simplify them, we must be vigilant to maintain their safety and effectiveness through continuing scrutiny in well constructed trials and ongoing audit. The very long-term sequelae of all of these endometrial surgical procedures is unknown and, particularly with the blind ablative techniques utilising different types of energy, it is important to follow-up those treated to ascertain subsequent rates of gynaecological malignancy.

The new generation ablative techniques, such as microwave, thermal balloon and others have been introduced to simplify endometrial ablation, but these techniques require strict evaluation. They are undoubtedly fast, probably less morbid techniques, that are easy to learn and have the potential to be undertaken in the out-patient setting. Unfortunately, like transcervical resection of the endometrium, none at present can guarantee amenorrhoea whilst the long-term sequelae are yet to be fully explored. Technical improvements hold the key to their future success. Decreasing instrument diameters to reduce cervical manipulation will increase their acceptability in the out-patient setting. Ensuring total endometrial destruction whilst maintaining strict energy safety levels remains the ultimate quest; although this can occasionally be achieved in a well prepared small regular cavity, it should ideally work on unprepared and irregular cavities. Once these newer ablative techniques are proven to be safe and effective, it opens up the possibility of a definitive one-stop, investigate and treat, menstrual clinic in the out-patient setting.

The impact of introducing ever new techniques seems to increase the number of procedures that are undertaken for menstrual dysfunction. Is this due to a lowering of the treatment threshold, the genuine introduction of more

**KEY POINTS FOR CLINICAL PRACTICE**

- Endometrial ablation is a proven safe treatment for women with heavy menstrual loss.

- Endometrial ablation should be offered as a treatment option by gynaecologists to all women who have completed their family, and who have a diagnosis of dysfunctional uterine bleeding.

- Second generation endometrial ablative techniques simplify and shorten the procedure, but the majority, excepting microwave ablation, have not been adequately evaluated in the context of randomised controlled trials comparing them to proven hysteroscopic techniques.

- Microwave and endothermal balloon ablation have the potential to allow acceptable and effective treatment in the out-patient setting.

- A significant reduction of the hysterectomy rate for dysfunctional uterine bleeding would be achieved if an ablation was used as first line surgical treatment.

advanced and acceptable treatments, or have women become less tolerant of menstruation? There is no evidence that the incidence of true menorrhagia has changed over the last 50 years, although as family sizes decrease the number of periods experienced by individual women are greater. We now know that health-related quality of life is significantly reduced in women with chronic heavy menstrual loss, and that it can be corrected by appropriate treatment. Women have become more informed of the therapeutic options available and to what is and is not perceived to be an acceptable degree of menstruation, through increased media coverage of women's issues. This enlightenment may have created an undercurrent of 'menstrual intolerance' in developed countries which is driving up demands for effective treatment modalities. If a safe, cheap out-patient treatment becomes available which can guarantee amenorrhoea, is it possible that we could witness an explosion of 'cosmetic' endometrial destruction, and, if so, is it wrong?

### References

1  Newrith R S, Amin H K. Excision of submucous fibroids under hysteroscopic control. Am J Obstet Gynecol 1976; 126: 91–94
2  De Cherney A, Polan M L. Hysteroscopic management of intrauterine lesions and intractable uterine bleeding. Obstet Gynecol 1983; 61: 392–397
3  De Cherney A, Diamond M P, Lavy G, Polan M L. Endometrial ablation for intractable uterine bleeding: hysteroscopic resection. Obstet Gynecol 1987; 70: 668–670
4  Magos A L, Baumann R, Turnbull A C. Transcervical resection of the endometrium in women with menorrhagia. BMJ 1989; 298: 1209–1212

5  Goldrath M H, Fuller T A, Segal S. Laser photovaporization of endometrium for the treatment of menorrhagia. Am J Obstet Gynecol 1981; 140: 14–19

6  Davis J A. Hysteroscopic endometrial ablation with the neodymium-YAG laser. Br J Obstet Gynaecol 1989; 96: 928–932

7  Garry R, Erian J, Grochmal S A. A multi-centre collaborative study into the treatment of menorrhagia by Nd-YAG laser ablation of the endometrium. Br J Obstet Gynaecol 1991; 98: 357–362

8  Magos A L, Baumann R, Lockwood G M, Turnbull A C. Experience with the first 250 endometrial resections for menorrhagia. Lancet 1991; 337: 1074–1078

9  Gannon M J, Holt E M, Fairbank J. A randomised trial comparing endometrial resection and abdominal hysterectomy for the management of menorrhagia. BMJ 1991; 303: 1362–1364

10  Dwyer N, Hutton J, Stirrat G M. Randomised controlled trial comparing endometrial resection with abdominal hysterectomy for the surgical treatment of menorrhagia. Br J Obstet Gynaecol 1993; 100: 237–243

11  Pinion S B, Parkin D E, Abramovich D R et al. Randomised trial of hysterectomy, endometrial laser ablation, and transcervical endometrial resection for dysfunctional uterine bleeding. BMJ 1994; 309: 979–983

12  O'Connor H, Broadbent J A M, Magos A L, McPherson K. Medical Research Council randomised trial of endometrial resection versus hysterectomy in management of menorrhagia. Lancet 1997; 349: 897–901

13  Crosignani P G, Vercillini P, Apolone G, De Giorgi O, Cortesi I, Meschia M. Endometrial resection versus vaginal hysterectomy for menorrhagia: Long-term clinical and quality of life outcomes. Am J Obstet Gynecol 1997; 177: 95–101

14  Bhattacharya S, Cameron I M, Parkin D E et al. A pragmatic randomised comparison of transcervical resection of the endometrium with endometrial laser ablation for the treatment of menorrhagia. Br J Obstet Gynaecol 1997; 104: 601–607

15  Vancaille T. Electrocoagulation of the endometrium with the ball end resectoscope. Obstet Gynecol 1989; 75: 425–427

16  McLucas B. Endometrial ablation with the rollerball electrode. J Reprod Med 1990; 35: 1055

17  Daniell J F, Kurtz B R, Ke R W. Hysteroscopic endometrial ablation using the rollerball electrode. Obstet Gynecol 1992; 80: 329

18  Garratt A M, Ruta D A, Abdalla M I, Russell I T. The SF-36 health survey questionnaire. II Responsiveness to changes in health status for patients with four common conditions. Qual Health Care 1994; 3: 186–192

19  Jenkinson C, Peto V, Coulter A. Measuring change over time: a comparison of results from a global single item of health status and the multi-dimensional SF-36 health status survey questionnaire in patients presenting with menorrhagia. Qual Life Res 1994; 3: 317–321

20  Cooper K G, Parkin D E, Garratt A M, Grant A M. A randomised comparison of medical and hysteroscopic management in women consulting a gynaecologist for treatment of heavy menstrual loss. Br J Obstet Gynaecol 1997; 104: 1360–1366

21  Coulter A, Kelland J, Long A et al. The management of menorrhagia. Effective Health Care Bull 1995; 9

22  Bradlow J, Coulter A, Brooks P. Patterns of Referral. London: Health Services Research Unit., Bulletin No. 9, 1992

23  Coulter A, Bradlow J, Agass M, Martin-Bates C, Tulloch A. Outcomes of referrals to gynaecology outpatient clinics for menstrual problems: an audit of general practice records. Br J Obstet Gynaecol 1991; 98: 789–796

24  Vessey M P, Villard-Mackintosh L, McPherson K, Coulter A, Yeates D. The epidemiology of hysterectomy: findings in a large cohort study. Br J Obstet Gynaecol 1992; 99: 402–407

25  Bridgeman S A. Increasing operative rates for dysfunctional uterine bleeding after endometrial resection. Lancet 1994; 344: 893

26  Coulter A. Trends in gynaecological surgery. Lancet 1994; 344: 1367

27  Armatage J, Quenby S, Granger K, Farquharson R. Trends in gynaecological surgery. Lancet 1994; 345: 129

28  Bicknell N, Earp J, Garrett J, Evans A. Gynaecologists' sex, clinical beliefs, and hysterectomy rates. Am J Public Health 1994; 84: 1649–1652

29  Scottish Hysteroscopy Audit Group. A Scottish audit of hysteroscopic surgery for menorrhagia: complications and follow up. Br J Obstet Gynaecol 1995; 102: 249–254

30  Overton C, Hargreaves J, Maresh M. A national survey of the complications of endometrial destruction for menstrual disorders: the MISTLETOE study. Br J Obstet Gynaecol 1997; 104: 1351–1359

31  Aberdeen Endometrial Ablation Trials Group. A randomised trial of endometrial ablation versus hysterectomy for the treatment of dysfunctional uterine bleeding: clinical, psychological and economic outcomes at four years. Br J Obstet Gynaecol 1999; 106: 360–366

32  O'Connor H, Magos A. Endometrial resection for the treatment of menorrhagia. N Engl J Med 1996; 335: 151–156

33  Sculpher M J, Bryan S, Dwyer N, Hutton J, Stirrat G M. An economic evaluation of transcervical endometrial resection versus abdominal hysterectomy for the treatment of menorrhagia. Br J Obstet Gynaecol 1993; 100: 244–252

34  Cameron I M, Mollison J, Pinion S B, Atherton-Naji A, Buckingham K, Torgerson D. A cost comparison of hysterectomy and hysteroscopic surgery for the treatment of menorrhagia. Eur J Obstet Gynecol Reprod Biol 1996; 70: 87–92

35  Sculpher M J, Dwyer N, Byford S, Stirrat G M. Randomised trial comparing hysterectomy and transcervical endometrial resection: effect on health related quality of life and costs two years after surgery. Br J Obstet Gynaecol 1996; 103: 142–149

36  Cooper K G, Grant A M, Garratt A M. The impact of using a partially randomised patient preference design when evaluating alternative managements for heavy menstrual bleeding. Br J Obstet Gynaecol 1997; 104: 1367–1373

37  Cooper K G, Parkin D E, Garratt A M, Grant A M. Two-year follow up of women randomised to medical management or transcervical resection of the endometrium for heavy menstrual loss: clinical and quality of life outcomes. Br J Obstet Gynaecol 1999; 106: 258–265

38  Coulter A, Peto V, Doll H. Patients' preferences and general practitioners' decisions in the treatment of menstrual disorders. Fam Pract 1994; 11: 67–74

39  Amso N A, Stabinsky S A, McFaul P, Blanc B, Pendley L, Neuwirth R. Uterine thermal balloon therapy for the treatment of menorrhagia: the first 300 patients from a multi-centre study. Br J Obstet Gynaecol 1998; 105: 517–523

40  Meyer W, Walsh B, Grainger D, Peacock L, Loffer F, Steege J. Thermal balloon and rollerball ablation to treat menorrhagia: a multicenter comparison. Obstet Gynecol 1998; 92: 98–103

41  Pittrof R, Majid S, Murray A. Transcervical endometrial cryoablation (ECA) for menorrhagia. Int J Gynaecol Obstet 1994; 47: 135–140

42  Gannon M J. Photodynamic therapy for menorrhagia. Trends Urol Gynaecol Sexual Health 1994; October: 16–20.

43  Sharp N C, Cronin N, Feldberg I, Evans M, Hodgson D, Ellis S. Microwaves for menorrhagia: a new fast technique for endometrial ablation. Lancet 1995; 346: 1003–1004

44  Cooper K G, Bain C, Parkin D E. A randomized trial comparing microwave endometrial ablation with transcervical resection of the endometrium. Br J Obstet Gynaecol 1998; 105: 25

45  Phipps J H, Smith T, Dymek P, Hesp R, Lewis B V. Validation of a method of treating menorrhagia by endometrial ablation. Clin Phys Physiol Measure 1992; 13: 273–280

46  Sharp N C, Hodgson D A, Feldberg I. Microwave endometrial ablation. An ultra-rapid simple treatment for menorrhagia: 3 years' experience. Br J Obstet Gynaecol 1998; 105: 106.

47  Higham J M, O'Brien P M S, Shaw R W. Assessment of menstrual blood loss using a pictorial chart. Br J Obstet Gynaecol 1990; 97: 734–739

48  Cooper K G, Pinion S B, Bhattacharya S, Parkin D E. The effects of the gonadotrophin releasing hormone analogue (goseralin) and prostaglandin E₁ (misoprostol) on cervical resistance prior to transcervical resection of the endometrium. Br J Obstet Gynaecol 1996; 103: 375–378

49  Lefler Jr HT. Premenstrual syndrome improvement after laser ablation of the endometrium for menorrhagia. J Reprod Med 1989; 34: 905–906

50  Gannon M J, Day P, Hammadieh N, Johnson N. A new method for measuring menstrual blood loss and its use in screening women before endometrial ablation. Br J Obstet Gynaecol 1996; 103: 1029–1033

51  Ferry J, Farnworth A, Webster M, Wren B. The efficacy of the pipelle endometrial biopsy

in detecting endometrial carcinoma. Aust N Z J Obstet Gynaecol 1993; 33: 76–78

52 Dwyer N A, Stirrat G M. Early endometrial carcinoma: an incidental finding after endometrial resection. Br J Obstet Gynaecol 1991; 98: 733–734

53 Colafranceschi M, Bettocchi S, Mencaglia L, van Herendael B J. Missed hysteroscopic detection of uterine carcinoma before endometrial resection: report of three cases. Gynecol Oncol 1996; 62: 298–300

54 Garry R. Endometrial ablation and resection: validation of a new surgical concept. Br J Obstet Gynaecol 1997; 104: 1329–1331.

55 Cooper K G, Bain C, Parkin D E. Comparison of microwave endometrial ablation and transcervical resection of the endometrium for treatment of heavy menstrual loss: a randomised trial. Lancet, November 1999: 354: 1859–1863

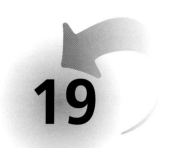

C. Jay McGavigan  Iain T. Cameron

# Medical therapy for menorrhagia

Menorrhagia is derived from Greek and literally means 'to burst forth monthly' (*mene*, the moon and *rhegnymi*, to burst forth). Heavy menstrual bleeding is now one of the main reasons for which women in developed societies seek medical advice. In a community survey of 521 women, 30% rated their menstrual loss as 'heavy', and 22% stated that heavy periods interfered with their life.[2] Today, women experience up to 10 times more menstrual cycles than their ancestors did. This may be attributed to the increased availability of effective contraception, decreased tolerance of the inconvenience of menorrhagia and higher expectations of the health service.

Hysterectomy, the traditional surgical treatment for menorrhagia, is only suitable for women who have no further wish to conceive. The operation itself is not without risk. Indeed, the National Confidential Enquiry into Perioperative Deaths in 1996–97 reported 7 deaths due to haemorrhage and/or infection in women who had a hysterectomy for benign disease.[3] Concerns about the 'invasiveness' of hysterectomy have led to the development of minimal access approaches, including endometrial resection and ablation, both as in-patient and, more recently, out-patient treatments.[4,5] But at least 1 in 5 women who undergo these procedures will require further surgery (repeat resection/ablation or hysterectomy) at a later stage[6] and, again, these approaches can only be used for women who have completed their families.

There continues to be a need, therefore, for effective medical therapies for menorrhagia.

**Dr C. Jay McGavigan** MBBBS, Clinical Research Fellow, University Department of Obstetrics and Gynaecology, The Queen Mother's Hospital, Yorkhill, Glasgow G3 8SJ, UK

**Prof. Iain T. Cameron** BSc MA MD FRCOG MRANZCOG, Professor of Obstetrics and Gynaecology, Princess Anne Hospital, Oxford Road, Southampton SO16 5YA, UK (for correspondence)

## PATHOPHYSIOLOGY

Menorrhagia may be secondary to underlying pathology such as fibroids, malignancy, infection or bleeding diatheses. In these instances, treatment can be directed towards the underlying cause. In the majority of cases, there is no demonstrable pathology and the disorder is termed dysfunctional uterine bleeding. Of these cases, 10–20% are associated with anovulation, especially at the extremes of reproductive life.

The precise cause of dysfunctional uterine bleeding is thought to lie at the level of the endometrium itself. Haemostasis during menstruation is achieved mainly by vasoconstriction, until the bleeding is finally checked by repair of the endometrial blood vessels in the first 7 days of the cycle.[7,8] A number of factors are thought to be involved in the local control of menstrual blood loss (Fig. 1),[9] and abnormalities in the prostaglandin and fibrinolytic systems in the endometrium have led to a rational medical approach to the treatment of menorrhagia in some women.

## OBJECTIVE ASSESSMENT OF MENSTRUAL BLOOD LOSS

The definition of menorrhagia as a menstrual blood loss greater than 80 ml each month arose from a large population study in Gothenberg in the early 1960s.[1] Women with a blood loss greater than 80 ml were in the upper 10th

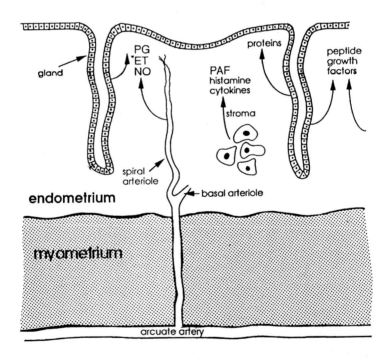

**Fig. 1** Local factors in the control of menstrual blood loss. The main cellular components of the endometrium (glandular epithelium, stroma and vascular endothelium) synthesize a wide variety of locally acting factors including prostaglandins, vasoactive agents, cytokines, endometrial proteins and peptide growth factors. PG, prostaglandin; ET, endothelin; NO, nitric oxide; PAF, platelet activating factor. Reproduced from Cameron and Norman[9] with permission.

centile of the population, and were considered to be at increased risk of iron deficiency anaemia. This study, and subsequent work from the UK, defined normal mean/median monthly menstrual blood loss as 30–40 ml.[1,10]

Assessment of blood loss in these population studies relied on the measurement of haemoglobin using the 'alkaline haematin' method.[11] Later work showed that 'blood' makes up less than half of the fluid loss experienced at the time of menstruation.[12] Furthermore, objective measurements have revealed that menstrual blood loss is less than 80 ml in over half of women complaining of heavy periods.[13,14] This is of direct relevance to clinical practice. Firstly, women with heavy periods who proceed to surgery, and whose blood loss is normal, are not having an operation to decrease their risk of iron deficiency anaemia. Secondly, part of the reason for the perception that medical treatment for menorrhagia is ineffective is that, in 50% of cases, the medical treatment is prescribed for women who do not actually have menorrhagia.

## MEDICAL TREATMENTS FOR MENORRHAGIA

The main classes of drugs used for the medical treatment of menorrhagia are antifibrinolytic agents, antiprostaglandins and hormonal therapies (Table 1). Ethamsylate, a medication believed to reduce capillary fragility, is not widely utilised, and has doubtful efficacy.[15]

### Antifibrinolytic agents

The endometrium possesses an active fibrinolytic system, and fibrinolytic activity is greater in the endometrium of women with menorrhagia than it is in the endometrium of women with menstrual blood loss in the normal range. Antifibrinolytic agents, such as tranexamic acid, provide a rational and effective treatment, reducing the degree of menstrual loss by about 50%. Comparative studies have shown that tranexamic acid is better at lowering menstrual flow than prostaglandin synthetase inhibitors, with reductions of 56% and 44% following tranexamic acid and 21% and 24% after flurbiprofen and diclofenac sodium, respectively.[16,17] Tranexamic acid reduced menstrual loss by 35–51% in women whose measured blood loss was less than 80 ml, and has also been shown to be effective in women with iatrogenic menorrhagia caused by the intra-uterine contraceptive device (IUCD).[17,18]

The incidence of adverse effects is related to the dose of drug prescribed. A third of women experience gastrointestinal side effects following treatment

**Table 1** Medical therapies for menorrhagia

| Antifibrinolytic agents | Tranexamic acid |
|---|---|
| Antiprostaglandins | e.g. Mefenamic acid |
| Hormonal treatments | Systemic progestagens (e.g. norethisterone)<br>Intra-uterine progestagens (LNG IUS)<br>Oestrogen/progestagen contraceptive pill<br>Danazol, GnRH analogues, gestrinone, tamoxifen |

with tranexamic acid, 3–6 g daily. As 90% of menstrual blood is lost in the first 3 days of full flow, dose-related side effects can be reduced by limiting the number of days on which the drug is taken to the first 3 or 4 days of the period. Serious side effects are uncommon, and may include intracranial thrombosis and central venous stasis retinopathy.[19] Early reports suggested that antifibrinolytic agents might be implicated in the pathogenesis of thrombo-embolic disease. However, histochemical studies failed to show suppression of fibrinolysis in superficial vein walls, using 3–4 g of tranexamic acid daily for 3 months.[20] In addition, no increase in the incidence of thrombo-embolic disease has been seen in women of reproductive age in Scandinavia, where tranexamic acid has been used since the early 1970s as a first line treatment for menorrhagia.[21] There is no clear evidence that tranexamic acid increases the risk of thrombo-embolic disease in women who are not already predisposed because of past history or a family history of thrombophilia.

Antifibrinolytic agents, therefore, represent a relatively effective first line treatment to reduce the degree of menstrual bleeding.

### Antiprostaglandins

Non-steroidal anti-inflammatory drugs (NSAIDs) remain a popular choice for the treatment of menorrhagia.[22] Their main mechanism of action is to decrease endometrial prostaglandin (PG) concentrations. The endometrium is a rich source of $PGE_2$ and $PGF_{2\alpha}$, and a number of studies have shown that PG concentrations are greater in the endometrium of women with menorrhagia, than they are in the endometrium of women with normal blood loss.[8,9]

The NSAID used most often for the treatment of menorrhagia is mefenamic acid. This agent consistently reduces menstrual blood loss by about 25% in three-quarters of women with menorrhagia.[23] Various studies have compared the efficacy of prostaglandin synthetase inhibitors with other treatment options. For example, menstrual blood loss was reduced by 24% and 20% in women with ovulatory dysfunctional uterine bleeding treated with mefenamic acid and norethisterone, respectively.[24] In a study of mefenamic acid and danazol, menstrual blood loss was reduced by 22% and 56%, however, the investigators concluded that mefenamic acid was a better initial treatment because it was cheaper and caused fewer side effects.[25]

Similar results have been reported after the use of other NSAIDs.[16,26] Of 14 women treated with mefenamic acid and naproxen, seven had a better response to mefenamic acid, whilst results were better after naproxen in two cases.[26]

The beneficial effect of mefenamic acid on menstrual blood loss (and other symptoms including dysmenorrhoea, headache, nausea, diarrhoea and depression) persists for several months. Mefenamic acid, 500 mg three times daily during menses, given for over a year to 83 women with a subjective complaint of menorrhagia, reduced menstrual blood loss from 66 ± 5 ml to 49 ± 10 ml at 6–9 months, and to 43 ± 5 ml at 12–15 months, an overall decrease in menstrual blood loss of 24%.[27]

In summary, mefenamic acid and related compounds may be effective first-line medical treatments for some women with menorrhagia. The degree of reduction of menstrual blood loss is not as great as it is with antifibrinolytic agents, but the NSAIDs have a lower side-effect profile in otherwise healthy women.

**Table 2** Mean (standard deviation) menstrual blood loss during two placebo cycles followed by two treatment cycles, in women randomized to receive norethisterone (5 mg, twice daily, days 19–26; $n = 21$) or tranexamic acid (1 g, four times daily, days 1–4; $n = 25$)

|  | Menstrual blood loss (ml) | |
|  | Norethisterone | Tranexamic acid |
| --- | --- | --- |
| Placebo cycle 1 | 178 (81) | 191 (90) |
| Placebo cycle 2 | 168 (91) | 159 (75) |
| Treatment cycle 1 | 195 (102) | 79*** (54) |
| Treatment cycle 2 | 220* (165) | 116** (112) |

The asterisks represent significant differences between placebo and treatment cycles: *$P = 0.26$; **$^P < 0.001$; ***$P < 0.0001$. Data extracted from Preston et al.[28]

## Hormonal therapies

### Systemic progestogens

Systemic progestogens, such as norethisterone and medroxyprogesterone acetate, offer a logical approach to the treatment of anovulatory dysfunctional uterine bleeding. However, most studies have shown that oral administration of these agents is not an effective therapy for the management of ovulatory dysfunctional uterine bleeding, if the drugs are given at low dose for short duration (5–10 days) in the luteal phase of the cycle (Table 2).[24,28,29] But norethisterone can be used to treat **ovulatory** menorrhagia if the drug is given at a higher dose for 3 weeks out of 4 weeks (5 mg three times daily from days 5 to 26 of the cycle; Table 3).[30,31]

### Intra-uterine progestogens

Whilst menstrual loss is increased after the insertion of inert or copper-containing IUCDs, blood loss is reduced if the device is impregnated with a progestogen.[32,33] The most recently described medicated device is the levonorgestrel intra-uterine system (LNG IUS; Mirena®). This delivers 20 µg of levonorgestrel to the endometrium every 24 h in a sustained release formulation that can last for up to 5 years. Direct administration of the progestogen to the uterus results in little systemic absorption.[34] Initial studies in 20 women with objective menorrhagia showed that menstrual blood loss decreased from a median of 176 ml before treatment to 24 ml at 3 months, and 5 ml at 12 months. Seven (35%) women were amenorrhoeic after 1 year.[34]

**Table 3** Objectively measured menstrual blood loss before and after treatment with norethisterone or the LNG IUS ($n = 22$ in each group)

|  | Menstrual blood loss (ml) | |
|  | Norethisterone | LNG IUS |
| --- | --- | --- |
| Control | 120 (82,336) | 105 (82,780) |
| Treatment cycle 1 | 46 (0,213) | 16 (0,62) |
| Treatment cycle 3 | 20 (4,137) | 6 (0,284*) |

Median blood loss is shown, with the range in brackets. *LNG IUS expelled spontaneously. Data extracted from Irvine et al.[31]

The efficacy of the LNG IUS for the treatment of menorrhagia has been compared with oral norethisterone and endometrial resection. A total of 44 individuals with objectively diagnosed menorrhagia were prescribed norethisterone (5 mg, three times daily from day 5 of the cycle for 21 days) or the LNG IUS.[31] Blood loss was measured before treatment and after 3 cycles. Menstrual blood loss was reduced to the normal range in both groups. There was no difference in the side-effect profile between the two groups, apart from intermenstrual spotting, which was seen in 53% of women treated with LNG IUS, but only 13% of those receiving the oral progestogen. However, this was not a major constraint to compliance in these women. Of those treated with LNG IUS, 80% chose to continue with this treatment at the end of the study, as opposed to 20% in the norethisterone group.

In another study, 70 premenopausal women with dysfunctional uterine bleeding were randomised to have the LNG IUS inserted or to undergo endometrial resection.[35] Blood loss was assessed semi-objectively and a general health questionnaire was completed after 12 months. Estimated blood loss was reduced by 79% and 89% in the LNG IUS and resection groups, respectively. Satisfaction with treatment was high – 85% and 94%. The LNG IUS would, therefore, appear to compare well with endometrial resection for the management of dysfunctional uterine bleeding, at least when assessed 12 months after the start of treatment.

The LNG IUS might also compare well with hysterectomy. An open, randomised study investigated the use of LNG IUS in women on the waiting list for hysterectomy.[36] Recruits were invited to have an IUS inserted 6 months prior to surgery or to continue with the form of medical treatment that they had been using. Of the women in the LNG IUS group, 64% (and 14% in the control group) chose to remove themselves from the waiting list for hysterectomy. Whilst there was a significant bias in this study, in that the control group were likely to be dissatisfied with a treatment option that had already been considered ineffective for them as a long-term solution, the LNG IUS might offer an acceptable alternative to hysterectomy for some women.

The main side effect associated with the LNG IUS is irregular breakthrough bleeding and spotting, particularly within the first few months after insertion of the system. Furthermore, 20% of women using the system will become amenorrhoeic within 1 year. These events must be discussed in detail prior to insertion of the system.

### The combined contraceptive pill

The combined oestrogen/progestogen contraceptive pill reduces menstrual blood loss by about 50%. Its main mechanism of action is thought to be endometrial suppression. It has long been recognised that women using the combined pill for contraception report reduced menstrual blood loss. This was confirmed objectively in 1967, in women with menorrhagia and normal controls.[37] Nevertheless, the combined pill was only prescribed by 11% of 518 general practitioners in a study of the treatment of menorrhagia in primary care.[22] It is likely that the combined pill has been unpopular for the treatment of menorrhagia because of concerns about arterial and thrombo-embolic disease, particularly in women over 35 years of age. However, age alone is not necessarily a contra-indication to the use of the low dose combined pill in the absence of smoking, obesity, other predisposing factors or a family history of thrombophilia.

### Danazol

Danazol is a synthetic androgen with anti-oestrogenic and antiprogestogenic activity. It inhibits the release of pituitary gonadotrophins, and has a direct suppressive effect on the endometrium. The drug was initially introduced as a medical treatment for endometriosis. It causes a significant reduction in menstrual blood loss, and usually results in amenorrhoea when prescribed at doses greater than 400 mg daily.[38] A high incidence of androgenic side effects has limited the use of danazol as a treatment option for women with gynaecological disease. Danazol is not a first-line treatment for menorrhagia. Its main use is as a short-term pre-operative adjunct, for example, to make the endometrium atrophic prior to endometrial resection.

### Antisteroids: gonadotrophin releasing hormone (GnRH) analogues, gestrinone and tamoxifen

Gonadotrophin releasing hormone (GnRH) analogues can be used to control menstrual loss by pituitary down-regulation and subsequent inhibition of cyclical ovarian activity. Ovarian suppression and amenorrhoea, with the associated problems of the hypo-oestrogenic state, including hot flushes, vaginal dryness and bone mineral loss (unless oestrogen/progestogen 'add-back' therapy is also used), is not a first-line option, but may have a place for the short-term treatment of women with intractable menorrhagia. As with danazol, GnRH analogues can be prescribed to suppress endometrial growth before transcervical endometrial resection or endometrial ablation. In addition, GnRH analogues can be given for 3–4 months to reduce the size of fibroids prior to myomectomy or hysterectomy.

Gestrinone is a synthetic derivative of 19-nortestosterone with anti-oestrogenic, antiprogestogenic and some androgenic activity. In a placebo-controlled study of 2.5 mg gestrinone twice weekly for 12 weeks in 19 women with objectively diagnosed menorrhagia, a marked reduction in MBL was seen in 5 individuals, and 10 became amenorrhoeic.[39] The drug was well tolerated, and all 19 women completed the 10 month study. Although not recommended as first-line therapy, gestrinone may have a role for some women with menorrhagia.

Anti-oestrogens have not been used widely to treat dysfunctional uterine bleeding, however one 23-year-old with menorrhagia due to myometrial hypertrophy was cured by 9 months treatment with tamoxifen.[40]

## CONCLUSIONS AND FUTURE PROSPECTS

Abnormalities of prostaglandin production and fibrinolysis in the endometrium of women with menorrhagia have led to the use of prostaglandin synthetase inhibitors or antifibrinolytic agents as a logical approach to medical therapy. Mefenamic acid and tranexamic acid have been used most often, and consistently reduce menstrual blood loss by about 25% and 50%, respectively. These agents are appropriate first-line drugs for the treatment of dysfunctional uterine bleeding. Fibrinolytic inhibitors appear to be more effective, but adverse gastrointestinal side-effects are more common. Synthetic progestogens may be of benefit in anovulatory dysfunctional bleeding, but they are only effective at reducing blood loss in women with ovulatory menorrhagia if given at high dose for three weeks out of four. The levonorgestrel intra-uterine system produces a marked reduction in menstrual loss and may offer an effective and acceptable alternative to oral treatments or surgery. Agents such as danazol or GnRH analogues result in marked reductions in menstrual blood loss, or amenorrhoea. These medications are not appropriate as first-line treatments or for long-term administration, but may have a place for short-term therapy in women with excessive menstrual loss who wish to avoid surgery, or as pre-operative adjuncts to endometrial resection, myomectomy or hysterectomy.

Future developments are likely to focus on local, reversible therapy delivered directly to the uterine cavity. At present, the most effective approaches to the medical treatment of menorrhagia induce a non-specific 'suppression' of the endometrium. A better understanding of the precise pathophysiology of dysfunctional uterine bleeding should lead to a more rational treatment plan. For example, specific treatment to promote vascular repair, or the correction of deficient local growth factor expression could provide novel therapeutic strategies in the new millennium for the management of this common clinical problem.

---

**KEY POINTS FOR CLINICAL PRACTICE**

- Heavy menstrual bleeding is one of the main reasons for which women in developed societies seek medical advice.

- Of women who complain of heavy periods, 50% have a measured menstrual blood loss within the normal range (< 80 ml per month). This should be remembered when choosing a management plan and interpreting the response to treatment.

- Mefenamic acid and tranexamic acid reduce blood loss by 25% and 50%, respectively. These drugs have relatively few side-effects and provide a good first-line therapy for some women.

- The oestrogen/progestagen pill reduces menstrual blood loss by 50%. It provides good cycle control and effective contraception.

- Oral norethisterone will reduce the degree of menstrual bleeding if prescribed at high dose for 3 weeks out of 4.

- The levonorgestrel intra-uterine system reduces menstrual blood loss by over 80% and may offer an acceptable alternative to other medical treatments and surgery. Breakthrough bleeding is common and is worst in the first few months after insertion of the system.

- Gonadotrophin releasing hormone analogues are not first line options, but have a place for the short-term treatment of women with intractable menorrhagia.

## References

1 Hallberg L, Hogdahl A M, Nilsson L, Rybo G. Menstrual blood loss – a population study. Acta Obstet Gynaecol Scand 1966; 45: 320–351

2 Gath D, Osborn M, Bungay G. Psychiatric disorder and gynaecological symptoms in middle aged women: a community survey. BMJ 1987; 294: 213–218

3 Anon. National Confidential Enquiry into Perioperative Deaths 1996–97. London: HMSO, 1998

4 Goldrath M. Hysteroscopic endometrial ablation. In: Cameron I T, Fraser I S, Smith S K. (eds) Clinical Disorders of the Endometrium and Menstrual Cycle. Oxford: Oxford University Press, 1998; 175–191

5 Soderstrom R M, Brooks P G, Corson S L et al. Endometrial ablation using a distensible multielectrode balloon. J Am Assoc Gynecol Laparosc 1996; 3: 403–407

6 Sculpher M J, Dwyer N, Byford S, Stirratt G M. Randomised trial comparing hysterectomy and transcervical endometrial resection: effect on health related quality of life and costs two years after surgery. Br J Obstet Gynaecol 1996; 103: 142–149

7 Markee J E. Menstruation in intraocular endometrial transplants in the rhesus monkey. Contrib Embryol 1940; 28: 219–308

8 Campbell S, Cameron I T. The origins and physiology of menstruation. In: Cameron I T, Fraser I S, Smith S K. (eds) Clinical Disorders of the Endometrium and Menstrual Cycle. Oxford: Oxford University Press, 1998; 13–30

9 Cameron I T, Norman J E. Endometrial biochemistry in menorrhagia. Prog Reprod Med 1995; 2: 267–279

10 Cole S K, Billewicz W Z, Thomson A M. Sources of variation in menstrual blood loss. J Obstet Gynaecol Br Commonwealth 1971; 78: 933–939

11 Hallberg L, Nilsson L. Determination of menstrual blood loss. Scand J Clin Lab Invest 1964; 16: 244–248

12 Fraser I S, McCarron G, Markham R, Resta T. Blood and total fluid content of menstrual discharge. Obstet Gynecol 1985; 65: 194–198

13 Fraser I S. Treatment of menorrhagia. Baillières Clin Obstet Gynaecol 1989; 3: 391–402

14 Cameron I T. Dysfunctional uterine bleeding. Baillières Clin Obstet Gynaecol 1989; 3: 315–327

15 Bonnar J, Sheppard B L. Treatment of menorrhagia during menstruation: randomised controlled trial of ethamsylate, mefenamic acid and tranexamic acid. BMJ 1996: 313: 579–582

16 Milsom I, Andersson J K, Andersch B, Rybo G. A comparison of flurbiprofen, tranexamic acid and a levonorgestrel releasing intrauterine contraceptive device in the treatment of idiopathic menorrhagia. Am J Obstet Gynecol 1991; 164: 879–883

17 Ylikorkala O, Viinikka L. Comparison between antifibrinolytic and antiprostaglandin treatment in the reduction of increased menstrual blood loss in women with intrauterine contraceptive devices. Br J Obstet Gynaecol 1983; 90: 78–83

18 Nilsson L, Rybo G. Treatment of menorrhagia with an antifibrinolytic agent, tranexamic acid. Acta Obstet Gynaecol Scand 1967; 46: 572–580

19 Snir M, Axer-Siegel R, Buckman G, Yassur Y. Central venous stasis retinopathy following the use of tranexamic acid. Retina 1990; 10: 181–184

20 Astedt B, Liedholm P, Wingerup L. The effects of tranexamic acid on the fibrinolytic activity of vein walls. Ann Chir Gynaecol 1987; 67: 203–205

21 Rybo G. Tranexamic acid therapy; effective treatment in heavy menstrual bleeding. Clinical update on safety. Therap Adv 1991; 4: 1–8

22 Coulter A, Kelland J, Peto V et al. Treating menorrhagia in primary care. An overview of drug trials and a survey of prescribing practice. Int J Technol Assess Health Care 1995; 11: 456–470

23 Anderson A B M, Haynes P J, Guillebaud J, Turnbull A C. Reduction in menstrual blood loss by prostaglandin synthetase inhibitors. Lancet 1976; i: 774–776

24 Cameron I T, Haining R, Lumsden M A, Reid Thomas V, Smith S K. The effects of mefenamic acid and norethisterone on measured menstrual blood loss. Obstet Gynecol 1990; 76: 85–88

25 Dockeray C J, Sheppard B L, Bonnar J. Comparison between mefenamic acid and danazol in the treatment of established menorrhagia. Br J Obstet Gynaecol 1989; 96: 840–844

26 Fraser I S, McCarron G. Randomised trial of two hormonal and two prostaglandin-inhibiting agents in women with a complaint of menorrhagia. Aust N Z J Obstet Gynaecol 1991; 31: 66–70

27 Fraser I S, McCarron G, Markham R, Robinson M, Smyth E. Long-term treatment of menorrhagia with mefenamic acid. Obstet Gynecol 1983; 61: 109–112

28 Preston J T, Cameron I T, Adams E J, Smith S K. Comparative study of tranexamic acid and norethisterone in the treatment of ovulatory menorrhagia. Br J Obstet Gynaecol 1995; 102: 401–406

29 Effective Health Care. The management of menorrhagia. Effective Health Care Bulletin 9, 1995

30 Fraser I S. Treatment of ovulatory and anovulatory dysfunctional uterine bleeding with oral progestogens. Aust N Z J Obstet Gynaecol 1990; 30: 353–356

31 Irvine G A, Campbell-Brown M B, Lumsden M A, Heikkila A, Walker J J, Cameron I T. Randomised comparative trial of the levonorgestrel intrauterine system and norethisterone for treatment of idiopathic menorrhagia. Br J Obstet Gynaecol 1998; 105: 592–598

32 Berqvist A, Rybo G. Treatment of menorrhagia with intrauterine release of progesterone. Br J Obstet Gynaecol 1983; 90: 255–258

33 Andersson J K, Odlind V, Rybo G. Levonorgestrel-releasing and copper-releasing (Nova-T) IUCDs during five years use: a randomised comparative trial. Contraception 1994; 49: 56–72

34 Andersson J K, Rybo G. Levonorgestrel-releasing intrauterine device in the treatment of menorrhagia. Br J Obstet Gynaecol 1990; 97: 690–694

35 Crosignani P G, Vercellini P, Mosconi P, Oldani S, Cortesi I, de Giorgi O. Levonorgestrel-releasing intrauterine device versus hysteroscopic endometrial resection in the treatment of dysfunctional uterine bleeding. Obstet Gynecol 1997; 90: 257–263

36 Lahteenmaki P, Haukkamaa M, Puolakka J et al. Open randomised study of use of levonorgestrel releasing intrauterine system as alternative to hysterectomy. BMJ 1998; 316: 1122–1126

37 Nilsson L, Solvell L. Clinical studies on oral contraceptives: a randomized double-blind, cross-over study of 4 different preparations. Acta Obstet Gynaecol Scand 1967; 46 (Suppl. 8): 1–31

38 Chimbira T H, Anderson A B M, Naish N, Turnbull A C. Reduction of menstrual blood loss by danazol in unexplained menorrhagia: a lack of effect of placebo. Br J Obstet Gynaecol 1980; 87: 1152–1158

39 Turnbull A C, Rees M C P. Gestrinone in the treatment of menorrhagia. Br J Obstet Gynaecol 1990; 97: 713–715

40 Fraser I S. Menorrhagia due to myometrial hypertrophy: treatment with tamoxifen. Obstet Gynecol 1987; 70: 505–506

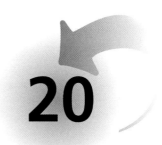

**20**

*Andreas J. Papadopoulos  Omer Devaja*
*John Cason  Kankipati S. Raju*

# The clinical implications of human papillomavirus infection in cervical carcinogenesis and emerging therapies

Cervical cancer is the second most common female malignancy world-wide. Despite advances in surgery, radiotherapy and chemotherapy treatment, overall survival for this disease has not changed in the last decade. The development of molecular biological techniques has resulted in a greater understanding of the aetiological role of human papillomavirus (HPV) infection in the oncogenesis of cervical cancer. This article aims to summarise recent developments in this field and discusses future prospects for improved diagnosis and, prevention and therapy.

## BACKGROUND

Cervical carcinoma is responsible for 466,000 deaths per year world-wide and is the leading cause of death in women aged 35–45 years.[1] During the past decade, there has been a greater understanding of the viral aetiology of this condition. Although infection by HPV alone does not appear to be sufficient for cancer development there is strong epidemiological evidence to suggest that HPV infection – most commonly types 16 and 18 – plays an important role in the development of pre-invasive lesions, cervical intra-epithelial neoplasia (CIN) and invasive cervical cancer. A recent multicentre study demonstrated

**Mr Andreas J. Papadopoulos** BSc MD MRCOG, Subspecialty Fellow, Department of Gynaecologic Oncology, Guys and St Thomas' Hospital, Lambeth Palace Road, London SE1 7EH, UK

**Dr Omer Devaja** MD MS PhD, Subspecialty Fellow, Department of Gynaecologic Oncology, Guys and St Thomas' Hospital, Lambeth Palace Road, London SE1 7EH, UK

**Dr John Cason** PhD, Senior Lecturer, The Richard Dimbleby Laboratory of Cancer Virology, UMDS Guys and St Thomas' Hospital, Lambeth Palace Road, London SE1 7EH, UK

**Miss Kankipati S. Raju** MD FRCOG, Director of Gynaecologic Oncology, Guys and St Thomas' Hospital, Lambeth Palace Road, London SE1 7EH, UK (for correspondence)

that HPV DNA was present in 93% of cancer specimens (range 75–100%)[2] and 94% of CNN lesions,[3–7] whilst in normal tissue (on cytological testing) a 43% detection rate has been observed.[2] It is the investigation of the mechanisms involved in the function of HPVs that has resulted in a greater understanding of the molecular events that contribute to the oncogenic process in cervical cancer. The influence of HPVs on cell transformation, primarily through the action of E6 and E7 oncoproteins, is well documented. As our knowledge of these viruses increases – and in particular viral oncogene function – so does the possibility of defining targets for prophylactic and therapeutic intervention.

## HUMAN PAPILLOMAVIRUSES

Papillomaviruses are widely distributed and infect both humans and animals. Although human and animal papillomaviruses share a similar genomic organisation they are species specific. Over 90 different types of HPVs have now been characterised. Although these different types are quite similar structurally, they demonstrate significant specificity with regard to the anatomical location of the epithelium they infect and the type of lesion that they produce. The majority are epitheliotropic and produce focal epithelial proliferations at the site of infection. In the female and male anogenital tract, approximately 30 different types of HPVs have been characterised and have been associated with a spectrum of anogenital diseases that range from condylomata acuminata to invasive cervical carcinoma. These associations between specific types of HPV and specific types of lesions have led to the classification of anogenital HPVs into three oncogenic-risk groups.[8] The low-risk group includes types 6, 11, 42, 43, and 44 and are commonly associated with benign lesions, condylomata acuminata, though they are occasionally found in low grade lesions (CIN 1). The intermediate oncogenic risk group is associated with high grade lesions (CIN 2 & 3) but are rarely detected in invasive anogenital cancers; this group includes types 33, 35, 39, 45, 51, 52 and 56. The high-oncogenic risk group includes types 16, 18 and 31, which are commonly detected in women with high grade lesions (CIN 2 & 3) or with invasive cancer of the cervix, vulva, penis or anus.

## GENOMIC STRUCTURE OF HUMAN PAPILLOMAVIRUSES

Papillomaviruses are DNA viruses with a double-stranded, circular DNA genome of approximately 8,000 base pairs of which only one strand codes for proteins. The viral genome is organised into three major regions: two protein-encoded regions (the early and late regions) and a non-coding up-stream regulatory region (URR).

The URR is a DNA segment of approximately 400 base-pairs, which contains binding sites for many different transcriptional repressors and activators. These include activator protein 1 (AP-1), keratinocytic-specific transcription factor 1 (KRF1), and nuclear factor (NF-I/CTF) as well as virally-derived transcriptional factors encoded by the early region. The URR regulates transcription from early and late regions and controls production of viral proteins and infectious particles.

The early region usually consists of 6 open reading frames (ORFs) E1, E2, E4, E5, E6, E7: ORFs are DNA segments that are transcriptional units and are capable of encoding for protein. Two of the early regions, E6 and E7, encode for oncoproteins E6 and E7, respectively; these are critical for viral replication as well as host cell immortalization and transformation.

The late region contains two separate ORFs named L1 and L2, which encode for viral capsid proteins. The L1 ORF encodes for the major viral capsid protein, which is highly conserved between different papillomavirus types. The L2-protein has considerably more sequence variation between HPV types than the L1 and has been used as a source for type-specific HPV antibodies.[9]

## VIRAL PROTEINS

Each early region encodes for the following corresponding proteins.

### E1 proteins

E1 ORF encodes for two separate proteins required for extrachromosomal DNA replication and completion of the viral life cycle. E1 proteins share structural similarities with the large T antigen of the Simian virus (SV40). These similarities suggest a common function for these proteins in the initiation of viral DNA replication.[10] Replication functions of the E1 gene product is derived primarily from studies of the bovine papillomavirus 1 genome (BPV-1). Analysis of E1-defective BPV-1 genomes have shown that mutations of the E1 gene result in increased levels of viral transcription and a corresponding increase in viral transformation activity.[11–13]

### E2 proteins

E2 ORF encodes for two separate proteins that together with E1, are required for extrachromosomal DNA replication. The full-length E2-encoded protein acts as a transcriptional activator that binds to specific DNA sequences in the URR to increase transcription of the early region; whereas a smaller E2-encoded protein inhibits transcription of the early region.[14] In the high risk HPVs, the smaller E2 protein can repress expression of the *E6* and *E7* genes by binding to E2-binding sites located near to the TATA box of the E6/E7 promoter. It most likely interferes with the assembly of the pre-initiation complex.[15,16]

### E4 protein

This protein appears to be important for viral maturation and replication of the virus and, like L1 and L2 capsid proteins, is expressed in later stages of infection when complete virions are assembled. In human keratinocytes, this protein induces the collapse of the cytokeratin network, suggesting that it may be involved in the release of the viral particles.[17] Collapse of the cytoplasmic cytokeratin network could also be responsible for the characteristic perinuclear clearing, or halos (koilocytosis) observed histologically in HPV infected cells.

### E5 protein

Its role in the viral life cycle is not fully understood. The E5 protein interacts with cell membrane receptors, such as those for epidermal growth factor (EGF) and, in BPVs, platelet derived growth factor (PDGF), and this may stimulate cell proliferation in HPV infected cells.[18] E5 has a weak transforming activity in several experimental systems.

### E6 protein

This is critical for viral replication as well as host cell immortalization. It appears to alter cell growth through its effect on the p53 protein which is an endogenous, cell-derived tumour-suppressor protein.

### E7 protein

This protein has high oncogenic activity and, by itself, can immortalise primary human keratinocytes, and in co-operation with the ras oncoprotein can transform primary rat cells in vitro.[19] Immortalisation of the keratinocytes by E7 protein is achieved through its interaction with the retinoblastoma protein (Rb).

## VIRAL ONCOPROTEINS AND CELL GROWTH

The primary site for HPV infection is the stratified squamous epithelia with viral capsid assembly occurring in the suprabasal cells undergoing terminal differentiation.[20] There is no viraemic phase during HPV infection. These factors appear to protect the HPV from the immune response. Early proteins are expressed throughout the epithelium, whilst the late proteins are only expressed in the upper layers. Whilst the episomal HPV DNA in benign lesions permits the expression of all viral genes, in cervical cancer just the E6 and E7 oncogenes are expressed. The reason for this difference is that in the latter case the viral DNA is linearised and integrated into the host DNA in such a way that just E6 and E7 ORFs are downstream of the viral promotor.

E6 and E7 proteins exert their action by forming complexes with cell proteins involved in cell cycle regulation, hence altering their normal function. The best understood of these viral/host protein interactions are those of E6 with p53[21] and E7 with pRb[22] (Fig. 1). The viral proteins affect the maintenance of normal cell growth by influencing the vital role played by p53 and pRb in controlling cell cycle progression. Both p53 and pRb act as negative regulators, or checkpoints, to prevent abnormal cell division. Loss of these regulatory pathways probably contributes to the development of many cancers.

### Interaction of E6 with p53

Although E6 proteins encoded by all genital HPV types can form a complex with p53,[23] only E6 proteins of the high risk HPV types have high affinity for p53 protein which results in its degradation. These E6 proteins form a complex with a cellular protein termed E6 associated protein (E6-AP), and the E6/E6-

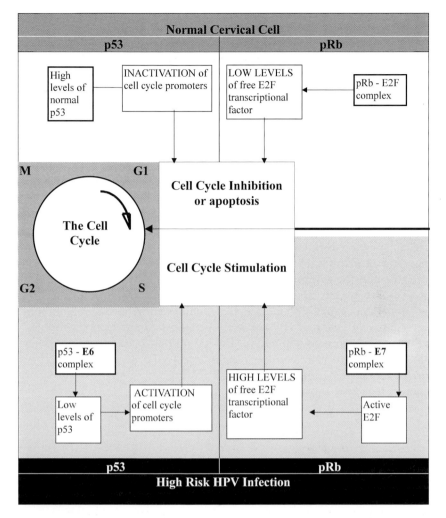

**Fig. 1** HPV infection and its effects on G1/S phase of the cell cycle. The effect of binding E6 and E7 to p53 and pRb, respectively. Top: a non-HPV infected cell and normal growth arrest. Below: the effect of HPV infection on controllers of the cell cycle.

AP complex causes degradation of p53 through an ubiquitin-dependant proteolytic pathway. Cells expressing high risk HPV E6 are, therefore, deprived of p53 tumour suppressor activities. This is supported indirectly by the observation that cervical cancers, unlike most other major epithelial malignancies, hardly ever show evidence of somatic p53 mutation.[24] It is only through an understanding of normal p53 function that the effect of the E6/p53 interaction can be fully appreciated. The p53 gene appears to play a major role in the cellular response to DNA damage, during which the *p53* gene is activated and p53 protein is overexpressed. Accumulation of wild-type p53 induces cell growth arrest in G1 phase of the cell cycle.[25,26] This temporary cessation of cell cycle progression allows DNA repair, or a more permanent solution is initiated namely programmed cell death by apoptosis.[27] The role of p53 is, therefore, thought to be in preventing the replication of damaged

DNA[28] and loss of this function is associated with the accumulation of genetic instability and potentially oncogenic mutations.[29] Recently, it has been reported that E6 can inhibit the action of p53 in an ubiquitin-independent manner.[30] Low risk E6 also alters p53 DNA binding and shows some ability to inhibit transcription, although activity in preventing the G1 arrest is not evident in studies carried out so far.[31] This interaction of E6 and p53 and role of p53 in cell cycle is summarised in Figure 1.

### Interaction of E7 with pRb

Several cell proteins have been shown to form complexes with E7, but interaction with pRb is one of the best understood. Like p53, pRb is a tumour suppressor protein whose function appears to be related to its ability to make complexes and control the activity of other cell proteins such as E2F, which functions as a transcription factor.[32] Control of transcription is a key mechanism by which progress through the cell cycle is regulated.[33] E2F appears to be involved in controlling the expression of several genes important for entry into the cell cycle and progression from G1 to S phase. Since the association between E2F and pRb prevents transcriptional activation of E2F, the interaction enables pRb to participate in the control of cell proliferation by preventing expression of E2F regulated genes. The transcription products of these genes are proteins required for DNA synthesis such as thymidine kinase, dihydrofolate reductase, DNA polymerase $\alpha$ as well as *c-myc* and *N-myc* proto-oncogenes. Binding of the E2F with pRb is precisely regulated through the action of the cyclin-dependent kinases at specific stages of the cell cycle.[26,34] E7 protein alters this precisely regulated cellular growth mechanism by binding to pRb. This causes the release of transcriptionally active E2F, which allows DNA replication (Fig. 1).

## FUTURE PROSPECTS

Advances in the field of molecular biology have led to new prospects in the diagnosis and treatment of precancerous and cancerous lesions of the cervix. HPV infection has a prevalence of 20–40% in sexually active women under 30 years of age;[35] however, the majority are self-limiting and do not result in smear abnormalities.

### Primary and secondary screening with HPV detection

Screening for cervical cancer and CIN pathology has generally revolved around cytology and the Papanicolaou smear. It has been shown that cervical cancer incidence rates fall in a screened population and this is directly in proportion to the number being screened and the length of the screening interval.[36] In addition, it is well recognised that there has been a drop in mortality from cervical cancer in those countries with a well organised and comprehensive screening programme. But screening programmes with cytology is not without pitfalls. Cytology has a relatively high false negative rate ranging from 16–36%, and the cost of screening programmes is relatively high; thus, there has been a need for another test which will augment results of cytology and reduce the cost.

Primary and secondary screening with combination of cytology and semiquantitative PCR for HPV detection of high risk types has been tested.[37–39] The initial problems with HPV testing related to poor analytic sensitivity and positive predictive values. However, recently the hybrid capture technique has demonstrated a high correlation between HPV detection and clinical disease with high clinical sensitivity.[40] This test can also measure the quantity of viral DNA in the sample. In addition, other investigators have demonstrated a relationship between the high risk HPV types, viral load and high grade CIN using this test.[39] In a recent study, HPV testing for 16, 18, 31, and 33 demonstrated that 44% of CIN 2 and CIN 3 lesions had negative cytology and were detected only by HPV testing.[41] In the older age group, Pap smears together with HPV DNA screening can detect more than 95% of patients with high grade lesions.[42–44] In another study, the risk of CIN 2/3 developing in Pap smear negative, but HPV-DNA positive, women during the 2 year period following screening was increased substantially compared to the HPV-DNA negative group (28% versus 3%).[38] In this study, the relative risk varied depending on the type(s) of HPV detected: multiple types including 16 and 18 – 49%; HPV 16/18 – 39%; and HPV 6/11 – 26%.

Initial results suggest that the incorporation of HPV testing into a screening programme could lead to an improvement in the positive predictive value of cytology. It is unlikely that it would replace cytology, as any advantage over smear cytology would depend on the fraction of true-HPV negative pre-cancers and treatable cancers detected by the Pap smear. However, there are indirect benefits to HPV testing including increased compliance and hence coverage through the development of self-tests.[45] In addition by changing screening strategy of current screening programmes through automation and quality control, the cost could be reduced.

## Non-antigen-specific therapies

Topical application of interferon-$\alpha$ and/or interferon-$\beta$ have been used with varying degrees of success,[46,47] but after initial enthusiasm there has been no major interest in this type of treatment. On the other hand, antisense HPV-16 E7 DNA oligonucleotides and inducible antisense HPV-18 E7 or E6 messenger RNA (mRNA) have been used to inhibit growth of cervical cancer cell lines in vitro[48] and in vivo.[49] Gene therapy offers some other possibilities but, at the moment, development of the vaccines seems to attract most of the attention.

## Vaccines in the treatment and prevention of cervical cancer

There is a clinical need for additional therapies in the management of cervical cancer as the efficacy of treatment with conventional therapy (surgery, radiotherapy and chemotherapy) has not altered significantly over the last decade. HPV is an established aetiological agent in cervical neoplasia, present in 95% of CIN 2 and CIN 3 lesions and invasive squamous cervical carcinoma, with type 16 being present in more than 50% of cases.[2] In addition, the importance of the immune response against HPV has been illustrated by the increased incidence of CIN in women with impaired immunocompetence (HIV, Hodgkin lymphoma, SLE, and organ transplantation). This has led to the concept of immunotherapy in the form of vaccines. Most of the work on vaccine development has been performed on experimental animals and only in recent years have phase I and II studies been conducted in humans. Currently, there are two types of vaccine strategies: prophylactic and therapeutic vaccines.

### Prophylactic vaccines

At present, it is thought that prophylactic vaccines would need to induce secreted, neutralising antibodies against the HPV capsid proteins L1, L2 or against cell surface binding receptor; and hence prevent viral entrance into the human keratinocytes.[50]

Capsid proteins of HPV (L1 and L2) co-assemble into virus-like particles (VLPs) when expressed at high levels in eukaryotic cells.[51] These VLPs appear to be morphologically identical to the intact virion except that they do not contain viral DNA,[52] and hence lack tumourigenic potential. Such VPLs have the ability to generate type-specific immune responses in animal models.[53,54]

Prophylactic vaccination should attempt to overcome the limitations of immunogenicity seen in natural infections by seeking to establish a secretory IgA mediated immunological barrier at the port of entry. It would also need to be multivalent; that is protect against different types of HPV, as 80% of HPV-induced cervical cancers contain HPV-16, 18, 31 or 45.[2] The requirements for such a prophylactic vaccine to prevent primary HPV-16 or other high risk types are that it should: (i) induce a high concentration of high-affinity neutralising antibodies to HPV capsid proteins in genital tract secretions; (ii) confer long-lasting immunity; (iii) be inexpensive and thermostable; (iv) be contained within a live vector so as to confer 'herd immunity' by spread of the vector via natural infection from vaccinated to non-vaccinated individuals; and (v) be administered at such a time that it is likely to have maximum efficacy.

### Therapeutic vaccines

A strategy for prevention of infection has its limitations, since even the most efficacious neutralising antibody response is unlikely to result in full immunity. Once inside the epithelial cell, HPV virions are likely to be safe from antibody interference. A vaccine should, therefore, stimulate cytotoxic T lymphocytes (CTL) directed against cytotoxic epitopes derived from intracellularly processed viral proteins. These proteins should be presented in the context of MHC class I alleles expressed by the host. The most attractive targets for immunotherapy are the oncoproteins E6 and E7, as these are the only HPV proteins expressed in cervical cancers. Animal studies have confirmed the feasibility of these approaches; both antibodies and tumour growth-inhibiting CTLs have been generated by vaccination against papillomaviruses. The E6 and/or E7 genes can be incorporated into target cells by transfection of naked DNA or infection with recombinant viral vectors. However, there are conceptual difficulties – these are oncogenes and the possibility of iatrogenic tumourigenesis cannot be ignored. A solution may be the use of mutant or altered forms of E6 or E7; however, this may impair the immune response. Viral vectors may well be the most efficient method of gene transfer but themselves may cause problems especially in the

**Table 1** Vaccine trials being undertaken investigating the feasibility of generating a HPV-specific immune response. (Patient numbers shown with initial study recruitment in italics and possible final numbers in normal text depending on study response.)

| Country of origin | Trial phase | HPV source | Patient nos *initial*/final | Disease type |
|---|---|---|---|---|
| Australia | I/II | Adjuvanted E7 protein | | Cervical cancer immuno-therapy |
| Australia (Tindle et al 1996)[61] | I | | 5 | Advanced disease |
| Europe (EORTC) | Multicentre II | r.vac/HPV | *18*/44 | Adjuvant to surgery and RRx I/IIA |
| Europe (The Netherlands) | I/II | Peptide based | 15 | Advanced disease |
| UK (Wales) | I/II | r.vac/HPV | 10 | CIN 3 |
| UK (Wales; Borysiewicz et al 1996)[58] | I | | 8 | Advanced disease |
| UK (Wales)/USA (NCI) | I/II | r. Vac/HPV | *14*/33 | Advanced/recurrent |
| USA (Norris Cancer Center) | I | Peptide | *20*/60 | CIN 2/3 (45), VIN (15) |
| USA (NCI) | I | Peptide – epitope | 15 | Recurrent/refractory disease |
| USA (NCI) | I/II | E6 & E7 peptides | 12 | Stage IV/recurrent III + residual after RRx III – residual after RRx |

EORTC, European Organisation for Research and Treatment of Cancer; NCI, National Cancer Institute; RRx, radiotherapy; r.vac/HPV, recombinant vaccinia/HPV; VIN, vulval intra-epithelial neoplasia.

immunocompromised patient. Alternatively E6 or E7 peptide epitopes may be utilised instead. Certain MHC class I restricted CTL epitope peptides, together with non-specific adjuvants, have demonstrated specific immunogenicity.[55,56] The entire E6 or E7 viral protein could be used to stimulate the immune response. Generally, soluble proteins result in a humoral response; however, newer adjuvants that specifically induce cell-mediated immune responses are being developed. Table 1 lists recent clinical trials in vaccine research.[57]

The first human trial of an HPV vaccine was reported from Cardiff (UK),[58] in June 1996. This illustrated that specific antibody and CTL responses could be induced by vaccinating with a recombinant vaccinia virus expressing the E6 and E7 proteins of HPV 16 and 18. However, vaccination results in the generation of CTLs against virally infected cervical cells may prove to be inappropriate since many tumours are down-regulated for the expression of MHC class I molecules.[59,60] CTLs only recognise peptide antigen presented on the cell surface in association with these molecules; therefore, their loss may contribute to immune evasion by the tumour.

An alternative treatment strategy involves immunotherapy using in vitro stimulation of CTLs from a patient with an HPV-expressed tumour with immunogenetic peptides of HPV. These stimulated CTLs are then expanded in vitro and subsequently transfused back into the same patient. This approach is less attractive due to high cost and complexity.

Nevertheless, immune intervention by vaccination in cervical cancer and intra-epithelial neoplasia remains an attractive prospect, and there are several on-going studies of HPV vaccines in Europe, US and Australia using different strategies. It is anticipated that, ultimately, prophylaxis for HPV infection will be achieved and therapeutic vaccination shown to be of use in preventing, delaying or eradicating recurrent disease in cervical cancer.

## CONCLUSIONS

Over the last decade, tremendous advances have been made in our understanding of the molecular biology of cervical cancer. We recognise that HPV is the primary aetiological agent for cervical carcinogenesis. We are also beginning to understand how interactions between cellular growth, regulatory proteins, and virally derived oncoproteins result in uncontrolled cell proliferation. Moreover, the identification and characterisation of specific genetic alterations in cervical cancers has begun. The rapid advances in molecular biology techniques will lead to a greater understanding of the molecular pathogenesis of cervical lesions and the possible implementation of these techniques in clinical practice. Results of new strategies using HPV vaccines are eagerly awaited and the next decade will probably witness this development.

### References

1  Sherris J D, Wells E S, Tsu V D, Bishop A. Cervical Cancer in Developing  Countries: A Situation Analysis. Working paper. Washington DC: The World Bank, 1993
2  Bosch F X, Manos M M, Munoz N et al (1995). Prevalence of human papilloma virus in cervical cancer: a worldwide perspective. International biological study on cervical cancer (IBSCC) Study group. J Natl Cancer Inst 1995; 87: 796–802
3  Morrison E A, Ho G Y, Vermund S H et al. Human papillomavirus infection and other risk factors for cervical neoplasia: a case-control study [see comment citations in Medline]. Int J Cancer 1991; 49: 6–13.1*
4  Becker T M, Wheeler C M, McGough N S et al. Contraceptive and reproductive risks for cervical dysplasia in southwestern Hispanic and non-Hispanic white women. Int J Epidemiol 1994; 23: 913–922
5  Munoz N, Bosch F X, de Sanjose S et al. Risk factors for cervical intraepithelial neoplasia grade III/carcinoma in situ in Spain and Colombia. Cancer Epidemiol Biomarkers Prev 1993; 2: 423–431
6  Olsen A O, Gjoen K, Sauer T et al. Human papillomavirus infection and cervical intraepithelial neoplasia grade II/III: a population-based case control study. Int J Cancer 1995; 61: 312–315
7  Schiffman M H, Bauer H M, Hoover R N et al. Epidemiologic evidence showing that human papillomavirus infection causes most cervical intraepithelial neoplasia. J Natl

Cancer Inst 1993; 85: 958–964

8   Lorincz A T, Reid R, Jenson A B, Greenberg M D, Lancaster W, Kurman R J. Human papillomavirus infection of the cervix: relative risk associations of 15 common anogenital types. Obstet Gynaecol 1992; 79: 328–337

9   Turek L P. The structure, function and regulation of papilloma viral genes in infection and cervical cancer. Adv Viral Res 1994; 44: 305–356

10  Seo Y S, Muller F, Lusky M et al. Bovine papilloma virus (BPV)-encoded E1 protein contains multiple activities required for BPV DNA replication. Proc Natl Acad Sci USA 1993; 90: 702–706

11  Lambert P F, Howely P M. Bovine papillomavirus type 1 E1 replication-defective mutants are altered in their transcriptional regulation. J Virol 1988; 62: 4009–4015

12  Schiller J T, Androphy E J, Lowy D R, Pfistner H. Identification of bovine papillomavirus E1 mutants with increased transforming and transcriptional activity. J Virol 1989; 63: 1775–1782

13  Sandler A B, Van de Pol S B, Spalholz B A. Repression of bovine papillomavirus type 1 transcription by the E1 replication protein. J Virol 1993; 67: 5079–5087

14  Ward P, Coleman D V, Malcom D B. Regulatory mechanisms of the papillomaviruses. Trends Genet 1989; 5: 97–98

15  Thierry F, Yaniv M. The BPV1-E2 trans-acting protein can be either an activator or a repressor of the HPV18 regulatory region. EMBO J 1987; 6: 3391–3397

16  Ramanczuk H, Howley P M. Disruption of either the E1 or the E2 regulatory gene of human papillomavirus type 16 increases viral immortalization capacity. Proc Natl Acad Sci USA 1992; 89: 3159–3163

17  Doorbar J, Ely S, Sterling J, McLean C, Crawford L. Specific interaction between HPV16 E1-E4 and cytokeratins results in collapse of the epithelial cell intermediate filament network. Nature 1991; 352: 824–827

18  Conrad M, Goldstein D, Andresson T, Schleger R. The E5 protein of HPV-6, but not HPV-16, associates efficiently with cellular growth factor receptors. Virology 1994; 200: 796–800

19  Bedell M A, Jones K H, Laminis L A. The E6-E7 region of human papillomavirus type 18 is sufficient for transformation of NIH 3T3 and rat-1 cells. J Virol 1987; 61: 3635–3640

20  Taichman L B, LaPorta R F(1987). The expression of papillomaviruses in human epithelial cells. In: Salzman N P, Howley P M. (eds) The Papavaviridae, vol 2. The Papillomaviruses. New York: Plenum, 1987; 109–139

21  Werness B A, Levine A J, Howely P M. Association of human papillomavirus types 16 and 18 E6 proteins with p53. Science 1990; 248: 76–79

22  Dyson N, Howely P M, Munger K, Harlow E. The human papillomavirus-16 E7 oncoprotein is able to bind to the retinoblastoma gene product. Science 1989; 243: 934–937

23  Crook T, Tidy J A, Vousden K H. Degradation of p53 can be targeted by HPV E6 sequences distinct from those required for p53 binding and transactivation. Cell 1991; 67: 547–556

24  Crook T, Wrede D, Tidy J A et al. Clonal p53 mutation in primary cervical cancer: association with human papillomavirus negative tumours. Lancet 1992; 339: 1070–1073

25  Lane D P. p53 and human cancers. BMJ 1994; 50: 582–599

26  Hartwell L, Katsan M B. Cell cycle control and cancer. Science 1994; 266: 1821–1828

27  Yonish-Rouach E, Resnitzky J, Lotem L. Wild-type p53 induces apoptosis of myeloid leukaemic cells that is inhibited by interleukin-6. Nature 1991; 352: 345–347

28  Lane D P. p53 guardian of the genome. Nature 1992; 358: 15–16

29  Livingstone L R, White A, Sprouse J et al. Altered cell cycle arrest and gene amplification potential accompany loss of wild type p53. Cell 1992; 70: 923–935

30  Molinari M, Milner J. p53 in complex with DNA is resistant to ubiquitin-dependent proteolysis in the presence of HPV-16 E6. Oncogene 1995; 10: 1849–1854

31  Foster S A, Demers G W, Etscheid B G, Galloway D A. The ability of human papillomaviruses E6 proteins to target p53 for degradation in vivo correlates with their ability to abrogate actinomycin D-induced growth arrest. J Virol 1994; 68: 5698–5705

32  Hamel P A, Gallie B L, Phillips R A. The retinoblastoma protein and cell cycle regulation. Trends Genet 1992; 8: 180–185

33  McKinney J D, Heintz N. Transcriptional regulation in the eukaryotic cell cycle. Trends Biochem Sci 1991; 16: 430–431

34 Nevins J R. Cell cycle targets of the DNA tumor viruses. Curr Opin Genet Dev 1994; 4: 130–134

35 Schiffman M H. Recent progress in defining the epidemiology of human papillomavirus infection and cervical neoplasia. J Natl Cancer Inst 1992; 84: 271–281

36 Laara E, Day N E, Hakama M. Trends in mortality from cervical cancer in the Nordic countries: association with organised screening programmes. Lancet 1987; ii: 1247–1249

37 Reid R, Greeneberg M D, Lorinz A et al. Should cervical cytologic testing be augmented by cervicography or human papillomavirus deoxyribonucleic acid detection. Am J Obstet Gynaecol 1991; 164: 1461–1471

38 Koutsky L A, Holmes K K, Critchlow C W et al. A cohort study of the risk of cervical intraepithelial neoplasia grade 2 or 3 in relation to papillomavirus infection. N Engl J Med 1992; 327: 1272–1278

39 Cox J T, Schiffman M H, Winzelberg A J, Patterson J M. An evaluation of human papillomavirus testing as a part of referral to colposcopy clinics. Obstet Gynecol 1992; 80: 389–395

40 Sun X W, Ferenczy A, Johnson D et al. Evaluation of the hybrid capture human papillomavirus deoxyribonucleic acid detection test [see comments]. Am J Obstet Gynecol 1995; 173: 1432–1437

41 Cuzick J, Szarewski A, Terry G et al. Human papillomavirus testing in primary cervical screening. Lancet 1995; 345: 1533–1536

42 Walboomers J M M, de Roda Husman A H, Van den Brule A J C, Snijders P J F, Meijer C J L M. Detection of genital human papillomavirus infections: critical review of methods and prevalence studies in relation to cervical cancer. In: Stern P L, Stanly M A (eds) Human Papillomavirus and Cervical Cancer. Oxford: Oxford University Press, 1994; 41–71

43 Meijer C J L M, Snijders P J F, Van den Brule A J C, Helmerhorst T H, Remmink A J, Walboomers J M M. Can cytological screening be improved by HPV screening? In: Monsenego J. (ed) Papillomavirus in Human Pathology. Paris: Ares-Serono Symposia Publications, 1995; 493–498

44 Walboomers J M M, Van den Brule A J C, Snijders P J F, Meijer C J L M. Analysis of genital HPV infections: clinical relevance. In: Van Krough G. (ed) HPV in Dermato-venerology. Boca Raton: CRC Press, 1995.

45 Given F T, Jones H W. Self administered cervical cancer screening. Clin Obstet Gynecol 1992; 35: 3–12

46 Einhorn N, Ling P, Strander H. Systemic interferon-alpha treatment of human codylomata acuminata. Acta Obstet Gynecol Scand 1983; 62: 245–287

47 Schonfeld A, Nitke S, Schattner A et al. Intramuscular human interferon-beta injections in treatment of condylomata acuminata. Lancet 1984; 1: 1038–1042

48 Storey A, Oates D, Banks I, Crawford I, Crook T. Anti-sense phosphorothioate oligonucleotides have both specific and non-specific effects on cells containing human papillomavirus type 16. Nucleic acids Research 1991; 19: 4109–4114

49 Hu G, Liu W, Hanania E G, Fu S, Wang T, Deisseroth A B. Suppression of tumorigenesis by transcription units expressing the antisense E6 and E7 messenger RNA (mRNA) for the transforming proteins of the human papillomavirus and the sense mRNA for the retinoblastoma gene in cervical carcinoma cells. Cancer gene therapy 1995; 2: 19–32

50 Christensen N D, Cladel N M, Reed C A (1995). Post-attachment neutralisation of papillomaviruses by monoclonal and polyclonal antibodies. Virology 1995; 201: 136–142

51 Kirnbauer R, Booy F, Cheng N, Lowy D R, Schiller J T. Papillomavirus L1 major capsid protein self-assembles into virus-like particles that are highly immunogenic. Proc Natl Acad Sci USA 1992; 89: 1280–1284

52 Kirnbauer R, Taub J, Greenstone H et al. Efficient self-assembly of human papillomavirus type 16 L1 and L1–L2 into virus-like particles. J Virol 1993; 67: 6929–6936

53 Breitburd F, Kirnbauer R, Hubbert N L et al. Immunization with virus-like particles from cottontail rabbit papillomavirus (CRPV) can protect against experimental CRPV infection. J Virol 1995; 69: 3959–3963

54 Suzich J A, Ghim S J, Palmer-Hill F J et al. Systemic immunization with human papillomavirus L1 protein completely prevents development of viral mucosal papillomas. Proc Natl Acad Sci USA 1995; 92: 11553–11557

55 Ressing M E, Sette A, Brandt R M et al. Human CTL epitopes encoded by human papilloma virus type 16 E6 and E7 identified through in vivo and in vitro

immunogenicity studies of HLA-A *0201-binding peptides. J Immunol 1995; 154: 5934–5943

56 Alexander M, Salgaller M, Celis E et al. Generation of tumour-specific T-lymphocytes from peripheral blood of cervical cancer patients by in-vitro stimulation with a synthetic HPV-16, E7 epitope. Am J Obstet Gynecol 1996; 175: 1586–1593

57 McNeil C. HPV vaccine treatment trials proliferate, diversify. J Natl Cancer Inst 1997; 89: 280–281

58 Borysiewicz L K, Fiander A, Nimako M et al. A recombinant vaccinia virus encoding human papillomavirus types 16 and 18, E6 and E7 proteins as immunotherapy for cervical cancer. Lancet 1996; 347: 1523–1526

59 Hiders C G, Houbiers J G, Krul E J, Fleuren G J. The expression of histocompatibility-related leukocyte antigens in the pathway to cervical carcinoma. Am J Clin Pathol 1994; 101: 5–12

60 Keating P J, Cromme F V, Duggan-Keen M et al. Frequency of down-regulation of individual HLA-A and -B alleles in cervical carcinomas in relation to TAP-1 expression. Br J Cancer 1995; 72: 405–411

61 Tindle R W. Human papillomavirus vaccines for cervical cancer. Curr Opinion Immunol 1996; 8: 643–650

Q. Davies  D. M. Luesley

# The future of surgery in gynaecological oncology

Whilst not blessed by clairvoyance, it is not difficult to predict the direction in which surgery will develop. One must accept, however, that prediction is fraught with the potential for error and given the rapid pace of change of technology that we have already witnessed this error could be substantial.

Despite this, what we have tried to do in this chapter is look into the next 10 years utilizing our current concepts of care and applying these concepts in concert with technology that is developing in parallel. Convention dictates that we should adopt a traditional 'tumour based' approach but we freely draw on the observations and applications that have occurred elsewhere in oncology.

## VULVAR CANCER

This tumour demonstrates more than any other in gynaecological oncology how changing thought processes have influenced care – from the blanket approach of radical vulvectomy to a spectrum of surgical and multimodality approaches has occurred over the last 10–15 years. There does not appear to have been any adverse effect on the outcome in terms of survival, yet the morbidity has been reduced. This has occurred without recourse to a series of randomised controlled trials, largely as a result of the rarity of the tumour but it does, to a certain extent demonstrate what can be achieved through basic clinical observational research.

### Radical vulvectomy

Radical vulvectomy with en bloc dissection of the inguino-femoral nodes as described by Taussig and Way in the 1940s improved 5-year survival from

**Dr Q. Davies** MRCOG, FRCS, Subspecialty Trainee, Department of Obstetrics and Gynaecology, City Hospital NHS Trust, Dudley Road, Birmingham B18 7QH, UK

**Prof. D. M. Luesley** MA MD FRCOG, Professor of Gynaecological Oncology, Department of Obstetrics and Gynaecology, City Hospital NHS Trust, Dudley Road, Birmingham B18 7QH, UK

20–25% to 60–70% and was established as the principal mode of treatment of vulvar cancer. However, this surgery has high morbidity with wound breakdown in up to 85% of patients.[1] As a result of this high morbidity, since the 1970s the trend has been towards more individualised treatment of vulvar cancer.

The triple incision technique was originally described in 1965 by Byron et al[2] but did not gain in popularity until Hacker et al[3] described 98 patients treated by the triple incision technique. Only 14% of patients had major wound breakdown and survival was comparable with radical vulvectomy.

Radical vulvectomy causes severe disfigurement and subsequent sexual dysfunction. The stimulus to less radical treatment of the primary lesion was the management of young women with microinvasive disease. In 1979, DiSaia et al[4] reported the complete preservation of sexual function in 17 of 18 patients who underwent wide local excision for small tumours which were no greater than 1 cm in diameter and less than 5 mm invasion. These patients also underwent bilateral inguinal node dissections.

The literature refers to a variety of different procedures as radical wide excision, with adequate excision margins varying from 1 cm to 3 cm. The types of excision include, hemivulvectomy for lateral lesions and anterior or posterior vulvectomy for lesions placed anteriorly or posteriorly. Risk of local recurrence is the main concern about using wide local excision . Ross and Ehrmann[5] reported multifocal disease in 20–28% of squamous cell carcinomas of the vulva. However, the microscopic metastases usually occurred in the close vicinity of the macroscopic tumour indicating the importance of an adequate excision margin. In a review of the literature on patients with stage 1 vulvar cancer, Hacker et al[6] demonstrated a local recurrence rate of 7% for 165 patients treated with radical local excision compared with 6% for 365 patients treated by radical vulvectomy. It is now generally accepted that a triple incision and less radical vulvar surgery are acceptable methods of treatment that have modified the management of vulvar cancer and reduced the morbidity with no apparent effect upon recurrence rates.

## The role of lymph node dissection in vulvar cancer

Current management of squamous carcinoma of the vulva includes radical inguino-femoral lymphadenectomy. Additional pelvic lymphadenectomy has, in general, been abandoned. Inguino-femoral lymph node status is definitely an important prognostic indicator and aids the planning of adjuvant radiotherapy. A 1986 report by the Gynecological Oncology Group demonstrated that, in patients with positive inguino-femoral nodes, adjuvant groin and pelvic radiotherapy improved survival compared with patients undergoing pelvic lymphadenectomy.[7] It has also been demonstrated that radiotherapy alone is not adequate treatment for the inguino-femoral region. A Gynecology Oncology Group study in which radiotherapy was substituted for bilateral inguinal lymphadenectomy was abandoned because of the high rate of recurrence in the irradiated patients.[8] This information strongly supports the use of inguino-femoral lymphadenectomy as part of treatment of patients with positive inguinal or femoral nodes. However, only 10–15 % of stage I–II vulvar cancers have positive nodes and require surgery and adjuvant radiotherapy, and bilateral inguinal lympadenectomy has a significant morbidity with a high risk of wound breakdown and chronic leg oedema.

In order to reduce the morbidity associated with treatment, the recent trend has been towards less radical inguinal node surgery. It is generally accepted that patients with small tumours (< 2 cm) that are laterally placed may be treated by unilateral lymphadenectomy because the risk of contralateral node involvement is 0.4%.[9] A more limited resection of the superficial inguinal lymph nodes has been proposed by DiSaia et al.[10] In 1979, they described removal of inguinal nodes superficial to the cribriform fascia associated with the long saphenous and superficial epigastric veins. These were then sent for frozen section and, if positive, a complete bilateral inguino-femoral lymphadenectomy was performed and this was shown to reduce the morbidity. However, when Stehman et al[11] used superficial inguinal lymphadenectomy in patients with early carcinoma of the vulva, 7.3% experienced recurrences compared with none in the control group. The validity of this study has been questioned because there were a number of midline lesions and there were twice as many poorly differentiated tumours in the group undergoing superficial lymphadenectomy. It is, therefore, not yet possible to conclude what role superficial lymphadenectomy has in these patients.

The principle of less radical lymphadenectomy is that the superficial inguinal nodes act as a sentinel group, that skip lesions to the deep nodes are rare and that the results are used as a prognostic indicator to guide further treatment, i.e. radical surgery and possible radiotherapy in patients who are node positive. This will reduce surgical morbidity in the patients who are node negative and currently undergo inguino-femoral lymphadenectomy. This idea has been taken further by attempts to identify 'sentinel' nodes pre-operatively. There are a number of techniques that have been proposed for this purpose. A dye, isosulphan blue, which is selectively taken up into the lymphatics may be injected into the leading edge of the tumour prior to groin incisions. The sentinel node is then identified by the bright blue colour of the dye and can be examined histologically prior to proceeding to radical dissection. Pilot studies of lymphoscintigraphy using injection of technetium-99 labelled colloid and an intra-operative gamma camera to identify sentinel nodes have been promising[12]. This is a technique that is already in widespread use in the management of breast cancer.[13] However, larger studies are necessary in order to prove the reliability of identifying a sentinel node in the management of carcinoma of the vulva. One other method that has been proposed is ultrasound scanning and fine needle cytology of suspicious nodes. This technique is operator dependent and also requires further evaluation with larger studies. These methods do have the great advantage that they can be evaluated in patients undergoing inguino-femoral lymphadenectomy without jeopardising the current management of the patients.

## The role of other treatment modalities

The treatment of vulvar cancer has been almost exclusively surgical. Radiotherapy has not been favoured as a primary treatment because of the poor tolerance of vulvar skin. More recent studies using high energy radiotherapy and modern techniques have been more encouraging. Boronow

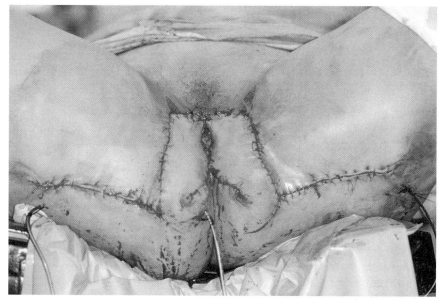

**Fig. 1** Appearance of the vulva after excision of a large tumour and reconstruction with rotational flaps.

has shown that radiotherapy in the treatment of locally advanced vulvar cancer can enable more limited and potentially sphincter preserving surgery to be performed.[14] Combined chemotherapy and radiotherapy has been increasingly used in a variety of squamous cancers. In particular, carcinoma of the anus and head and neck, but more recently it has been shown to be beneficial in cervical cancer. Chemoradiotherapy may have an important role in sphincter preserving surgery in advanced carcinoma of the vulva.[15]

### Reconstructive surgery in vulvar cancer

There is likely to be increased demand for vulvar reconstruction in the future as a result of public pressure in order to reduce surgical morbidity and as a result of increased emphasis on cosmesis. Rhomboid flaps, rotational skin flaps (Fig. 1) and V–Y flaps are relatively simple surgical procedures that can usually be performed by an appropriately trained gynaecological oncologist and have an important role in perineal reconstruction.[16,17] These techniques are particularly important if there is peri-anal involvement with vulvar cancer, and their use may result in less wound dehiscence, less vaginal stenosis, less sexual dysfunction and less urinary problems.[18] If larger defects require closure rectus abdominus or gracilis musculocutaneous flaps may be employed,[19,20] and these will require the involvement of plastic surgeons.

### The future in vulvar cancer

We must see the role of surgery for vulvar cancer within a multidisciplinary context. We should start to move away from the idea that surgery is, by necessity, the first choice and radiotherapy with or without chemotherapy be employed if surgery cannot. This mechanistic approach is often at odds with disease biology. Recent work in vulvar cancer has demonstrated the feasibility and advantages of a planned combined approach. These new treatment combinations and non radical approaches require systematic and prospective evaluation before they are introduced into widespread practice. The progressive centralisation of oncology facilities provides an ideal structure and opportunity for the first time to implement controlled trials and protocols in this rare disease.

## CERVICAL CANCER

One must accept that, despite our best efforts at prevention, there will still be cases of invasive cancer of the cervix to manage. In developed societies, the number will be less, perhaps falling to a level similar to that of vulvar cancer and, thus, hopefully benefiting from the centralisation of cancer care. What is necessary now is to move away from our ideas of a 'Wertheims' type procedure or radiotherapy and apply the knowledge that we have gained from other cancers, vulva, head and neck and breast cancer in particular. For early cervical cancers (1a to 1bI) our current therapies are largely effective with 5-year survival rate of 97–100%; thus, any advancement must be in terms of reduction of morbidity. Although the death rate from cervical cancer is falling, there has been an increase in the incidence of cervical cancer in young women between 25–34 years who are more likely to want to retain their fertility.

### Treatment choices in early cervical cancer

There is general acceptance in the UK that conisation of the cervix is adequate treatment for stage 1aI cervical cancer[21] and that simple hysterectomy is adequate treatment for stage 1aII.[22,23] Most clinicians would also accept that, if the cancer has been adequately excised by conisation in a young patient with stage 1aII cervical carcinoma, a hysterectomy is not mandatory for squamous lesions if the patient wishes to retain her fertility, but careful follow-up is necessary. The role of conservative management in the treatment of early adenocarcinomas of the cervix is more controversial because of the difficulties in defining microinvasion, its potential for skip lesions and the absence of a reliable method of follow-up.

For stage 1b carcinoma of the cervix, the standard treatment is either radical hysterectomy (Wertheims type) and pelvic lymphadenectomy or pelvic radiotherapy. Both of these treatments produce good survival results but both render the patient sterile and are often associated with significant morbidity. The choice between the two forms of treatment is usually dependent upon their side effect profile. Potential side effects of surgery include, haemorrhage, urinary tract fistulae, bladder dysfunction, lymphocysts and febrile morbidity. Radiotherapy may cause ovarian failure, vaginal shortening, urinary, rectosigmoid and small bowel complications. In general, younger fit patients tend to undergo operative treatment more commonly whereas older less fit patients will tend to be selected for radiotherapy. Direct comparison of the side effects is not possible because of this inherent case selection and the fact that surgical treatment eliminates patients with advanced disease from the surgical group. Much of our information on the side effects and complications is based on data from the 1970s and 1980s and the population of patients being operated on and the methods of administration of radiotherapy have changed since that time. One side effect of radiotherapy that makes it less attractive to young women is ovarian failure, but this problem could be reduced by performing laparoscopic ovarian transposition prior to treatment. The incidence of ovarian metastases being less than 1% in squamous cell carcinoma of the cervix[24] and in adenocarcinoma ovarian metastases have been demonstrated to only be present in post-menopausal women, in patients with positive nodes or in patients with obvious macroscopic ovarian disease.[25]. It is, therefore, probably unnecessary to perform oopherectomy in young premenopausal women with cervical cancer.

The standard surgical procedure for the treatment of stage 1b cervical carcinoma is a Class III radical hysterectomy, as described by Piver et al,[26] and pelvic lymphadenectomy. In this procedure, extensive resection of paracervical and parametrial tissues occurs. The ureters and bladder are completely mobilised from the paracervical tissue. The necessity for such radical surgery and its potential urinary tract morbidity in patients with stage 1bi squamous cervical cancer less than 2 cm in diameter has been questioned. This group of patients has a very good prognosis (97.6%) when treated by a class III radical hysterectomy. There is some evidence to suggest that this group of patients would be equally well treated by modified radical hysterectomy[27] without compromising survival but lowering the associated morbidity.[28]

Larger 1b tumours (> 6 cm) present a management dilemma because radiotherapy is not as effective as in smaller tumours of the same stage because of the inability of the intracavitary source to penetrate all of the tumour. However, if treated primarily by surgery, a high percentage will require subsequent postoperative radiotherapy thus committing them to the combined morbidity of both forms of treatment. Larger doses of external beam radiotherapy or extrafascial hysterectomy have been advocated to improve survival, but surgery has not been proven to offer improved survival or reduced risk of pelvic recurrence.

## The role of lymph node sampling

Whilst pelvic lymphadenectomy provides important prognostic information and patients with stage 1b carcinoma of the cervix who have tumour metastases in the pelvic lymph nodes have a 55–60% 5-year survival compared with an overall survival of 85–90%.[29] Studies suggest that 15% of patients with stage 1 cancer of the cervix will have lymph node metastases.[30] Adjuvant radiotherapy is usually recommended for patients with tumour in the lymph nodes. It is self evident that the pelvic lymphadenectomy will only benefit therapeutically those patients with involved lymph nodes. In addition, adjuvant radiotherapy has not been proven to improve survival, although it does significantly reduce local pelvic recurrence.[31,32] No survival benefit has been demonstrated for patients with stage 1B and 2A carcinoma undergoing lymphadenectomy and radiotherapy to the pelvic nodes as compared with a group of patients undergoing radiotherapy alone, but the complication rates are higher for combined treatment.[33]

The role of pelvic and para-aortic lymphadenectomy in patients being treated primarily with radiotherapy is controversial. In North America, surgical lymph node staging is required before entry of patients into most Gynecologic Oncology Group clinical studies. The GOG also noted that the complication rate was 12% if a transperitoneal approach was used compared with only 4% if a retroperitoneal approach was used.[34]

## New approaches in surgery for cervical cancer

There has been a renewed interest in the vaginal approach to the surgical treatment of cervical cancer as a result of the development of laparoscopic pelvic lymphadenectomy.[35,36] This procedure combined with Schauta's radical vaginal hysterectomy offers the potential for laparoscopically assisted treatment of early cervical cancer. Laparoscopic techniques can be applied to pelvic lymphadenectomy and para-aortic lymph node dissections and despite initial concerns about the risk of injury to bladder, bowel, ureter and pelvic vessels complication rates have been low in a number of series. Childers et al[37] observed no significant complications in 61 cases whilst Querleu et al[38] observed 7 complications, of which 6 were vascular injuries and all were repaired laparoscopically. Survival in patients treated laparoscopically appears to be comparable with open surgery.

This form of treatment has been taken further by Dargent et al[39] and Shepherd et al,[40] who have developed a modification of radical vaginal hysterectomy (radical trachelectomy; Fig. 2). This technique provides adequate local excision for small volume stage 1B carcinoma of the cervix but enables the preservation of fertility. Shepherd et al reported 10 cases of whom one required postoperative radiotherapy and another completion radical hysterectomy, but three live births have resulted. All patients also underwent laparoscopic pelvic

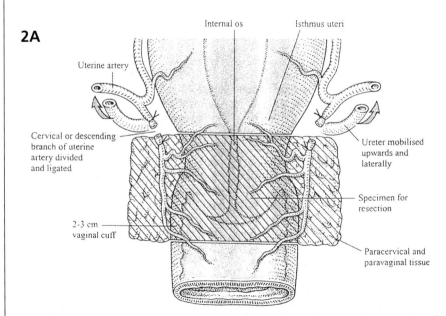

**2A**

Internal os   Isthmus uteri

Uterine artery

Cervical or descending branch of uterine artery divided and ligated

Ureter mobilised upwards and laterally

Specimen for resection

2-3 cm vaginal cuff

Paracervical and paravaginal tissue

**Fig. 2** The technique used for radical trachelectomy. (**A**) Area of tissue for resection (shaded) including cervix and upper vagina with paracervical and paravaginal tissues up to the level of the uterine isthmus. (*continued on next page*)

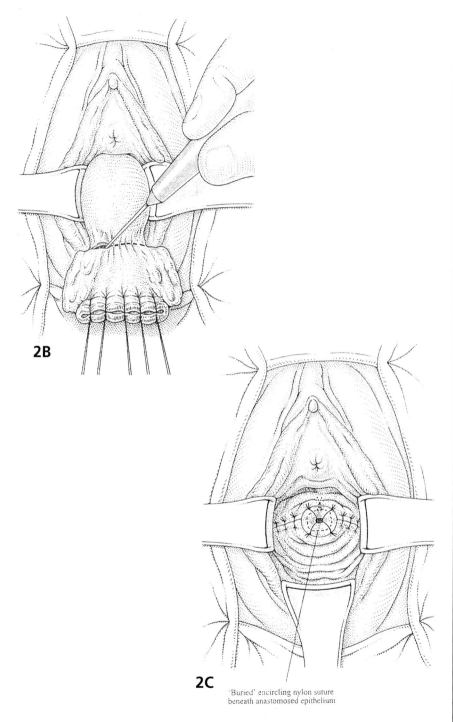

**2B**

**2C**

'Buried' encircling nylon suture
beneath anastomosed epithelium

**Fig. 2** The technique used for radical trachelectomy. (**A**) Area of tissue for resection
(shaded) including cervix and upper vagina with paracervical and paravaginal tissues
up to the level of the uterine isthmus. (**B**) Transection of the specimen of the level of
the uterine isthmus using cutting diathermy. (**C**) Vaginal–isthmic re-anastomosis.
Reproduced with the permission of the *British Journal of Obstetrics and Gynaecology*
from Shepherd et al.[40]

lymphadenectomy or extraperitoneal lymphaedenectomy. The development of more conservative surgery is particularly important in the context of an increase of 77% in the incidence of invasive carcinoma of the cervix in young women aged between 25–34 years.

### Multimodality approach

The complementary roles of radiotherapy and surgery in the management of cervical cancer have already been discussed and there are some areas in which a collaborative approach will be necessary to determine or reassess the relative roles of these two treatment modalities. In particular, in the management of young women with stage 1Bi or stage 1Bii disease in whom the best treatment is likely to be decided upon on an individual patient basis based on the relative complications and side effects of the treatment modalities. More recently, the role of neo-adjuvant chemotherapy has been further investigated and been shown to improve survival in bulky stage 1bii and advanced cervical cancer.[41,42]

## ENDOMETRIAL CANCER

As the majority of patients present with early stage disease, endometrial cancer is generally perceived as being reasonably straight forward to manage and to have a good outcome. However, the overall outcome is only marginally better than for carcinoma of the cervix, and there are some areas of great controversy in its management, which are currently being investigated.

### Choice of surgery

Patients with endometrial cancer are often obese and it is, therefore, very important to have adequate access at the time of operation; in these patients a midline incision is recommended. In practice in the UK, a wide variety of procedures are performed from TAH and BSO through TAH with a vaginal cuff to radical hysterectomy. When the cervix is involved, a radical hysterectomy is required but, if the disease is believed to be confined to the uterus, a total abdominal hysterectomy and bilateral salpingo-oopherectomy is sufficient to ensure adequate excision. However, for complete staging, peritoneal washings should be taken and pelvic and para-aortic lymphadenectomy are options that will be discussed in the next section. Alternatively, if the patient is unfit for surgery, external beam radiotherapy may be administered prior to performing a total abdominal hysterectomy.

### Role of lymphadenectomy

Whilst lymphadenectomy is indicated in cases of endometrial cancer in which the lymph glands are macroscopically enlarged, the role of lymphadenectomy in early endometrial cancer is unclear. No randomised surgical trials have been reported on the use of pelvic lymphadenectomy in endometrial cancer. In the US, lymphadenectomy is performed routinely and where the lymph nodes are negative radiotherapy is avoided; but, in the UK, lymphadenectomy is not generally performed as a method of assessing prognosis. This may be partly due to the lack of consensus on the appropriate use of adjunctive radiotherapy in early endometrial cancer. Only one randomised trial of adjuvant radiotherapy has been published by Aalders et al in 1980.[43] In this study, patients receiving intracavitary vault therapy alone were compared with patients receiving external beam radiotherapy in addition to the intracavitary treatment. Whilst this study failed to show a survival advantage for patients receiving external beam radiotherapy, the combined approach did appear to give lower pelvic recurrence rates (1.9% versus 6.9%). The Gynecologic Oncology Group has recently completed a study randomising patients to receive radiotherapy or not, but the results have not yet been published. The 2-year survival for all patients with stage 1 disease as defined by surgical staging is 97% and it is unlikely that adjuvant external beam radiotherapy would improve this survival. There is also some evidence to suggest that patients who undergo pelvic node sampling do better than those who do not. Kilgore et al[44] reported 649 patients in a case control study and demonstrated that patients who had undergone pelvic lymph node sampling had significantly better survival than those who had no node sampling. However, this may have been due to the planning of adjuvant treatment and there may have been selection bias for patients having lymph node sampling. In the UK, there are no consistent criteria for designating patients as high risk or low risk and there is no agreement on which patients should receive adjuvant radiotherapy. Both the issue of adjuvant radiotherapy and that of lymphadenectomy are currently being addressed in a multicentre MRC trial – the ASTEC study – into which all patients with early endometrial cancer should be entered.

## New treatments

The development of laparoscopic techniques has resulted in renewed interest in vaginal hysterectomy as a method of treatment for endometrial cancer in combination with laparoscopic lymphadenectomy. There have been a number of studies suggesting this is a safe alternative that may result in reduced length of hospital stay, improved quality of life and significant cost savings.[45–47] The main concerns about laparoscopic lymphadenectomy have been the risk of injury to bowel, bladder and ureters, the potential for port site metastases and the long-term survival, as compared with patients treated by open laparotomy which has already been discussed with reference to cervical cancer. One early study in endometrial cancer by Melendez et al[48] suggests that this is a safe procedure and that, while operating time and conversion rate to laparotomy decrease with the experience of the surgeon, the ability to detect metastases and the complication rate appear to be unrelated to the experience of the surgeon. The overall complication rate in this study was 4% (two enterotomies, two cystotomies, and a transected ureter). The role of laparoscopic lymphadenectomy in endometrial cancer is likely to depend upon the establishment of a role for lymph node sampling in endometrial cancer, but the technique appears to have a sound basis for use in selected cases.

One experimental approach to the management of endometrial cancer has been the conservative and fertility preserving approach to patients with well differentiated carcinoma by treatment with megestrol acetate or combined megestrol and tamoxifen. There are only case reports of this form of treatment by Kimming et al[49] and there are no long term data for survival and recurrence rates.

## Multimodality approaches

The treatment of all patients with endometrial cancer can potentially involve both surgery and radiotherapy it is important that the role of these two treatment modalities is tailored to meet the requirements of the individual patient, and that there is good communication between the specialists involved in planning the treatment and the patient who is being treated. It should be established what the aims of treatment are for each patient, i.e. palliation or cure.

## OVARIAN CARCINOMA

The objective of surgery for ovarian carcinoma has for many years been to either remove all of the cancer or, in cases where residual macroscopic disease is inevitable, to optimally 'debulk' the tumour. It is unclear whether or not this approach for advanced disease improves the outcome.

The evidence for maximal surgical effort in advanced disease was presented by Griffiths,[50] who reported improved survival of patients in whom 'optimal' debulking was achieved. However, there are no randomised controlled trials to confirm this concept and the improved outlook in patients who have undergone optimal debulking surgery may be as a result of tumour biology rather than the surgery. Despite newer surgical techniques enabling increasingly radical surgery and the increased acceptance of radical surgery there has been no significant improvement in the survival of patients with advanced ovarian cancer.[51] In addition, a meta-analysis of observational studies in patients with advanced ovarian cancer demonstrated that the type of chemotherapy was the main influence on survival and cytoreductive surgery had minimal effect.[52] Whilst there is no question that patients with early disease or significant symptoms that may only be relieved by surgical treatment should undergo laparotomy, the place of this operation as a routine in advanced disease is less certain. Indeed, surgery may delay the administration of chemotherapy in such a manner as to adversely affect the patients prognosis. *The Confidential Enquiry into Peri-operative Deaths (1994–1995)*[53] highlighted the need for multidisciplinary discussion and the potential use of scanning and guided biopsy to assess pelvic masses.

It is becoming apparent that gynaecological oncologists must address the issue of how to provide sensible cytoreduction along with symptomatic relief. What is 'appropriate' surgical effort in the management of ovarian carcinoma? Clearly, a high proportion of patients with early ovarian carcinoma are 'cured' without recourse to chemotherapy. Patients with advanced ovarian cancer fall into two categories:

1. Patients in whom maximum surgical effort can achieve elimination of all macroscopic disease without increasing the risk of death or significant morbidity or significantly delaying chemotherapy.

2. Patients in whom maximum surgical effort is still not going to result in elimination of all macroscopic disease or in whom it is going to result in unacceptable risk of mortality and morbidity.

The only prospective randomised trial to demonstrate a benefit for surgery in advanced ovarian cancer has been for interval debulking surgery in patients with advanced disease.[54] It would seem appropriate to consider interval debulking in the second group of patients after initial cytoreduction by chemotherapy. This does not mean that radical surgery is never appropriate in this group of patients: it may be appropriate for symptom control or for prevention of the onset of imminent problems, e.g. bowel obstruction. Some would advocate radical surgery removing all peritoneal deposits of tumour in all patients with advanced disease.[55] However, this is performed at the cost of a high morbidity and the role of this type of ultraradical surgery in advanced ovarian cancer is still not clear. It is likely that, in the future, greater efforts will need to be made pre-operatively to assess patients with suspected ovarian carcinoma and to establish the appropriateness of radical surgery.

The diagnosis of ovarian carcinoma can be reliably confirmed by means of CT scanning and cytology of ascitic taps or scan guided fine needle biopsy of pelvic or omental masses.

There have been a number of papers proposing neo-adjuvant chemotherapy prior to definitive cytoreductive surgery in patients with advanced ovarian carcinoma. Surwit et al[56] reported 29 patients treated with neo-adjuvant chemotherapy prior to surgery and concluded that it offered the same survival as primary cytoreductive surgery, but with only one operative procedure (Table 1). Schwartz et al[57] described the management of 59 patients with advanced malignancy compatible with ovarian carcinoma as diagnosed by CT scan and cytology or histology. These patients all received neo-adjuvant chemotherapy and their survival was not statistically different from a group of patients treated by conventional primary cytoreductive surgery and chemotherapy. Of the 59 patients, 41 subsequently underwent cytoreductive surgery. It is proposed that randomised prospective trials are required to compare conventional treatment with neo-adjuvant chemotherapy and to

**Table 1** The evidence for neo-adjuvant chemotherapy in advanced ovarian cancer

| Reference | No of patients | Stage | Surgery | Median survival |
|-----------|----------------|-------|---------|-----------------|
| Schwartz et al[57] | 59 | IIIc/IV | Debulking after chemo | 12 months |
| Surwit et al[56] | 29 | IIIc/IV | Debulking after chemo | 22.5 months |
| Vergote et al[61] | 41 | III/IV | IDS | 24.8% at 3 years |
| Jacob[62] | 22 | IIIc/IV | IDS + SLL | 16 months |
| | 22 | IIIc/IV | Primary debulk + debulk at SLL | 19.3 months |
| | 18 | IIIc/IV | Primary surgery, relaparotomy + debulk at SLL | 18 months |

IDS, interval debulking surgery; SLL, second look laparotomy; chemo, chemotherapy.

determine the effect on quality of life and cost/benefit outcomes. The EORTC Gynaecological Cancer Co-operative Group is currently randomising patients for a comparison of primary cytoreductive surgery and pre-operative chemotherapy.

In the UK, development of neo-adjuvant chemotherapy regimens will be dependent upon satisfactory pre-treatment assessment of patients. There are two potential methods – CT scan evaluation and guided biopsies – which would require increased involvement of radiologists, but has been demonstrated as being an effective method of assessing the extent of disease.[58] It would also be important to ensure that CT films were properly reviewed prior to biopsy because of the potential for seedling along the track of the biopsy converting a stage 1 carcinoma into a stage 3.

An alternative to CT scan assessment would be open laparoscopy which has been shown to be an effective method of assessing operability and of safely obtaining a biopsy; however, it does have a significant risk of causing port site metastases (13%).[59] Minimal access surgery may have a number of other roles in the management of ovarian carcinoma. Patients who have been incompletely staged at laparotomy may have further assessment including para-aortic node biopsy performed laparoscopically.

Laparoscopic surgery may also be appropriate for early stage disease in young women who wish to retain their fertility. Conservative surgery may or may not be appropriate for young women with early stage epithelial tumours, but it is definitely the correct management in cases which may be germ cell tumours, since these are very chemosensitive and fertility may be retained in these women. If radical surgery is not appropriate, then these patients are candidates for laparoscopic staging. In this very young group of patients, the cosmetic advantages of laparoscopic surgery may be more important but this does not mean that the standard of surgical treatment should be compromised to achieve a better cosmetic result. Germ cell tumours are rare and should, if possible, be treated in cancer centres with a particular interest in gynaecological cancers. The main concerns about laparoscopic surgery in ovarian cancer are the potential complications, in particular vascular injuries, the risk of dissemination of tumour by rupture of an ovarian tumour (thus converting stage 1a disease into stage 1c) and the risk of port site metastases.

Surgery is likely to continue to have a prophylactic role in women at high risk of ovarian cancer. Whilst there are very few women with an identifiable gene that suggests that they are at high risk, there are a large number of women who have a family history of ovarian cancer. The key to the future of surgery in these patients is finding better ways of assessing the individual's risk of developing ovarian cancer and improving non-invasive screening techniques.

## SURGICAL PALLIATION

This is a relatively new topic to appear in surgical texts on cancer care for a number of reasons. The word palliate means to alleviate without curing which seems superficially to be at odds with the basic surgical principles of oncology. However, in practice, attempts to cure by surgery often end in failure to cure, but may, nevertheless, provide significant palliation.[60] Palliative care is multidisciplinary, it is not usually surgically led and surgery is often seen as being invasive, traumatic and expensive. There has also been very little research into the palliative role of surgery either at relapse or in failed attempts at curative surgery.

Surgical palliation has a number of specific roles, but a key decision in deciding that surgery is appropriate is to predict the survival of a patient. Since we are often unable to accurately predict the survival time or to objectively measure the quality of life, it is very important to involve the patient and their family in the decision making process. The situations in which surgery may seem the most obvious choice are: (i) gastrointestinal obstruction; (ii) fistulae; (iii) renal tract obstruction; and (iv) localised mass related symptoms.

## Gastrointestinal obstruction

Loop ileostomy may be beneficial in patients with large bowel obstruction, for instance in ovarian carcinoma. This is a quick procedure, has a rapid recovery and alleviates symptoms; although stomas can be problematic, this does not appear to be the case in appropriately selected patients who are given adequate support and stoma care. It is, of course, essential to ensure that the small bowel is functioning before proceeding. In patients with gastric outlet obstruction, percutaneous gastrostomy may relieve symptoms and can be performed without a general anaesthetic.

## Fistulae

These may affect both the urinary and gastrointestinal tracts in gynaecological cancers and can cause very distressing symptoms for the patient. They are particularly common in patients who have had radiotherapy and, in these circumstances, are more difficult to close. However, there are a number of surgical interventions that may alleviate the symptoms of fistulae. Ureteral fistulae may be stented, urinary diversion by ileal conduit or ureterostomy may alleviate the symptoms of a vesico-vaginal fistula and large bowel fistulae may be defunctioned by either an ileostomy or colostomy.

## Renal tract obstruction

The alleviation of renal tract obstruction by surgery is rarely justified in patients with advanced disease unless they are awaiting potentially curative treatment. However there may be circumstances in which surgery is appropriate, e.g. when an ovarian mass is causing urinary retention

## Localised masses

An ovarian mass may cause significant pressure symptoms which may be amenable to salvage surgery, but these patients must be carefully selected. Recurrent vulvar cancer can cause significant pain and unpleasant discharge. Wide excision of such masses, even if skin grafting is necessary, can provide valuable palliation.

# NEW TECHNOLOGIES THAT ARE LIKELY TO INFLUENCE CHANGE

The greatest influences are likely to occur in imaging and image-guided biopsy and in improved understanding of disease behaviour through molecular prognostication. The latter may also prove to be of value in the prediction of response to current and future adjuvant therapies. The short to medium term future is unlikely to hold any promise for curing cancer by medical means (single or combined approaches), we must however continue to develop integrated strategies that extract the best of what we have and minimize the damage to individuals and health service alike.

# EVIDENCE AND THE DEVELOPMENT OF SURGERY

Up until now, surgical procedures appear to have, for the most part, escaped the rigours of proof of effect. It is unlikely that this state of affairs will be acceptable in the future yet, at the same time, clinicians must face the very real problems of how to recruit patients into surgically based clinical trials. The problems are not insignificant, but one might hope that the re-organised infrastructure of cancer care and a growing awareness amongst patients and the potential patients of the value of taking part in clinical trials will only serve to facilitate the production of a far more robust evidence base than that which currently prevails.

## References

1  Podratz K C, Symonds R E, Taylor W F. Carcinoma of the vulva: analysis of treatment failures. Am J Obstet Gynecol 1982; 143: 340–347
2  Byron R L, Mishell D R, Yonemoto R H. The surgical treatment of invasive carcinoma of the vulva. Surg Gynecol Obstet 1965; 121: 1243–1251
3  Hacker N F, Leuchter R S, Berek J S et al. Radical vulvectomy and bilateral lymphadenectomy through separate groin incisions. Obstet Gynecol 1981; 58: 574–579
4  DiSaia P H, Creasman W T, Rich W M. An alternate approach to early cancer of the vulva. Am J Obstet Gynecol 1979; 133: 825–832
5  Ross M J, Ehrmann R L. Histologic prognosticators in stage 1 squamous cell carcinoma of the vulva. Obstet Gynecol 1987; 70: 774–784
6  Hacker N F, van der Velden J. Conservative management of early vulvar cancer. Cancer 1993; 71: 1673–1677
7  Homesley H D, Bundy B N, Sedlis A, Adcock L. Radiation therapy versus pelvic lymph node resection for carcinoma of the vulva with positive groin nodes. Obstet Gynecol 1986; 68: 733–740
8  Keys H. Gynecological Oncology Group randomised trials of combined technique therapy for vulvar cancer. Cancer 1993; 71: 1691–1696
9  Hacker N F. Current treatment of small vulvar cancers Oncology 1990; 4: 21–25
10 DiSaia P J, Creasman W T, Rich W M. An alternative approach to early cancer of the vulva. Am J Obstet Gynecol 1979; 133: 825–830
11 Stehman F B, Bundy B N, Dvoretsky P M, Creasman W T. Early stage I carcinoma of the vulva treated with ipsilateral superficial inguinal lymphadenectomy and modified radical hemivulvectomy. A prospective study of the Gynecologic Oncology Group. Obstet Gynecol 1992; 79: 490–497
12 Terada K Y, Coel M N, Ko P, Wong J H. Combined use of intraoperative lymphatic mapping and lymphoscintigraphy in the management of squamous cell cancer of the vulva. Gynecol Oncol 1998 ; 70: 65–69
13 Veronesi U, Paganelli G, Galimberti V et al. Sentinel-node biopsy to avoid axillary dissection in breast cancer with clinically negative lymph-nodes. Lancet 1997; 349: 1864–1867

14  Boronow R C, Hickman B T, Reagan M T, Smith A, Steadham R E. Combined therapy as an alternative to exenteration for locally advanced vulvovaginal cancer. II: results, complications and dosimetric and surgical considerations. Am J Clin Oncol 1987; 10: 171

15  Thomas G, Dembo A, Depetrillo A et al. Concurrent radiation and chemotherapy in vulvar carcinoma. Gynecol Oncol 1989; 34: 263–267

16  Hoffman M S, Lapolla J P, Roberts W S, Fiorica J V, Cavanagh D. Use of local flaps for primary anal reconstruction following perianal resection for neoplasia. Gynecol Oncol 1990; 36: 348–352

17  Tateo A, Tateo S, Bernasconi C, Zara C. Use of the V-Y flap for vulvar reconstruction. Gynecol Oncol 1996; 67; 203–207

18  Landoni F, Proserpio M, Maneo A, Cormio G, Zanetta G, Milani R. Repair of the perineal defect after radical vulvar surgery: direct closure versus skin flaps reconstruction. A retrospective comparative study. Aust N Z J Obstet Gynaecol 1995; 35: 300–304

19  Chun J K Behnam A B, Dottino P, Cohen C. Use of the umbilicus in reconstruction of the vulva and vagina with a rectus abdominis musculocutaneous flap. Ann Plast Surg 1998; 40; 659–663

20  Burke T W, Morris M, Roh M S, Levenback C, Gershenson D M. Perineal reconstruction using single gracilis myocutaneous flaps. Gynecol Oncol 1995; 57: 221–225

21  Morgan P R, Anderson M C, Buckley C H et al. The Royal College of Obstetricians and Gynaecologists micro-invasive carcinoma of the cervix study: preliminary results. Br J Obstet Gynaecol 1993; 100; 664–668

22  Buxton E J, Luesley D M, Wade-Evans T, Jordan J A. Residual disease after cone biopsy: completeness of excision and follow-up cytology as predictive factors. Obstet Gynecol 1987; 70: 529–532

23  Jones W B, Mercer G O, Lewis J L, Rubin S C, Hoskins W J. Early invasive carcinoma of the cervix. Gynecol Oncol 1993; 51: 26–32

24  Toki N, Tsukamoto N, Kaku T et al. Microscopic ovarian metastasis of the uterine cervical cancer. Gynecol Oncol 1991 ;41: 46

25  Brown J V, Fu Y S, Berek J S. Ovarian metastases are rare in stage 1 adenocarcinoma of the cervix. Obstet Gynecol 1990; 76: 623

26  Piver M S, Rutledge F, Smith P J. Five classes of extended hysterectomy for women with cervical carcinoma. Obstet Gynecol 1974; 44: 265–272

27  Magrina J F, Goodrich M A, Lidner T K et al. Modified radical hysterectomy in the treatment of early squamous cervical cancer. Gynecol Oncol 1999; 72: 183–186

28  Magrina J F, Goodrich M A, Weaver A L, Podratz K C. Modified radical hysterectomy: morbidity and mortality. Gynecol Oncol 1995; 59: 277–282

29  Burghardt E, Pickel H, Haas J, Lahousen M. Prognostic factors and operative treatment of stages 1B and 2B cervical cancer. Am J Obstet Gynecol 1987; 156: 998

30  Alvarez R D, Potter M E, Soong S J et al. Rationale for using pathologic tumor dimensions and nodal status to subclassify surgically treated stage 1B cervical cancer patients. Gynecol Oncol 1991; 43: 108–112

31  Soisson A P, Soper J T, Clarke-Pearson D L et al. Adjuvant radiotherapy following radical hysterectomy for patients with stage 1B and 2A cervical cancer. Gynecol Oncol 1990; 37: 390–395

32  Kinney W K, Alvarez R D, Reid G C. Value of adjuvant whole pelvis irradiation after Wertheims hysterectomy for early stage squamous carcinoma of the cervix with pelvic nodal metastasis: a matched–control study. Gynecol Oncol 1989; 34: 256–262

33  Perez C, Camel H, Kao M. Randomised study of preoperative radiation and surgery or irradiation alone in the treatment of stage 1B and 2 A carcinoma of the uterine cervix: final report. Gynecol Oncol 1987; 27: 129–140

34  Weiser E B, Bundy B N, Hoskins W J et al. Extraperitoneal versus transperitoneal selective para-aortic lymphadenectomy in the pretreatment surgical staging of advanced cervical carcinoma (A Gynecologic Oncology Group Study). Gynecol Oncol 1989; 33: 283–289

35  Dargent D. A new future for Schauta's operation through pre-surgical retro peritoneal pelviscopy. Eur J Gynecol Oncol 1987; 8: 292

36  Querleu D, Leblanc E, Castelain B. Laparoscopic pelvic lymphadenectomy. Am J Obstet Gynecol 1991; 164: 579–581

37  Childers J M, Hatch K D et al. Laparoscopic para-aortic lymphadenectomy in gynecologic malignancies. Obstet Gynecol 1993; 82: 741–747

38  Querleu D, Leblanc E, Chapters 12 and 25. In: Gomel V, Taylor P J (eds) Diagnostic and Operative Gynecologic Laparoscopy. New York: Mosby, 1995

39  Dargent D, Brun J L, Roy M, Mathevet P, Remi I. La trachelectomie elargie(TE): une alternative a l'hysterectomie radicale dans le traitement des cancers infiltrants developes sur la face externe du col uterin J Obstet Gynecol 1994; 2: 285–292

40  Shepherd J H, Crawford R A F, Oram D H. Radical trachelectomy: a way to preserve fertility in the treatment of early cervical cancer. Br J Obstet Gynaecol 1998; 105: 912–916

41  Keys H M, Bundy B N, Stehman H et al. Cisplatin, radiation and adjuvant hysterectomy compared with radiation and adjuvant hysterectomy for bulky stage 1b cervical carcinoma. N Engl J Med 1999; In press

42  Rose P G, Bundy B N, Watkins E B et al. Concurrent cisplatin based radiotherapy and chemotherapy for locally advanced cervical cancer. N Engl J Med 1999; In press

43  Aalders J, Abeler V, Kolstad P, Onsrud M. Postoperative external irradiation and prognostic parameters in stage I endometrial carcinoma: clinical and histopathologic study of 540 patients. Obstet Gynecol 1980; 56: 419–426

44  Kilgore L C, Partridge E E, Alvarez R D et al. Adenocarcinoma of the endometrium: survival comparisons of patients with and without pelvic node sampling. Gynecol Oncol 1995; 56: 29–33

45  Childers J M, Hatch K, Surwit E A. The role of laparoscopic lymphadenectomy in the management of cervical carcinoma. Gynecol Oncol 1992: 47: 38–43

46  Holub Z, Voracek J, Shomani A. A comparison of laparoscopic surgery with an open procedure in endometrial cancer. Eur J Gynaecol Oncol 1998; 19: 294–296

47  Spirtos N M, Schlaerth J B, Gross G M, Spirtos T W, Schlaerth A C, Ballon S C. Cost and quality of life analyses of surgery for early endometrial cancer: laparotomy versus laparoscopy. Am J Obstet Gynecol 1996; 174: 1795–1799

48  Melendez T D, Childers J M, Nour M, Harrigill K, Surwit E A. Laparoscopic staging of endometrial cancer: the learning experience. J Soc Laparoendosc Surg 1997; 1: 45–49

49  Kimming R, Strowitzki T, Muller-Hocker J et al. Conservative treatment of endometrial cancer permitting subsequent triplet pregnancy. Gynecol Oncol 1995; 58: 255–257

50  Griffiths C T, Parker L M, Fuller A F. Role of cytoreductive surgical treatment in the management of advanced ovarian cancer. Cancer Treat Rep 1979; 63: 235–240

51  Eisenkop S C, Nalick R H, Wang H, Teng N H. Peritoneal implant elimination during cyto-reductive surgery for ovarian cancer: impact on survival. Gynecol Oncol 1993; 51: 224–229

52  Hunter R W, Alexander N D E, Soutter W P. Meta-analysis of surgery in advanced ovarian carcinoma: is maximum cytoreduction an independent determinant of prognosis? Am J Obstet Gynecol 1992; 166: 504–511

53  The National Confidential Enquiry into Perioperative Deaths, 1994/95 Report. Published September 1997.

54  van der Berg M E L, van Lent M, Buyse M et al. The effect of debulking surgery after induction chemotherapy on the prognosis in advanced epithelial ovarian cancer. N Engl J Med 1995; 332: 629–634

55  Eisenkop S M, Friedman R L, Wang H J. Complete cytoreductive surgery is feasible and maximises survival in patients with advanced epithelial ovarian cancer. A prospective study. Gynecol Oncol 1998; 69: 103–108

56  Surwit E, Childers J, Atlas M et al. Neoadjuvant chemotherapy for advanced ovarian cancer. Int J Gynecol Cancer 1996; 6: 356–361

57  Schwartz P E, Chambers J T, Makuch R. Neoadjuvant chemotherapy for advanced ovarian cancer. Gynecol Oncol 1994; 53: 33–37

58  Nelson B E, Rosenfeld A T, Schwartz P E. Preoperative abdominopelvic computed tomographic prediction of optimal cytoreduction in epithelial ovarian carcinoma. J Clin Oncol 1993; 11: 166–172

59  van Dam P A, Decloedt J, Tjama W, Vergote I B. Diagnostic laparoscopy to assess oper-ability of advanced ovarian cancer: a feasibility study. Eur J Gynaecol Oncol 1997; 18: 272–273

60  Blythe J G, Wahl T P. Debulking surgery: does it increase the quality of survival? Gynecol Oncol 1982; 14: 396–408

61  Vergote I, De Wever I, Tjalma W, Van Gramberen M, Decloedt J, Van Dam P. Neoadjuvant chemotherapy or primary debulking surgery in advanced ovarian carcinoma: a retrospective analysis of 285 patients. Gynecol Oncol 1998; 71: 431–436

62  Jacob J H, Gershenson D M, Morris M, Copeland L J, Burke T W, Wharton J T. Neoadjuvant chemotherapy and interval debulking for advanced epithelial ovarian cancer. Gynecol Oncol 1991; 42: 146-150

*Anil Sharma  Robert Fox  John Richardson*

# 22

# Hereditary cancer syndromes in gynaecology: an opportunity for prevention

## Cancer – the size of the problem

Cancer has overtaken heart disease as the leading cause of death in Britain with mortality from cancer now accounting for one quarter of all deaths.[1] Each year, more than 300,000 men and women in the UK are found to have cancer and more than half die of their disease.[2] Of the survivors, a large proportion suffer long-term morbidity much of which is treatment induced. It is a sad statistic that trends in mortality over the past three decades show that there has been little improvement in crude deaths rates for all the major cancers with the sole exception of stomach cancer,[2] and the reason for this decline is not known.

## Gynaecological cancer – treatment survival rates static

Gynaecological cancer (excluding breast cancer) accounts for about 10% of new cancer cases in women and 12% of cancer deaths. Public anxiety about gynaecological cancer in some senses even outweighs these poor statistics such that the burden of fear dominates some women's lives. Aside from the recent successes of the restructured cervical cytology programme on death rates from cervical cancer,[3] the last 20 years has seen little improvement in the survival rates for ovarian, endometrial and vulval cancers.

## Hereditary cancer syndromes – a new opportunity

The concept of cancer as a genetic disorder resulting from accumulative genetic cellular damage (sporadic mutations) has long been recognised; the p53 mutation

**Mr Anil Sharma** MB MRCOG MRANZCOG, Senior Specialist Registrar, Directorate of Obstetrics, Gynaecology and Paediatrics, Taunton and Somerset Hospital, Taunton TA1 5DA, UK

**Mr Robert Fox** MD MRCPI MRCOG, Consultant Gynaecologist, Directorate of Obstetrics, Gynaecology and Paediatrics, Taunton and Somerset Hospital, Taunton TA1 5DA, UK (for correspondence)

**Mr John Richardson** FRCS FRCOG, Consultant Gynaecologist, Directorate of Obstetrics, Gynaecology and Paediatrics, Taunton and Somerset Hospital, Taunton TA1 5DA, UK

is thought to be involved in about 50% of cases of sporadic ovarian cancer.[4] It is now thought that some tumours result from inherited (germline) mutations and that these account for 5–10% of cases of ovarian cancer and perhaps 3% of endometrial cancer.[5] Identification of these familial cancer syndromes offers a new opportunity to benefit individual patients, but might also lead to considerable harm. It is important, therefore, for clinicians to be both aware of the range of genetic syndromes, which may otherwise pass unrecognised through their clinics, and to grasp what is appropriate in terms of investigation and treatment. The aim of this paper is to review the current state of our knowledge and to explore management strategies. In addition to this, we shall briefly outline the principles of cancer prevention and the genetics of tumour formation, high-lighting the potential advantages and pitfalls of any genetic testing programme.

## CANCER PREVENTION – GENERAL PRINCIPLES

### Cancer – the need for prevention

In 1992, the UK Government's *Health of the Nation* document set out clear objectives to reduce ill health and death caused by certain tumours. The development of methods for prevention of cancer and early diagnosis were central to public policy initiatives on reduction of cancer death rates, as much as, if not more so, than research into novel treatments for established disease. Because any individual cancer is relatively rare and because primary prevention programmes are not without risk and expense, these strategies often depend on identification of high-risk groups for cost-effectiveness and to limit adverse events. Techniques such as gene analysis for mutations are playing an increasing role in risk assessment, but currently such testing is restricted to those with a significant family history.

### Methods of prevention

Cancer prevention programmes may adopt a primary approach (avoid cancer arising), or secondary methods (the early detection of cancer in asymptomatic cases). There are four main methods for primary prevention of cancer: (i) avoidance of known carcinogens; (ii) chemoprophylaxis; (iii) the detection of a pre-malignant phase of the disease; and (iv) removal of apparently healthy non-vital organs in high-risk individuals.

Limiting exposure to known environmental agents may be directed at the population at large, such as anti-smoking, healthy-eating, and safe-sex campaigns, or be more specific as with health and safety regulations for regulating handling of known industrial carcinogens and exposure to radio-active sources. Detection of pre-malignant disease is limited to a small number of cancers but includes the national cervical cytology programme. Examples of elective removal of healthy (pre-diseased) non-vital organs are mastectomy, oophorectomy and colectomy. The option of endocrine therapy (chemopro-phylaxis) is being developed for hormonally sensitive tissues such as breast and ovary.

Clearly primary methods represent an ideal, but many tumours do not have known trigger agents and they occur in low-risk people with no pre-malignant

**Table 1** Theoretical problems of early diagnosis screening programmes for cancer prevention

Longer death (if prognosis not altered)
False reassurance (with false negative test result)
Pre-test anxiety
Unnecessary post-test anxiety (with false positive test result)
Unnecessary medical intervention and morbidity (with false positive test result)
Morbidity of the screening test
Capital outlay and running costs (diversion of funding from other healthcare projects)

*Adapted from Austoker[6]*

phase. Furthermore, surgical prophylaxis, such as oophorectomy, is often not suitable for younger women and yet a need exists for something to be done. Early diagnosis is then the only method of hoping to modify disease progression before symptoms develop. The theoretical advantages of early-disease screening methods includes improved prognosis, less radical treatment and decreased iatrogenic morbidity, and re-assurance for those with negative tests. Examples of such screening methods include mammography and ovarian ultrasound. The stitch-in-time philosophy of secondary prevention is not without problems however (Table 1), perhaps the most sobering of which is that early detection may simply mean a longer death (Fig. 1). It is essential, therefore, that any screening programme is shown conclusively to fulfil the criteria for screening set out by the World Health Organization.[7]

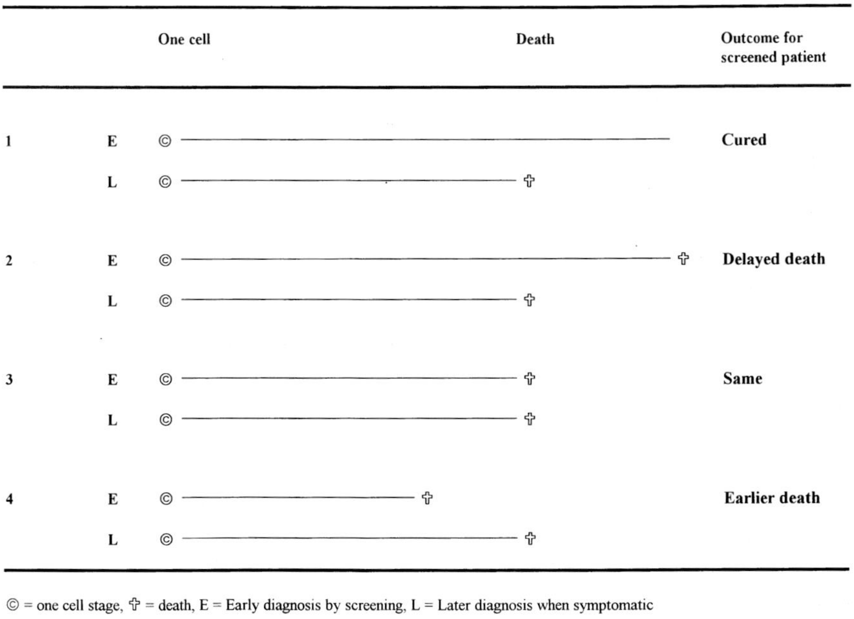

| | | One cell | Death | Outcome for screened patient |
|---|---|---|---|---|
| 1 | E | © ——————————————————— | | Cured |
| | L | © ——————————— ✝ | | |
| 2 | E | © ——————————————————————— ✝ | | Delayed death |
| | L | © ——————————— ✝ | | |
| 3 | E | © ——————————— ✝ | | Same |
| | L | © ——————————— ✝ | | |
| 4 | E | © ——————— ✝ | | Earlier death |
| | L | © ——————— ✝ | | |

© = one cell stage, ✝ = death, E = Early diagnosis by screening, L = Later diagnosis when symptomatic

**Fig. 1** Time-line chart of the four possible outcomes of screening for cancer (one cell to death).

## GENETICS OF CANCER

### Tumour genes

Cancer usually arises as a result of one or more mutations in genes concerned with the regulation of cell growth (proto-oncogenes and tumour suppressor genes) or DNA repair (mismatch repair genes). Environmental factors such as smoking, viruses, industrial chemicals and sunlight commonly play a part in the development of sporadic cancers by causing damage to the genome (somatic mutations such as p53 in sporadic ovarian cancer); but, more rarely, tumours arise as a result of inherited (germline) mutations such as the BRCA1 and BRCA2 gene mutations which confer a greatly increased risk of breast and ovarian cancers. The nature and action of tumour genes is beyond the scope of this chapter and has been well reviewed by Jacobs.[8]

### Ethical and psychological problems of genetic testing

Testing for gene mutations is not a simple matter particularly if the condition generally occurs many years later, may lead to death, and cannot be prevented effectively. All of this will be compounded if there is uncertainty about whether the condition will arise or not (variable penetrance). As well as causing dilemmas for the individual requesting advice, if the test result is positive it raises difficult issues for the counsellor and client as to the ethics of informing, or not, other relatives. Asymptomatic individuals will have widely different reactions to being approached by a clinical genetics' specialist; is ignorance bliss or is knowledge power?[9] In addition to any reaction the individual might have, family dynamics may change with expressions of anger and guilt being common; occasionally even perverse emotions arise, such as delight at the misfortune of sibs in those with negative test results. Clearly, then, genetic counselling demands great expertise in dealing with individuals and families, both the imparting of facts clearly and the management of differing emotional reactions. Psychological support is probably as important as the giving of information. Perhaps more so if the latter is done ineptly.

### Principles of advising individuals with possible cancer syndromes

The process begins with data collection. A family tree should be constructed with the aid of the proband client. This information is often vague, not necessarily accurate and so must be supplemented with detail from hospital records whenever possible. Information such as the age at onset, site of origin and histological type should all be determined whenever possible. The histology is particularly important, as syndromes are often tissue-specific; the familial association of one epithelial cancer and one granulosa cell tumour is of much less significance than two cases of epithelial cancer.

Once the basic family details have been collated, the next stage is to consider whether a hereditary syndrome is likely or not. In some families, the pattern will be clearly against there being a genetic basis to the disease and then general advice about cancer risk and healthy living is all that is appropriate. Some may find it difficult to accept that familial association of single cases of 4 unrelated tumours is sporadic clustering. Moreover, many women with a family history consistent with a genetic cancer syndrome will also have nothing more than chance clustering; a strong familial history does not necessarily indicate hereditary disease. For those in whom a syndrome does seem likely, the counsellor should offer to discuss estimates of life-time cancer risk and methods of prevention. Computer software is now available to provide precise information based on large studies (e.g. Cyrillic).

## Laboratory testing for gene mutations

With advances in molecular biology, tumour genes have been searched for, found and cloned. Some of this basic science is now being applied to clinical medicine. Like any other clinical method, gene testing is not without problems and rigorous criteria need to be applied. This starts by defining the nature of the family history according to an agreed standard such as the Amsterdam criteria for HNPCC (see below) as general population screening is not yet advisable. The client must be fully informed of the implications of both positive and negative results, including non-medical issues such as dealing with prospective life partners, implications for child-rearing, and applying for life insurance. It is helpful if the patient sees both outcomes as useful.

Gene testing must be undertaken in context and BRCA1 results without knowledge of the gene status of affected relatives are difficult to interpret. For this reason, it is of value to store samples from living affected relatives, as testing for genes as yet unknown may become available in the future.

Any discussion should include an acknowledgement that our understanding of genetic cancer is at a rudimentary stage. For instance, it is highly likely that not all genes/gene mutations responsible for breast cancer are yet known. It is also important to emphasise to patients from the outset that laboratory testing is complex and may take some time. BRCA1, for instance, is a massive gene encoding for an 1800 amino acid chain. The gene has numerous mutations and the investigation of a single family consumes an enormous amount of laboratory manpower and resources.

# HEREDITARY BREAST/OVARY CANCER SYNDROMES (HBOC)

## Disease background

The increased risk of ovarian cancer in women with an affected blood relative has long been recognised. More recently, Lynch reported evidence of a familial association between ovarian and breast cancers.[10] Both tumours are relatively common and, in many families, the association of these tumours will represent nothing more than co-incidence; but it is now known that, in a high proportion of cases, a strong association of breast and/or ovarian cancers within a family is the manifestation of a genetic disorder. It has been estimated that about 10% of breast and 7% of ovarian cancers have an inherited basis. BRCA1 and BRCA2 mutations are thought to account for 75% and 10% of familial ovarian cancer, respectively.[11] HNPCC (see below) probably accounts for about another 3–5%. Almost certainly some genetic syndromes have not been identified. It is not yet clear if there is a major site-specific ovarian cancer syndrome or not.

Most information is known about the recently identified genes BRCA1 and BRCA2,[12,13] and most of our discussion will centre around these two syndromes. Loci for these genes have been mapped to chromosomes 17q21 (*BRCA1*) and 13q12 (*BRCA2*) and the natural alleles have been cloned.[12,13] In all, over 100 mutations have been identified. They behave as autosomal dominant genes with high penetrance but with some variation of expression. It is thought that about 1 in 800 Caucasian women are carriers for BRCA1,[11] but there is racial variation and in Ashkenazi Jews the prevalence is 1 in 50.[14]

Most BRCA1 mutations confer a predisposition to both breast and ovarian cancer. As yet, less is known of the ovarian cancer risk in women with BRCA2 but it does seem to be substantially increased.[15] The precise chance and type of tumour development within a specific family might also depend on the location of the mutation and possibly other unknown factors.[16] For BRCA1 mutations, the life-time risk of breast and ovarian cancer is about 80% and 40%, respectively, compared with an 11% risk of sporadic breast cancer and about a 1% risk of sporadic ovarian cancer in the UK.[15,17]

## Breast cancer in HBOC

### Level of risk

When counselling patients, it should be remembered that the risks of breast and ovarian cancer quoted are derived from families which have met stringent criteria for autosomal dominant inheritance of cancer predisposition and that these selection criteria may have given a slanted view of risk.[18] The cumulative risks of breast cancer associated with BRCA1 and BRCA2 mutation carriers has been estimated to be 80% by the age of 70 years.[15,17] The chance of early disease is even more striking; by 50 years of age the risk of breast cancer in BRCA1 mutation carriers is 51% and 28% for BRCA2 compared with a 2% risk in the general population.[19] Those with a BRCA mutation who have had breast cancer are estimated to have a 64% risk of developing a tumour in the other breast. Incidentally, male carriers of BRCA2 mutations have an approximate 7% life-time risk for breast cancer.

### Clinical action

Breast disease is not within the realm of most gynaecologists and our discussion will, therefore, be brief. The options for women with a known BRCA1/BRCA2 mutation include primary chemoprophylaxis, mammography, and prophylactic bilateral mastectomy. Primary chemoprophylaxis using tamoxifen has proved ineffective and this disappointment was compounded by an increased rate of abnormal vaginal bleeding and endometrial tumours amongst uses. Preliminary data suggest that raloxifene, a new highly-selective oestrogen receptor modulator, reduces breast cancer risk in postmenopausal women as well as preventing osteoporosis.[20] In addition, it has no effect on endometrium. Raloxifene has not been tested in women with genetic breast/ovary cancer risk, but, in the future, it might prove extremely valuable for such women who undergo oophorectomy. X-ray mammography is now proven to reduce the chance of death from breast cancer in women beyond 50 years and newer data suggest it is also effective in younger women.[21] The consensus view for women with BRCA is to start mammography at 35 years but it should be borne in mind that the effect on breast cancer death rates in the general population is relatively modest; most studies have shown a 10–20% change in age-specific mortality.

The value of prophylactic mastectomy is uncertain. One recent paper has suggested that it is effective,[22] but currently, most commentators believe that there is insufficient evidence for or against prophylactic mastectomy,[23] and further studies are needed. The effectiveness of the procedure is limited by the presence of residual breast tissue and cancer is well documented even after radical procedures. In addition to questions about the efficacy of mastectomy for the prevention of breast cancer, decision making is made complex by the unpredictable effects on body image and sexual partnerships. Although these effects might be limited by reconstructive surgery, mastectomy remains a far from ideal method of prevention for many women regardless of its efficacy.

## Ovarian cancer in HBOC

### Level of risk

BRCA1 mutation carriers who have had breast cancer are estimated to have a cumulative risk of ovarian cancer of 40% by 70 years of age and for BRCA2 it is 27%. A much greater proportion of tumours in women with BRCA mutations are of the serous type. The prognosis for these tumours is not significantly different from sporadic cases.[24]

### Clinical action

Primary prevention depends on chemoprophylaxis or oophorectomy. Chemoprophylaxis is a proven method of preventing ovarian cancer and appears to be particularly useful for women who have not completed their family. The combined oral contraceptive pill substantially reduces the risk of ovarian cancer with prolonged use in the general population,[25] and this effect has now been shown in BRCA1 mutation carriers also; OCP use for more than 6 years reduces the risk of ovarian cancer by 60% and without increasing the rate of breast cancer.[26] Women at genetic predisposition to ovarian cancer should, therefore, be offered the combined oral contraceptive pill certainly until such time as prophylactic oophorectomy becomes more appropriate.

Technically, prophylactic oophorectomy (PO) is a relatively simple procedure with a low rate of surgical morbidity. Some have conclusively stated that women with a proven family history of hereditary ovarian cancer should be offered prophylactic oophorectomy.[27] It is not without problems, however, perhaps the most taxing of which are the timing in relation to the menopause and the use of HRT. Given the high-chance of ovarian cancer amongst BRCA mutation carriers, it seems likely that there will be health gain from PO but this has not been conclusively shown and the possibility remains that the longer term risks of a surgical menopause may outweigh the risks of leaving the ovaries *in situ* for premenopausal women. With our current state of knowledge, it does seem logical to advise that oophorectomy is appropriate once the menopause has been reached but it must not be forgotten that these women still run a 2–4% risk of primary peritoneal cancer.[28,29] For premenopausal women undertaking PO, the crucial issue is that of whether or not to use HRT, which has been reported to give a relative risk of breast cancer of 1.3 with greater than 5 years' use – an increase in diagnosis of breast cancer by 2.3% for each year of use.[30] For this reason, some have suggested that BRCA1 or BRCA2 mutation carriers should not have HRT even if they have had a prophylactic oophorectomy.[31] The problems of PO before the menopause, therefore, are of acute and chronic menopausal symptoms (including loss of libido), premature bone mineral loss, and possibly increased rates of cardiovascular disease. To this list can be added a possible further increase in the risk of breast cancer if conventional HRT is used. If oophorectomy is chosen by the woman, peritoneal washings should be taken for cytology and the peritoneal cavity should be inspected in detail for occult tumours. In addition, care should be taken to examine for extra-ovarian nodules of ovarian tissue along the embryological tract. Lynch and colleagues have suggested the procedure should be performed laparoscopically. They also advised that it is combined with hysterectomy to simplify hormone replacement therapy,[32] but this would greatly add to the chance of major and minor surgical morbidity. Hysterectomy does seem a more logical if the woman has had breast cancer and is receiving adjuvant tamoxifen.

Options for HRT after oophorectomy include standard $E_2/P$ regimens, tibolone, and raloxifene. We do not yet know which is best for symptoms and which is safest for health. Raloxifene appears to be promising because of its beneficial effect on the breast, but it will not control some of the acute menopausal symptoms. Tibolone may prove to be valuable for this. It has oestrogenic, progestogenic and androgenic properties and compares favourably with oestrogens in reducing climacteric symptoms. This includes an excellent effect on libido which may be very important in younger women after castration. It prevents bone mineral loss and, like raloxifene, it does not stimulate postmenopausal atrophic endometrium. Currently there is no evidence of tibolone use in BRCA1 and BRCA2 mutation carriers.

The only other option for prevention is screening for early ovarian cancer but our knowledge of this is at a far more rudimentary stage than for mammography. Serum CA12-5 measurement and transvaginal ultrasonography (TVS) have been assessed alone, and in combination, for the general female population and found to be ineffective. Currently, the UKCCCR is studying CA12-5/TVS screening for high-risk women. The initial findings are encouraging, with a higher proportion of women with stage I disease, but the data are not yet conclusive.[25] It has to be remembered that the very nature of the disease means it is not an ideal example for screening. There is no known pre-malignant phase and ovarian cancer metastasises early and widely by transcoelomic migration. This, together with the lack of effective treatment for advanced disease, means that, overall, the prognosis is poor (20% 5-year survival). As with mammography, therefore, it seems improbable that screening for early ovarian cancer will eliminate the chance of death from the disease. Conversely, it seems highly likely there will be disproportionate number of false positive test results because the ultrasound findings are not reliable (Fig. 2). As a consequence, a large proportion of women will suffer unnecessary anxiety and morbidity from surgical procedures to confirm or refute the diagnosis.

## Other cancers in HBOC

### Level of risk

By the age of 70 years, BRCA1 mutations confer a 4-fold increased risk of colon cancer in men and women, and men have a 3-fold increased risk of prostate

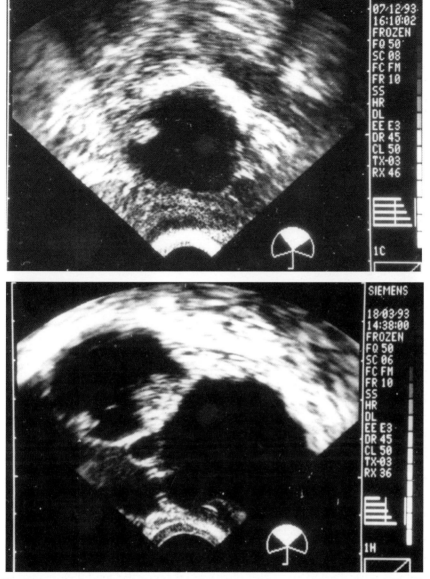

**Fig. 2** Transvaginal ultrasound images of the ovary demonstrating the unreliability of the method for ovarian cancer screening. Image (**A**) shows a small unilocular cyst with one small intra-locular nodule – against expectations this was a cancer. Image (**B**) shows a multiloculated mass with solid areas – against expectations this was a benign lesion.

cancer.[34] There are insufficient data for those with BRCA2 mutations but there are suspicions of a weak association with pancreas, prostate and colon cancers.

### Clinical action

BRCA1 mutation carriers should be informed of a possible increased risk of colorectal cancer. Some authorities advise annual faecal occult blood testing, but this is too insensitive; regular colonoscopy is suggested by most groups though the optimal frequency for screening has not yet been agreed.

## Overview of HBOC syndromes

Genetic ovary/breast cancers syndromes account for a small, but significant, proportion of these tumours. BRCA1 and BRCA2 mutations probably account for the large majority of genetic breast and ovarian cancers. Identification of these syndromes is now with us. Strategies exist for primary prevention of breast and ovarian cancer; these are not ideal, partly because of the conflicting needs of the two tumour types, particularly with reference to HRT, and also because of the morbidity of mastectomy and oophorectomy. The very nature of secondary prevention with mammography and ovarian screening suggest that they are unlikely to provide a complete answer unless the false positive rate is reduced and the treatment of early established tumours becomes much simpler and much more effective.[25]

# COLON/ENDOMETRIUM/OVARY CANCER SYNDROMES (HNPCC)

## Disease background

The hereditary non-polyposis colorectal cancer syndrome (HNPCC) stems from a germline mutation of one of five mismatch repair genes (MSH2, MLH1, PMS1, PMS2 and MSH6).[35] Mutations MSH2 and MLH1 are implicated in 90% of families.[35] This syndrome is quite distinct from familial adenomatous polyposis coli in which numerous benign polyps line the bowel from early life. Two variants of HNPCC have been described (Lynch I and Lynch II). Both syndromes are characterised by a hereditary predisposition to colorectal cancer. In Lynch I, the cancer risk is site-specific but with Lynch II there is also an excess risk of several other solid malignancies including endometrial and ovarian cancers.[36] The syndrome is defined by the Amsterdam criteria (Table 2),[35] and many laboratories will only undertake testing if these criteria are fulfilled. It is now widely acknowledged that these criteria are restrictive, however, and that they exclude about 20% of families with HNPCC.[37]

## Colon cancer in HNPCC

### Level of risk
There is a greatly increased risk of colorectal cancer (around 75% by age 65 years).[38] About 70% of tumours are proximal to the splenic flexure. There is also an early age of onset (around 45 years) and an excess of synchronous and metachronous primaries. Overall, HNPCC is thought to account for about 5–10% of colon cancer cases.[39]

**Table 2** Amsterdam criteria for HNPCC

| |
|---|
| Verified colorectal cancer (CRC) in three of more relatives |
| CRC involving at least two generations |
| One or more case of CRC diagnosed before 50 years |
| Familial adenomatous polyposis excluded |

## Clinical action

This has been reviewed well by Burke and colleagues.[40] It is widely agreed that colorectal cancer in both its sporadic and hereditary forms commonly arises in pre-cancerous adenomatous polyps. Colonoscopy (with endoscopic resection) is advised by most authorities to screen for polyps (and early colon cancer) in individuals with HNPCC. The optimum screening interval is not known. Some have advocated barium studies instead of colonoscopy because of lower cost,[41] but this has not gained widespread acceptance.[42] The effect of colonoscopy on incidence of and mortality from colorectal cancer in these individuals is as yet unclear, but preliminary data are encouraging.[43] Prophylactic colectomy, which is the mainstay of treatment for familial adenomatous polyposis, has been raised as possible method of prevention for HNPCC,[40] but once again its value has not been defined. The beneficial effects of chemoprophylaxis with drugs such as sulindac and aspirin and the beneficial effects of life-style modifications (diet, exercise, cessation of cigarette smoking) have been established for the general population and evidence is gathering for an effect in those with an inherited predisposition to colorectal cancer.[44] There are preliminary data linking $E_2$-based HRT with a lower risk of colorectal cancer in postmenopausal women, but this has not been studied in women with HNPCC mutations.

## Endometrial cancer in HNPCC

### Level of risk

Endometrial cancer is the second commonest tumour in HNPCC families with a 30–39% cumulative risk by age 70 years in proven cases compared with 3% in the general population.[45] Endometrial cancers outnumber colorectal cancers in those with the MSH6 mutation. The endometrial tumours occur about 15 years earlier than the usual peak of 65 years seen in sporadic cases. The natural history of the disease is unclear and it not known whether there is a pre-malignant phase (endometrial hyperplasia) or not. The comparative prognosis for sporadic and hereditary tumours has not been described.

### Clinical action

Annual screening is recommended commencing at age 25–35 years using a combination of transvaginal ultrasound (for endometrial thickness) and endometrial biopsy.[40] Although these give sensitivity in combination of well over 90% in symptomatic postmenopausal women,[46] their efficacy in premenopausal women needs further evaluation. Hysteroscopy is another option for screening. Once child-bearing is complete, hysterectomy should be discussed with the patient. Many women wish surgical prophylaxis and hysterectomy is likely to be highly efficacious for endometrial cancer prophylaxis in HNPCC. The advantage of hysterectomy is not simply that it might prevent death from endometrial malignancy, but also that it avoids exposure to radiotherapy which will have adverse effects on bowel. Progestogens are thought to help prevent endometrial cancer in women with unopposed oestrogen states, but this may not apply to women with HNPCC who are ovulatory.

## Ovarian cancer in HNPCC

### Level of risk

Ovarian cancer occurs with a cumulative life-time risk of approximately 9% in

Lynch II syndrome women.[47] Lynch's data for HNPCC families give a mean age for developing ovarian cancer as 43 years, about 15 years less than that for non-hereditary cancer.[45] The prognosis for established tumours appears to be no different from that of sporadic cases.

*Clinical action*
The role for screening for ovarian cancer with TVS/CA12-5 in HNPCC is unresolved. However, given the much lower risk than for BRCA mutations, it is likely to give a more adverse false positive/true positive profile and currently screening is not recommended outside of clinical trials. Given that many women will choose prophylactic hysterectomy, prophylactic bilateral oophorectomy must also be considered. As before, the menopause brings additional problems (see HBOC section) and there might be a case for delaying PO until after the menopause even if the woman opts for hysterectomy much before this time.

## Overview of HNPCC

HNPCC is less common than HBOC but in some ways it is of greater importance to the gynaecologist because the options for screening and prevention are not so hindered by possible adverse effects on the breast. However, any benefit from gynaecological intervention may be limited by non-genital tract tumours.

## POLYCYSTIC OVARIAN DISEASE

### Disease background

Polycystic ovarian disease (PCOD) is syndrome of ovarian disorder with a very diverse clinical presentation including menstrual disorder, hirsutism, anovulatory infertility and recurrent miscarriage. It is extremely common with perhaps as many as 20% of women having polycystic ovaries at scan.[48] The underlying pathophysiology is complex, but PCOD is now known to be commonly associated with a metabolic disorder characterised by insulin resistance, hyperinsulinaemia and a tendency to diabetes and cardiovascular disease in later life (reviewed by Fox[49]). Ovarian physiology is modulated by insulin, and hyperinsulinaemia is thought to disrupt steroidogenesis in the granulosa and theca cell compartments. In many families, PCOD appears to have a hereditary basis,[50] and it seems that this may reflect a genetic predisposition to insulin resistance.[51]

### Carcinogenesis and PCOD

It has been recognised for many years that women with PCOD have an increased risk of endometrial adenocarcinoma. Conventional thought has argued that the association between PCOD and endometrial cancer is the consequence of anovulation; oestrogen unopposed by progesterone acting on the endometrium to promote proliferation, hyperplasia and, ultimately, neoplasia. Recently there has been evidence to suggest that women with

PCOD also have an increased chance of breast and ovarian cancers.[52,53] The reason for these associations is likely to be complex with a variety of factors playing a role, but the key factor might be an acceleration in cell division rates secondary to hyperinsulinaemia.[54] It is known that women with severe PCOD have evidence of excessive growth of bone (pseudoacromegaly) and skin (acanthosis nigricans).[55,56] True acromegaly due to growth hormone excess is also associated with growth disorder and an increased chance of colonic tumours.[57] It is possible, therefore, that tumour development in PCOD is a reflection of an effect of hyperinsulinaemia, or altered production of other growth factors, such as IGF-1, on cellular growth. This theory is consistent with observations on cancer risk and dietary excess; non-smoking related solid tumours being more common in adults with obesity.[58] The biological basis for this observation is not known, but it has been suggested that an increased rate of cell turnover induced by insulin and other growth factors in response to dietary excess increases the chance for sporadic mutation during mitosis (more cell division, more opportunity for mismatch errors), and that these, in turn, lead to malignant transformation of tissues. The common link between PCOD and dietary excess both promoting tumour formation would be hyperinsulinaemia, one related to abnormalities of insulin receptor function and the other to carbohydrate intake.

## Ovarian cancer in PCOD

### Level of risk

The authors of two early case series speculated that women with PCOD might be at greater risk of ovarian tumours.[59,60] A recent population-based case-control study identified a 2.5-fold increased risk of epithelial cancer of the ovary in women with the syndrome.[52] A study of the prevalence of PCOD in women with strong family history of ovarian cancer showed no excess compared with female controls (Fox and Richardson, personal observation) confirming that the excess risk of ovarian cancer in PCOD is relatively modest.

### Clinical action

Because the risk is only moderately increased, it is unlikely that ovarian cancer screening with transvaginal ultrasonography and/or CA12-5 would be of benefit (see above) but perhaps should be undertaken prior to commencement of ovulation induction therapy for medico-legal purposes. One possible option to reduce the risk of ovarian cancer in this group of women would be to use the oral contraceptive pill, which may be indicated in any case for hirsutism or menstrual disorder. Women with PCOD are also probably more likely to request hysterectomy for menstrual disorder and that gives the opportunity for prophylactic oophorectomy, but this has not been subjected to careful clinical trial for this particular indication.

## Breast cancer in PCOD

### Level of risk

A study of causes of death in women with PCOD revealed a standardised mortality ratio for breast cancer of 1 in 48.[53] Again, this is a relatively modest increase and further study is required to clarify this further. More precise indicators of the excess and information on the mean age at presentation are needed.

### Clinical action

The women should be encouraged to enter any national breast-screening programme (mammography), but because the excess risk is likely to be low, prophylactic mastectomy is not indicated.

## Endometrial cancer in PCOD

### Level of risk

Those with long-standing oligo-amenorrhoea are at the greatest risk of endometrial cancer such that the association between pre-menopausal and PCOD is particularly strong.[61] One study of endometrial sampling of 50 pre-menopausal anovulatory women with PCOD showed that 2 had hyperplasia.[62] The life-time risk of endometrial cancer for these women is not known, but the excess risk is likely to extend well into the menopause.[63]

### Clinical action

There is no national screening for endometrial cancer, but a known history of PCOD should be considered a risk factor when deciding on the need for endometrial sampling in women with menstrual disorder. It has always been assumed that the cause of endometrial neoplasia in women with PCOD is unopposed endogenous oestrogen, and that exogenous progestogen therapy is likely to prevent the development of hyperplasia and neoplasia in as much as it does so in women taking oestrogen-based HRT. This has not been conclusively shown, however, and it is worrying to note that insulin has effects on endometrial tissue suggesting that chronic anovulation may not be the sole cause.[64] Nevertheless, given the apparent safety of cyclical progestogen therapy, it does not seem unreasonable to advise this for women with infrequent or absent periods. For those with menorrhagia or contraceptive needs, the levonorgestrel intra-uterine system (LNG-IUS) might usefully combine control of menstrual loss and protection against endometrial cancer.

## Overview of PCOD

There are theoretical reasons to suspect that women with PCOD have an increased risk of cancer related to hyperinsulinaemia and accelerated cell growth/division. Given that PCOD is an extremely common condition and that, in many cases, there is a clear inherited component, it is potentially an important cause of familial cancer. The increased risk of ovarian cancer with PCOD appears to be relatively modest, however, such that it appears to be an uncommon cause of familial ovarian cancer. Moreover, the apparently modest increased chance of ovarian cancer means that current screening policies are unlikely to be of benefit. Use of the OCP is likely to be of benefit in preventing cancer, but this should be considered carefully given the possible increased risk of breast cancer. Care should be exercised when considering the type and duration of ovulation induction in women with anovulatory infertility related to PCOD. It seems quite possible that there is an increased chance of breast

**Table 3** Rare hereditary tumour syndromes (breast and ovary)

| Syndrome | Cancer predisposition | Other features |
| --- | --- | --- |
| Cowden disease | Ovary and thyroid (follicular) | Mucocutaneous lesions and uterine fibroids |
| Gorlin's syndrome | Ovary (thecoma and sarcoma), skin (BCC) & brain | Dental cysts, high forehead, and falx calcification |
| Ataxia-telangiectasia | Breast and skin (SCC) | Ataxia/telangiectasia. Asymptomatic hetero'tes also |
| Ollier's disease | Ovary (granulosa cell) | Osteochondromatosis |
| Peutz-Jeghers disease | Ovary (granulosa cell) and breast | Mucosal freckles and GI hamartomatous polyps |
| Torre-Muir* | Breast, GI and GU tracts, and skin | Sebaceous adenomas |

Adapted from Kasprzak et al.[31]
*Now thought to be a variant of HNPCC

cancer in women with PCOD, but the level of the risk is not precisely known. Standard breast screening should be encouraged, but early screening and prophylactic mastectomy are not indicated on the basis of current data. Care should perhaps be exercised when considering sex-steroid therapy. Endometrial cancer is undoubtedly a feature of PCOD and the risk does not stop at the menopause. Routine screening is not yet known to be of value. Progestogen therapy has not been conclusively shown to prevent cancer in this particular circumstance, but, given that it is cheap and well tolerated, it use should be considered for women with oligo-amenorrhoea.

## RARE CANCER SYNDROMES IN GYNAECOLOGY

An ever-increasing number of cancer syndromes are being recognised in women. Many are extremely rare and the cancer risk for each condition is generally not as high as for BRCA and HNPCC syndromes. This applies particularly to the unusual types of ovarian tumours, such as granulosa cell tumours and ovarian sarcomas, and, although the relative risk is greatly increased, the absolute chance of the tumour arising remains very low. We have listed them here for completeness (Table 3). Gorlin's disease is of interest for obstetricians because the luteinised thecomas may present in pregnancy with accelerated hypertension secondary to renin secretion by the tumour.[65]

## CONCLUSIONS

Current developments in molecular genetics will not only help our understanding of cancer biology but will allow improved diagnosis of hereditary cancer syndromes. The public is gradually becoming more aware of these cancer syndromes, but at a stage when our understanding of their nature and natural history is still very limited. The theoretical advantage to affected individuals is the benefit to be gained from preventive therapies, but any such treatments must be based on evidence and not speculation how ever logical they may seem. Well-organised studies are needed and it is essential that such research not only looks at cancer death rates but also at the effects of management on the general physical and psychological well-being of patients. What is already clear is that gene testing is a double-edged sword and, for this reason alone, clinical geneticists must remain central to care of such patients.

Despite our incomplete knowledge, some public health experts believe the case for ovarian cancer prevention clinics has been made.[66] In general terms, however, it should not be forgotten that hereditary cancer syndromes are rare, and that, although any advances in their diagnosis and treatment might have a big impact on the lives of the individuals affected, the effect on cancer death rates overall is likely to be very small. Given that for the general female population lung cancer is now the commonest cause of cancer death, reducing the prevalence of cigarette smoking is likely to be the simplest and most effective measure for the prevention of cancer for some years to come.

## References

1 Mayor S. Cancer is main cause of death in Britain. BMJ 1998; 316: 571

2 Austoker J. Cancer prevention: setting the scene. BMJ 1994; 308: 1415–1420

3 Quinn M, Babb P, Jones J et al. Effect of screening on the incidence of and mortality from cancer of cervix in England: evaluation based on routinely collected statistics. BMJ 1999; 318: 904–908

4 Marks J, Davidoff A M, Kerns B J et al. Over expression of the p53 mutation in ovarian cancer. Cancer Res 1991; 51: 2979–2984

5 Claus E B, Schwartz P E. Familial ovarian cancer. Cancer 1995; 76: 1998–2003

6 Austoker J. Screening for ovarian, prostatic, and testicular cancers. BMJ 1994; 309: 315–320

7 Wilson J M, Junger G. Principles and practice of screening for disease. WHO Public Health Paper. Geneva: WHO, 1968; 34

8 Jacobs I. The impact of molecular genetics in gynaecological cancer. In: Studd J. (ed) Progress in Obstetrics and Gynaecology, vol 13. Edinburgh: Churchill Livingstone, 1997; 421

9 Wilcke J T. Late onset genetic disease: where ignorance is bliss, is it folly to inform relatives? BMJ 1998; 317: 744–747

10 Lynch H T, Krush A J. Carcinoma of the breast and ovary in three families. Surg Gynecol Obstet J 1971; 133: 644–648

11 Ford D, Easton D F, Peto J. Estimates of the gene frequency of BRCA1 and its contribution to breast and ovarian cancer incidence. Am J Hum Genet 1995; 57: 1457–1462

12 Miki Y, Swensen J, Shattuck-Eidens D et al. A strong candidate for the breast and ovarian cancer susceptibility gene BRCA1. Science 1994; 266: 66–71

13 Wooster R, Bignell G, Lancaster J et al. Identification of the breast cancer susceptibility gene BRCA2. Nature 1995; 378: 789–792

14 Fitzgerald M G, Macdonald D J, Krainer M et al. Germ-line BRCA1 mutation in Jewish and non-Jewish women with early-onset breast cancer. N Engl J Med 1996; 334: 143–149

15 Ford D, Easton D F, Stratton M et al. Genetic heterogeneity and penetrance analysis of the BRCA1 and BRCA2 genes in breast cancer families. Am J Hum Genet 1998; 62: 676–689

16 Gayther S A, Warren W, Mazoyer S et al. Germline mutations of BRCA1 in breast/ovary cancer families: evidence for a genotype/phenotype correlation. Nat Genet 1995; 11: 428–433

17 Easton D F, Ford D, Bishop D T, The Breast Cancer Linkage Consortium. Breast and ovarian cancer incidence in BRCA1 mutation carriers. Am J Hum Genet 1995; 56: 265–271

18 Burke W, Daly M, Garber J et al. Recommendations for follow-up care of individuals with an inherited predisposition to cancer II: BRCA1 and BRCA2. JAMA 1997; 277: 997–1003

19 Ford D, Easton D F. The genetics of breast and ovarian cancer. Br J Cancer 1995; 72: 805–812

20 Cummings S R, Norton L, Eckert D et al. Raloxifene reduces the risk of breast cancer and may decrease the risk of endometrial cancer in postmenopausal women. JAMA 1999; 281: 2189–2197

21 Alexander F E, Anderson T J, Brown H K et al. 14 years of follow-up from the Edinburgh randomised trial of breast cancer screening. Lancet 1999; 353: 1903–1908

22 Hartman L C, Schaid D J, Lods J E et al. Efficacy of bilateral mastectomy in women with a family history of breast cancer. N Engl J Med 1999; 340: 77–84

23 Fentiman I S. Prophylactic mastectomy: deliverance or delusion? BMJ 1998; 317: 1402–1403

24 Rubin S C, Benjamin I, Behbakht K et al. Clinical and pathological features of ovarian cancer in women with germline mutations of BRCA1. N Engl J Med 1996; 335: 1413–1416

25 Hankinson S E, Colditz G A, Hunter D, Spencer T L, Rosner B, Stampfer M J. A quantitative reassessment of oral contraceptive use and risk of ovarian cancer. Obstet Gynecol 1992; 80: 708–714

26 Narod S A. Risch H, Moslehi R et al. Oral contraceptives and the risk of hereditary ovarian cancer. N Engl J Med 1998; 339: 424–428

27 Kerlikowske K, Brown J S, Grady D G. Should women with familial ovarian cancer undergo prophylactic oophorectomy? Obstet Gynecol 1992; 80: 700–707

28 Tobacman J K, Greene M H, Tucker M A, Costa J, Kase R, Fraumeni Jr J F. Intra-abdominal carcinomatosis after prophylactic oophorectomy in ovarian-cancer-prone families. Lancet 1982; ii: 795–797

29 NIH Consensus Development Panel on Ovarian Cancer. Screening, treatment and follow-up. JAMA 1995; 273: 491–497

30 Beral V, Collaborative Group on Hormonal Factors in Breast Cancer. Breast cancer and HRT: collaborative re-analysis of data from 51 epidemiological studies of 52705 women with breast cancer and 108411 women without breast cancer. Lancet 1997; 350: 1047–1059

31 Kasprzak L, Foulkes W, Shelling A. Hereditary ovarian carcinoma. BMJ 1999; 318: 786–789

32 Lynch H T, Casey M J, Lynch J, White T E K, Godwin A K. Genetics and ovarian carcinoma. Semin Oncol 1998; 25: 265–281

33 Jacobs I. Screening for ovarian cancer – a pilot randomised controlled trial. Lancet 1999; 353: 1207–1210

34 Ford D, Easton D F, Bishop D T, Narod S A, Goldgar D E, The Breast Cancer Linkage Consortium. Risks of cancer in BRCA1 mutation carriers. Lancet 1994; 343: 6920–695

35 Pal T, Flanders T, Mitchell-Lehman M et al. Genetic implications of double primary cancers of the colorectum and endometrium. J Med Genet 1998; 35: 978–984

36 Aarnio M, Mecklin J P, Aaltonen L A et al. Lifetime risk of different cancers in hereditary nonpolyposis colorectal cancer (HNPCC) syndrome. Int J Cancer 1995; 64: 430–433

37 Aaltonen L A, Salovaara R, Kristo P et al. Incidence of hereditary nonpolyposis colorectal cancer and the feasibility of molecular screening. N Engl J Med 1998; 338: 1481–1487

38 Aarnio M, Mecklin J P, Aaltonen L A et al. Lifetime risk of different cancers in hereditary nonpolyposis colorectal cancer (HNPCC) syndrome. Int J Cancer 1995; 64: 430–433

39 Lynch H T, Lanspa S J, Boman B M et al. Hereditary nonpolyposis colon cancer – Lynch syndromes I and II. Gastroenterol Clin North Am 1988; 17: 679–712

40 Burke W, Petersen G, Lynch P et al. Recommendations for follow-up care of individuals with an inherited predisposition to cancer: I. Hereditary nonpolyposis colon cancer. JAMA 1997; 277: 915–919

41 Ferruci J F. Screening for colon cancer: programs of the American College of radiology. Am J Radiol 1993; 160: 999–1003

42 Charatan F B. US recommends screening for colon cancer. BMJ 1997; 314: 396

43 Vasen H F, Nagengast F M, Meera Khan P. Interval cancers in HNPCC. Lancet 1995; 345: 1183–1184

44 Giardello F M, Hamilton S R, Krush A J et al. Treatment of colonic and rectal adenomas with sulindac in familial adenomatous polyposis. N Engl J Med 1993; 328: 1313–1316

45  Watson P, Lynch H T. Extracolonic cancer in HNPCC. Cancer 1993; 71: 677–685

46  Van den Bosch T, van den Vael A, van Schouboreck D et al. Combining vaginal ultrasonography and office endometrial sampling in the diagnosis of endometrial disease in postmenopausal. Obstet Gynecol 1995; 85: 349–352

47  Marra G, Boland C R. Hereditary nonpolyposis colorectal cancer. J Natl Cancer Inst 1995; 87: 1114–1125

48  Polson D W, Wadsworth J, Adams J, Franks S. Polycystic ovaries – a common finding in normal women. Lancet 1988; i: 870–872

49  Fox R. Polycystic ovarian disease and insulin resistance: pathophysiology and wider health issues. In: Studd J. (ed) Progress in Obstetrics and Gynaecology, vol 11. Edinburgh: Churchill Livingstone, 1995; 341

50  Hague W, Adams J, Reeders S, Peto T E, Jacobs H S. Familial polycystic ovaries: a genetic disease. Clin Endocrinol 1988; 29: 593–606

51  Fox R. Prevalence of a positive family history of type 2 diabetes in women with PCOD. Gynecol Endocrinol 1999; 13: 390–392

52  Schildkraut J M, Schwingl P J, Bastos E, Evanoff A, Hughes C. Epithelial ovarian cancer risk among women with polycystic ovary syndrome. Obstet Gynecol 1996; 88: 554–559

53  Pierpoint T, McKeigue P M, Isaacs A J, Wild S H, Jacobs H S. Mortality in women with polycystic ovary syndrome. J Clin Epidemiol 1998; 51: 581–586

54  Kaaks R. Nutrition, hormones and breast cancer: is insulin the missing link? Cancer Control 1996; 7: 569–571

55  Fox R, Wardle P G, Clarke L, Hull M G R. Acromegaloid bone changes in severe polycystic ovarian disease: an effect of hyperinsulinaemia? Br J Obstet Gynaecol 1991; 98: 410–411

56  Barbieri R L, Ryan K J. Hyperandrogenism, insulin resistance and acanthosis nigricans. Am J Obstet Gynecol 1983; 147: 90–101

57  Jenkins P J, Fairclough P D, Richards T et al. Acromegaly, colonic polyps and carcinoma. Clin Endocrinol 1997; 47: 17–22

58  Albanes D. Energy balance, body size and cancer. Crit Rev Oncol Hematol 1990; 10: 283–303

59  Hutchison J R, Taylor H B, Zimmerman E A. The Stein-Leventhal syndrome and coincident ovarian neoplasms. Obstet Gynecol 1966; 28 700–703

60  Babaknia A, Calfopoulos P, Jones H W. The Stein-Leventhal syndrome and coincidental ovarian tumours. Obstet Gynecol 1976; 47: 223–224

61  Jackson R L, Dockerty M D. The Stein-Leventhal syndrome: analysis of 43 cases with reference to association with endometrial cancer. Am J Obstet Gynecol 1957; 73: 161–173

62  Fox R. Polycystic ovarian disease: ultrasound and endocrine studies. MD Thesis, University of Bristol. 1992

63  Nagamani M, Hannigan E V, Dinh T V, Stuart C A. Hyperinsulinaemia and stromal luteinisation of the ovaries in postmenopausal women with endometrial cancer. J Clin Endocrinol Metab 1988; 67: 144–148

64  Randolph J F, Kipersztok S, Ayers J W, Ansbacher R, Peegal H, Menon K M. The effect of insulin on aromatase activity in isolated human endometrial glands and stroma. Am J Obstet Gynecol 1987; 157: 1534–1539

65  Fox R, Eckford S, Hirschowitz L, Browning J J, Lindop G. Refractory gestational hypertension due to a renin-secreting ovarian fibrothecoma associated with Gorlin's syndrome. Br J Obstet Gynaecol 1994; 101: 1015–1016

66  Campbell H, Mackay J, Porteous M. The future of ovarian cancer clinics: no longer research – now a clinical need. BMJ 1995; 311: 1584–1585

**23**

*John Bidmead  Linda D. Cardozo*

# Surgery for genuine stress incontinence

Stress incontinence is a distressing symptom that has a major impact on a woman's quality of life. It has proved difficult to accurately establish its true incidence; however, even the most conservative estimate is that one in ten women will suffer from genuine stress incontinence (GSI) at some time. In the past, many women have suffered in silence, accepting incontinence as an inevitable consequence of childbearing and ageing. This situation has now changed dramatically; more women are coming forward requesting treatment at an earlier stage anticipating prompt and effective management.

In recent years the management of women with GSI has undergone a number of significant changes: new types of surgical treatment are being developed which aim to offer good long-term results with reduced hospital stay and a quicker return to normal activity.

This article outlines some of the changes that have taken place in recent years and the alternatives to traditional surgery for stress incontinence which are being developed.

## PATHOPHYSIOLOGY

Genuine stress incontinence is defined as the involuntary loss of urine when the intravesical pressure exceeds the intra-urethral pressure in the absence of detrusor activity.[1]

The exact pathophysiology of GSI remains unclear. A number of theories have been proposed to explain the mechanism although, with a condition as widespread as GSI, it is probable that no single theory will account for all cases.

**Mr John Bidmead** MBBS MRCOG, Subspecialty Trainee in Urogynaecology, Department of Urogynaecology, King's College Hospital, 8 Devonshire Place, London W1N 1PB, UK

**Prof. Linda D. Cardozo** MD FRCOG, Professor of Urogynaecology, King's College School of Medicine and Dentistry, Denmark Hill, London SE5 8RX, Consultant Gynaecologist, King's College Hospital, 8 Devonshire Place London W1N 1PB, UK (for correspondence)

Enhorning proposed that GSI resulted from displacement of the bladder neck from within the intra-abdominal pressure zone. Some doubt has been cast on this by a number of authorities including Enhorning himself.[2]

The action of the pubo-urethral ligaments and endopelvic fascia in supporting the urethra, thereby allowing effective transmission of intra-abdominal pressure rises, has been proposed by DeLancey[3] and Zacharin.[4] Both suggest that the connective tissue supporting the urethra and bladder neck acts as a 'hammock', supporting the urethra and allowing effective transmission of intra-abdominal pressure.

The role of the urethral sphincter mechanism in maintaining continence during raised intra-abdominal pressure is unclear, although the intrinsic sphincter certainly contributes to the overall maintenance of continence. Blavais and Olsen have suggested a classification of GSI, dividing it into three types:[5] type I, where there is hypermobility of the bladder neck; type II, where bladder neck hypermobility is less marked and urethral sphincter failure more apparent; and type III, where the urethra is fixed with failure of the intrinsic sphincter. In practice, a fixed scarred urethra is usually seen only after previous surgery or radiotherapy and the majority of cases of primary GSI form a spectrum consisting of a variable combination of poor bladder neck support and impaired urethral sphincter function.

The exact pathophysiology of GSI remains unknown, although the failure of pressure transmission theory remains the most popular. To a certain extent, this is supported by the success of bladder neck repositioning techniques. However, the fact that retropubic operations are effective does not necessarily imply a pathophysiological mechanism.

## MANAGEMENT

Conservative management should be the first line of treatment in any age group. It has few complications, it in no way compromises future surgery and it may even enhance the results of surgical treatment. It is unreasonable to resort to surgical management of what is, after all, a non-life-threatening condition without a trial of conservative therapy. Conservative management is also appropriate in women who are too frail or medically unfit for surgery, for women who have not completed childbearing and for 6 months post partum or during breast feeding.

Pelvic floor physiotherapy with or without the use of electrical stimulation is the mainstay of conservative management of GSI. Many studies have shown excellent results, although it is clear that closely monitored therapy by a physiotherapist, interested and experienced in this area, is necessary. Vague instructions to 'do pelvic floor exercises' are ineffective and may be counterproductive. At least 30% of women are unable to perform these exercises correctly without tuition.[6] Gardner and Fonda[7] state that urinary incontinence in an older age group of patients can be cured or significantly improved in 60% of cases with conservative measures. Unfortunately, this fact is often ignored. Dougherty et al[8] showed that 16 weeks of pelvic floor exercise produced a significant improvement in urinary incontinence.

The use of prosthetic devices in the management of GSI is a relatively recent innovation. A number of devices are available some intra-urethral, others intravaginal or occlusive. They can be valuable in the conservative management of women who do not wish, or are unfit for, surgical intervention or whilst awaiting surgery. Such devices may allow women to return to a normal level of activity or sport without resorting to surgery. There is now a wide range of continence devices from which to choose; they may not suit all women but, nevertheless, they are a valuable addition to the range of therapeutic options.

## SURGICAL TECHNIQUES FOR TREATMENT

As outlined above, two main types of pathology are thought to contribute to genuine stress incontinence; namely urethral hypermobility and intrinsic sphincter deficiency.[9] Both conditions may exist in the same woman.[10] In those women with urethral hypermobility, operations that re-position the bladder neck, such as the retropubic urethropexies, needle suspensions, sling procedures and anterior colporrhaphy will have a high success rate, at least initially.[11]

In women with mainly intrinsic sphincter deficiency, the defect is not in urethral pressure transmission but due to poor urethral closure which results from scarring from previous surgery, childbirth or neurological injury. Maximal urethra closure pressure may be low.[12] In these women, operations to re-position the bladder neck are likely to have a higher failure rate as the bladder neck may already be optimally positioned.[13] In this situation, procedures to enhance urethral sphincter function, such as peri-urethral bulking agents and slings (perhaps tensioned so as to be more obstructive than where there is urethral hypermobility) would be more appropriate.

In addition, the expectations, physical activity and medical fitness of a woman are also important factors. Needle suspension or peri-urethral injection may be appropriate for a frail 80-year-old, but give poor long-term results in a 40-year-old who wishes to take aerobics classes again. There is clearly a need to tailor the available surgical techniques to suit each individual woman.

Over 150 operative procedures for treatment of stress incontinence have been described. While many of these are modifications of similar interventions, the fact that so many variations have been described reflects uncertainty over the most effective surgical treatment of this condition.

The situation was clarified when Jarvis examined published results of various continence operations in a meta-analysis in 1994,[14] the results of which are summarised in Table 1.

**Table 1**  Objective cure rates for first procedure and recurrent incontinence

| Procedure | Mean (%) first procedure | Mean (%) recurrent incontinence |
|---|---|---|
| Bladder buttress | 67.8 | Not available |
| Marshall-Marchetti Krantz | 89.5 | Not available |
| Burch colposuspension | 89.8 | 82.5 |
| Bladder neck suspension | 86.7 | 86.4 |
| Slings | 93.9 | 86.1 |
| Injectables | 45.5 | 57.8 |

From Jarvis 1994.[14]

| Procedure | Cure rate at 24–47 months(%) | Cure at over 48 months (%) | *De novo* postoperative urgency (%) | Voiding difficulties (%) |
|---|---|---|---|---|
| Retropubic suspensions | 84 | 84 | 11 | 5 |
| Transvaginal suspensions | 65 | 67 | 5 | 5 |
| Anterior repair | 85 | 61 | Not available | Not available |
| Sling procedures | 82 | 83 | 8 | 8 |

Following this meta-analysis and a further systematic review by Black and Downs in 1996,[15] it became clear that a suprapubic approach to bladder neck elevation gave improved results compared to a vaginal repair combined with a buttress procedure. Alternative techniques still have a place in management of GSI. Injectables may be useful where the urethra is scarred and fixed or in patients for whom low operative morbidity is a priority. The same is also true for needle suspension procedures. Suburethral sling operations give good results in both primary and secondary incontinence; but, due to their higher complication rates, they are most often reserved for recurrent incontinence.

The American Urological Association also published a report on surgical management of female stress urinary incontinence.[16] This was a further review of published series and re-inforces the results of the studies by Jarvis and by Black, Retropubic suspensions and slings appear to give better success rates compared to anterior vaginal repair and needle suspension procedures. The results of this report are summarised in Table 2.

## THE PLACE OF PRE-OPERATIVE URODYNAMIC INVESTIGATION

Controversy still surrounds the need for urodynamic assessment prior to surgery and some gynaecologists and urologists are prepared to undertake surgery without prior investigation. While it is reasonable to offer a short trial of conservative therapy based on clinical history and examination it would be unwise to undertake **any** major surgical intervention without thorough pre-operative investigation and evaluation. Surgical treatment of GSI should be no exception to this rule.

Although urodynamics are not perfect they remain the mainstay of urodynamic diagnosis. Jarvis demonstrated that an experienced clinician made the correct urodynamic diagnosis only 65% of the time when relying on clinical history and examination alone.[17] The symptom of stress incontinence may be produced by detrusor instability in the absence of anatomical disorder; bladder neck surgery will not lead to any improvement in symptoms and is in fact likely to worsen the underlying detrusor instability.

The presence of detrusor instability pre-operatively has been shown to have a major impact on the success of colposuspension. Stanton et al demonstrated a significantly reduced cure rate in such patients compared to those with genuine stress incontinence, (43% compared to 83%).

Khullar et al have suggested that ambulatory urodynamics detect a greater proportion of patients with detrusor instability pre-operatively.[18] Using this technique it was possible to detect DI in 30% of patients with a laboratory diagnosis of GSI prior to colposuspension. Postoperatively, all these patients developed irritative bladder symptoms.

Where detrusor instability and urethral sphincter incompetence co-exist, it is the current practice in the urogynaecology department at Kings College to treat detrusor instability, before surgery, using anticholinergic medication and to re-assess urodynamically once irritative bladder symptoms are controlled, before considering surgical treatment of stress incontinence.

Pre-operative urodynamic studies also allow the assessment and prediction of voiding dysfunction. This allows adequate preparation of women at high risk of postoperative voiding difficulties; counselling can be provided and clean intermittent self catheterisation (CISC), taught prior to surgery.

While clinical diagnosis may often be correct in detecting GSI, the value of pre-operative urodynamics in helping to predict outcome and prevent inappropriate surgery is undeniable. Both clinically and medico-legally, it is becoming increasingly difficult to justify surgical intervention without thorough urodynamic investigation.

## FACTORS AFFECTING THE OUTCOME OF SURGERY

Some factors are important in predicting outcomes in all types of surgery. Monga and Stanton[19] demonstrated that a MUCP of less then 20 cm water predicted a worse outcome, but only in those patients with previous failed continence surgery.

Age appears to have an influence on the failure rate of continence procedures in general. Hilton showed a decrease in success with increasing age likely to be due to atrophic tissue changes with poorer healing, combined with the normal loss of urethral closure pressure that occurs with age. These changes may be partly reversible with preoperative oestrogen replacement.

The tensile strength of collagen may also influence the results of surgery. Those patients with weaker collagen are likely to have earlier failure. Currently, interest in collagen status is growing, but it is not possible to predict results based on collagen biopsy at present.

## IMPORTANCE OF THE PRIMARY PROCEDURE

When examining the results of all operations used for GSI, it becomes clear that the highest success rates are found with primary procedures. (Slings are a possible exception to this rule as most of the case series of sling techniques concern their use in recurrent incontinence.) There is an increased risk of postoperative detrusor instability with successive operations, presumably due to increased denervation. Complication rates rise as, with each successive operation, dissection becomes more difficult and wound infections and haematoma formation become more likely. Sphincter function may be adversely affected by denervation. This is not to say that secondary surgery cannot have reasonable success rates, but it is clear that a woman's best chance of long-term cure is with the first operation. In the light of this, it is no longer appropriate to perform an operation with lower morbidity, such as an anterior colporrhaphy, first, then proceed to a needle suspension and finally when this fails to attempt a sling procedure.

The first operation performed should be that which offers the greatest chance of long-term cure.

## MEASUREMENT OF SURGICAL OUTCOME

One of the difficulties of assessing any continence procedure has been the choice of a suitable outcome measure. Obtaining data on objective cure rates requires invasive investigations such as urodynamics which, although vital in clinical studies, are impractical in the majority of women undergoing routine surgery. However, subjective cure rates may not give an accurate picture of the efficacy of a particular technique.

A useful method of assessing outcomes, which has recently gained some popularity, is in measuring the effect of a procedure on quality of life before and after incontinence surgery with the means of validated and disease-specific quality of life questionnaires.[20] This allows relatively easy collection of a women's own assessment of subjective results in a standardised form. Assessment of the result of surgery for GSI is complicated, simple cure of stress leakage is not sufficient as the occurrence of postoperative voiding problems and urinary urgency and frequency may have a profound influence on the outcome of surgery. Objective testing in the form of videocysto-urethrography (VCU), which is the current 'gold standard' objective measure or by using standardised Pad tests can provide objective evidence of cure. However VCU is a somewhat blunt instrument and it is acknowledged that the results of VCU and symptoms may not always correlate.[21]

Subjective results, in the form of a woman's symptoms recorded by the surgeon, have, therefore, formed an additional source of information regarding the outcome of surgery. There are a number of obvious flaws in this method of assessing subjective results. Women may feel inhibited discussing the outcome of recent surgery with the surgeon who undertook the operation and may report the absence of symptoms when this is not the case. Surgeons, on the other hand, may tend to interpret results over optimistically.

## WHO SHOULD PERFORM SURGERY?

A recent study undertaken by Black et al involved 38 gynaecologists and 11 urologists in the North Thames region from 18 units, using four different operations and in a group of women who may or may not have had pre-operative urodynamic assessment.[22,23] A total of 442 women having surgery for stress incontinence were recruited over an 18-month period. Pre-operative and postoperative data were obtained both from surgeons and women themselves. The results of this survey showed a marked discrepancy between previously reported results and the reports of women in the study, only 28% of whom reported subjective cure. It was also apparent that surgeon's perception of results differed from those of their patients, surgeons considered the outcome successful in 85% of cases. Each surgeon will, on average, have operated on 9 women over the 18-month period.

Results appear to be better after thorough pre-operative assessment, by surgeons with special interest and training in this area and in a unit where appropriately trained, experienced and motivated staff are available to provide support as part of a multidisciplinary team. Throughout medicine, there is now growing recognition that concentration of treatment in sub-specialist units, with appropriate facilities and ancillary staff, gives the opportunity to improve outcomes in many areas. The treatment of stress incontinence, a benign condition, but one that has a major impact on the lives of many women, appears to be an area where treatment in special interest units can markedly improve the outcome. It is, therefore, questionable whether continued management of this condition by generalist gynaecologists and urologists is in the best interests of women. In the light of this, it important that any unit performing surgery for GSI has a regular audit of the results of surgery and should be able to give women an up-to-date estimate of the results of surgery in that unit and not those extrapolated from published series.

## ECONOMIC ASPECTS OF SURGERY

In the current climate of the National Health Service, economic, as well as clinical, considerations apply to the selection of procedure for GSI. The cost-benefit relationship of any procedure needs to be taken closely into account before a new operation is adopted. A number of factors come into play; the cost of disposable equipment versus the cost of re-sterilisation is a particular area of interest in relation to minimal access surgery. Operating time is also expensive and long procedures may not be economically justifiable. The increased costs of hospital in-patient treatment, however, act strongly in favour of procedures with a minimal in-patient stay. The economic impact of any treatment to society in terms of the length of time that a woman is unable to work or look after her family following operative treatment is also an important consideration. This aspect of laparoscopic surgery has also generated much discussion, Kholi et al found that, despite a shorter in-patient stay, costs of laparoscopic procedures were higher than a traditional approach.[24]

However, the cost of unsuccessful continence surgery to society in terms of a woman's reduced capacity to work or look after her family as well as the cost of continence pads and, not least, the effect of reduced quality of life on a woman's family and relationships should not be forgotten. Berman and Kreder carried out an economic analysis of peri-urethral injection of collagen compared to sling insertion in 1997.[25] They found that sling surgery was more expensive, at $10,382, than peri-urethral injection of collagen, at $4,996 per case. Despite this, the cure rates of 71.4% and 27.7%, respectively, made sling surgery far more cost-effective.

Lastly, the cost of any necessary further treatment, medical or surgical, which results from failure or complications of surgery need to be taken into account. The high costs of repeated surgery, incontinence pads and long-term anti-cholinergic medication mean that relatively minor differences in efficacy and cost of primary surgical techniques may assume much greater economic importance.

## SURGICAL TECHNIQUES

### Retropubic cyto-urethropexies (MMK and Burch colposuspension)

A suprapubic approach to surgical elevation of the bladder neck was first described by Marshall-Marchetti and Krantz in 1949.[26] This was initially reported in incontinent male patients following radical prostatectomy. The retropubic space is entered via a low transverse suprapubic incision. the urethra and bladder neck are dissected free and sutures taken to include the para-urethral tissues, urethral wall and attached to the periosteum of the superior ramus.

Subjective cure rates of 90% have been reported but objective cure rates may be lower.

The major complication of the Marshall-Marchetti Krantz procedure is osteitis pubis with a reported frequency of 5–7%. Due to the problem of osteitis pubis and the technical difficulty of retaining sutures in the periosteum, Burch[27] described an alternative retropubic approach in 1961.

Burch suggested that the urethra and bladder could be supported by elevation of the paravaginal tissue to the ipsilateral ileopectineal ligament and this technique, after modification, has become widely used today (Fig. 1). Two to four sutures of no. 1 PDS (polyglycolic acid) or Ethibond are inserted into the para-vaginal fascia. These are then inserted into the ipsilateral ileopectineal ligament. The initial suture is placed at the level of the bladder neck and subsequent sutures about 1 cm proximal. Once all the sutures have been positioned, each lateral fornix is elevated allowing the sutures to be tied without tension (Fig. 2), it is the practice of some surgeons to leave these sutures quite lax.[28]

### Postoperative complications

Voiding difficulties are not uncommon following Burch colposuspension. They are particularly common in patients with flow rates of less than 15 ml/s or

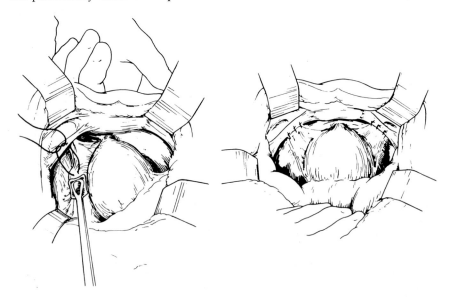

**Fig. 1** While the vaginal fornix is elevated, sutures are placed in the paravaginal fascia and secured to the ileopectineal ligaments.

**Fig. 2** When the sutures on each side have been placed, the vagina is elevated and the sutures tied. From Stanton S L, Tanagho E A. (eds) Surgery of Female Incontinence, 2nd edn. Heidelberg: Springer, 1986; with permission.

maximum voiding detrusor pressure below 15 cmH$_2$O. Between 12–25% of women are reported to suffer delayed voiding postoperatively and 11–20% have increased residual volumes and reduced flow rates when measured at 3 months postoperatively.[29] In a recent study by Smith and Cardozo[30] of 100 women undergoing colposuspension, 21% experienced significant voiding difficulties for up to 6 months following their surgery, although this persisted beyond 6 months in only 2% in women identified pre-operatively as likely to suffer voiding problems.

Hilton and Stanton[31] performed postoperative urodynamic studies on women 3 months after colposuspension and found highly significant reduced flow rates and increased voiding pressure.

Enterocele and rectocele formation is thought to occur as a result of elevation of the anterior vaginal wall creating a posterior defect and causing intra-abdominal pressure to be transmitted directly to the posterior vaginal wall. The incidence of postoperative posterior compartment defects is estimated to be 7–17%.[32] It is not clear whether these represent new defects or merely a pre-existing defect becoming symptomatic once the support of the anterior vaginal wall has been rectified.

### *De novo* detrusor instability

It has been shown that detrusor instability arises de novo in 12–18.5% of women postoperatively.[33] It occurs more commonly following previous contin-ence surgery. It seems likely that a number of cases reflect pre-existing detrusor instability not detected at cystometry pre-operatively. In addition, it has been suggested that damage to the autonomic nerve supply occurs during lateral displacement of the bladder at operation.[34]

### Results of Burch colposuspension

Burch originally reported success rates of 100%; however, objective cure rates determined on the basis of postoperative urodynamic testing are usually lower. Hilton and Stanton[35] reported a 90% objective cure rate and Stanton and Cardozo[36] and Galloway[37] an 84% cure rate. A comparison of published results is shown in Table 3.

A recent prospective study of colposuspension after previous failed surgery demonstrated a 79% objective cure rate at 9 months compared to a 96% objective

Table 3  Objective results of colposuspension

| Reference | No. of patients | Continent (%) | Follow-up (months) |
|---|---|---|---|
| Stanton and Cardozo 1979[29] | 25 | 84 | 4 |
| Mundy 1983[38] | 26 | 73 | 12 |
| Stanton 1984[39] | 60 | 83 | 12 |
| Galloway 1987[37] | 50 | 84 | 6 |
| Stanton 1976[40] | 32 | 80 | 6–30 |
| Milani 1985[41] | 44 | 79 | > 12 |
| Cardozo and Cutner 1992[42] | 100 | 80 | 6-12 |
| Herbertsson 1993[43] | 72 | 90.3 | 84–144 |
| Jarvis meta-analysis 1994[14] | 2300 | 84.3 | > 12 |

**Table 4** Results of colposuspension as a secondary procedure

| Reference | Objectively continent (%) | Follow-up (months) |
|---|---|---|
| Stanton 1984[39] | 65 | 60 |
| Galloway 1987[37] | 63 | 54 |
| Stanton and Cardozo 1979[40] | 77 | 12 |
| Jarvis meta-analysis 1994[14] | 82.5 | > 12 |
| Cardozo 1999[44] | 79 | 9 |

cure rate for women having a primary procedure performed in the same unit by the same surgeon.[44] The complication rates and percentages of women with postoperative voiding difficulties were not significantly different. This demonstrates that primary procedures give higher success rates but also that colposuspension is still useful as a secondary procedure (Table 4).

## Laparoscopic colposuspension

As laparoscopic surgery has become increasingly used in gynaecological practice, interest in the use of this technique has grown. In theory, a laparoscopic colposuspension should provide the long-term success rates of an open colposuspension with low morbidity and short in-patient stay. If this were possible, it would prove attractive to patient, surgeon and manager alike.

A number of variations in technique have been described using an extra-peritoneal approach or a transperitoneal approach. The use of standard suture materials or clips and prolene or mersilene mesh have also been described. Extensive discussion of the techniques of laparoscopic colposuspension is beyond the scope of this chapter.

Many authors have reported results of laparoscopic colposuspension, Liu[45] in particular has reported results of 107 patients with a 97% short-term cure rates. However, only two randomised trials comparing laparoscopic and open approaches have been published to date. A randomised trial by Su et al[46] examined objective success rates at one year and demonstrated a statistically significant difference. The study showed an 84% cure with laparoscopic colposuspension and a 95.6% cure with traditional colposuspension. However, the longest running randomised trial of laparoscopic versus open colpo-suspension by Burton[47] shows a disappointing 40% failure rate in the laparo-scopic group compared to 15% in the open group after 3 years (Table 5).

**Table 5** Short to medium term results of laparoscopic colposuspension

| Reference | Cure at 3 months (%) | Cure at 12 months (%) | Cure at over 2 years (%) |
|---|---|---|---|
| Lobel and Sand | 89 | 86 | 69 |
| Ross[48] | 98 | 93 | 89 |
| Burton[47] | 73 | Not available | 60 |
| Su[46] | 80 | Not available | Not available |

## Complications of laparoscopic colposuspension

Operative morbidity has been extensively studied, intra-operative blood loss appears similar although febrile morbidity and length of hospital stay are both higher in the open colposuspension group.[49]

The incidence of urinary tract injury is higher with the laparoscopic approach. Published series are few, but two reports of ureteric injury (a very unusual occurrence at open surgery with only 15 cases reported in the literature[50]), suggest that the risk of lower urinary tract injury may be much greater with a laparoscopic approach.[51,52]

The major drawback of minimal access techniques is the relatively long learning curve taken to gain proficiency in order to be able to perform laparoscopic Burch colposuspension. While laparoscopic colposuspension offers some promise for reducing operative morbidity, it has yet to be shown that it offers an acceptable alternative to an open procedure and further evaluation with a register of surgeons performing the technique has been proposed.[53]

At present, although laparoscopic colposuspension appears to offer low morbidity and early return to work, the poorer long-term results and higher rate of urinary tract injury suggest that the open approach remains preferable. However, as more surgeons with previous experience in incontinence surgery are adopting a laparoscopic approach, objective cure rates appear to improve suggesting that the skills required are those of both an experienced laparoscopic surgeon together with experience of open incontinence procedures.

At the time of writing, a large multi-centre randomised trial of laparoscopic and open colposuspension funded by the MRC is underway. This will eventually provide definitive evidence of the role of laparoscopic surgery in this area.

## Slings

Sling procedures with many different modifications have been used for almost 100 years in the treatment of female incontinence. Initially, strips of fascia and muscle were used to compress the urethra.[54-57] In 1942, Aldridge described his sling procedure, which can be recognised as the predecessor of modern sling techniques.[58] Aldridge proposed that his technique should be used as a primary technique, in women where previous surgery had failed and, particularly, where sphincter function was compromised.[59] Since Aldridge's description, a number of modifications have been described. The common feature of sling operations is the use of a strip of material, which is passed completely beneath the urethra or bladder neck and anchored to a point on the abdominal wall

Sling insertion, utilising a combined vaginal and abdominal approach, a vaginal approach alone or a suprapubic technique alone, with blind dissection beneath the urethra and bladder base, have all been described. However, there is no definitive evidence to suggest which surgical approach is superior; it is the choice of material and tension which appear to most influence the outcome of sling surgery (Fig. 3).

## Sling materials

The Aldridge sling requires a large abdominal incision and creation of a defect in the rectus fascia, which increases the surgical morbidity. In addition, women

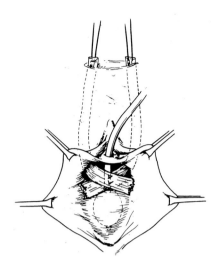

**Fig. 3** Suburethral sling. Strips of fascia or synthetic material are passed beneath the bladder neck and attached to the rectus aponeurosis. From Hurt W G. (ed) Urogynaecologic Surgery. London: Aspen, 1993; with permission.

with stress incontinence may have connective tissue that is inherently weak leading to poorer long-term results.[60,61] Previous abdominal surgery may also cause difficulty in obtaining a sufficient length of good quality undamaged fascia from this site.

### Natural sling materials

To circumvent the problems of using abdominal wall fascia, use of a strip of autologous fascia lata was proposed by Price in 1933.[62] Fascia lata can be obtained in an 18–20 cm long strip, with the use of a fascial stripper and is thicker and stronger than abdominal aponeurosis. However, a second operative site is created with a concomitant increase in operative morbidity. The operative time is also increased, as fascia must be first harvested and prepared before proceeding with colporrhaphy and sling insertion.[63]

Allogenic fascia provides similar results to autologous grafts without the donor site morbidity and potential complications associated with intra-operative harvesting of the graft and good results have been reported using these materials.[64,65] Allografts are either fresh frozen or freeze-dried, both of which effectively destroy their antigenicity.[66] To minimise the risk of viral infection, graft material is sterilised and processed reducing the graft to an acellular fibrous mesh and inactivating any viral agents. The risk of HIV transmission from soft tissue allografts has been estimated at 1 in $8 \times 10^6$.[67]

Porcine dermis has also been described as an alternative allogenic sling material[68,69] and Lyodura, (homologous lyophilized dura mater) has been used with comparable results to other natural sling materials.[70,71] As with human fascia lata, the process of preservation and sterilisation renders the tissue non-immunogenic and should destroy any viral particles.

### Synthetic sling materials

Another approach reducing the complications of graft harvesting has been to use synthetic sling materials. While synthetic materials are easily available, all share the disadvantage of local tissue reaction leading to persistent local infection or erosion.[72]

The use of medical grade Silastic strips, re-inforced with Dacron fibres, has been described by Stanton et al and Korda.[73,74] The Silastic material was reported to produce little fibrosis and subsequent scarring allowing easy removal and revision surgery. However, longer term follow-up shows an 11% incidence of sling erosion and a high rate of de-novo detrusor instability.[75]

Mersilene was first used in vaginal sling surgery in 1962 in the form of a narrow ribbon, but this was discontinued as a result of a high incidence of postoperative obstruction and urethral transection.[76,77] Moir first described the use of a thin, open weave, mesh in 1968.[78] A broad strip of mesh is laid loosely beneath the bladder base and urethra.[79]

Polypropylene mesh ('Marlex' CR Bard) was described by Morgan in 1970.[80] The technique differs slightly from a standard sling in that a broad 'hammock' of mesh is placed beneath the bladder neck and urethra and anchored to Cooper's ligaments rather than the aponeurosis.

Gore-tex was introduced as a synthetic material for suburethral sling procedures as it was relatively inert and has been extensively used as a vascular prosthesis.[81] Good results using Gore-tex have been reported in the short-term,[82] and it has been widely used, particularly in the US. However, it is associated with the highest published erosion and infection rates of any synthetic sling material.

## Results of sling surgery

Assessing the outcomes of sling techniques is complicated as many series consist of women who have undergone, at least one, and in some cases many, previous failed incontinence operations.

Jarvis[14] in a meta-analysis of all surgery for stress incontinence found an objective cure rate of 85.3% and a subjective cure rate of 82.4%. These figures agree closely with the results of the American Urological Association[16] who report an overall subjective cure rate of 82%.

**Table 6** Summary of the results of sling procedures

| Sling material | Author | Primary or secondary surgery | Follow up | Objective cure |
|---|---|---|---|---|
| Autologous rectus fascia | Carr et al[84] | 78% secondary | 22 months | 90% |
| Autologous fascia lata | McLennan et al[85] | 67% secondary | | 87% (subjective) |
| Cadaveric fascia lata | Handa et al[65] | Mixed | 6–12 months | 79% |
| Porcine dermis | Hilton[86] | Secondary | 3 months | 90% |
| Lyodura | Iosif[87] | Mixed | 1–5 years | 92% (subjective) |
| Silastic | Chin & Stanton[75] | 84% secondary | 5 years | 69% |
| Mersilene | Young et al[88] | Mixed | 13 months | 93% |
| Gore-tex | Weinberger & Ostergard[8] | Secondary | 38 months | 61% |
| Marlex | Morgan et al[96] | mixed | 5 years | 77.4% |

Few long-term results of sling techniques are available. The failure of a sling procedure is most likely to become apparent in the first 6 months, and this is probably due to degeneration of fascia or failure of anchoring sutures.[83]

From those long-term studies available, it appears that sling operations successful after 6 months are likely to remain successful for many years (Table 6).

## Voiding difficulties following sling procedures

The relatively high incidence of voiding difficulties following sling surgery has been one of the most significant factors preventing more widespread use of this technique.[90]

Recently, the importance of avoiding excessive sling tension has been recognised[91] There is a trend for slings to be placed under less tension, or even completely loose, and this may reduce the incidence of voiding dysfunction. Appell reports only 2% of women required long-term CISC with fascial slings placed under minimal tension.[92]

## Detrusor instability following sling procedures

Many of the published series relate to a group of women who have undergone numerous previous unsuccessful operations and it has been shown that the incidence of detrusor instability in this group is, in any case, higher than in women undergoing a first operation for genuine stress incontinence.[93] The reported incidence of postoperative symptoms of urge incontinence varies widely, from 3–30%.

## Sling release techniques

Over-elevation of the urethra and bladder neck is associated with a high incidence of voiding difficulties. A number of techniques for avoiding and correcting excessive sling tension have been advocated. Various intra-operative techniques to gauge correct sling tension have been described, including measurement of Q-tip angle, intra-operative UPP and cystoscopy, although there is no convincing evidence that they correctly determine appropriate sling tension. Avoiding excess tension appears to rely mainly on the experience of the surgeon.

When obstruction occurs postoperatively, simple urethral dilation has been suggested which may produce temporary relief but also progressive worsening of the obstruction due to peri-urethral fibrosis.[94,95] Trans-urethral resection[96] or incision of the bladder neck[97] may fail, as the sling is extra-luminal.

Transvaginal urethrolysis has been described[98] and Stanton[99] described transvaginal division of the sling material. Ghoniem et al[100] advanced this by incising the suburethral portion of the sling and then using a patch of vaginal epithelium to reunite the two ends.

## Graft erosion

Problems related to erosion of the sling material, either through the vagina or urethra, appear to be encountered almost exclusively with synthetic sling materials. Although the incidence of such problems is low, graft erosion can pose a formidable management problem with persistent vaginal discharge, vesicovaginal fistula formation and fibrosis and destruction of the urethral sphincter.

Some conclusions can be drawn about the likelihood of such problems and the characteristics of graft materials most likely to lead to erosion. A chronic inflammatory response occurs due to either the inherent tissue reaction of the material itself, or more probably due to chronic infection

Gore-tex has been associated with a high rate of local infection and sling removal of up to 23% in some studies.[101] It appears that its micro-porous structure inhibits in-growth of fibrous tissue and provides inaccessible areas for bacterial colonisation and chronic infection.

Marlex and Mersilene have a large open weave mesh, which allows free in-growth of fibrous tissue. However, non-healing of the vaginal wall appears to be a particular problem with Marlex and is reported as occurring in 7%[102] and 6.2%[103] of cases. Low rates of erosion and mesh removal of 2.5% have been ascribed to the open weave, flexibility and thinness of Mersilene mesh. Estimating the true incidence of synthetic sling related problems is complicated by the fact that many problems related to erosion may not become apparent until relatively late, 1–4 years postoperatively. From those publications available, the incidence of significant problems associated with synthetic materials (excluding Gore-tex) appears to be in the region of 1–6%.

Interestingly, where sling erosion and infection have necessitated resection or division of the sling material, continence is often maintained, re-inforcing the view that it is the lateral fibrosis induced by the sling that provides urethral support rather than the sling material itself.[75]

## The tension free vaginal tape (TVT) procedure

This relatively new technique is based on the premise that stress incontinence results from failure of the pubo-urethral ligaments in the mid-urethra,[104,105] which led to the proposal of 'an integrated theory for the maintenance of female stress incontinence'.[106–108] In this model, continence is maintained at the mid-urethra and not at the bladder neck.

The TVT procedure uses a knitted prolene mesh tape placed at the mid-urethra.[109] The tape is inserted via a small vaginal incision using two 6 mm trochars, due to the weave of the tape it is self-retaining. This can be performed under local or regional anaesthesia, allowing the position of the tape to be adjusted during a series of coughs. The aim is to have the tape lying free at rest (hence 'tension free') and to only exert sufficient pressure on the urethra during a cough to prevent leakage of urine. To date, over 15,000 TVT tapes have been inserted in Europe alone.

Ulmsten[110] reported an 84% cure rate with no long-term voiding difficulties or *de novo* detrusor instability. A multicentre study carried out in six centres in Sweden on women with no previous surgery for incontinence showed a 91% cure rate after one year.[111] The most recent results from Ulmsten et al demonstrate an 86% objective cure after 3 years.[112] Other groups using this device have also begun to report their results with similar outcomes but a relatively high rate (8%) of bladder injury.[113,114] Hilton and Ward have recently published results from 50 women, 40% of whom had previously undergone at

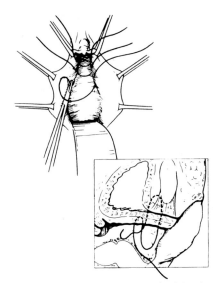

**Fig. 4** Technique of anterior colporrhaphy for GSI From Thompson J D, Rock J A. (eds) TeLinde's Operative Gynaecology, 7th edn. New York: JB Lippincott, 1992; with permission.

least one incontinence operation. Their results show an 88% objective cure rate as a primary procedure and 75% as a secondary procedure; however, 4 women in this study developed long-term voiding difficulties and required CISC.[115]

Currently, large-scale randomised trials comparing the TVT and open colposuspension are underway in the UK and Europe

### Anterior colporrhaphy

Vaginal plastic procedures, the forbears of the modern anterior colporrhaphy, were first described by Schultz as a treatment for anterior vaginal prolapse in 1888[116] and modified by a number of authors, most notably Kelly.[117,118] Kelly described the excision of a portion of anterior vaginal wall and plication of the paravesical tissue, at the bladder neck, and paravaginal fascia as a primary treatment for GSI. This technique was further developed by Pacey in 1949, who described plication of the pubococcygeous and cardinal ligaments to support the bladder and anterior vaginal wall.[119] Until recently, anterior colporrhaphy was widely used as a primary treatment for GSI (Fig. 4).

Bergman et al studied the effect of colposuspension, needle suspension and anterior colporrhaphy and found that, while cure rates were similar at 3 months, there was a marked reduction in the proportion of women remaining cured at 1 year with the anterior repair and needle suspension.[120] Van Geelen et al followed two groups of women, clinically and urodynamically, who were undergoing colposuspension or anterior repair for primary stress incontinence. This study again showed a marked deterioration in the cure rate over 5 years with the anterior repair but a much less marked fall in the colposuspension group.[121] The results of these studies are summarised in Table 7. Following these studies and the meta analyses by Jarvis and Black, the relatively poor medium to long-term cure rates have lead increasingly to the use of alternative procedures.

Many would now advocate that anterior colporrhaphy should be reserved for treatment of prolapse alone. However, in a frail elderly woman whose main symptoms are of prolapse but with mild GSI, insertion of 'Kelly' or 'Pacey' buttress sutures to the bladder neck may be appropriate. The procedure has a

**Table 7** Results of comparative studies of anterior colporrhaphy

| Author | | Cure rate at 3 months (%) | Cure rate at 1–2 years (%) | Cure rate at 5 years (%) |
|---|---|---|---|---|
| Bergman[120] | Needle suspension | 84 | 65 | Not available |
| | Anterior repair | 82 | 72 | Not available |
| | Colposuspension | 92 | 91 | Not available |
| Van Geelen[121] | Anterior repair | 74 | 44.6 | 31 |
| | Colposuspension | 100 | 85 | 75 |

low morbidity and relatively little postoperative pain allowing early mobilisation and discharge from hospital. The technique may also be useful in the presence of a very large cystocele which may be difficult to repair in any other way. A Stamey procedure or peri-urethral injection may be added if GSI is more marked with little increase in morbidity.

Recently, the high recurrence rate after anterior colporrhaphy and the narrowing and scarring of the vagina produced have lead to some dissatisfaction with the results and growing interest in alternative techniques of vaginal prolapse repair.

The paravaginal repair was first described by White in 1909[122] as a vaginal operation. Paravaginal repair may also be performed abdominally. In recent years, this technique has gained popularity as a method for repairing cystocele due to lateral detachment of the vaginal connective tissue. Via a vaginal or abdominal approach, the paravaginal tissue is re-attached to the fascia of the pelvic side wall with a series of non-absorbable sutures. In a series of 800 repairs, a satisfactory result in over 95% has been quoted by Richardson.[123] This technique may usefully be used to extend a Burch colposuspension to include repair of a cystocele. Good early results of paravaginal repair in the treatment of GSI have been reported although the long-term result appears poorer and similar to those of anterior repair.[124]

## Needle suspension

The first description of a needle bladder neck suspension was by Pereyra in 1959.[125] He described the use of a long needle to suspend sutures from the vagina to the fascia of the anterior abdominal wall. Originally these sutures were of wire but, because these wire loops eventually cut through the vaginal wall, the suture material was changed to prolene in a series of modifications culminating in 1982.[126]

In 1973, Stamey described the use of specially developed needles to suspend nylon sutures from the para-urethral tissues to the anterior abdominal fascia. Originally buffers of woven Dacron were recommended to prevent the sutures cutting through weak paravaginal tissue (Fig 5).

Raz, in 1981,[127] suggested extending the dissection laterally and including paravaginal tissue within the helical suture. Many authors have suggested further variations in technique; Mundy[128] recommended inserting sutures vaginally with cystoscopy only after suture placement and Jarvis, after a review of the literature in 1995,[129] concluded that the use of the cystoscope had little effect on

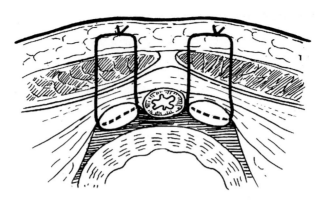

**Fig. 5** Cross section showing Dacron buffers supporting the paravaginal tissue and sutures suspended from the rectus sheath. From Karram M M. In: Hurt W G. (ed). Clinical Urogynaecology. London: Aspen, 1992; with permission.

the outcome. Hilton suggested Silastic rather than Dacron buffers to reduce the infection rate.[130]

During the 1980s, needle suspensions were commonly undertaken because they are easy to perform and it was considered unlikely that they would compromise the results of future surgery should it be required. In addition, the short hospital stay and low complication rate seemed attractive.

### Complications of needle suspension

Most of the published series give little data on the number and type of complications associated with needle suspension, although these are usually described as 'few'. Stamey in his original paper described no infections when using monofilament sutures. Hilton and Mayne in a series of 100 cases report no wound or buffer infections using Silastic buffers (although one buffer was passed vaginally), a 3% urinary tract infection rate and one deep vein thrombosis. Only in one case in this series was the blood loss over 200 ml. Shah[131] found a higher incidence of postoperative bleeding (12%) after Pererya procedures compared to Stamey, but a 13% Silastic buffer infection rate after Stamey procedures.

In general, the peri-operative complication rates for needle suspension procedures appear consistently low, although certainly not negligible; the commonest is infection of the buffers.

### *De novo* detrusor instability

Of particular importance in any procedure to correct stress incontinence is the incidence of *de novo* detrusor instability with a 15% incidence reported following Burch colposuspension.[132] Hilton and Mayne[130] and Shah and Holder[131] found no evidence of *de novo* detrusor instability whilst Mundy[128] found an increase.

The variation amongst these results may well to be due to technique; in general, bladder neck suspension appears to improve pressure transmission to the urethra without causing obstruction and with a low incidence of voiding difficulties and detrusor instability.

## Short-term results of needle suspensions

Stamey reported an initial cure rate of 91% at 6 months; however, these figures have not been supported by studies with longer follow-up.[136] Leach and Raz reported 94% continence rates after at least 2 year follow-up of the modified Raz procedure performed as a secondary continence procedure.[137]

In women over the age of 65 years, Peattie and Stanton reported a 61% objective cure rate.[138]

In 100 women considered unsuitable for colposuspension, Hilton and Mayne[7] conducted a close urodynamic and clinical follow-up over 4 years. They showed an objective cure rate of 83% 3 months after a Stamey procedure but medium-term subjective cure rates of 53% in patients under 65 years and 76% in older patients.

## Longer term results of needle suspension

O'Sullivan et al[139] conducted a questionnaire based survey at intervals following surgery. Immediately postoperatively, 70% were dry and 15% much improved; after 1 year these figures were 31% and 28%, respectively but after 5 years only 18% were dry.

Kevelighan et al,[140] in a study of 259 patients who underwent Stamey procedure at St James' Hospital, Leeds from 1985 to 1995, used life table analysis to assess long-term results. The subjective cure rates were 45% at 2 years, 18% at 4 years and only 6% at 10 years.

Thus, the published data suggest that needle suspensions have reasonable success rates at least approaching those of colposuspension initially.[141] Compared to a suprapubic procedure, the morbidity is low although not negligible.

The poorer long-term results are predictable when examining the mechanical properties of the tissues and materials used. Monofilament sutures and buttresses or anchoring sutures have been selected to minimise the 'cheese-wiring' effect of a single suture under tension in sub-optimal tissues. Monofilament sutures, however, are notorious for their tendency to fail, particularly at stress multiplier sites, such as knots or areas of damage. The minimally invasive nature of these procedures also means that little permanent fibrosis occurs. It may be that alternative suture materials would prolong the efficacy of these procedures and provide a more valuable alternative in the management of stress incontinence.

## Bone anchors and needle suspension techniques

A number of commercial kits for performing bone anchored bladder neck suspension procedures are available. The 'Vesica' technique marketed by Boston Medical consists of a device used to anchor the abdominal end of the sutures into the pubic bone; a number of other similar kits are available. A vaginal epithelial patch is used to buttress the vaginal end of the suture. Appell et al report 94% cure at 12 months using this technique,[142] although in a series of 77 women one required re-operation for an infected bone anchor. The advantage of these techniques is that, like a traditional needle suspension procedure, they have relatively low surgical morbidity and faster recovery with very good short-term results; however, the high cost of some of the commercially available kits obviates any economic advantage.

While bone anchoring may increase the strength of the abdominal end of the suture attachment, the use of a vaginal epithelial patch is not dissimilar to the techniques used by Raz[143,144] and Peyrera[145] and this remains a potential weak spot. In addition, the suture material used is still subject to sudden stress-related failure.

Whether the use of bone anchoring will improve the very poor long-term results of the traditional needle suspension techniques remains to be seen, although examination of the surgical principles involved suggests that they may not. Some longer-term reports are now being published showing medium-term failure rates similar to those of the needle suspensions;[146] they also introduce the possibility of osteomyelitis.[147] Although no randomised trials comparing the use of bone anchors exist, over 45,000 kits have been sold in the US. Long-term follow-up will reveal whether these techniques live up to their initial promise.

The use of bone anchoring devices in recently developed procedures avoids potential weakness at the rectus fascia. However, where the cause of failure is known, it appears to be more often due to paravaginal tissue failure or stress fracture of the monofilament suture. In the majority of cases, the cause of failure is not known but it remains to be seen whether the long-term results of the minimally invasive bone anchoring procedures, which still rely on a monofilament suture, will be similarly poor.

Initial enthusiasm for needle suspension procedures has been tempered by their much poorer long-term results when compared to alternative procedures. However, the apparently low rates of voiding difficulty and *de novo* detrusor instability together with their low morbidity make these procedures more suitable for women where these are areas of concern. They would seem to have a place in patients unsuitable or unfit for suprapubic surgery and perhaps in the elderly woman where long-term results may be better and low operative morbidity carries greater weight than long-term objective cure.

### Injectable peri-uriurethral bulking agents

The use of injectable peri-urethral bulking agents is gaining popularity both in Europe and in North America, although the technique was first described by Murless, using phenol, as long ago as 1938.[148]

The mechanism of continence achieved after peri-urethral injection is not well defined. It is thought that peri-urethral bulking achieves better apposition of urethral epithelium without an increase in obstruction, although some authors report obstructive features following peri-urethral injection.[149] As peri-urethral injectables act by co-apting the urethral mucosa and increasing urethral closure pressure it has been suggested that they would be particularly suitable for women with stress incontinence due to intrinsic sphincter deficiency.

Injections may be made either transurethrally via a cystoscope or peri-urethrally under cystoscopic control (Fig. 6). A number of small studies published in abstract form have attempted to determine the best route but, in general, either technique seems to give equivalent results and the route of injection is governed by the surgeons preference.[150]

Although peri-urethral injectables as a primary procedure are popular in the US, in our experience it is unusual to find women with low maximum

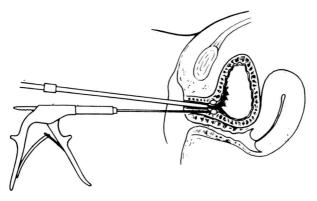

Fig. 6 Para-urethral placement of bulking agent under cystoscopic guidance.

urethral closure pressure due to intrinsic sphincter deficiency presenting for a primary continence procedure.

It has also been suggested that peri-urethral bulking agents may have a place in the treatment of women who wish to have further children.[151] In general, the medium to long-term results of this form of treatment are poor and, while it is claimed that injection has no effect on future surgery, it is possible that fibrosis, from repeated injections, may lead to a decline in intrinsic sphincter function. For this reason, use of this technique as a primary procedure should only be as part of a controlled trial with long-term follow up.

## Materials used for peri-urethral injections

A number of materials have been used for peri-urethral injection. The ideal material would be completely inert, cheap, easy to inject and free from long-term complications, yet provide long-lasting results.

Teflon was the first widely used peri-urethral injectable material. Lopez et al[152] reported a series of 128 women treated over 27 years with cure rates of up to 61%. Teflon was found to produce dense fibrous tissue and a granulomatous reaction leading to urinary obstruction, urethral erosion and severe problems with any subsequent surgery. Teflon has also been shown to migrate from the injection site to local lymph nodes, lung and brain in post-mortem studies.[153,154] As a result of these problems, Teflon is now rarely used. However, the encouraging initial results led to the use of alternative materials.

Autologous fat has been reported as a urethral bulking agent. It has the advantage of being cheap and easy to obtain. However, fat is rapidly phagocytosed and, while initial results may be reasonable, longer term results are disappointing[155] and this technique is now little used. A recent report of fatal fat embolism following peri-urethral fat injection casts further doubt on the use of this material.[156]

One of the most common materials used currently is gluteraldehyde cross-linked bovine collagen (GAX collagen; BARD, Crawley, UK). This has not been shown to have any side effects due to migration, but does produce a local inflammatory response in which injected collagen is replaced with endogenous collagen.[157] Due to the inflammatory response produced by GAX collagen and the resorption of this material, repeated injections may be necessary to sustain continence.[158] Cure rates in published case series vary from 7%[159] to 83%.[160] However, most studies report cures in the region of 40–60%.[161,162]

Another widely used injectable material consists of micronised silicone rubber particles suspended in a non-silicone carrier gel.[163] This is currently marketed as Macroplastique (Uroplasty, Reading, UK). The larger particle size of this material makes migration and displacement less likely and, in addition, the inert nature of the material makes a local inflammatory reaction less problematic. The silicone particles are designed to act as a bulking agent with local inflammatory response removing the carrier gel, encapsulating the silicon in fibrin and replacing the gel with collagen fibres. Cure rates reported with Macroplastique are similar to those with GAX.[164] Only one non-randomised trial to compare GAX with Macroplastique has been published.[165]

Other peri-urethral injectable materials have become available, including alternative extracts of bovine collagen, carbon coated silicon particles, bone and ceramic materials and silicon balloons inflated after positioning in the peri-urethral tissues; however, there are insufficient data at present to compare these new materials.

## Complications

Complications from peri-urethral injection are uncommon. Urinary infection may occur in some 20% of women (Contigen data sheet). Some studies report that postoperative *de novo* detrusor instability is rare[166] while others report a rate of 39%.[162] The lack of long-term data on the use of Macroplastique means that the long-term effects of peri-urethral injection with this material cannot be assessed. GAX collagen has the complication of hyper-sensitivity to bovine collagen which appears to occur in approximately 3% of women.[167]

Injectable materials are expensive; however, the short in-patient stay and convalescent period required reduces the cost initially in comparison with open surgery, although the need for subsequent re-injection dramatically increases the expense of these techniques. Peri-urethral bulking agents are undoubtedly useful in the treatment of GSI and may be particularly beneficial in the treatment of intrinsic sphincter deficiency. They are invaluable in the treatment of secondary incontinence in women who have undergone multiple failed procedures or after radiotherapy where the urethra is fixed and scarred, a group of patients for whom other techniques have high morbidity and poor results.

## Management of intractable stress incontinence

Unfortunately for a small number of women, stress incontinence may persist even after a number of surgical treatments. This does not mean that nothing further can be done to improve their quality of life. Life-style modifications, such as restriction of fluid and modification of activities, may help and provision of appropriate modern pads can be invaluable. The advice and support of a continence advisor is particularly useful in this situation. Continence devices may be particularly useful for this group of women an enable return to a more normal life-style.

However, for some women, more radical solutions may be necessary in the form of artificial sphincters or urinary diversion. Artificial sphincters were first used in women over 25 years ago. The artificial sphincter consists of an inflatable cuff placed around the urethra to provide occlusion with a reservoir to allow deflation and an activating mechanism often sited within the labia. Use of artificial sphincters has been proposed as a primary procedure for women with intrinsic sphincter failure but, due to problems with cuff erosion and mechanical failure, they are most often used when other surgical options have failed.[5] Urinary diversion has also been used to allow women to regain continence. The simplest form of diversion is into a segment of ileum brought to the abdominal wall to drain directly into a stoma bag. Continent reservoirs have been developed using the Mitrofanoff principle, which may allow emptying by intermittent catheterisation. None of these techniques are without complications and they are generally only applicable as a last resort.[168]

## CONCLUSIONS

Over the last 100 years, our understanding of the mechanisms of female stress incontinence has increased and continues to do so. Our knowledge of the efficacy of the variety of surgical methods available has also increased. The relative cure rates along with the morbidity of these techniques have become more clearly defined. This allows the tailoring of treatment to suit the individual woman depending on life-style, expectation and medical fitness.

However, there is still a need to expand our knowledge and expertise in this area. More information is required on the economics of surgery for stress incontinence, together with information on the effect of the various types of surgery on women's quality of life in addition to objective measures of cure. New techniques offering reduced morbidity continue to be developed and need careful evaluation before widespread use.

In 1987 Blavais stated that:

*With modern techniques of diagnosis and careful tailoring of the surgical treatment to the underlying physiological derangement...a cure rate of at least 90% should be the accepted standard for the treatment of stress incontinence in women.*

Continued research and development is needed if we are to be able to offer this, and better, to all women with GSI.

---

**KEY POINTS FOR CLINICAL PRACTICE**

- Stress incontinence is a distressing condition which affects a significant number of women. Effective management can improve the quality of these women's lives
- Conservative management should be offered to all women with GSI. Where conservative therapy has failed, surgical treatment can provide good results for the majority of women
- A wide range of surgical procedures are available for GSI. Thorough pre-operative assessment should enable surgery to be tailored to suit the needs of an individual woman
- The outcome of surgical treatment may be improved if investigation and treatment are carried out in a unit with an interest in stress incontinence, able to provide the services of a multi-disciplinary team during investigation, surgery and postoperative support

## References

1  Abrams P, Blaivas J G, Stanton S L, Andersen J T. The standardisation of terminology of lower urinary tract function. Br J Obstet Gynaecol 1990; 97 (Suppl 6): 1–16

2  Enhorning G. Simultaneous recording of intravesical and intraurethral pressure. Acta Chir Scand 1961; 276: 1–68

3  DeLancy J. Structural support of the urethra as it relates to stress urinary incontinence: the hammock hypothesis. Am J Obstet Gynecol 1994; 170: 1713–1723

4  Zacharin R F. Abdomino-perineal suspension in the management of recurrent stress incontinence of urine – a 15 year experience. Obstet Gynecol 1983; 62: 644–654

5  Blavais J G, Olsson C A. Stress incontinence: classification and surgical approach. J Urol 1998; 39: 727–731

6  Laycock J. The Investigation and Management of Urinary Incontinence in Women. London: RCOG Press, 1995

7  Gardner J, Fonda D. Urinary incontinence in the elderly. Disabil Rehabil 1994; 16: 140–148

8  Dougherty M, Bishop K, Mooney R, Gimotty P, Williams B et al. Graded pelvic muscle exercise. Effect on stress urinary incontinence. J Reprod Med 1993; 38: 684–691

9  Chaliha C, Williams G. Peri-urethral injection therapy for the treatment of stress incontinence. Br J Urol 1995; 76: 151–155

10  Nitti V W, Combs A J. Correlation of valsalva leak point pressure with subjective degree of stress urinary incontinence in women. J Urol 1996; 155: 281–285

11  Stanton S L, Williams J E, Ritchie D. The colposuspension operation for urinary incontinence. Br J Obstet Gynaecol 1976; 83: 890–895

12  McGuire E J, Fitzpatrick C, Wan J et al. Clinical assessment of urethral sphincter function. J Urol 1993; 150: 1452–1454

13  Sand P K, Bowen L W, Panganiban R, Ostergaard D R. The low pressure urethra as a factor in failed retropubic urethropexy. Obstet Gynecol 1987; 69: 399–402

14  Jarvis G J. Surgery for stress incontinence. Br J Obstet Gynaecol 1994; 101: 371–374

15  Black N A Downs S H The effectiveness of surgery for stress incontinence in women: a systematic review. Br J Urol 1996; 78: 497–510

16  Leach G, Dmochowski R, Appell R, et al. Female stress urinary incontinence guidelines. Panel summary report on surgical management of female stress urinary incontinence. J Urol 1997; 158: 875–880

17  Jarvis G J, Hall S, Stamp S et al. An assessment of urodynamic examination in incontinent women. Br J Obstet Gynecol 1980; 87: 893–896

18  Khullar V et al Ambulatory urodynamics: a predictor of de-novo detrusor instability after colposuspension. Neurourol Urodyn 1994; 13: 443–444

19  Monga A, Stanton S L. Predicting outcome of colposuspension – a prospective evaluation. Neurourol Urodyn 1997; XX: 354–355

20  Kelleher C J, Cardozo L D, Khullar V, Salvatore S. A new questionnaire to assess the quality of life of urinary incontinent women. Br J Obstet Gynaecol 1997; 104: 1374–1379

21  Jarvis G J, Hall S, Stamp S, Millar D R, Johnson A. An assessment of urodynamic examination in incontinent women. Br J Obstet Gynaecol 1980; 87: 893–896

22  Black N, Griffiths J, Pope C, Bowling A, Abel P. Impact of surgery for stress incontinence on morbidity: cohort study. BMJ 1997; 315: 1493–1498

23  Hutchings A, Griffiths J, Black N. Surgery for stress incontinence: factors associated with a successful outcome. Br J Urol 1998; 82: 634–641

24  Kholi N et al. Open compared with laparoscopic colposuspension. A cost analysis. Obstet Gynecol 1997; 90: 411–415

25  Berman C, Kreder K. Comparative cost analysis of collagen injection and facia lata sling cystourethropexy for the treatment of type III incontinence in women. J Urol 1997; 157: 122–124

26  Marshall-Marchetti A A, Krantz K E. The correction of stress incontinence by simple vesico-urethral suspension. Surg Gynecol Obstet 1949; 88: 509–518

27  Burch J C. Urethrovesical fixation to Cooper's ligament for correction of stress incontinence, cystocele and prolapse. Am J Obstet Gynecol 1961; 81: 281–290

28  Tanagho E A. Colpocystourethropexy: the way we do it. J Urol 1976; 116: 751–753

29  Stanton S L, Cardozo L D, Williams J E, Ritchie D, Allan V. Clinical and urodynamic

features of failed incontinence surgery in the female. Obstet Gynecol 1978; 51: 515–520

30  Smith R N, Cardozo L D. Early voiding difficulties after colposuspension. Br J Urol 1997; 160: 911–914

31  Hilton P, Stanton S L. A clinical and urodynamic assessment of the Burch colposuspension for genuine stress incontinence. Br J Obstet Gynaecol 1983; 90: 934–939

32  Burch J C. Coopers ligament urethrovesical suspension for urinary stress incontinence. Am J Obstet Gynecol 1968; 100: 764–772

33  Alcalay M, Monga A, Stanton S L. Burch colposuspension: a 10–20 year follow up. Br J Obstet Gynaecol 1995; 102: 740–745

34  Cardozo L D, Stanton S L, Williams J E. Detrusor instability following surgery for GSI. Br J Urol 1979; 58: 138–142

35  Hilton P, Stanton S L. A clinical and urodynamic assessment of the Burch colposuspension for genuine stress incontinence. Br J Obstet Gynaecol 1983; 90: 934–939

36  Stanton S L, Cardozo L D. A comparison of vaginal and suprapubic surgery in the correction of incontinence due to urethral sphincter incontinence. Br J Urol 1979; 51: 497–499

37  Galloway N T M, Davies N, Stephenson T P. The complications of colposuspension. Br J Urol 1987; 60: 122–124

38  Mundy A R. A trial comparing the Stamey bladder neck suspension procedure with colposuspension for stress incontinence. Br J Urol 1983; 55: 687–690

39  Stanton S L. Urethral Sphincter Incompetence in Clinical Gynaecologic Urology. St Louis: Mosby, 1984; 169–192

40  Stanton S L, Williams J E, Ritchie B. The colposuspension operation for urinary stress incontinence. Br J Obstet Gynaecol 1976; 83: 890–895

41  Milani R, Scambrio S et al. MMK procedure and Burch colposuspension in the surgical treatment of female stress incontinence. Br J Obstet Gynaecol 1985; 68: 1050–1053

42  Cardozo L D, Cutner A. Surgical management of stress incontinence. Contemp Rev Obstet Gynaecol 1992; 4: 36–41

43  Herbetsson G, Iosif C S. Surgical results and urodynamic studies 10 years after retropubic colpocystouretropexy Acta Obstet Gynecol Scand 1993; 72: 298–301

44  Cardozo L D, Hextall A, Bailey J, Boos K. Colposuspension after previous failed continence surgery. A prospective observational study. Br J Obstet Gynaecol 1999; 106: 340–344

45  Liu C Y, Paek W. Laparoscopic retropubic colposuspension (Burch procedure). J Am Assoc Gynecol Laparosc 1993; 1: 31–35

46  Su T, Wang K, Hsu C, Wei H, Hong B. Prospective comparison of laparoscopic and traditional colposuspensions in the treatment of genuine stress incontinence. Acta Obstet Gynecol Scand 1997; 76: 576–582

47  Burton G. A three year prospective randomised urodynamic study comparing open and laparoscopic colposuspension. Neurourol Urodyn 1997; XX: 353-354

48  Ross J W. Multichannel urodynamic evaluation of laparoscopic Burch colposuspension for GSI. Obstet Gynecol 1998; 91: 55–59

49  Lyons T L, Winner W K. Clinical outcomes with laparoscopic and open Burch procedures for urinary stress incontinence. J Am Assoc Gynecol Laparosc 1995; 2: 193–198

50  Virtanen H S et al. Ureteral injuries in conjunction with Burch colposuspension. Int Urogynecol J 1995; 6: 114–118

51  Aslan P, Woo H. Ureteric injury following laparoscopic colposuspension. Br J Obstet Gynaecol 1997; 104: 266–268

52  Deitz H P et al. Ureteric injury following laparoscopic colposuspension. Br J Obstet Gynaecol 1997; 104: 1217

53  Smith A R B, Stanton S L. Laparoscopic Colposuspension. Br J Obstet Gynaecol 1998; 105: 383–384

54  Goebell R G. Zur operativen Behandlung der incontinenz der mannlichen harnrohre. Gynakol Urol 1910; 2: 187

55  Stoeckel W. Uber die verwendung der muculi pyramidales bei der operativen behadlung der incontinentia urinae. Gynakol Urol 1917; 41: 11

56  Frangheim P. Zur operativen behanlung der incontinenz. Verhandlung der Deutsche Gesellschaft für Chirurgie, 43rd Congress, 1914; 149

57 Wheeless C R, Wharton L, Dorsey J, TeLinde R. The Goebell-Stockel operation for universal cases of urinary incontinence. Am J Obstet Gynecol 1977; 128: 546

58 Aldridge A H. Transplantation of fascia for the relief of urinary incontinence. Am J Obstet Gynecol 1942; XX: 398–411

59 Jeffcoate T N A. Results of Aldridge sling operation for stress incontinence. J Obstet Gynecol Br Empire 1956; 63: 36–39

60 Ulmsten U, Ekman G, Giertz G, Malstrom A. Different biochemical composition of connective tissue in continent and stress incontinent women. Acta Obstet Gynecol Scand 1987; 66: 455–457

61 Landon C R, Smith A R B, Crofts C E, Trowbridge E A. Biomechanical properties of connective tissue in women with stress incontinence of urine. Neurourol Urodyn 1989; 8: 369–370

62 Price P B. Plastic operations for incontinence of urine and of faeces. Arch Surg 1933; 26: 1043–1048

63 Kaplan S A, Santarosa R P, Te A E. Comparison of fascial and vaginal wall slings in the management of intrinsic sphincter deficiency. Urology 1996; 47: 885–889

64 Wright E J, Iselin C E, Carr L K. Pubovaginal sling using cadaveric allograft. J Urol 1998; 169: 1312–1316

65 Handa V, Jensen J, Germain M, Ostergaard D. Banked human fascia lata for the suburethral sling procedure: a preliminary report. Obstet Gynecol 1996; 88: 1045–1049

66 Buck B E, Malinin T I. Human bone and tissue allografts: preparation and safety. Clin Orthop 1994; 303: 8–17

67 Buck B E, Resnick L, Shah S M, Malini N. Human immunodeficiency virus cultured from bone; implications for transplantation. Clin Orthop 1990; 251: 249–253

68 Jarvis G J, Fowlie A. Clinical and urodynamic assessment of the porcine dermis bladder sling in the treatment of genuine stress incontinence. Br J Obstet Gynaecol 1985; 92: 1189–1191

69 Iosif C S. Porcine corium sling in the treatment of urinary stress incontinence. Arch Gynecol 1987; 240: 131

70 Faber P, Beck L, Heindreich J. Treatment of urinary stress incontinence with the lyodura sling. Urol Int 1978; 33: L117

71 Rottenburg R, Weil A, Brioschi P et al. Urodynamic and clinical assessment of the lyodura sling operation for urinary stress incontinence. Br J Obstet Gynaecol 1985; 92: 829–834

72 Horbach N S. Suburethral sling procedures. In: Ostergard D R, Bent A E. (eds) Urodynamics and Urogynaecology: Theory and Practice, 3rd edn. Baltimore: Williams and Wilkins, 1991; 449–458

73 Stanton S L, Brindley G S, Holmes D M. Silastic sling for urethral sphincter incompetence in women. Br J Obstet Gynaecol 1985; 92: 747–750

74 Korda A, Peat B, Hunter P. Silastic slings for female incontinence. Int Urogynecol J 1990; 1: 66–69

75 Chin Y K, Stanton S L. A follow up of silastic sling for genuine stress incontinence. Br J Obstet Gynaecol 1995; 102: 143–147

76 Williams T J, Te Linde R W. The sling operation for urinary incontinence using Mersilene ribbon. Obstet Gynecol 1962; 19: 241–245

77 Melnick I, Lee R. Delayed transection of the urethra by Mersilene tape. Urology 1976; 8: 580–581

78 Moir J C. The gauze hammock operation. J Obstet Gynaecol Br Commonwealth 1968; 75: 1–13

79 Kersey J, Martin M R, Mishra P. A further assessment of the gauze hammock operation for recurrent stress incontinence. Br J Obstet Gynaecol 1988; 95: 382–385

80 Morgan J E. A sling operation using Marlex polypropylene mesh, for treatment of recurrent stress incontinence. Am J Obstet Gynecol 1970; 106: 369

81 Horbach N S, Blanco J S, Ostergard D R. A suburethral sling procedure with PTFE for the treatment of genuine stress incontinence in patients with low urethral closure pressure. Obstet Gynecol 1988; 71: 648–652

82 Barbalias G A, Liatsikos E N, Athanasopoulos A. Gore-tex sling urethral suspension in type III female urinary incontinence: clinical results and urodynamic changes. Int Urogynecol J 1997; 8: 344–350

83 Jarvis G J. Stress incontinence. In: Mundy A R, Stephenson T P, Wein A J. (eds) Urodynamics; Principles, Practice & Application, 2nd edn. New York 1994: Churchill Livingstone, 1994; 299–326

84 Carr L, Walsh P, Abraham V, Webster G. Favourable outcome of pubovaginal slings for geriatric women with stress incontinence. J Urol 1997; 157: 125–128

85 McLennan M, Melick C, Bent A. Clinical and urodynamic predictors of delayed voiding after fascia lata suburethral sling. Obstet Gynecol 1998; 98: 608–612

86 Hilton P. A clinical and urodynamic study comparing the Stamey bladder neck suspension and suburethral sling procedures in the treatment of genuine stress incontinence. Br J Obstet Gynaecol 1989; 96: 213–220

87 Iosif C S, Sling operation for urinary incontinence. Acta Obstet Gynecol Scand 1985; 64: 187–190

88 Young S B, Rosenblatt P L, Pingeton D M, Howard A, Baker S P. The Mersilene mesh suburethral sling: a clinical and urodynamic evaluation. Am J Obstet Gynecol 1995; 173: 1719–1726

89 Weinberger M, Ostergaard D. Long-term clinical and urodynamic evaluation of the polytetrafluoroethylene suburethral sling for treatment of genuine stress incontinence. Obstet Gynecol 1995; 86: 92–96

90 Horbach N S. Suburethral sling procedures. In: Ostergard D R, Bent A E. (eds) Urogynecology and Urodynamics, 3rd edn. Philadelphia: Williams and Wilkins, 1991; 413–421

91 Blaivas G, Jacobs B. Pubovaginal fascial sling for the treatment of complicated stress urinary incontinence. J Urol 1991; 145: 1214–1218

92 Appell R. Primary slings for everyone with genuine stress incontinence? The argument for... Int Urogynecol J 1998; 9: 249–251

93 Cardozo L D, Stanton S L, Williams J E. Detrusor instability following surgery for GSI. Br J Urol 1979; 58: 138–142

94 Zimmern P, Hadley H, Leach G, Raz S. Female urethral obstruction after Marshall Marchetti-Krantz operation. J Urol 1987; 138: 517

95 Beck R, McCormick B, Nordstrom L. The fascia lata sling procedure for treating recurrent stress incontinence of urine. Obstet Gynecol 1988; 72: 699–703

96 Morgan J, Farrow G, Stewart F. The Marlex sling operation for the treatment of recurrent stress incontinence: a sixteen year review. Am J Obstet Gynecol 1985; 151: 224–226

97 Moloney P, Fenster H. Bladder neck incision for relief of obstruction after anti-incontinence surgery. Int J Urogynecol 1993; 4: 68

98 McGuire E, Leston W, Wang S. Transvaginal urethrolysis after obstructive urethral suspension procedures. J Urol 1989; 142: 1037–1038

99 Stanton S L. Silastic sling for urethral sphincter incompetence in women. Br J Obstet Gynaecol 1985; 92: 747

100 Ghoniem G, Elgamasy A. A simplified surgical approach to bladder outlet obstruction following pubovaginal sling. J Urol 1995; 154: 181–183

101 Bent A E, Ostergard D R, Zwick-Zaffuto M. Tissue reaction to expanded polytetrafluoroethylene suburethral sling for urinary incontinence: clinical and histologic study. Am J Obstet Gynecol 1993; 169: 1198–1204

102 Bryans F E. Marlex gauze hammock sling operation with Cooper's ligament fixation in the management of recurrent urinary stress incontinence. Am J Obstet Gynecol 1979; 133: 292–294

103 Drutz H P, Buckspan M, Flax S, Mackie L. Clinical and urodynamic re-evaluation of combined abdomino-vaginal Marlex sling operation for recurrent stress urinary incontinence. Int Urogynecol J 1990; 1: 70–73

104 Petros P, Ulmsten U. An integral theory on female urinary incontinence. Experimental and clinical considerations. Acta Obstet Gynecol Scand 1990; 69 (Suppl): 153.

105 Petros P, Ulmsten U. An integral theory and its method for the diagnosis and management of female urinary incontinence. Scand J Urol Nephrol 1993; 151: 1–93

106 Petros P, Ulmsten U. Urethral pressure increase on effort originates from within the urethra, and continence from musculovaginal closure. Neurourol Urodyn 1995; 14: 337–350

107 Petros P, Ulmsten U. Role of the pelvic floor in bladder neck opening and closure: I

Muscle forces. Int Urogynecol J 1997; 8: 74–80

108 Petros P, Ulmsten U. Role of the pelvic floor in bladder neck opening and closure: II Vagina. Int Urogynecol J 1997; 8: 69–73

109 Petros P, Ulmsten U. Intravaginal slingplasty. An ambulatory surgical procedure for treatment of female urinary stress incontinence. Scand J Urol Nephrol 1995; 29: 75–82

110 Ulmsdten U, Henriksson L, Johnson P, Varhos G. An ambulatory surgical procedure under local anaesthesia for treatment of female urinary incontinence. Int Urogynecol J 1996; 7: 81–86

111 Ulmsten U, Falconer C, Johnson P et al. A multicentre study of tension-free vaginal tape (TVT) for surgical treatment of stress urinary incontinence. Int Urogynecol J 1998; 9: 210–213

112 Ulmsten U, Johnson P, Rezapour M. A three year follow up of TVT for surgical treatment of female stress incontinence. Br J Obstet Gynaecol 1999; 106: 345–350

113 Nilsson C G. The TVT procedure for the treatment of female stress urinary incontinence. Acta Obstet Gynecol 1998; 168: 34–37

114 Riva D et al. Tension free vaginal tape for the therapy of SUI: early results and urodynamic analysis. Neurourol Urodyn 1998; 17: 351–352

115 Ward K, Hilton P. TVT early experience. Int Urogynecol J 1998

116 Schultze B S. Operative Heilung der urethralen Incontinenz beim Weibe. Cor-Bl d allg arztl Ver v. Thuringen, Weimar 1888; 17: 289

117 Kelly H A. Incontinence of urine in women. Urol Cutan Rev 1913; 17: 291–297

118 Kelly H A, Dumm W. Urinary incontinence in women, without manifest injury to the bladder. Surg Gynecol Obstet 1914: XX: 444–450

119 Pacey K. The pathology and repair of genital prolapse. J Obstet Gynaecol Br Empire 1949; 56: 1–15

120 Bergman A, Ballard C, Koonings P. Comparison of three different surgical procedures for genuine stress incontinence. Am J Obstet Gynecol 1989; 160: 1102–1106

121 Van Geelen J, Theeuwes A, Eskes T, Martin C. The clinical and urodynamic effects of anterior vaginal repair and colposuspension. Am J Obstet Gynecol 1988; 159: 137–144

122 White G R. Cystocele. JAMA 1909; 53: 1707

123 Richardson A C. Paravaginal repair. In: Benson J T. (ed) Female Pelvic Floor Disorders. New York: Norton, 1992; 280–287

124 Shull B, Baden W B. A six year experience with paravaginal defect repair for stress urinary incontinence. Am J Obstet Gynecol 1989; 160: 1432–1440

125 Pereyra A J. A simplified surgical procedure for the correction of stress incontinence in women. West J Surg 1959; 67: 223–226

126 Pereyra A J. Lebherz T B. Pubourethral supports in perspective: modified Pererya procedure for urinary incontinence. Obstet Gynecol 1982; 59: 643–648

127 Raz S. Modified bladder neck suspension for female stress incontinence. Urology 1981; 17: 82–84

128 Mundy A R. A trial comparing Stamey bladder neck suspension with colposuspension for the treatment of stress incontinence. Br J Urol 1983; 55: 687–690

129 Jarvis G J. Long needle bladder neck suspension for GSI: Does endoscopy influence results? Br J Urol 1995; 76: 467–469

130 Hilton P, Mayne C. The Stamey endoscopic bladder neck suspension: a clinical and urodynamic investigation including actuarial follow up over four years. Br J Obstet Gynaecol 1991; 98: 1141–1149

131 Shah P J, Holder P D. Comparison of Stamey and Pererya-Raz bladder neck suspensions. Br J Urol 1989; 64: 481–484

132 Cardozo L D, Stanton S L, Williams J E. Detrusor instability following surgery for genuine stress incontinence. Br J Urol 1979; 51: 204–207

133 to 135 (deleted)

136 Stamey T A. Endoscopic suspension of the vesical neck for urinary incontinence in females: a report of 203 consecutive patients. Ann Surg 1980; 192: 465–471

137 Leach G E, Raz S. Modified Pererya bladder neck suspension after previously failed anti-incontinence surgery. Urology 1984; 23: 359–362

138 Peattie A B, Stanton S L. The Stamey operation for correction of genuine stress incontinence in the elderly woman. Br J Obstet Gynaecol 1989; 96: 983–986

139 O'Sullivan D C, Chilton C P, Munson K W. Should Stamey colposuspension be our primary surgery for stress incontinence? Br J Urol 1995; 75: 457–460

140 Kevelighan E, Aagaard J, Jarvis G J. The Stamey endoscopic bladder neck suspension – a 10 year follow up. ICS Annual Meeting 1997. Neurourol Urodyn 1997

141 Stanton S L, Cardozo L D. Results of colposuspension for incontinence and prolapse. Br J Obstet Gynaecol 1979; 86: 693–697

142 Appell R A, Rackley R R, Dmochowski R R. Vesica percutaneous bladder neck stabilisation. J Endourol 1996; 10: 221–225

143 Raz S. Modified bladder neck suspension for female stress incontinence. Urology 1981; 17: 82–84

144 Raz S, Siegel A, Short J, Synder J. Vaginal wall sling. J Urol 1989; 141: 43–46

145 Pereyra A J. A simplified surgical procedure for the correction of stress incontinence in women. West J Surg 1959; 67: 223–226

146 Schultheiss D, Hofner K, Oelke M et al. Percutaneous bladder neck suspension with bone anchors: an improvement in the therapy of female stress urinary incontinence. Neurourol Urodyn 1998; 17: 457–458

147 Maktov T G, Hejna Coogan C L. Osteomyelitis as a complication of vesica percutaneous bladder neck suspension. J Urol 1998; 160: 1427

148 Murles B C. The injection treatment of stress incontinence. J Obstet Gynaecol Br Empire 1938; 45; 67–73

149 Stricker P, Haylen B. Injectable collagen for type three female stress incontinence: the first 50 Australian patients. Med J Aust 1993 158: 89–91

150 Appell R, Goodman J, McGuire E. Multi centre study of periurethral and transurethral injection of GAX collagen in female urinary incontinence. Int Urogynecol J 1989: 1: 41

151 Carr L K, Herschorrn S. Periurethral collagen injection and pregnancy. J Urol 1996; 155: 1037

152 Lopex E A, Padron F O, Patsias G, Polytarno V A. Trans-urethral polytetrafluoroethylene in female patients with urinary incontinence. J Urol 1993; 150: 856–858

153 Ferro M A, Smith J H, Smith P J. Peri-urethral granuloma: unusual complication of Teflon peri-urethral injection. Urology 1988; 31: 422–423

154 Rames R A, Irenson I. The migration of polytef paste to the lung and brain following intra-vesicle injection for the correction of reflux. Pediatr Surg Int 1991; 6: 239–240

155 Santarosa R P, Blaivas J G. Periurethral injection of autologous fat for the treatment of sphincteric incontinence. J Urol 1994: 151; 607–611

156 Currie I, Drutz H, Deck J, Oxorn D. Adipose tissue and lipid droplet embolism following periurethral injection of autologous fat: case report and review of the literature. Int Urogynecol J 1997; 8: 377–380

157 Kligman A M, Armstrong R C. Histological response to intra-dermal zyderm and zyplasy (gluteraldehyde cross-linked) collagen in humans. J Dermatol Surg Oncol 1986; 12: 351–357

158 Monga A K, Robinson D, Stanton S L. Peri-urethral collagen injections for genuine stress incontinence: a two year follow-up. Br J Urol 1995; 76: 156–160

159 Homer Y, Kawabe K, Kageyama S et al. Injection of gluteraldehyde cross-linked collagen for urinary incontinence. Two year efficacy by self-assessment. Int J Urol 1996; 155: 124–127

160 Faerber G J. Endoscopic collagen injection therapy in elderly women with type one stress urinary incontinence. J Urol 1996; 155: 512–514

161 Eckford S D, Abrams P. Para-urethral collagen implantation for female stress incontinence. Br J Urol 1991; 68: 586–589

162 Khullar V, Cardozo L D, Abbott D, Anders K. GAX collagen in the treatment of urinary incontinence in elderly women: a two year follow-up. Br J Obstet Gynaecol 1997; 104: 96–99

163 Macroplastique Implants Technical Overview. Maastricht, The Netherlands: Uroplasty BV, 1995

164 Adile B et al. Macroplastique implant for the treatment of type three urinary stress incontinence: one year follow-up. Presented at the International Urogynecology Association Meeting: Kuala Lumpur, Malaysia 1995

165 Fischer M, Szabo N, Durer A. Endoscopic implantation of collagen or microparticulate silicone for the treatment of female urinary incontinence. Presented at the ICS Meeting, Australia 1995

166 Monga A K, Robinson D, Stanton S L. Peri-urethral collagen injections for genuine stress incontinence: a two year follow-up. Br J Urol 1995; 76: 156–160

167 Appel R A. Collagen injection therapy for urinary incontinence. Urol Clin North Am 1994; 21: 177–182

168 Mitrofanoff P. Cystostimie continente transappendiculare dans la travail des vessies neurologique. Chir Pediatr 1980; 21: 297

G.J. Jarvis

# 24

# Treatment of detrusor instability and urge incontinence

The normal human bladder is essentially a dual function organ and the major anatomical component of this organ is the bladder muscle, the detrusor. The bladder must relax during the filling phase, as evidenced by relaxation and extension of the bladder muscle and must contract during the micturition phase, as evidenced by a shortening of the bladder muscle. During the storage phase, the detrusor relaxation is associated with an increase in bladder volume without a co-existing increase in intravesical pressure. During the voiding phase, the intravesical pressure increases and when that pressure exceeds the maximal urethral closure pressure, urine flows.

A detrusor which relaxes during the storage phase is termed compliant and such a bladder is termed stable. Conversely, the bladder in which the detrusor contracts involuntarily, either naturally or during provocation, during the filling phase is termed unstable. The clinical condition is termed detrusor instability, otherwise known as the unstable bladder. By convention, this condition should be distinguished from involuntary detrusor contraction as a result of gross interruption of the nervous system, such as occurs with spinal injury, where the anatomical loss of an inhibiting influence upon detrusor contractility is termed detrusor hyper-reflexia. These principles have been adopted by the International Continence Society who define detrusor instability as 'the condition in which the detrusor is shown objectively to contract, either spontaneously or on provocation, during bladder filling, whilst the subject is attempting to inhibit micturition'.[1]

It is clear that the International Continence Society definition is a urodynamic one since it uses the word objective. As described below, under certain circumstances, it is acceptable to consider that the condition is present on clinical grounds.

**Mr Gerry J. Jarvis** MA BM BCh FRCSE FRCOG, Consultant in Obstetrics and Gynaecology, St James's University Hospital, Leeds LS9 7TF, UK

The prevalence of detrusor instability has been assessed from various studies. It is generally accepted that somewhere between 5–25% of all women between the ages of 15–65 years leak urine involuntarily and a figure of 14% would be generally accepted.[2] Urodynamic studies suggest that approximately 42% of women with urinary incontinence have detrusor instability either alone or in combination with other disorders.[3] Thus, it may be estimated that 6% of adult women have detrusor instability.

## AETIOLOGY OF DETRUSOR INSTABILITY

Since our understanding of the pathophysiology of detrusor instability is imperfect, no single explanation is available for the condition in all patients. This may also be compounded by the observation that not all detrusor instability has the same aetiology but, rather, different aetiological factors condense into the same pathway to produce the same end result.

In the child, it is a normal physiological observation that the detrusor is unstable and, as the child learns to inhibit detrusor contraction, bladder control becomes established. It is likely, therefore, that at least some patients with an unstable bladder should be considered as having a variation upon normal physiology rather than the presence of a pathological condition. This may relate particularly to nocturnal enuresis with satisfactory day-time control of the bladder and the increase in the prevalence of detrusor instability in the elderly population. In a study of a cohort of women aged 20–95 years, maximum bladder capacity decreased with increasing age, the capacity at first desire to void increased with increasing age, and the prevalence of detrusor instability increased. It may, therefore, be that with increasing age there is a combination of decreased voluntary bladder capacity, decreased sensation and decreased central nervous system inhibition.[4]

The basic micturition reflex involves afferent nerves from the bladder, the spinal cord, the brain stem, the descending fibres of the spinal cord, and an efferent connection to the detrusor.[5] Above the brain stem lie multiple controlling areas which inhibit, amplify, and fine-tune this reflex activity, the cerebral cortex being considered the most important of these. These observations may explain the co-existence of detrusor instability with certain neurological disorders including Parkinson's disease and multiple sclerosis.[6]

In some patients the aetiology includes bladder outflow obstruction and in others psychoneurotic features.[7]

It has long been known that following prostatectomy, a significant portion of men with previous bladder instability convert to bladder stability suggesting that the removal of an outflow obstruction reverses instability.[8] Of more relevance to the gynaecologist is the evidence that women with a stable bladder and genuine stress incontinence who undergo otherwise successful surgery for their genuine stress incontinence may develop detrusor instability, including incontinence from this condition. It is an unfortunate truism that those operations which are the most successful in relieving genuine stress incontinence are the most obstructive and the ones associated with the highest postoperative incidence of both voiding disorder and *de novo* detrusor instability. Thus, the incidence of *de novo* instability is in the region of 1% following an anterior colporrhaphy, 5.8% after endoscopic bladder neck suspension, and 10% following either colposuspension or sub-urethral sling surgery.[9] Since it is likely that detrusor instability if present pre-operatively will be aggravated by bladder neck surgery, one of the indications for pre-operative urodynamic assessment is the recognition that the detrusor is stable.

There is accumulating evidence that detrusor instability may have psychogenic features, at least in some women. This evidence does not allow the conclusion that the instability is psychogenic since the alternative explanation that those who are susceptible to psychogenic disorders are also susceptible to detrusor instability fits the available evidence.

Several authors have drawn attention to the association by the patient to the onset of her symptoms with either a strong emotive event or the presence of interesting related triggers such as the sound of running water.[10] Others have shown that women with detrusor instability have a higher neuroticism score on formal testing than do women with genuine stress incontinence.[11] Behavioural forms of therapy, as discussed below, are very effective methods of treatment whilst those trials which have included a control arm have demonstrated a strong placebo effect in the region of 25% (see below).

Albeit unusually, it must always be considered whether the detrusor instability in a given patient is due to intravesical pathology which has increased the afferent impulses from the bladder. Thus, a history must include a formal urological history with particular emphasis on the presence or absence of haematuria or dysuria, and microscopy of urine for the identification of red blood cells which may indicate pathology such as a bladder tumour.

There is current interest surrounding the hypothesis that detrusor instability may not be due to an increased motor nerve activity but rather relate to an abnormality of the detrusor smooth muscle itself with evidence of partial denervation which is manifest by a resulting increased excitability and ability for the spread of electrical activity between cells.[7] Such an excitable predisposition may occur with alteration in both presynaptic and postsynaptic receptors and the presence of peptides, such as vasoactive intestinal polypeptide, which can act as a neuromodulator and increase the muscular response to a given chemical, predominantly cholinergic, stimulus.[7] This increased excitable state may also occur in the presence of free radicals, such as nitric oxide and substance P, or the presence of increased concentrations of both potassium and calcium ions in the tissue fluid of the urothelium.[12]

It is important for the pathophysiology of detrusor instability to be investigated further, and with greater clarity, since the abnormalities identified may lead to the production of more effective pharmacological agents together with a realistic expectation of the efficacy of those which exist currently.

## CLINICAL FEATURES AND INVESTIGATION

The classical symptoms associated with detrusor instability include any or all of frequency, nocturia, urgency, urge incontinence, stress incontinence, nocturnal enuresis and incontinence at orgasm. Not all of these clinical features must be present for a presumed diagnosis to be made and it is of particular importance to note that the symptom of stress incontinence will occur in 26% of women with an unstable bladder but without genuine stress incontinence, whilst the symptom of urge incontinence will occur in 37% of women with genuine stress incontinence but with an unstable bladder.[3] Should the patient complain of urgency and urge incontinence but no stress incontinence and if there are no other features of urological disease, then it is reasonable for there to be a presumptive diagnosis made of detrusor instability and empirical therapy may commence without the need for urodynamic investigation.

Such a patient will almost certainly have an unstable bladder. If the symptoms include both urge incontinence and stress incontinence, however, then a clinical diagnosis cannot be made with any realistic accuracy and under such circumstances a urodynamic assessment should be performed before a decision is made upon treatment options. The simplest and most useful urodynamic investigation – in order to distinguish between detrusor instability and genuine stress incontinence – is a filling cystometrogram. Since a cystometrogram is an invasive procedure, all women should have a sterile mid-stream urine investigation prior to instrumentation and, furthermore, urinary infection may invalidate the results of urodynamic investigation.

A frequency–volume chart may be suggestive of the diagnosis of detrusor instability by identifying frequent voiding of relatively small volumes of urine but is not diagnostic. In those women in whom a cystometrogram is not diagnostic of any pathology, as may happen in somewhere between 4–8% of all investigations, either the filling cystometrogram should be repeated or an ambulatory test be performed which will detect detrusor instability in up to 65% of patients in whom a static cystometrogram was normal.[14]

Despite these investigations, there will be some patients who have the clinical features of detrusor instability yet a stable bladder but, generally, a first desire to void at relatively low bladder capacity and a reduced maximum cystometric capacity. This condition is generally termed primary vesical sensory urgency and, in this situation, cystoscopy should be performed to avoid chronic inflammatory conditions of the bladder, such as interstitial cystitis or chronic cystitis, although cystoscopy itself is not indicated in the routine management of detrusor instability.

## TREATMENT

There is no single treatment modality which should be considered as the first choice of treatment over all others in this condition. There are several reasons for holding this view. No single therapy is universally efficacious and a balance of benefit with side effects and cost (for in-patient treatment) is required. The assessment of efficacy from the scientific literature is sometimes difficult, since not all studies use the same outcome measures and, indeed, in some studies it can be exceedingly difficult to understand the percentage of patients who have been significantly improved or even made continent. It is likely that there is selection and publication bias in studies with those studies giving the better results being offered for and accepted for publication. Randomised trials are few, although increasing. Results tend to be analysed in the short-term rather the intermediate and long-term. The placebo effect is significant. In the author's experience, some patients are satisfied with explanation and re-assurance and do not then wish to pursue treatment. It is against this background that the available treatment modalities must be assessed following which the author gives a personal view on a treatment algorithm.

The size of the placebo effect in treating detrusor instability should not be under-estimated. Whilst most studies which have identified a placebo effect have estimated a figure of between 20–25% for significant improvement, a well-known study of two so-called active agents against placebo demonstrated that the placebo arm carried the greatest success rate, this being 47%.[15]

## Treatment options

The major treatment options for detrusor instability are drug treatment, behavioural forms of therapy, electrical stimulation, and surgery.

### Drug treatment

*Oestrogen.* Although there is good evidence for the benefit of oestrogens in treating non-specific lower urinary tract symptoms in post-menopausal women, especially complaining of frequency, urgency and dysuria, there is no convincing evidence that oestrogen is superior to placebo in reducing incontinence in women who have proven detrusor instability.[16]

*Propantheline.* Since the primary innervation of the detrusor is by the sympathetic nervous system, and since the major neurotransmitter at the neuro-muscular junction is acetylcholine, it is logical that anticholinergic drugs with antimuscarinic activity should be used in this condition. Unfortunately, the non-specific mode of action is associated with other anti-muscarinic side effects, including dry mouth, blurred vision, tachycardia and constipation. Propantheline is a quarternary ammonium analogue of atropine and has both antimuscarinic and antinicotinic properties, acting on the neuromuscular junction. Given orally in a dose which ranges from 15 mg four times a day up to 90 mg four times a day, it has a relatively modest benefit in improving somewhere between 30–48% of patients but associated with some 19% of patients finding the drug's side effects to be unacceptable.[17] Emipronium carageanate is an anticholinergic agent derived from seaweed and, whilst not available in the UK, is available in Ireland and Europe. The place of this drug in clinical practice is difficult to elucidate, given that various trials demonstrate an improvement in anywhere between 0–79% of patients in a dose of up to 2000 mg per day.[3]

*Flavoxate.* Flavoxate hydrochloride is a musculotropic agent, that is it acts directly as a smooth muscle relaxant competing with acetylcholine at the neuromuscular junction. The drug is of modest efficacy with results demonstrating a benefit of between 0–58%, although there is evidence that increased dosage of 1200 mg per day may be more effective than the more conventional 600 mg per day. The side effects are the same as those of anticholinergic drugs.[18]

*Oxybutynin.* This was the first truly effective agent in the drug treatment of detrusor instability. It is a tertiary amine with musculotropic, anticholinergic, and local anaesthetic effects. It is convincingly superior to placebo with improvement rates occurring in 57–69% of patients in the usual dose of 15 mg daily, although up to 30 mg daily may be prescribed. Efficacy must be balanced against side effects, with nausea and constipation reported in up to 14% of patients, a dry mouth in up to 88% of patients, whilst 7.5% of patients discontinued therapy because of side effects. In those patients who have detrusor instability co-existing with a voiding disorder, intravesical administration is effective.[17,19,20] Until recently, oxybutynin has been considered the drug treatment of choice for detrusor instability.

*Tolterodine.* This is a relatively new antimuscarinic agent developed specifically for the treatment of detrusor instability. It is said to have an equal affinity and specificity for the muscarinic receptors of the bladder yet less affinity for muscarinic receptors elsewhere.[21] Such findings suggest that tolterodine may be equally effective to oxybutynin in reducing bladder contractions, yet have a lower range of adverse effects. There have now been 4 randomised trials which have compared oxybutynin with tolterodine. All trials show similar results and one such trial reports a 71% reduction in the number of incontinence episodes in women receiving oxybutynin compared with a 47% reduction with tolterodine and a 19% reduction with placebo. Dry mouth was reported in 86% of women with oxybutynin, 50% with tolterodine and 21% with placebo, whilst withdrawals due to adverse effects occurred in 17% of women receiving oxybutynin, 12% with placebo and 8% with tolterodine.[21,22] The authors conclude 'tolterodine represents a promising alternative for the effective long-term treatment of the over-active bladder, overcoming many of the limitations of existing antimuscarinic agents'.

*Propiverine.* This is a new bladder antispasmodic agent with both anti-cholinergic and calcium-channel blocking properties. A previous calcium-channel blocking agent had been in clinical use and, whilst effective, was withdrawn because of a low but, nevertheless real, incidence of cardiac adverse events especially in elderly patients. Although there is little information available in the peer-reviewed journals, the manufacturer's data claim 'overall improvements in clinical symptoms were noted in 83% of those given propiverine, 79% taking oxybutynin and 68% of the placebo controls'.[23] There is clearly a need for further randomised studies.

*Tricyclic antidepressants.* The tricyclic antidepressants potentiate the bladder relaxant effect of the sympathetic nervous system whilst having anticholinergic properties and central sedative effects. This last effect makes them particularly useful for patients in whom nocturia is a problem. Using either imipramine in dosages of 50–150 mg at night or amitriptyline in dosages of 25–75 mg at night, nocturia and nocturnal enuresis have been reduced by up to 74%, whilst 10% of patients complain of drowsiness and 20% experience postural hypotension.[24]

*Antidiuretic hormone analogues.* Synthetic vasopressin (DDAVP) is a peptide hormone which can be administered either intranasally or in tablet form. It has a potent antidiuretic effect increasing the permeability in the distal convoluted tubules and the collecting ducts of the kidney, thereby increasing fluid re-absorption and decreasing urine output. Clearly such an agent can only be taken as a way of altering the diurnal production of urine and, hence, it is useful under specific circumstances. Patients must understand that the benefit whilst taking the drug must be balanced by another period of the day where there will be increased urinary production. It should be particularly useful, therefore, for nocturia or nocturnal enuresis. It is relatively contra-indicated in the presence of coronary artery disease. It is superior to placebo in reducing the number of episodes of either nocturia or bed-wetting.[25]

### Behavioural therapy

The basis of behavioural therapy is that a patient with an intact nervous system can be taught to 're-learn' to be able to inhibit a detrusor contraction. Such therapy includes bladder re-training (sometimes called bladder drill), biofeedback, hypnotherapy, and acupuncture.

**Bladder drill.** This is a simple but effective technique for the treatment of idiopathic detrusor instability. The rationale of bladder drill is to make patients aware of the problem and enlist their help in treatment by using behavioural therapy and a structure regimen. It is generally held that bladder drill is more effective on an in-patient basis than an out-patient basis, perhaps because the patients are withdrawn from their own environment and placed in a situation where their major daily task is to concentrate upon their treatment. A frequently used regimen can be broken into the following components:

1  *Exclude pathology*
2  *Admit to hospital*
3  *Explain rationale to patient*
4  *Instruct to void every 1.5 h during the day. The patient must not void between these times; she must wait or be incontinent*
5  *The voiding interval is increased by half hourly increments when the initial goal is achieved and the process repeated*
6  *The patient should have a normal fluid intake*
7  *The patient should keep her own intake and output chart. It is considered that the increasing volumes of urinary output at increasing intervals act as a reinforcement reward*
8  *The patient should receive praise and encouragement on reaching her daily targets*

Using such a regimen, some 90% of patients became continent compared with 23% in a control group.[26] Similar success rates have been recorded by other authors, but there is a relapse rate of up to 40% within 3 years of treatment.[27] However, such relapse could be treated by re-admission.

**Biofeedback.** This is a technique by which a patient is made aware of an autonomic function using visual or auditory signals in order to demonstrate the strength of that autonomic function. It has been used, for instance, as a way of demonstrating the level of systolic blood pressure. In a study of 27 patients with detrusor instability, 81% were improved following several 1 h sessions of biofeedback using both audible and visual signals of detrusor activity. This type of treatment requires a great deal of input from motivated doctors and nurses, but may represent a useful treatment option in specialist centres.[28,29]

*Hypnotherapy.* Since it is likely that there is a psychogenic element in the aetiology of this condition, it is not surprising that hypnosis may be an effective, but time-consuming, form of treatment. In a series involving 63 incontinent women receiving 12 sessions of hypnosis over a 1 month period of time, 58% of patients became free of symptoms, 28% improved, whilst 14% remained unchanged.[30] Although the results of this study have not been substantiated by further studies, hypnotherapy must be regarded as a potential treatment option when the facilities are available.

*Acupuncture.* Traditional Chinese acupuncture has been used in a small series of patients in whom 69% were improved (with only a single patient 'cured').[31] Acupuncture is thought to act by increasing the levels of endorphins and enkephalins in the cerebrospinal fluid. Further studies in peer-review journals are required before this therapy can be recommended.

*Maximal electrical stimulation.* Different types of electrical stimulation have been tried in both the treatment of detrusor instability and genuine stress incontinence. The logic of this treatment is that stimulation of afferent fibres results in activation of the inhibitory pathways restoring detrusor inhibitory reflexes. The efficacy of such treatment has to be based upon reported cohort studies in the absence of randomised trials. The electrodes used for stimulation include intravaginal and intra-anal as well as transperineal stimulation of the pudendal nerve. Using such techniques, some 70% of patients are subjectively improved and, interestingly and perhaps surprisingly, there were no withdrawals with the technique being universally acceptable.[32] In a comparative trial of maximum electrical stimulation to oxybutynin, similar results are obtained in both arms.[33] In a study which compared surface neuromodulation with a sham stimulation, active therapy reduced the mean maximum height of detrusor contractions whilst sham therapy had no discernible effect.[34]

### Surgery

Although the primary treatment for detrusor instability is non-surgical, various surgical techniques have been used. Some have not stood the test of time, whereas others are indicated when the patient's symptoms are sufficient for her to wish further treatment yet non-surgical treatment has failed.

Several forms of treatment have been tried and either have limited efficacy or have not withstood the test of time. These treatments include urethral dilatation, vaginal denervation, bladder denervation, and transvesical phenol injections.

*Urethral dilatation.* This is an empirical treatment which is relatively free of side effects so long as the dilatation is not over-zealous. In one study, some 23% of patients were relieved of symptoms but it is not clear whether this represents a true beneficial effect of treatment or whether it actually represents a placebo effect (26).

*Vaginal denervation.* This has been advocated, although the results, whilst encouraging, have never been subject to widespread use or recent evaluation.[35,36]

*Bladder denervation by bladder transection.*   This was advocated as a way of reducing, dramatically, the afferent and efferent supplied from and to the bladder but complete bladder denervation is neither desirable, otherwise voiding could not occur, nor possible since the nerves run with the blood supply. Given that this is a significant size surgical procedure, the initial 'cure' rate of 74% was disappointingly only 19% after 5 years giving the procedure a very limited place in clinical practice.[37]

*Transvesical phenol injection.*   This was advocated, injecting 10 ml of 6% aqueous phenol into the trigone, midway between the ureteric orifices, in order that it should dissipate through the subtrigonal nerve plexus. Although the initial results seemed encouraging with 76% of patients being continent, longer term results show that only 2% of patients had any benefit at one year and there have been reports of fistula formation related to sloughing of the trigone.[38–40] This procedure cannot be advocated for clinical use.

There are two surgical procedures which do have a place in clinical practice in patients in whom conservative therapy has failed, these being prolonged cystodistension under regional block, and augmentation cystoplasty.

*Prolonged cystodistension.*   Prolonged hydrostatic bladder distension produces ischaemic nerve damage when the intravesical pressure is maintained part-way between systolic and diastolic blood pressure using a fluid column. This technique is based on treatment previously described for carcinoma of the bladder. A 2 h period of distension is considered appropriate and there is a need for adequate pain relief, hence the use of an epidural or spinal blockade rather than prolonged general anaesthesia. The initial results demonstrated that 70% of 20 patients with refractory detrusor instability became continent, this initial improvement being maintained over the intermediate term.[41] In a more recent series of 29 patients, 6 had 'marked improvement' and 8 'some improvement'.[42] In an overview of the results, some 50% of patients showed significant improvement following this technique.[43] The major complication of the procedure is bladder rupture, which occurs in up to 8% of patients. Fortunately, the bladder rupture tends to be extraperitoneal, rather than intraperitoneal, and the bladder tends to heal spontaneously after prolonged catheter drainage.[43] This technique should be considered as an alternative to the major surgical procedure of augmentation cystoplasty.

*Augmentation cystoplasty.*   the technique of clam augmentation ileocysto-plasty was first described by Bramble. The technique involves almost complete bisection of the bladder in the coronal plane down as far as the ureters on either side and then insertion of an isolated vascular loop of ileum approximately 25 cm in length to restore bladder integrity.[44] Other authors have demonstrated that 90% of the patients undergoing this treatment became continent, although 25% had some degree of voiding disorder and 15% required clean intermittent self-catheterisation.[45] Patients who are counselled for this procedure must balance the benefits with the potential risk of the development of malignant disease within the enteric segment, especially on the anastomotic site. It is known that there is a 5% risk of adenocarcinoma arising in ureterosigmoidostomies where the colonic mucosa is exposed to nitrosamines in the urine.[46] It is not clear whether this statistic is applicable to the small bowel used in the clam and there have been isolated reports of adenocarcinoma arising in the ileal segment but such reports tend to have occurred in patients whose original pathology was tuberculosis.[47] The true risk in the ileal segment following surgery for idiopathic detrusor instability has to be stated as unknown, but theoretically real, and such patients must understand the risk before undergoing such surgery and should be subject to annual cystoscopy in the absence of symptoms and immediate cystoscopy should haematuria occur.

## Algorithm for treatment

Given the range of treatments and the balance between efficacy and side effects, there is no single treatment which should take precedent over all others nor is there a single treatment plan which could be universally adopted. Much will depend not only upon that which is available locally, but upon the wishes of the patient and upon the results of previous therapy.

In this author's practice, the patient is re-assured once other pathology has been excluded and an explanation of the unstable given. The majority of patients require therapy and this author would choose drug therapy in the first instance on the grounds that it is cheap, easy to administer, and larger number of patients can be treated over unit time compared with the more efficacious, but more effective, behavioural therapies. This author's first line choice of drug is oxybutynin. The patients are then reviewed after 6 weeks of therapy. If symptoms have improved and side effects are absent, then either the treatment can be continued or the dosage increased. If side effects have inhibited compliance with the treatment, or the treatment has been relatively ineffective, then either tolterodine or propiverine is prescribed. Should these drugs be ineffective, then either flavoxate or probanthine is used. In specific circumstances, especially nocturia or nocturnal enuresis, imipramine or DDAVP is prescribed.

In patients who remain symptomatic, admission is offered for bladder drill. Bladder drill could be augmented by drug therapy should there have been some improvement with drugs but side effects or dosage regimens mean that the maximum dose of drug for a given patient has been reached. Should bladder re-training fail, patients are offered prolonged cystodistension under epidural. Should this treatment work but relapse, re-treatment is offered. Should this treatment not work then patients are counselled concerning the pros and cons of a clam ileocystoplasty with special emphasis being laid upon the risk of malignant change.

Unfortunately, there remain a group of patients who will not be made continent yet instability will probably be aggravated by the use of an indwelling catheter. Such patients require the assistance of a Continence Nurse Adviser in order to find appropriate methods by which their incontinence can be managed using pads and devices, details of which are outside the range of this chapter.

## Longer term results

Unfortunately, many of the treatments described above even though of limited efficacy in the short-term are even less effective in the intermediate term.

Patients successfully treated with drug therapy or bladder drill may relapse in time. In one series, some 40% of patients had relapsed within 3 years.[27] In a study of 256 women with detrusor instability treated by various modalities and assessed between 6–12 months after treatment, whilst only 5.5% were completely free of all symptoms, a further 48% were significantly improved, 40.5% were unchanged and 6% were worse.[48] The need to develop more effective long-term therapy, or the ability to repeat therapy in relapse are major requirements for current practice.

## CONCLUSIONS

Detrusor instability is a common and unpleasant condition and, whilst benign, many patients find that their quality of life is severely restricted by this condition. There is a need to exclude underlying pathology, in as much as that is possible, and a need to consider accurate diagnosis by urodynamic assessment.

The choice of treatment depends to some degree on the patient's expectations. Different treatments carry different efficacy and different side effects and complication and it is important to explore which symptoms the patient wishes to have treated as opposed to make an assumption. Given discussion with the patient, the choice of treatment may become clearer. When conservative treatment has failed, and the patient is sufficiently distressed by her symptoms, surgical intervention may be required; but, under such circumstances, a urodynamic confirmation of diagnosis is mandatory.

The outlook for patients with detrusor instability has improved recently with additional drugs becoming available, but there is still the need for more efficacious pharmacological agents.

---

**KEY POINTS FOR CLINICAL PRACTICE**

- Detrusor instability is a common condition causing considerable distress
- Consider underlying pathology
- Urodynamic assessment should be performed if there is no evidence of underlying pathology and symptoms include more than frequency, nocturia, urgency, or urge incontinence

- Drug treatment is probably the first line treatment with oxybutynin as the most efficacious agent followed by tolterodine and propiverine

- Behavioural forms of therapy, especially bladder drill should be considered for those in whom drug therapy has failed

- Prolonged cystodistension under epidural should be considered in those in whom easier treatment options have failed

- Clam ileocystoplasty is an effective procedure but carries an unquantified risk

---

*References*

1  Bates P, Bradley W E, Glen F et al. First report of the standardisation of terminology of lower urinary tract function. Br J Urol 1976; 48: 39–42

2 Brocklehurst J C. Urinary incontinence in the community. BMJ 1993; 306: 832–834

3 Jarvis G J. The management of urinary incontinence. In: Jarvis G J (ed) Obstetrics and Gynaecology. Oxford: Oxford University Press, 1994; 260–299

4 Collas D M, Malone-Lee J G. The effect of age on lower urinary tract symptoms. Int Urogynaecol J 1996; 7: 24–29

5 de Groat W C. A neurological basis for the over-active bladder. Urology 1997; 50 (suppl 6A): 36–52

6 Bosch J L R H. The over-active bladder: current aetiological concepts. Br J Urol 1999; 83 (suppl 2): 7–9

7 Brading A F, Turner W H. The unstable bladder: towards a common mechanism. Br J Urol 1994; 73: 3–8

8 Abrams P H, Farrar D J, Turner-Warwick R. The results of prostatectomy. J Urol 1979; 121: 540–542

9 Jarvis G J. Surgery for genuine stress incontinence. Br J Obstet Gynaecol 1994; 101: 371–374

10 Macauley A J. Psychiatric aspects in the unstable bladder. In: Freeman Mulvern (eds). London: Wright, 1988; 38–44

11 Hafner R J, Stanton S L, Gui J. A psychiatric study of women with urgency and urge incontinence. Br J Urol 1977; 49: 211–214

12 Hohlbrugger G. Urinary potassium and the over-active bladder. Br J Urol, 1999; 83 (suppl 2): 22–28

13 Wise B. Detrusor instability and hyper-reflexia. In: Cardozo L D. (ed) Urogynecology. New York: Churchill Livingstone, 1997; 287–306

14 Webb R J, Griffiths C J, Ramsden P D. Ambulatory monitoring in low compliance neuropathic bladder function. J Urol 1992; 148: 1477–1481

15 Meyhoff H H, Gerstenberg T C, Nordling J. Placebo – the drug of choice in female motor urge incontinence. Br J Urol 1983; 55: 34–37

16 Cardozo L D. Detrusor instability – current management. Br J Obstet Gynaecol 1990; 97: 463–466

17 Thuroff J W, Bunk E B, Ebner A. Randomised double-blind multicentre trial of treatment of frequency, urge and incontinence related to detrusor hypersensitivity. J Urol 1991; 145: 813–817

18 Chapple C R, Parkhouse H, Gardener C. Double-blind placebo-controlled study of flavoxate in the treatment of idiopathic detrusor instability. Br J Urol 1990; 66: 491–494

19 Moisey C U, Stephenson T P, Brendler C B. The urodynamic and subjective result of treatment of detrusor instability with oxybutynin. Br J Urol 1980; 52: 472–475

20 Moore K H, Hay D M, Imrie A E et al. Oxybutynin hydrochloride in the treatment of female idiopathic detrusor instability. Br J Urol 1990; 66: 479–485

21 Abrams P, Freeman R, Anderstrom C et al. Terodiline a new antimuscarinic agent. Br J Urol 1998; 81: 801–810

22 Abrams P, Larsson G, Chapple C et al. Factors involved in the success of antimuscarinic treatment. Br J Urol 1999; 83 (suppl 2): 44–47

23 Monthly Index of Medical Specialties, September 1994; 6

24 Castleden C M, Dufnim C M, Gulati R S. Double-blind study of imipramine and placebo for incontinence due to detrusor instability. Age Aging 1986; 15: 299–302

25 Ramsden P D, Hindmarsh J R, Price D A et al. DDAVP for adult enuresis. Br J Urol 1982; 54: 256–258

26 Jarvis G J, Millar D M. Controlled trial of bladder drill for detrusor instability. BMJ 1980; 281: 1322–1323

27 Holmes D M, Stone A R, Barry P R et al. Bladder training – 3 years on. Br J Urol 1983; 55: 660–664

28 Cardozo L D, Abrams P H, Stanton S L et al. Idiopathic detrusor instability treated by biofeedback. Br J Urol 1978; 50: 521–523

29 Holmes D M, Plevnik S, Stanton S L. Bladder neck electrical conductance in the treatment of detrusor instability with feedback. Br J Obstet Gynaecol 1989; 96: 321–326

30 Freeman R M, Baxby K. Hypnotherapy for incontinence caused by detrusor instability. BMJ 1982; 284: 1831-1834

31 Philp T, Shah P J R, Worth P H L. Acupuncture in the treatment of bladder instability. Br J Urol 1988; 61: 490-493

32 Jonasson A, Larsson B, Pschera H et al. Short-term maximal electrical stimulation. Gynaecol Obstet Invest 1990; 30: 120–123

33 Wise B G, Cardozo L D, Cutner A et al. Maximal electrical stimulation – an acceptable alternative to anticholinergic therapy. Int Urogynecol J 1992; 3: 270

34 Bower W F, Moore K H, Adams R D et al. A urodynamic study of surface neuromodulation versus sham in detrusor instability and sensory urgency. J Urol 1998; 160: 2133–2136

35 Ingleman-Sundberg A. Partial bladder denervation for detrusor dyssynergia. Clin Obstet Gynaecol 1978; 21: 279–305

36 Warrell D W. Vaginal denervation of the bladder nerve supply. Urol Int 1977; 32: 114–116

37 Mundy A R. Detrusor instability. Br J Urol 1988; 62: 393–397

38 Ewing R, Bultitude M I, Shuttleworth K E D. Subtrigonal phenol injection for urge incontinence secondary to detrusor instability in females. Br J Urol 1982; 54: 689–692

39 Rosenbaum T P, Shah P J R, Worth P H L. Transtrigonal phenol. Neurol Urodyn 1988; 7: 294–295

40 Cameron-Strange A, Millard R J. Management of refractory detrusor instability by transvesical phenol injection. Br J Urol 1988; 62: 323–325

41 Dunn M, Smith J C, Ardran G M. Prolonged bladder distension as a treatment of urgency and urge incontinence of urine. Br J Urol 1974; 46: 645–652

42 Lloyd S N, Lloyd S M, Rogers K et al. Is there still a place for prolonged bladder distension? Br J Urol 1992; 70: 382–386

43 Wall L L. Urinary incontinence due to detrusor instability. Obstet Gynaecol Surv 1990; 45: 1S–47S

44 Bramble F J. The treatment of adult enuresis and urge incontinence by enterocystoplasty. Br J Urol 1982; 54: 693–696

45 Mundy A, Stephenson T P. Clam ileocystoplasty for the treatment of refractory urge incontinence. Br J Urol 1985; 57: 541–546

46 Husmann D A, Spence H M. Current status of tumour of the bowel following ureterosigmoidostomy. J Urol 1990; 144: 607–610

47 Stone A R, Davis N, Stephenson T P. Cancer associated with augmentation cystoplasty. Br J Urol 1987; 60: 236–238

48 Kelleher C J, Cardozo L D, Khullar V. A medium term analysis of the subjective efficacy and treatment of women with detrusor instability. Br J Obstet Gynaecol 1997; 104: 988–993

*James Drife*

# 25

# The effect of hormones on the breast

The human breast has two components, glandular tissue and fatty stroma, each of which is sensitive to ovarian steroids. The stroma is one of the most oestrogen-sensitive tissues of the body, at least at the onset of puberty. Cyclical breast changes in response to the ovarian cycle continue during reproductive life, and both the stroma and the glandular tissue remain sensitive to exogenous steroids after the menopause.

Even in the UK, where most women with breast disease are referred to surgeons, the effects of hormones on the breast are important to obstetricians and gynaecologists. The hormonal changes of pregnancy result in lactation. Gynaecologists may be consulted about mastalgia or galactorrhoea. A woman's choice of contraception or hormone replacement therapy may be affected by breast side-effects or concern about breast cancer risk

## CHILDHOOD AND PUBERTY

### Normal development

Embryonic and fetal development is the same in both sexes. The 'milk streaks' – bands of tall epithelial cells – appear before the 6th week and disappear by the 10th week, leaving only the nipple area.[1] About the 15th week, 15–20 ducts begin to form – a process independent of hormonal control. Differentiation of cell types begins during intra-uterine life, and differentiation of basal cells into myo-epithelial cells appears to be completed before birth.[2]

At birth, lobules may be present and colostrum secretion may be stimulated by the withdrawal of placental sex steroids. The lobules regress after birth. During childhood, the ductal system keeps pace with general body growth, though the breast is capable of responding to hormones.

**Prof. James Drife**, MD FRCOG FRCPS FRCSE, Division of Obstetrics and Gynaecology, D floor Clarendon Wing, Leeds General Infirmary, Belmont Grove, Leeds LS2 9NS, UK

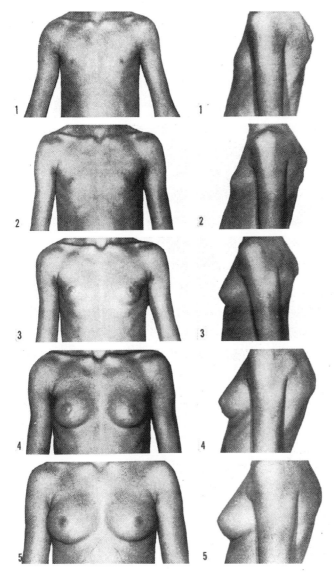

**Fig. 1** Stages of breast development at puberty. Reproduced with the permission of Blackwell Science Ltd from Marshall and Tanner.[3]

Breast development is the first sign of puberty, beginning at a mean age of 11 years and being completed at a mean age of 15.5 years. The five phases[3] are: (i) pre-adolescent elevation of the nipple; (ii) protrusion of a small 'breast hill' and an increase in the diameter of the areola; (iii) further growth of the nipple; (iv) accelerated growth of subareolar tissues; and (v) the mature breast (Fig. 1). These stages are correlated with plasma oestradiol levels.[4] Prolactin levels do not increase greatly at puberty. Ovulation does not normally occur until several months after the menarche and breast development is well advanced before progesterone is first secreted.

At the end of puberty, the stroma is fully developed, but only partial development of the glandular component has occurred, compared with that required for lactation.[1] By far the greater part of the volume of the non-lactating breast is made up of fibrous tissue and fat, the function of which is unclear. It seems to have nothing to do with lactation. Morris[5] has suggested that its purpose is to signal to the male that the female is sexually mature, and that it is analogous to the hormone-sensitive perineal stroma of the apes.

The juxtaposition of this stroma and the mammary gland itself may be an accident of evolution which has important consequences. Adipose tissue contains aromatase, which catalyses the synthesis of oestrogen.[6] Local interaction between adipose cells and glandular epithelium may occur,[7] similar to that hypothesised between adipose tissue and breast cancer cells.[8,9] Within lobules, the extracellular matrix and the basement membrane also regulate differentiation of glandular cells.[10]

### Inadequate breast development

In 97% of normal children, breast development has begun by the 14th birthday. If not, investigation is required. Hypergonadotrophic hypogonadism (due, for example, to ovarian dysgenesis) should be distinguished from hypogonadotrophic hypogonadism. If treatment is needed, it should aim to mimic the timescale of normal puberty, which can take 3–5 years to complete. This means beginning with a small dose of ethinyloestradiol, less than 5 µg daily if possible, for about 6 months, and increasing the dose as slowly as possible.[11] Conventional adult regimens should not be started until 2 years from the beginning of treatment. If the oral contraceptive pill is given too soon, breast development is confined mainly to the nipple and areolar area, and will remain incomplete.

If puberty has been otherwise normal but breast development is unsatisfactory, endocrine treatment is unlikely to be of benefit.

### Early or excessive breast development

Breast development before age 8 years may be a sign of precocious puberty or premature thelarche. In precocious puberty, breast development is followed by other signs of puberty. Full investigation is required. Treatment with gonadotrophin releasing hormone analogue can reduce breast size.

Premature thelarche is breast development without other signs of puberty. Breast enlargement tends to regress in cases of early onset; but, in patients in whom thelarche occurred after the age of 2 years, the breasts remain enlarged until other signs of puberty occur – usually at the normal age but sometimes earlier. The condition may be unilateral, and it is important to avoid surgery in such cases.[12]

## REPRODUCTIVE LIFE

### The normal menstrual cycle

During the normal ovarian cycle, changes occur in both components of the breast.

*Stroma*
Many women report a feeling of fullness in the premenstrual phase of the cycle. Several studies have measured breast volume with serial X-rays, plaster casts,

water displacement or ultrasound, and all have demonstrated that breast volume is greatest in the second half of the cycle.[13] The increase is of the order of 20%. As major histological changes do not occur, it seems that this change is due to oedema. During the normal cycle there are changes in the amount of fluid retained in body tissues, but the overall change in body weight is no more than 1 kg in most women, and the degree of oedema in the breast is, therefore, not merely a reflection of generalised fluid retention.

Thermography has shown increased vascularity of the breast during the week before menstruation. Pickles,[14] using a baroplethysmographic method, found that blood flow in the breast increased during the luteal phase to a maximum just before menstruation, and then fell to its lowest point at about the 10th day of the cycle. This leads to a detectable change in breast temperature. Distortion of this 'heat cycle', detected by a thermometric brassière, may be of use in screening for breast cancer.[15,16]

## Glandular tissue

The effects of the menstrual cycle on breast epithelium have been a source of debate since 1922, when it was claimed that the corpus luteum causes sprouting of the breast ductules.[17] Three years later, it was suggested that the apparent cyclic pattern was due to age differences between the cases, and subsequent investigators concluded that the numbers of lobules or acini do not change during the cycle.[18]

It was then suggested that cyclical changes may differ before and after first pregnancy. Parous women have greater numbers of breast lobules and a greater density of ductules within lobules. Nulliparous women have greater numbers of clear vacuolated basal cells. During the menstrual cycle; however, only slight cellular changes occur. The height of the ductule epithelium is greater in the luteal phase and this cyclical change is slightly more obvious among parous than nulliparous women.[17,19]

The numbers of mitotic figures in breast biopsies were quantified by Anderson,[20] and mitoses appeared to be more plentiful in the luteal phase of the cycle. Apoptosis (cell death) was also quantified in this study, and the peak followed 3 days after the peak in the number of mitoses.

Masters[21] examined the uptake of labelled thymidine by samples of normal breast tissue in organ culture, and compared this with the day of the cycle on which the biopsy was obtained. Label uptake – an indicator of the 'S' (synthesis) phase of the cell cycle – was greatest in the luteal phase of the ovarian cycle. The effect is more striking when the results are plotted according to the last (not the first) day of the menstrual cycle, thus synchronising the luteal phases: there is a linear increase in the uptake of label, indicating that progesterone has an effect on normal breast epithelium (Fig. 2).

More recently, using breast epithelial cells obtained from volunteers by repeated fine needle aspiration biopsy, studies on Ki-67/MIB-1 (an antibody to a nuclear antigen present in proliferating cells) have confirmed that the percentage of proliferating cells increases during the luteal phase compared with the proliferative phase, and that proliferation is correlated with serum levels of progesterone.[22] Bcl-2 (a protein which prevents apoptosis) in lobular epithelial cells shows maximal expression in mid-cycle, when apoptosis is least prevalent, and a sharp decline in the late luteal phase, as the incidence of apoptosis rises.[23]

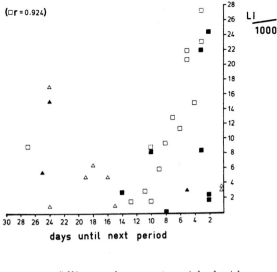

**Fig. 2** Effect of ovarian cycle on cell turnover in the 'resting' breast. LI is labelling index, the proportion of cells taking up labelled thymidine; from Drife.[17]

Studies of steroid receptors have shown that oestradiol stimulates cell proliferation and synthesis of progesterone receptors in luminal epithelial cells. Cells positive for oestrogen receptor (ER) are distributed evenly thoughout the epithelium. Dividing cells are separate from those expressing steroid receptors (though often in close proximity), suggesting that cell proliferation is controlled by paracrine factors released from ER-positive cells.[24]

The effect of the cell cycle on breast surgery is controversial. It has been reported that premenopausal patients with breast cancer and positive axillary nodes operated on during the luteal phase had a significantly better prognosis than patients operated on during the follicular phase.[25] This finding has been attributed to chance but it has also been supported and further research is needed.[26]

## Pregnancy

Breast tenderness usually begins at 5–6 weeks and the breast enlarges and becomes more vascular. Hytten[27] found that the main increase in volume occurs in the middle of pregnancy, and that subsequent milk yield correlates better with the increase than with total breast volume, i.e. with the proliferation of the glandular component, not with the volume of fat and stroma.

In the first 3–4 weeks, there is increased ductular sprouting, which continues until halfway through pregnancy, after which there is proliferation of ductules and hypertrophy of existing lobulo-alveolar structures. The amount of stroma is relatively decreased. In the third trimester, the breast consists mainly of enlarged lobules with only a little supporting tissue, and differentiation and maturation of the secretory cells occur.[1]

Thus histological development correlates with the steady increases in oestrogen, progesterone, prolactin and placental lactogen during pregnancy, and not with the early rise in chorionic gonadotrophin. In animal studies, single hormones cannot produce complete breast development, which probably requires synergism between ovarian steroids, prolactin, growth hormone, insulin and cortisol. The view that oestrogens stimulate duct growth while progesterone produces lobulo-alveolar development was in vogue before the importance of prolactin was realised. Whether placental lactogen has a role in stimulating mammary development is not known.

## Lactation

During the first 3–5 days after parturition, the breast produces colostrum, a yellowish fluid rich in immunoglobulin, particularly IgA, which is important in the transfer of passive immunity to the neonate. After this, the concentration of protein falls and that of lactose and fat rises. The histological structure of the breast remains static during lactation, with the alveolar cells having the typical appearance of actively secreting epithelium. The alveoli are surrounded by a basket-shaped network of myo-epithelial cells which are the effector organ in the suckling reflex. Stimulation of the nipple and areola produces oxytocin release from the posterior pituitary by a neuronal pathway involving the supra-optic and paraventricular nuclei of the hypothalamus. Oxytocin acts on the myo-epithelial cells to stimulate contraction and they are said to be 10–20 times more sensitive to oxytocin than myometrial cells.

The endocrine control of lactation has two aspects: initiation and maintenance. Prolactin is essential for initiating lactation, but other hormones, such as oestrogen, are also necessary. Progesterone is thought to have an inhibitory effect, and initiation of lactation is brought about partly by the removal of this inhibition when progesterone levels fall. Maintenance of lactation requires both suckling and adequate levels of prolactin. Other hormones, such as insulin and growth hormone, also seem to play a part. Oestrogen and progesterone are not necessary and indeed may suppress lactation. Ovarian activity is suppressed during full lactation by neural stimuli: it seems that suckling inhibits the production of gonadotrophin-releasing factor by the hypothalamus.

Lactation problems and their management are outside the scope of this chapter.

## Involution

If suckling is discontinued for more than 48 h, milk synthesis and secretion rapidly begin to decrease. Surges of oxytocin and prolactin no longer occur and there is a gradual fall in plasma prolactin levels. Within the breast, retained secretion distends the alveoli and may rupture the alveolar wall.[1] The epithelial cells are flattened and intracellular lysosomal enzymes are induced to remove secretory material. Phagocytic cells migrate into the alveolar lumen, secretion is removed and the alveolar wall desquamates. Myo-epithelial cells are the least

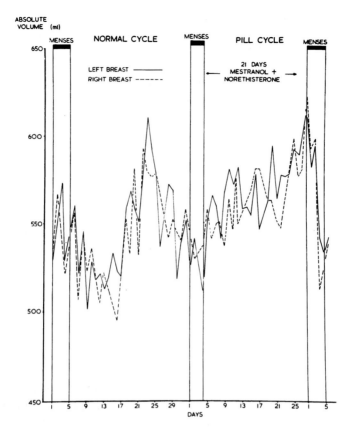

**Fig. 3** Change in breast volume in normal and oral contraceptive-controlled cycles. Reproduced with the permission of the *British Medical Journal* from Milligan et al.[13]

affected by the disorganisation of involution. Fibrous tissue re-grows and the last stage is the reappearance of fatty tissue. The process may last 3–12 months, depending on whether lactation is stopped suddenly or gradually.

## Oral contraceptive pill

### Stroma

During a cycle controlled by the combined oral contraceptive (COC) an increase in breast volume occurs in most women, similar to that in the normal cycle (Fig. 3). Breast volume may increase by up to 20% during the 3 weeks on the COC, and falls during the pill-free week.[13] As in the normal cycle, this seems to be due to changes in the breast stroma.

### Epithelium

Data on the effects of exogenous steroids on the glandular epithelium itself are few. Anderson[28] found an increase in mitotic activity in COC-controlled cycles that reaches a peak at day 25 of the artificial cycle: there is also a peak in apoptosis at day 28 of the cycle. Neither the mitotic response nor the apoptotic response seems to be related to the 'potency' of the steroids in the COC, as assessed by their effect on other organs. Masters studied DNA synthesis in a small number of COC-users: it seemed to be towards the lower end of the range seen in normally cycling women, and in the small number of specimens examined there was no evidence of cyclical activity.[17]

These studies indicate that the COC mimics the effect of the normal cycle on mammary glands. In Anderson's studies,[28] the breasts of nulliparous women were very responsive to COC use, whereas the breasts of parous women were almost unaffected. The effect also depended on the oestrogen content of the COC: low-oestrogen COCs produced a level of stimulation similar to that in the normal cycle, but higher oestrogen COCs produced higher levels of stimulation.

## Mastalgia

Benign breast disease is outside the scope of this chapter, but mastalgia is a symptom that may present to the gynaecologist. In a US study,[29] 69% of women at an obstetrics and gynaecology clinic reported regular premenstrual discomfort and 36% had consulted a health care provider about the symptoms. Mastalgia was moderate to severe in 11%. It interfered with usual sexual activity in 48% and with work activity in 8%. In a British study of severe mastalgia,[30] the median age of onset of breast pain was 36 years and the mean duration was 12 years. Women with cyclic mastalgia often have other symptoms of the premenstrual syndrome.[31]

### Pathophysiology
Breast pain may be cyclical, non-cyclical or extramammary. Extramammary causes include angina, cholelithiasis, cervical spondylitis and Tietze's syndrome (pain in a costochondral junction, which can be treated by injection of lignocaine and hydrocortisone). Non-cyclical pain can be difficult to treat and, since it may be associated with breast cancer, careful examination and follow-up – with mammography, if appropriate – are necessary. Non-cyclical mastalgia may persist beyond the menopause.[30]

Cyclical breast pain is one of the commonest components of the premenstrual syndrome. Hormone levels show little difference between women with severe cyclical mastalgia and normal women. For 85% of sufferers, re-assurance that the condition is benign will allow them to tolerate their pain. If treatment is required, the woman should be asked to chart the pattern and severity of the pain over a 3-month interval.

### Treatment
Many women with mastalgia have been labelled 'neurotic', but in most this label is unjustified. Treatments have included exclusion diets and antibiotics, but there is no evidence that bacterial 'mastitis' underlies most benign breast disease. Vitamins are widely prescribed but seem to exert a placebo effect only. There is no evidence that women with mastalgia retain more body water in the pre-menstrual phase than normal controls, and diuretics are no more effective than placebo. Progestogens are advocated by some, but as progesterone deficiency has not been demonstrated in women with cyclical mastalgia it is not surprising that they too are no more effective than placebo.

Drugs which have been assessed for mastalgia include danazol, bromocriptine, anti-oestrogens such as tamoxifen, and evening primrose oil. In trials,[32] danazol 200 mg/day produced an improvement in 70% of cases of cyclical and 30% of cases of non-cyclical mastalgia; with bromocriptine the figures were 47% and 20%, respectively, and with evening primrose oil, 45% and 27%. Placebo improved 20% of cases of cyclical and 9% of cases of non-cyclical mastalgia. Tamoxifen (20 mg/day) produces an improvement in over 70% of cases, but is not licensed for this indication.[33] Severe mastalgia runs a chronic relapsing course, often requiring repeated drug treatments.[30]

## MENOPAUSE AND POST-MENOPAUSE

With the fall in circulating ovarian steroids at the menopause, there is a reduction in the amount of lobular and alveolar structures, and ultimately only fat, connective tissue and mammary ducts remain. The amount of stroma is not reduced. It has been claimed that this process begins around the age of 35 years and speeds up after 45 years, though the hormonal reason for this is obscure.

Studies in monkeys have shown that hormone replacement therapy (HRT) prevents the postmenopausal atrophy of mammary lobules, and suggest that proliferation of lobules is greater with combined HRT than with oestrogen-only HRT.[34] Studies of cell turn-over rates in postmenopausal women undergoing breast surgery did not confirm this, however.[35] Turn-over rates were unaffected by age or duration of menopause, or by HRT, either oestrogen-only or combined, but both types of HRT increased the amount of progesterone receptor. Nevertheless, cell turn-over rates were much lower than in similar studies of the premenopausal breast, suggesting a possible attenuation of sensitivity to oestradiol-induced proliferation in the post-menopausal breast. Belgian researchers, studying topical application of hormone-containing gels to the breast, reported that oestrogen caused an increase in the number of cycling epithelial cells and that this was reduced by progestogen.[36]

The composition of the adipose tissue also changes at the menopause. Levels of the protein CD36 are lower in adipocytes from postmenopausal as compared to premenopausal women,[37] suggesting a reduced ability to transport or store fatty acids. Within adipocytes, oestrone and oestradiol levels are lower in postmenopausal women than in premenopausal women: levels are related to the body mass index and are raised by HRT.[38]

## EPIDEMIOLOGY OF BREAST CANCER

The role of hormones and antihormones in the treatment of breast cancer is outside the scope of this chapter, which will confine itself to the role of sex hormones in the aetiology of the disease. Many other factors influence a woman's risk of developing breast cancer[39] – for example, the country in which she lives, her family history and the age at which she has her first full term pregnancy. Nulliparous women and women who have never breast-fed are at increased risk of breast cancer. Among women who have borne children, there is a linear relationship between the age at first live birth and the risk of breast cancer: the later child-bearing begins, the less is its protective effect. A first live-birth after the age of 32 years seems to increase a woman's risk of breast cancer. The reason for the steady reduction in the protective effect of first pregnancy is unclear.

## Ovarian activity

The menstrual history is also important. An early menarche is a risk factor for subsequent breast cancer and so is a late menopause. The risk is decreased by a late menarche and by an early menopause, either natural or surgical. The fact that the total duration of ovarian activity is related to the risk of breast cancer implicates natural ovarian hormones in the initiation or promotion of the disease.

A relatively small variation in the age at menarche can be important. A girl whose menarche occurs before the age of 13 years has twice the risk of subsequently developing breast cancer than a girl whose menarche occurs after this age. The early establishment of ovulatory cycles seems to be the important factor.[39] The effect is most marked in women aged 32 years or less at diagnosis of cancer, but age at menarche may still have a substantial effect on risk later in life, even at age 70 years. This indicates that breast cancer has a long latency and its occurrence may reflect patterns of hormone exposure many years previously.

At the other end of reproductive life, it takes a greater variation to achieve the same effect: a woman who has her menopause after age 55 years has double the risk of breast cancer compared to a woman whose menopause occurs before age 44 years. This difference between the effects of menarche and menopause suggests that the breast tissue is less sensitive to variations in ovarian steroids later in life than around the menarche.

## Oral contraceptive pill

There have been many case-control studies of the effect of COCs on breast cancer risk, and their results have been somewhat contradictory. No studies have suggested that the COC has a protective effect against breast cancer (in contrast to its clear protective effects against cancers of the ovary and the endometrium). Some studies have shown no adverse effect. Others have shown an increase in breast cancer risk in women who took the COC at an early age, but have concluded that in the middle of reproductive life – between the ages of 25 and 39 years – the COC has no effect on risk.[40]

In 1996, the data from a total of 54 epidemiological studies were re-analysed by an international collaborative group.[41] The results provided strong evidence for two main conclusions. First, while women are taking COCs and in the 10 years after stopping there is a small increase in the relative risk (RR) of having breast cancer diagnosed, the RR being 1.24 in current users and falling to 1.07 5–9 years after stopping. Second, there is no significant excess risk of having breast cancer diagnosed 10 or more years after stopping COC use. Breast cancers in COC users tended to be less advanced clinically than those diagnosed in non-users.

These conclusions applied to women from all countries and ethnic groups, and to those with or without a family history of breast cancer. Duration of COC use and age at first use had little additional effect. Women who began COC use before age 20 years had higher relative risks while using COCs and in the 5 years after stopping than women in older age groups, but breast cancer in this age group is very rare.

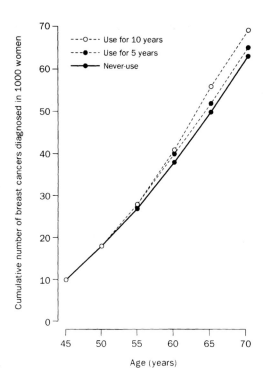

**Fig. 4** Age-related risk of breast cancer according to duration of use of hormone replacement therapy. Reproduced with the permission of The Lancet Ltd from Collaborative Group on Hormonal Factors in Breast Cancer.[44]

This study also concluded that the dose and type of hormone within the COCs had little additional effect. Nevertheless, it is worth pointing out that the median year of cancer diagnosis in the original studies ranged from 1976 to 1992. Bearing in mind the long latent period of breast cancer, many of the women must have been taking COCs before low-dose formulations were introduced. It is possible that the long-term effects of currently used COC formulations are less than those described in Collaborative Group's report. Further epidemiological studies are required to assess the effect of modern low-oestrogen COCs on breast cancer risk, in view of the evidence (mentioned above) that low-oestrogen COCs stimulate the breast less than high-dose formulations.[28]

## Postmenopausal hormone replacement therapy

Postmenopausal HRT differs from the COC in that exogenous hormones are being taken by women who otherwise would be subject to little if any endogenous hormonal stimulation. The adverse effect of a late natural menopause on breast cancer risk is a reason for concern about the effect of HRT. On the other hand, the possible age-related reduction in hormonal sensitivity of mammary tissue is a reason for optimism. The steroid dosages in HRT are low, but, nevertheless, HRT and low-dose COCs are more similar in bioequivalence than most people think.

There have been many epidemiological studies of the relation between HRT and breast cancer risk.[42,43] In 1997, the Collaborative Group published a re-analysis of the data from 51 studies involving over 150,000 women.[44] They concluded that the risk of having breast cancer diagnosed is increased in women using HRT and rises with increasing duration of use (Fig. 4). The effect disappears about 5 years after cessation of HRT use. Of the many factors that might affect the relationship between HRT and breast cancer risk, only body weight had a material effect, the increase in risk being greater for women of lower weight.

Women with a family history of breast cancer may be particularly concerned about the safety of HRT. One meta-analysis of 5 studies has suggested that there may be a further increase in risk among women who have a first-degree relative with breast cancer,[43] but another meta-analysis concluded that neither family history of breast cancer nor a previous history of benign breast disease alters the relationship between HRT and breast cancer risk.[42]

Because in the breast, unlike the endometrium, progesterone has a stimulatory effect on cell growth, combined HRT could carry more risk than 'unopposed' (oestrogen-only) HRT. Most of the epidemiological studies so far have examined the effect of unopposed oestrogen therapy, and the data at present are inadequate to tell whether or not the addition of progestogen increases the risk. Nevertheless, the results from the first 4 studies to include combined HRT have not given cause for serious concern, with the relative risk being 1.13 for combined therapy.

### HRT after breast cancer

Standard teaching is that HRT is contra-indicated for a woman who has had breast cancer, because of concern that oestrogen may stimulate proliferation of residual cancer cells. Some women, however, may be very troubled by symptoms of oestrogen withdrawal and it was suggested several years ago[45] that the decision on HRT should be taken on an individual basis and that 'oestrogen could be considered for those women who have been adequately treated for early stage breast cancer when there is no evidence of disease progression after 1 to 2 years'. A more recent consensus conference[46] emphasised the need for further research, particularly regarding relief of symptoms, but agreed that 'an informed woman, knowing all the potential benefits and risks of oestrogen, could choose to take oestrogen and may be supported in that decision'.

## CONCLUSION

After many years of controversy and intermittent alarms about the effects of the COC and HRT, we now have a clearer understanding of their risks. Neither seems to have a lasting effect on breast cancer risk many years after cessation of use. The COC may cause a small increase in risk among users and recent ex-users, but it remains uncertain whether this conclusion applies to currently used low-dose preparations. The risk associated with HRT is small, but steadily increases with duration of use. The biggest difficulty, therefore, is faced by women who wish to continue HRT indefinitely. Advising women about these risks requires an understanding of the effects of the normal menstrual cycle, and an ability to balance the risks and benefits of exogenous hormones.

## References

1  Dawson E K. A histological study of the normal mamma in relation to tumour growth. Edinb Med J 1934; 41: 653–682 and 1935; 42: 569–598 and 633–660

2  Anbazhagan R, Osin P, Bartkova J, Nathan B, Lane B, Gusterson BA. The development of epithelial phenotypes in the human fetal and infant breast. J Pathol 1998; 184: 197–206

3  Marshall W A, Tanner J M. Puberty. In: Davis J A, Dobbing J. (eds) Scientific Foundations of Paediatrics. London: Heinemann, 1974

4  Apter D. Serum steroids and pituitary hormones in female puberty: a partly longitudinal study. Clin Endocrinol 1980; 12: 107–120

5  Morris D. The Naked Ape. London, Jonathan Cape, 1967

6  Simpson E R, Merrill J, Hollub A J, Graham-Lorence S, Mendelson C R. Regulation of estrogen biosynthesis by human adipose cells. Endocrine Rev 1989; 10: 136–148

7  Brodie A, Lu Q, Nakamura J. Aromatase in the normal breast and breast cancer. J Steroid Biochem Mol Biol 1997; 61: 281–286

8  Simpson E R, Mahendroo M S, Means G D et al. Aromatase cytochrome P450, the enzyme responsible for estrogen biosynthesis. Endocrine Rev 1994; 15: 342–355

9  Miller W R, Mullen P, Sourdaine P, Watson C, Dixon J M, Telford J. Regulation of aromatase activity within the breast. J Steroid Biochem Mol Biol 1997; 61: 3–6

10  Bissell M J. Glandular structure and gene expression: lessons from the mammary gland. Ann NY Acad Sci 1998; 842: 1–6

11  Brook C G D. Management of delayed puberty. BMJ 1985; 290: 657–658

12  Styne D M. New aspects in the diagnosis and treatment of pubertal disorder. Pediatr Clin North Am 1997; 44: 505–529

13  Milligan D, Drife J O, Short R V. Changes in breast volume during normal menstrual cycle and after oral contraceptives. BMJ 1977; iv: 494–496

14  Pickles V R. Blood-flow estimations as indices of mammary activity. J Obstet Gynaecol Br Emp 1953; 60: 301–311

15  Simpson H W, McArdle C, Pauson A W, Hume P, Turkes A, Griffiths K. A non-invasive test for the precancerous breast. Eur J Cancer 1995; 31: 1768–1772

16  Bjarnason G A. Menstrual cycle chronobiology: is it important in breast cancer screening and therapy? Lancet 1996; 347: 345–346

17  Drife J. The effects of parity and the menstrual cycle on the normal mammary gland and their possible relationship to malignant change. MD Thesis, University of Edinburgh, 1981

18  Haagensen C D Diseases of the Breast, 3rd edn. Philadelphia: Saunders, 1986

19  Drife J O. Evolution, menstruation and breast cancer. In: Bulbrook R D, Taylor D S. (eds) Commentaries on Research in Breast Cancer. New York: Liss, 1979; 1–23

20  Anderson T J, Fergusson D J P, Raab G M. Cell turnover in the 'resting' human breast: influence of parity, contraceptive pill, age and laterality. Br J Cancer 1982; 46: 376–382

21  Masters J R W, Drife J O, Scarisbrick J J. Cyclic variation of DNA synthesis in human breast epithelium. J Natl Cancer Inst 1977; 58: 1263–1265

22  Soderqvist G, Isaaksson E, von Schoultz B, Carlstrom K, Tani E, Skoog L. Proliferation of breast epithelial cells in healthy women during the menstrual cycle. Am J Obstet Gynecol 1997; 176: 123–128

23  Spencer S J, Cataldo N A, Jaffe R B. Apoptosis in the human female reproductive tract. Obstet Gynecol Surv 1996; 51: 314–323

24  Clarke R B, Howell A, Patton C S, Anderson E. Dissociation between steroid receptor expression and cell proliferation in the human breast. Cancer Res 1997; 57: 4987–4991

25  Veronesi U, Luini A, Mariani L et al. Effect of menstrual phase on surgical treatment of breast cancer. Lancet 1994; 343: 1545–1547

26  Fentiman I S, Gregory W M, Richards M A. Effect of menstrual phase on surgical treatment of breast cancer. Lancet 1994; 344: 402

27  Hytten F E. Clinical and chemical studies in human lactation VI: the functional capacity of the breast. BMJ 1954; i: 912–915

28 Anderson T J, Battersby S, King R J B, McPherson K, Going J J. Oral contraceptive use influences resting breast proliferation. Hum Pathol 1989; 20: 1139–1144

29 Ader D N, Browne M W. Prevalence and impact of cyclic mastalgia in a United States clinic-based sample. Am J Obstet Gynecol 1997; 177: 126–132

30 Davies E L, Gateley C A, Miers M, Mansel R E. The long-term course of mastalgia. J R Soc Med 1998; 91: 462–464

31 Goodwin P J, Miller A, Del Giudice M E, Ritchie K. Breast health and associated premenstrual symptoms in women with severe cyclic mastopathy. Am J Obstet Gynecol 1997; 176: 998–1005

32 Pye J K, Mansel R E, Hughes L E. Clinical experience of drug treatments for mastalgia. Lancet 1985; ii: 373–377

33 Fentiman I S, Caleffi M, Brame K, Chaudary M A, Hayward J L. Double-blind controlled trial of tamoxifen therapy for mastalgia. Lancet 1986; i: 287–288

34 Cline J M, Soderqvist G, von Schoultz E, Skoog L, von Schoulz B. Effects of hormone replacement therapy on the mammary gland of postmenopausal cynomolgus macaques. Am J Obstet Gynecol 1996; 174: 93–100

35 Hargreaves D F, Knox F, Swindell R, Potten C S, Bundred N J. Epithelial proliferation and hormone receptor status in the normal post-menopausal breast and the effects of hormone replacement therapy. Br J Cancer 1998; 78: 945–949

36 Foidart J M, Colin C, Denoo X, Desreux J, Beliard A, Fournier S, de Lignieres B. Estradiol and progesterone regulate the proliferation of human breast epithelial cells. Fertil Steril 1998; 69: 963–969

37 Abbadia Z, Vericel E, Mathevet P, Bertin N, Panaye G, Frappart L. Fatty acid composition and CD36 expression in breast adipose tissue of premenopausal and postmenopausal women. Anticancer Res 1997; 17: 1217–1222

38 O'Brien S N, Anandjiwala J, Price T M. Differences in the estrogen content of breast adipose tissue in women by menopausal status and hormone use. Obstet Gynecol 1997; 90: 244–248

39 Henderson I C. Risk factors for breast cancer development. Cancer 1993; 71: 2127–2140

40 Schlesselman J J. Oral contraceptives and breast cancer. Am J Obstet Gynecol 1990; 163: 1379–1387

41 Collaborative Group on Hormonal Factors in Breast Cancer. Breast cancer and hormonal contraceptives: collaborative reanalysis of individual data on 53 297 women with breast cancer and 100 239 women without breast cancer from 54 epidemiological studies. Lancet 1996; 347: 1713–1727

42 Colditz G A, Egan K M, Stampfer M J. Hormone replacement therapy and risk of breast cancer: results from epidemiologic studies. Am J Obstet Gynecol 1993; 168: 1473–1480

43 Persson I. Hormone replacement therapy and the risk of postmenopausal breast cancer. In: Studd J, Asch R. (eds) Annual Progress in Reproductive Medicine. Carnforth: Parthenon, 1993; 301–310

44 Collaborative Group on Hormonal Factors in Breast Cancer. Breast cancer and hormone replacement therapy: collaborative reanalysis of data from 51 epidemiological studies of 52 705 women with breast cancer and 108 411 women without breast cancer. Lancet 1997; 350: 1047–1059

45 Lobo R A. Oestrogen replacement after treatment for breast cancer? Lancet 1993; 341: 1313–1314

46 Santen R, Pritchard K, Burger H. The consensus conference on treatment of estrogen deficiency symptoms in women surviving breast cancer. Obstet Gynecol Surv 1998; 53: S1–S83

S. A. Beardsworth  D. W. Purdie  C. E. Kearney

**26**

# Selective oestrogen receptor modulators

## EVOLUTION

The menopause, strictly defined as the ending of the monthly reproductive cycle, is the outward manifestation of ovarian failure. Exhaustion of primordial follicles leads to an order of magnitude, or 10-fold decline in circulating oestradial to a median of about 50–80 pmol/l, a level below that found in many healthy age-matched men. Were the functions of oestradiol confined to the reproductive arena, no problems would ensue. Fertility over fifty is desired by few; but those functions are now known to range far beyond the regulation of ovulation, implantation and adaptation to pregnancy. The oestrogens have been accorded central roles in the normal function of the cardiovascular, skeletal, central nervous and immune systems – to name but four. Indeed, the anatomical locations of the oestrogen receptors – of which there are at least three – and the known physiological activities of these steroid hormones grow virtually by the month. In summary, the oestrogens and their receptors comprise such a useful signalling system that they can, and they have been, recruited to a plethora of roles provided always that these do not compromise their prime function in reproduction, which is heavily protected and conserved. Thus, the occurrence of a mid-life climacteric with loss of the oestrogen producing granulosa and theca cells which once lined the follicles, deprives oestrogen-consuming systems of an essential element of their daily economy. It has long been a goal of developmental pharmacology to discover,

**Dr S.A. Beardsworth** MRCOG, Clinical Research Fellow, Centre for Metabolic Bone Disease, HS Brocklehurst Building, Hull Royal Infirmary, 220–236 Anlaby Road, Hull HU3 2RW, UK

**Prof. D.W. Purdie** MD FRCOG FRCP(E), Head of Clinical Research, Centre for Metabolic Bone Disease, HS Brocklehurst Building, Hull Royal Infirmary, 220–236 Anlaby Road, Hull HU3 2RW, UK (for correspondence)

**Dr C.E. Kearney** MRCOG, Clinical Research Fellow, Centre for Metabolic Bone Disease, HS Brocklehurst Building, Hull Royal Infirmary, 220–236 Anlaby Road, Hull HU3 2RW, UK

or to synthesise, an oestrogen replacement which would restore oestrogenic activity to the systems which require it, while not returning the woman to a quasi-menstrual cycle with the breast changes, uterine cycling and the symptomatic and pathological consequences which such cycling may bring in its train.

Two prior therapeutic advances gave hope for future selective oestrogen action. It had once been thought that the action of adrenalin proceeded through a unitary receptor pathway until Black[1] confirmed a suggestion by Alquhist that the adrenoreceptor might be dual. The result, after considerable research, was cardioselective β-adrenergic blockade. Similarly, there was the puzzling observation that antihistamines failed to suppress histamine-induced gastric HCl production. Again, the reason was tracked to the histamine receptor being dual and the result again was a significant therapeutic advance with cimetidine.[2] So it was to prove with oestrogens, our increasing awareness of complexity in oestrogen receptor structure and function coming with the realisation that such complexity was not an obstacle but a major therapeutic opportunity. These developments in pharmacology dove-tailed with the clinical requirements for an oestrogen which would side-step the two principal difficulties reported by patients receiving conventional oestrogen, both of which relate to engagement of the oestrogen receptor at reproductive sites. These difficulties are unwanted vaginal bleeding as a result of endometrial stimulation and the increased risk of breast cancer associated with prolonged oestrogen exposure.[3] This created a requirement for a compound with a beneficial bone, cardiovascular and neurological profile without adverse effects on the reproductive tissues of breast and uterus. The ideal oestrogen is not yet with us, but a start has been made on the road to its development.

## MOLECULAR PHARMACOLOGY

The precise mechanism by which the oestrogens and their non-steroidal SERM analogues achieve their tissue specific activity remains unclear. However, the recent identification of ERβ and greater understanding of its functional relationship to ERα, has lead to a recent re-evaluation of oestrogen and anti-oestrogen signalling and physiology.

### The oestrogen receptors

For many years, the mechanisms of oestrogen receptor (ER) action seemed relatively simple. It was believed that all actions of oestrogen were mediated by a single high-affinity ER, located within target cell nuclei. However, as our appreciation of the diverse actions of oestrogen grew, it became clear that certain tissues such as bladder and ovary, though clearly affected by oestrogen, appeared to lack the receptors needed for this response. The discovery of ERβ, first in the rat[4] and then in the human[5] and mouse,[6] revealed much more complex and diverse oestrogen signalling pathways.

ERα consists of 595 amino acids and has been divided into distinct structural domains. In particular, domains responsible for ligand binding, DNA recognition, and at least two regions which are required for transcriptional activity – activating function-1 (AF1), located towards the amino terminus, and activating function-2 (AF2), contained within the ligand binding domain.[7] In the absence of oestradiol, the transcriptionally inactive ER is located in target cell nuclei in a large macromolecular complex associated with several heat-shock proteins.[8] Upon interaction with the ligand, the receptor undergoes a conformational change with displacement of these inhibitory proteins.[9,10] The receptor then spontaneously dimerises and acquires the ability to interact, as a homodimer, with specific DNA response elements located within the regulatory regions of target genes.[11] Exactly how the promoter-bound receptor initiates the activity of RNA polymerase is still unknown. It is known that the activated complex co-operates with an array of co-activators and co-repressors that may or may not be tissue specific.

Although ERβ may have unique activities in oestrogen responsive tissues, there is a high degree of amino acid sequence similarity between the two proteins[5] that suggests that their general mechanism of action is as described above. ERβ consists of 477 amino acids and there is a 58% amino acid homology between the two receptors in the ligand binding domain and the AF2 core sequences are identical. The main differences between the amino acid sequence of the two receptors occur towards the amino terminus, the region of the protein that contains the AF1 in ERα.[5] Thus it may be that ERβ does not contain a functional AF1.

Expression of ERβ has been observed in a variety of tissues. The highest levels have been found in the granulosa cells of the ovary, but significant expression has also been seen in uterus, Fallopian tube, bladder, pituitary, heart, lung, breast, bone and brain.[4,12–14]. Comparison of the patterns of expression of the two receptors suggests that each receptor subtype may perform specific biological function. However, in tissues where ERα and ERβ are co-expressed, the two receptors might physically interact to form heterodimers or act as targets of independent signalling pathways.[13] The higher affinity that ERα has for oestradiol over ERβ[5] suggests that an independent signalling pathway via ERα homodimers would dominate but would depend on the relative number of receptors present.

It has been determined that all ER ligands (including the selective oestrogen receptor modulators) interact with the common ligand binding domain (LBD) within both ERα and ERβ, efficiently displacing the heat-shock proteins and promoting association of the ER with target DNA. Thus, the tissue selectivity is not due solely to the existence of more than one ER.

## The activation functions

Both activation functions (AF-1 and AF-2) appear to operate in a cell-specific manner and, depending on the cell and promoter context, it was found that the requirement for these activation functions varied.[15] In some contexts, one specific AF would be required, while in others, either AF would be sufficient. Sometimes, both would be needed. In contexts where AF2 is required, either alone or with AF1, the selective oestrogen receptor modulator (SERM) tamoxifen functions as an ER antagonist.[7,16,17]. However, in contexts where AF1 alone is required, tamoxifen functions as a partial agonist manifesting about 40% the agonist activity of oestradiol. These in vitro mechanistic distinctions have not, as yet, been shown to occur in vivo. However, the triphenylethylene derived SERMs droloxifene, toremifene, clomiphene, and nafoxidine all

A

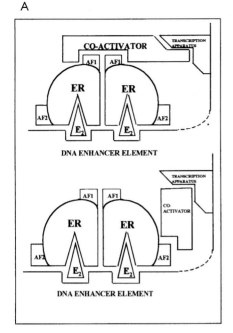

B

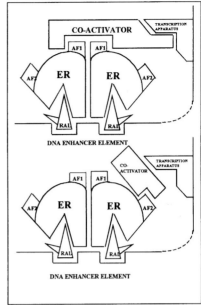

**Fig. 1** Schematic representation of the dimerised oestrogen receptor with oestrogen (A) and raloxifene (B). Both oestrogen and raloxifene will initiate RNA polymerase in cells that require AF1 alone for the promoter bound receptor to engage the transcription apparatus (top). However, in cells where AF2 is required, either alone or in addition to AF2, only oestrogen will initiate transcription and raloxifene will behave as an antagonist (bottom).

display agonist activity in the uterus and antagonist activity in the breast and all function as cell-specific AF1 agonists in vitro.[7,18]

The concept of SERMs being AF2 antagonists was further strengthened when the crystal structure of the ligand-binding domain (LBD) was demonstrated with either oestradiol or raloxifene in the ligand binding site.[19] As anticipated, the backbone of raloxifene concisely binds to the appropriate amino acids that bind oestradiol into the LBD. However, the alkylaminoethoxy side chain projects out of the hydrophobic pocket and displaces helix 12 of the ER. This displacement interferes with the recruitment of co-activators to AF2. Thus, in ERα, when both AF1 and AF2 are present the effect of SERMs will be variable, while in ERβ, until it is proven that AF1 subsists, it should be assumed that SERMs will cause a major loss of function (Fig. 1).

## DNA enhancer elements

The possibility that different DNA enhancer elements may play a role in the tissue selectivity of SERMs has been demonstrated in vitro. The SERMs tamoxifen and raloxifene had the opposite effect on transcriptional activation caused by oestradiol at ERβ with two different DNA enhancer types, the classical oestrogen response element (ERE) and the AP1 system. In addition, with ERα and the ERE the SERMs caused no transcriptional activation while oestradiol

**Table 1** Differential ligand activation of oestrogen receptors ERα and ERβ with different DNA enhancer types

|  | ERα with ERE | ERα with AP1 | ERβ with ERE | ERβ with AP1 |
|---|---|---|---|---|
| Oestrogen | +++ | +++ | +++ | 0 |
| Tamoxifen | 0 | +++ | 0 | +++ |
| Raloxifene | 0 | + | 0 | +++ |
| Control | 0 | 0 | 0 | 0 |

did. This suggests that AF2 is required for the homodimers of both receptors to engage the ERE and cause transcriptional activation. Finally, with ERα and the AP1 enhancer element transcriptional activation occurred with all three ligands, though to a much lesser extent with raloxifene.[20] This last finding cannot be explained by AF2 antagonism alone and clearly demonstrates that we are still some distance from completely explaining the molecular pharmacology of the SERMs (Table 1).

However, the complex signalling physiology of the ER with at least two and possibly three distinct receptor isoforms of different ligand affinity co-existing in many tissues, the existence of at least two activating factors and at least two DNA enhancer elements and the increasing number of co-activators and co-repressors leaves ample scope for the pharmacological evolution of tissue selective ER modulation.

## FIRST GENERATION SERMS: TAMOXIFEN

The scientific basis of selective oestrogen receptor modulation was born out of research in the late 1970s into the 'anti-oestrogens' clomiphene and tamoxifen, at a time when the structure and function of the presumed unitary cytosolic oestrogen receptor was poorly understood. Though one may argue which of tamoxifen and clomiphene was the first SERM to be discovered, it is clear that the former has a therapeutic profile closer to the ideal (Table 2).

A failed contraceptive, tamoxifen has proved useful as adjuvant therapy in the treatment of breast cancer. Indeed, its therapeutic ability to reduce the incidence of contralateral breast tumours by 40%[21] has recently been shown to complement its ability to reduce the incidence of primary breast cancer in individuals considered to be at high-risk.[22] Initially, there were significant concerns that this anti-oestrogenic activity on breast might be associated with osteoporosis and an increased incidence of heart disease. The first evidence

**Table 2** Clinical profile of oestrogen, tamoxifen, raloxifene and the ideal SERM

|  | Oestrogen | Tamoxifen | Raloxifene | The ideal |
|---|---|---|---|---|
| Bone | + | + | + | + |
| Breast | + | – | – | – |
| Uterus | + | + | – | – |
| CHD risk | + | + | + | + |
| VTE risk | + | + | + | – |
| Menopausal symptoms | + | – | – | + |
| Urogenital atrophy | + | 0 | ? | + |
| Cognitive function | + | ? | ? | + |

that this might not be the case was published in 1984.[23] As part of a NASA funded project, ovariectomised rats treated with clomiphene (a mix of *cis*- and *trans*-isomers) surprisingly failed to develop x-ray changes in trabecular bone indicating a decrease in bone mineral content. The ability of tamoxifen (a pure *trans*-isomer) to produce stabilisation of bone loss in ovariectomised rats was first demonstrated in 1987 by Jordan[24] and then further confirmed in women taking tamoxifen for 5 years.[25] Tamoxifen's oestrogen-like actions were also observed in its effect on hepatic lipoprotein metabolism. Tamoxifen decreases total cholesterol, LDL cholesterol, apolipoprotein B, fibrinogen levels and platelet counts.[26,27]. Despite having no effect on HDL cholesterol and actually increasing triglyceride levels, this apparently favourable lipid profile may, in part, explain the reduction in risk of myocardial infarction reported in tamoxifen users.[28] From this mixed picture of oestrogen agonist and antagonist actions was born the concept that these agents might be of tissue-specific oestrogens, their activities being consequent on differential modulation of the oestrogen receptor. However, a factor limiting the use of tamoxifen for indications other than the adjuvant chemotherapy of breast cancer proved to be the question of uterine safety. As early as 1985, a link between endometrial carcinoma and tamoxifen was suspected[29] and was borne out by the large National Surgical Adjuvant Breast and Bowel Project, in which the estimated annual risk of endometrial cancer was 8 times that seen in non-users.[30]

These concerns gave impetus to the development of other 'anti-oestrogen' breast cancer treatments. However, published data on these second generation SERMs are scarce and data on their use in humans are almost exclusively restricted to the benzothiophene, raloxifene. Other SERMs more closely related to the triphenylethylene, tamoxifen, are currently in phase III trials but only raloxifene has a license for use in the EU and the US. The licensed indication in Europe is 'the prevention of non-traumatic vertebral fractures in postmeno-pausal women considered to be at risk of osteoporosis'. As a result, most of the clinical data that exist for SERMs relate to raloxifene.

## BONE

### Animal data

Raloxifene's potential as a SERM was first recognised in 1987 by Jordan during his work with tamoxifen. He showed that raloxifene, then known as keoxifene, mitigated the decrease seen in the femur ash density of ovariectomised rats. This reduction in bone loss was similar to that seen with oestradiol benzoate but, in contrast, was not associated with an increase in uterine wet weight.[24] In 1994, these bone data were confirmed in the femur, tibia and vertebrae of ovari-ectomised Sprague-Dawley rats given ethynyl oestradiol, raloxifene or con-trol.[31,32] These latter reports used the more accurate assessments of bone density computed tomography (CT), single photon absorptiometry (SPA) and dual energy X-ray absorptiometry (DEXA). At all three sites, raloxifene reduced the bone loss seen after oophorectomy. The magnitude of this effect was indistin-guishable from that of oestradiol at the femur and tibia but was slightly less than that seen with oestradiol at the vertebrae. In addition, both treatments preserved bone strength at the femoral neck and partially preserved bone strength at the lumbar spine.[32] Raloxifene also prevented cancellous osteopenia as well as the changes in radial growth and bone resorption that are seen in the rat following oophorectomy. Thus, in the rat model, it appeared that raloxifene had potent oestrogenic activity.[33]

### Human data

In 1996, these findings were confirmed in postmenopausal women by Draper.[34] A group of 251 healthy postmenopausal women were randomly assigned to either placebo, conjugated oestrogens or raloxifene at doses of 200 and 600 mg/day (considerably higher than the now licensed dose of 60 mg/day) for 8 weeks. Markers of bone resorption, urinary pyridinoline cross-links, and of bone formation, serum alkaline phosphatase and serum osteocalcin, were significantly reduced and reached normal premenopausal levels in all but the placebo group. There were no significant differences between raloxifene and oestradiol in this reduction in markers of bone turnover. In a longer prospective study of 601 healthy postmenopausal women reported by Delmas et al, patients were randomly assigned to placebo, or raloxifene at doses of 30, 60 and 150 mg/day for 24 months.[35] Bone mineral density (BMD) was assessed at lumbar spine and total hip every 6 months by dual energy X-ray absorptiometry (DEXA). Over the 2 years, the BMD of the placebo group fell by 0.8% at both lumbar spine and total hip, while in the raloxifene 60 mg/day group the BMD at both sites increased by 1.6%. In a further study, 143 postmenopausal women with established osteoporosis were randomly assigned to placebo or raloxifene 60 and 120 mg/day for 1 year.[36] Both groups received calcium and vitamin-D supplementation. Bone mineral density was measured at lumbar spine, total hip and radius every 6 months by DEXA. By 12 months, the placebo group had lost 0.7% of their total hip BMD while the raloxifene 60 mg/day group had gained 0.95%. A similar though more dramatic effect was seen at the ultradistal radius. At lumbar spine the control group increased their BMD by 0.96% while the raloxifene group had an increase of 1.78%. Though a greater improvement than placebo, this increase did not achieve statistical significance.

Thus, the data suggest that by reducing bone turn-over raloxifene is effective at preventing bone loss in both healthy postmenopausal women and in women who already have established osteoporosis. Clearly, though, the critical end-point is fracture prevention. The Multiple Outcome of Raloxifene Evaluation (MORE) study addressed this in approximately 7,700 women randomly assigned to placebo or raloxifene 60 and 120 mg/day. The data from this study, now of 4 years' duration, remains largely unpublished. However, some data have been presented in abstract form and show a 40–60% reduction in the incidence of both new and recurrent vertebral fractures in the raloxifene treated women compared to their placebo treated controls.[37]

## UTERUS

### Animal data

Jordan's original paper demonstrated that while oestradiol caused significant increases in the uterine wet weight of ovariectomised rats, raloxifene produced only a small increase.[24] Black and Turner[31,32] confirmed these finding. Oestradiol returned the uterine weight of an ovariectomised rat to that of a sham operated control while raloxifene, even at doses of 10 mg/kg, produced little to no increase in uterine weight. Perhaps of more significance was the complete absence of change in uterine epithelial height and stromal eosinophilia observed in the raloxifene treated groups. This was in marked contrast to the oestradiol treated group who developed epithelial heights and stromal eosinophilia comparable to that in the sham operated controls.

### Human data

In Draper's study, an endometrial biopsy was performed at baseline and on completion of the 8 weeks.[34]. These were read independently and blindly. The biopsies were then graded on a system of standard criteria for oestrogen-induced proliferation. The biopsies of subjects treated with raloxifene showed no change in their grading over the 8 weeks while both the placebo and oestradiol groups showed a statistically significant increase in their grading over the course of the study. The uterine effects of raloxifene were assessed every 6 months by Delmas et al[35] using transvaginal ultrasonography to determine the double-thickness of the endometrium. The median base-line thickness was 1.9–2.0 mm and remained unchanged in all groups throughout the study. Lufkin et al,[36] using a similar method to assess uterine stimulation, found raloxifene had no effect at either 60 or 120 mg/day. These clinical findings are again confirmed by unpublished data from the MORE study where the incidence of vaginal bleeding in the raloxifene treated women is very small at 2.3% in the raloxifene 60 mg/day group and was no different from the 2.4% seen in the placebo treated controls.

The lack of uterine stimulation is essential for patient acceptability to treatment, but the farther-reaching possibility of raloxifene reducing the incidence of endometrial carcinoma is as yet unproven. Two years of the MORE study produced only 8 cases of endometrial cancer in all groups[38] with a relative risk in the raloxifene treated groups of 0.50 (CI, 0.1–2.0). No conclusion can be drawn from these data.

## CARDIOVASCULAR SYSTEM

As with the uterus, the effect of SERMs on clinical cardiovascular endpoints is unknown. There have been no published data with regard to myocardial infarction and angina in the second generation SERMs. The unpublished data from the MORE study are equivocal with a relative risk of myocardial infarction in the raloxifene 60 mg/day group of 1.34 (CI, 0.64–2.83). However, if myocardial infarction and ischaemia are considered, then the relative risk is 0.73 (CI, 0.50–1.07). Clearly further data are required. However considerable data exists on raloxifene and other SERMs' effects on the surrogate markers of cardiovascular risk such as the lipid profiles, coagulation factors and atherogenesis.

### Lipid profiles

It has been recognised for some time that the SERM tamoxifen produces a lipid profile presumed to be favourable and that the incidence of myocardial infarction is reduced in tamoxifen users. In ovariectomised Sprague-Dawley rats the second generation SERMs produced a reduction in serum cholesterol levels akin to that seen with oestradiol.[31] These initial data were expanded in Draper's study using high doses of raloxifene for just 8 weeks. This group demonstrated a significant reduction in both total cholesterol and LDL cholesterol in the raloxifene, compared to placebo, treated women. HDL cholesterol, however, was unchanged.[34]. Almost identical findings have been reported by Delmas in women taking raloxifene for 2 years at more conventional doses.[35] They also reported that, unlike oestradiol which increases serum triglycerides, raloxifene caused no significant change from placebo. Most recently in a study comparing the effects of oestradiol and raloxifene on markers of cardiovascular risk in healthy postmenopausal women, Walsh et al confirmed all these findings.[39] In addition, they demonstrated that raloxifene favourably altered several markers of cardiovascular risk. Specifically, raloxifene: (i) reduced the levels of LDL cholesterol, fibrinogen and lipoprotein(a); (ii) did not raise triglyceride levels; and (iii) raised HDL(2) cholesterol levels. However, in contrast to oestradiol, raloxifene had no effect on HDL cholesterol and apolipoprotein-A1 levels and a lesser effect on HDL(2) cholesterol and lipoprotein(a) levels.

### Atherosclerosis

Thus, the effect of raloxifene on markers of cardiovascular risk is closer to the pattern previously reported with tamoxifen than that seen with oestradiol and this pattern does appear to reduce the incidence of myocardial infarction[28] and the number of hospital admissions for cardiac disease.[40] Raloxifene has also been shown to reduce the aortic accumulation of cholesterol in ovariectomised cholesterol-fed rabbits. The raloxifene treated rabbits had 66% of the aortic atherosclerosis found in the placebo treated rabbits. This was more than the oestrogen treated rabbits who only had 33% of the aortic atherosclerosis.[41] These effects are only partially explained by the recognised changes in lipid profiles and probably represent a direct action of raloxifene on vessel walls. It may be that these effects are endothelium-dependent and receptor-independent involving increased levels of nitric oxide. Whatever the mechanism, there remains a possibility that raloxifene and other second generation SERMs will decrease the incidence of cardiovascular disease but clinical endpoint data are still awaited.

## BREAST

### Animal data

Initially it was hoped that raloxifene might prove to be an alternative to tamoxifen in the fight against the recurrence of breast cancer. In vitro studies with MCF-7 breast tumour cells[42] proved raloxifene to be a more potent inhibitor of cell proliferation than tamoxifen. In other oestrogen-dependent cell lines (47-DN and ZR 75-1) tamoxifen and raloxifene were equally potent.[43,44]

In vivo, however, tamoxifen is consistently more effective. Raloxifene does appear to reduce tumour load in DMBA (dimethylbenzanthracene) induced rat tumours which are dependent on an intact pituitary and not typical of human breast cancer.[45] The nitrosomethylurea (NMU) induced tumour is oestrogen dependent and, once again, raloxifene does reduces tumour load but to a lesser degree than tamoxifen.[46] However, phase II clinical trials in women with metastatic breast cancer refractory to tamoxifen showed no response to raloxifene and so further treatment trials were not instigated.[47]. Idoxifene, a second generation SERM with a closer chemical structure to tamoxifen, continues to be investigated as an alternative adjuvant breast cancer treatment. The action of raloxifene in **normal** breast tissue, though, may prove important. It has been shown that raloxifene caused mammary gland regression in intact adult rats.[48].

### Human data

Thus the action of raloxifene on the breast has engendered much interest in therapeutic trials of raloxifene. In the MORE study at the 33 month data analysis point, women treated with raloxifene had a 70% lower risk of developing invasive breast cancer (RR 0.30, 95% CI 0.16–0.52). This is primarily due to an 87% reduction in the risk of developing an oestrogen receptor positive tumour (ER+).[38] More recently, Jordan presented a meta-analysis of 10,575 postmenopausal women who had taken raloxifene in a clinical trial setting.[49] After a median follow-up of 40 months, the breast cancer rate was reduced from 3.8/1000 patient years in the placebo group to 1.7/1000 patient years in the raloxifene treated group. These results have prompted the American Surgical Adjuvant Breast and Bowel Project to compare tamoxifen and raloxifene in women at high risk of breast cancer. This study (STAR) started in 1999 and will last 5–10 years.

Women fear breast cancer more than any other single disease and hence any treatment that may reduce the risk is to be welcomed. However, it is important to note that the existing data are from a low-risk population and that the long-term consequences of treatment need to be evaluated before embarking on prescription in the postmenopausal population. Perhaps more importantly, the precise mechanism for this reduction in risk needs to be understood. Do the SERMs truly prevent or only repress ER+ breast cancers? If the latter is the case, then there is at least a theoretical possibility of rebound following cessation of therapy and trial work will have to contain a post-treatment surveillance period of appropriate length and rigour.

## CLINICAL APPLICATIONS

### The future

If the initial data concerning breast, endometrial and cardiovascular protection are substantiated and they remain free from unforeseen major side effects, the SERMs could become a therapeutic option for many postmenopausal women. Indeed, as our ability to manipulate the oestrogen receptor increases, their use could expand into the premenopausal woman with possible uses in the treatment of leiomyoma, endometriosis, menorrhagia and contraception. However, though the current SERMs are not genotoxic nor carcinogenic, there does appear to be a potential for teratogenicity, with a low incidence of hydrocephalus and ventricular septal defect of the heart in rabbits taking raloxifene. This will need to be addressed prior to their use in potentially fertile women.

The effect of SERMs on other organs and tissues that contain the oestrogen receptors remains to be defined. Clearly of interest will be the effect of SERMs in the brain, eye, immune system, bowel, bladder and vagina. Although all these areas appear to benefit from oestrogen replacement, there are, at present, little or no data with regard to the SERMs activity. However, all the second generation SERMs currently available or under trial, have no effect on the commonest menopausal vasomotor symptom of hot sweats and flushes. Indeed unpublished data from the MORE study reveal that the incidence of hot sweat and flushes is 8.7% in the raloxifene treated women compared to 5.4% in the placebo treated women. Both these incidences increase the closer the woman is to her menopause. This increase in incidence of hot sweats and flushes, however, rarely results in a discontinuation of therapy, but it does mean that the current second generation SERMs will not be a replacement for oestrogen replacement therapy.

## The present

The licensed use for the only currently available second-generation SERM, raloxifene, is for the prevention of non-traumatic vertebral fracture in postmenopausal women at risk of osteoporosis. Thus, if the principal problem facing a patient in the perimenopausal years is the vasomotor and psychological disturbances which may attend oestrogen deficiency, it is clear that the conventional HRT preparations based on native oestradiol should retain the major role in arresting bone loss while abrogating symptoms of oestrogen deficiency. A standard 12 week trial of a licensed HRT preparation will take the patient through the start-up syndrome of oestrogen re-introduction, and will allow an accurate assessment as to which, if any, of the symptoms presented are amenable to oestrogen replacement. Thereafter, residual symptoms may be tackled using other appropriate means. HRT would be given from menopause with its mean age of 51 years, through to the end of the sixth decade, when ovarian function may be safely assumed to have ceased. This HRT could then be replaced with a receptor modulator, which would continue the beneficial bone and cardiovascular effects of oestradiol while sparing the patient the effects of breast or uterine stimulation. The increasing availability of bone densitometry with its ability to stratify osteoporosis risk will allow more precise targeting of SERMs on those whose risk of future fracture can be shown to be above an agreed threshold.

The advent of the SERMs also provides a welcome increase in choice for the postmenopausal women who wishes protection from osteoporosis but is unable or unwilling to take conventional HRT. However one should be aware that, certainly with raloxifene, there is an increased incidence of thrombo-embolic phenomena. This incidence, 28 per 100,000, is similar to that reported with conventional HRT.[50–52] Thus it should be used with caution in women with a recognised thrombophilia or a past personal or family history of confirmed venous thrombosis. There are no data as to whether the other second generation SERMs will share this predilection.

All the SERMs currently available or on trial are taken once a day orally. Raloxifene has a half-life of 1 day and is rapidly metabolised by the liver into metabolites that do not bind to the oestrogen receptor. In contrast, idoxifene, another second generation SERM in trial, is slowly metabolised and has a half-life of some 36 days. They all appear to be a safe and well tolerated. The commonest side effects reported are the already mentioned increase in hot sweats and flushes, leucorrhoea and leg cramps. However, these are usually described as mild and do not significantly affect continuation of therapy.

## CONCLUSION

In summary, we are embarked upon an interesting and potentially rewarding journey. Ultimately, all menopausal women should be counselled by a member of the primary care group with attention being paid to the suitability or otherwise of oestrogen replacement for that individual woman. Not all women need or want oestrogen replacement, but all should be considered for it. That replacement should initially be in the form of a conventional steroidal oestrogen with a later switch, if indicated, to a selective oestrogen designed to protect those organ systems where oestrogen deficiency impairs function. Ultimately, a range of SERMs may become available so that the practitioner may precisely target those systems where risk of malfunction or disease is most likely. The arrival of the first licensed SERM, bleed-free and breast-safe as it appears to be, is but one step on what will be a long and challenging road.

*References*

1  Black J W, Stephenson J S. Pharmacology of a new adrenergic beta-receptor-blocking compound (Nethalide). Lancet 1962; ii: 311–314
2  Black J W, Duncan W A M, Durant C J, Ganellin C R, Parsons E M. Definition and antagonism of histamine $H_2$-receptors. Nature 1972; 236: 385–390
3  Purdie D W, Steel S A, Howey S, Doherty S M. The technical and logistical feasibility of population densitometry using DXA and directed HRT intervention: a 2-year prospective study. Osteoporos Int 1996; 11 (Suppl. 3): S31–S36
4  Kuiper G G J M, Enmark E, Pelto-Huikko M, Nilsson S, Gustafsson J-A. Cloning of a novel estrogen receptor expressed in rat prostate and ovary. Proc Natl Acad Sci USA 1996; 93: 5925–5930
5  Mosselman S, Polman J, Dijkema R. ERβ: identification and characterization of a novel human estrogen receptor. FEBS Lett 1996; 392: 49–53
6  Tremblay G B, Tremblay A, Copeland N G et al. Cloning, chromosomal localization and functional analysis of the murine estrogen receptor β. Mol Endocrinol 1997; 11: 353–365
7  Tzuckerman M T, Esty A, Santiso-Mere D et al. Human estrogen receptor transcriptional capacity is determined by both cellular and promoter context and mediated by two functionally distinct intramolecular regions. Mol Endocrinol 1994; 8: 21–30
8  Smoth D F, Toft D O. Steroid receptors and their associated proteins. Mol Endocrinol 1993; 7: 4–11
9  Beekham J M, Allan G F, Tsai S Y, Tsai M-J, O'Malley B W. Transcriptional activation by the estrogen receptor requires a conformational change in the ligand binding domain. Mol Endocrinol 1993; 7: 1266–1274
10  McDonnell D P, Nawaz Z, O'Malley B W. In situ distinction between steroid receptor binding and transactivation at a target gene. Mol Cell Biol 1991; 11: 4350–4355
11  Kumar V, Chambon P. The estrogen receptor binds tightly to its responsive element as a ligand-induced homodimer. Cell 1988; 55: 145–156
12  Kuiper G G J M, Carlsson B, Grandien K et al. Comparison of the ligand binding specificity

and transcript tissue distribution of estrogen receptors α and β. Endocrinology 1997; 138: 863–870

13  Onoe Y, Miyaura C, Ohta H, Nozawa S, Suda T. Expression of estrogen receptor beta in rat bone. Endocrinology 1997; 138: 4509–4512

14  Li X, Scwartz PE, Rissman EF. Distribution of estrogen receptor β-like immunoreactivity in rat forebrain. Neuroendocrinology 1997; 66: 63–67

15  Cowley S M, Hoare S, Mosselman S, Parker M G. Estrogen receptors α and β form heterodimers on DNA. J Biol Chem 1997; 272: 19858–19862

16  McDonnell D P, Lieberman B A, Norris J. Development of tissue-selective estrogen receptor modulators. In: Baird D T, Schutz G, Krattenmacher R (eds) Organ-selective Actions of Steroid Hormones, vol 16. Berlin: Springer, 1995: 1–28

17  McDonnell D P, Clemm D L, Imhof M O. Definition of the cellular mechanisms which distinguish between hormone and anti-hormone activated steroid receptors. Semin Cancer Biol 1994; 5: 503–513

18  McDonnell D P, Clemm D L, Herman T, Goldman M E, Pike J W. Analysis of estrogen receptor function in vitro reveals three distinct classes of antiestrogens. Mol Endocrinol 1995; 9: 659–669

19  Brzozowski A M, Pike A C W, Dauter Z et al. Molecular basis of agonism and antagonism in the oestrogen receptor. Nature 1997; 389: 753–758

20  Paech K, Webb P, Kuiper G J M et al. Differential ligand activation of estrogen receptors ERα and ERβ at AP1 sites. Science 1997; 277: 1508–1510

21  Early Breast Cancer Trialists Collaborative Group. Effects of adjuvant tamoxifen and of cytotoxic therapy on mortality in early breast cancer. An overview of 61 randomized trials among 28,896 women. N Engl J Med 1988; 319: 1681–1692

22  Ault A, Bradbury J. Experts argue about tamoxifen prevention trial. Lancet 1998; 351: 1107

23  Beale P T, Misra L K, Young R L, Spjut H J, Evans H J, LeBlanc A. Clomiphene protects against osteoporosis in the mature ovariectomized rat. Calcif Tissue Int 1984; 36: 123–125

24  Jordan V C, Phelps E, Lindgren J U. Effects of anti-estrogens on bone in castrated and intact female rats. Breast Cancer Res Treat 1987; 10: 31–35

25  Love R D, Barden H S, Mazess R B, Epstein S, Chappell R J. Effect of tamoxifen on lumbar spine bone mineral density in post-menopausal women after five years. Arch Intern Med 1994; 154: 2585–2588

26  Love R R, Wiebe D A, Newcomb P A et al. Effects of tamoxifen on cardiovascular risk factors in postmenopausal women. Ann Intern Med 1991; 115: 860–864

27  Love R R, Surawicz T S, Williams E C. Antithrombin III, fibrinogen and platelet number changes with adjuvant tamoxifen therapy. Arch Intern Med 1991

28  McDonald C C, Stewart H J. Cardiac and vascular morbidity of tamoxifen. Breast 1995; 4: 246

29  Killackey M A, Hakes T B, Pierce V K. Endometrial adenocarcinoma in breast cancer patients receiving antiestrogens. Cancer Treat Rep 1985; 69: 237–238

30  Fischer B, Constantino J P, Redmond C K. Endometrial cancer in tamoxifen treated breast cancer patients: findings NSABP B-14. J Natl Cancer Inst 1994; 86: 527–537

31  Black L J, Sato M, Rowley E R et al. Raloxifene (LY139481 HCl) prevents bone loss and reduces serum cholesterol without causing uterine hypertrophy in ovariectomized rats. J Clin Invest 1994; 93: 63–69

32  Turner C H, Sat M, Bryant H U. Raloxifene preserves bone strength and bone mass in ovariectomized rats. Endocrinology 1994; 135: 2001–2005

33  Evans G, Bryant H U, Magee D, Sato M, Turner R T. The effects of raloxifene on tibia histomorphometry in ovariectomized rats. Endocrinology 1994; 134: 2283–2288

34  Draper M W, Flowers D E, Huster W J, Neild J A, Harper K D, Arnaud C. A controlled trial of raloxifene (LY139481) HCl: impact on bone turnover and serum lipid profile in healthy postmenopausal women.

35  Delmas P D, Bjarnason N H, Mitlak B H et al. Effects of raloxifene on bone mineral density, serum cholesterol concentrations and uterine endometrium in postmenopausal women. New Engl J Med 1997; 337: 1641–1647

36  Lufkin E G, Whitaker M D, Nickelsen T et al. Treatment of established postmenopausal osteoporosis with raloxifene: a randomized trial. J Bone Miner Res 1998; 13: 1747–1754

37  Ettinger B, Black D, Cummings S R et al. Raloxifene reduces the risk of incident

vertebral fractures: 24-month interim analyses. Osteoporos Int 1998; 8 (Suppl. 3): OR23

38 Cummings S R, Norton L, Eckert S et al. Raloxifene reduces the risk of breast cancer and may decrease the risk of endometrial cancer in postmenopausal women: two-year findings from the multiple outcomes of raloxifene evaluation trial. Proceedings of the American Society of Clinical Oncology 34th annual meeting; May 1998; Philadelphia, PA: WB Saunders/Mack Printing Group; 1998; 2a Abstract 3

39 Walsh B W, Kuller L H, Wild R A et al. Effects of raloxifene on serum lipids and coagulation factors in healthy postmenopausal women. JAMA 1998; 279: 1445–1451

40 Rutqvist L E, Mattsson A, for the Stockholm Breast Cancer Study Group. Cardiac and thrombo-embolic morbidity among postmenopausal women with early stage breast cancer in a randomized trial of adjuvant tamoxifen. J Natl Cancer Inst 1993; 85: 1398–1406

41 Bjarnason N H, Haarbo J, Byrjalsen I, Kauffman R F, Christiansen C. Raloxifene inhibits aortic accumulation of cholesterol in ovariectomized, cholesterol-fed rabbits. Circulation 1997; 96: 1964–1969

42 Wakeling A E, Valcaccia B. Non-steroidal antioestrogens – receptor binding and biological response in rat uterus, rat mammary carcinoma and human breast cancer cells. J Steroid Biochem 1984; 20: 111–120

43 Witznitzer I, Benz C. Tamoxifen vs. LY156758 for treatment of human breast and prostate cancer in vitro. Breast Cancer Treat Res 1983; 3: 305

44 Labrie F, Poulin R, Simard J et al. Interactions between estrogens, androgens, progestins and glucocorticoids in ZR-75-1 human breast cancer cells. Ann NY Acad Sci 1990; 595: 130–148

45 Wakeling A E, Valcaccia B. Antioestrogenic and antitumour activities of a series of non steroidal antioestrogens. J Endocrinol 1983 ;99: 455–464

46 Gottardis M M, Jordan V C. Antitumor actions of keoxifene and tamoxifen in the N-nitrosomethylurea-induced rat mammary carcinoma model. Cancer Res 1987; 47: 4020–4024

47 Buzdar A U, Marcus C, Holmes F, Hug V, Hortobagyi G. Phase II evaluation of LY156758 in metastatic breast cancer. Oncology 1988; 45: 344–345

48 Clemens J A, Bennet D R, Black L J, Jones C D. Effects of a new anti-estrogen, keoxifene (LY156758), on growth of carcinogen-induced mammary tumors and on LH and prolactin levels. Life Sci 1983; 32: 2869–2875

49 Jordan V C, Glusman J E, Eckert S et al. Incident primary breast cancers are reduced by raloxifene: integrated data from multicentre, double-blind, randomised trials in ~12,000 postmenopausal women. Proceedings of the American Society of Clinical Oncology 34th annual meeting; May 1998; Philadelphia, PA: WB Saunders/Mack Printing Group; 1998; 122a Abstract 466

50 Daly E, Vessey M P, Hawkins M M, Carson J L, Gough P, Marsh S. Risk of venous thromboembolism in users of hormone replacement therapy. Lancet 1996; 348: 977–980

51 Jick H, Derby L E, Myers M W, Vasilakis C, Newton K M. Risk of hospital admission for idiopathic venous thromboembolism among users of postmenopausal oestrogens. Lancet 1996; 348: 981–983

52 Grodstein F, Stampfer M J, Goldhaber S Z et al. Prospective study of exogenous hormones and risk of pulmonary embolism in women. Lancet 1996; 348: 983–987

*David M. Semple  Michael J. A. Maresh*
*E. F. Nigel Holland*

# Audit and colposcopy

The introduction of clinical governance by the present UK Government in its recent *White Paper*[1] on the National Health Service is both exciting and challenging. Clinical governance with its emphasis on quality has the potential to lead to significant improvements in the health service, if funded properly. Quality is now expected to pervade all aspects of health care and the National Health Service Cervical Screening Programme (NHSCSP) is no exception. Quality must be seen to be at the heart of the agenda of the NHSCSP particularly in view of the recent well-publicised events that have damaged its credibility. A programme of quality assurance (QA) needs to be developed if the public, and a very sceptical media, are to put their faith into the programme. These schemes must be developed both locally and nationally and must include all aspects of the screening programme.

Medical audit was initially introduced into NHS practice[2] as a method to improve the quality of medical care. However, with the change to multidisciplinary clinical audit,[3] it has been used as a tool to improve quality both within medicine and the allied professions. This chapter addresses areas within the cervical screening programme where audit may have an effect. The authors try to look at the role of clinical audit within the NHSCSP, in particular colposcopy, and whether it is a suitable mechanism whereby the quality of the NHSCSP can be evaluated.

## CLINICAL AUDIT

The Secretary of State for Health, in the *White Paper* on the NHS[1] states *'all patients in the National Health Service are entitled to high quality care.... The variations*

**Mr David M. Semple** MRCOG, Specialist Registrar in Obstetrics and Gynaecology, Department of Gynaecology, Liverpool Women's Hospital, Crown Street, Liverpool L8 7SS, UK (for correspondence)

**Mr Michael J. A. Maresh** MD FRCOG, Consultant Obstetrician and Gynaecologist, St Mary's Hospital for Women and Children, Whitworth Park, Manchester M13 0JH, UK

**Mr E. F. Nigel Holland** MD MRCOG DipVen, Consultant Gynaecologist, Warrington District General Hospital, Lovely Lane, Warrington WA5 1QG, UK

*that have grown up in recent years must end'*. Variations in the provision of health care are inevitable and occur between countries, regions, hospital trusts and even between clinicians within the same hospital department. Differences in hospital catchment areas, resources and staffing will inevitably lead to differences in clinical practice. This is not necessarily indicative of poor practice, providing a quality service is delivered with appropriate standards being practised and maintained. The NHSCSP is certainly subject to variations in practice.[4] It involves a multi-disciplinary team which includes smear-takers, cytologists, histopathologists and colposcopists, as well as nursing and clerical staff. The NHSCSP also crosses the boundary between primary and secondary care and, as such, variations are again inevitable. However, when this results in practice falling below accepted quality standards, patient's lives may be put at risk, and this cannot be acceptable. Problems with the NHSCSP have been evident in the last few years with incidents where the programme has been seen to fail patients. In one example, a large number of women had smears wrongly reported as false negative, and subsequently some of these patients have died of cervical cancer and others have had to undergo radical surgery and radiotherapy.[5] This adverse publicity damages confidence in the programme. Colposcopy is an integral component of the NHSCSP and is no exception to unfavourable media reports as highlighted recently with the alleged problems about one hospital colposcopy service where inadequate treatment was used. It is, therefore, vital that a service, which carries so much public expectation and is under so much scrutiny, is able to demonstrate that mechanisms for internal quality control already exist or are currently being developed.

The issues surrounding quality in health care are very complicated; nonetheless, quality is considered vitally important by the current government as is evident by the concept of clinical governance. Maxwell[6] broke down the idea of quality into six components: (i) effectiveness; (ii) efficiency; (iii) equity; (iv) access; (v) acceptability; and (vi) appropriateness. Within any clinical service, conflict between these components is inevitable, and the challenge to health service workers is how best to achieve an acceptable and achievable balance. Methods of quality evaluation are difficult but the introduction of audit into the NHS in 1991 was seen as one such method. Audit was defined as 'the systematic, critical analysis of the quality of medical care, including the procedures used for the diagnosis and treatment, the use of resources and the resulting outcome for the patient'.[7] Audit has been described[7] as 'the third clinical science, with its own theories, techniques and literature' and that, if undertaken in the correct fashion, 'has the potential to deliver substantial benefits to patients and health professionals'.[7] However, the value of clinical audit has been questioned by some authorities[8,9] who argue the evidence that audit with all its financial implications has not actually achieved what it set out to do, namely benefit the patient.

## NATIONAL HEALTH SERVICE CERVICAL SCREENING PROGRAMME

The ultimate aim of the NHSCSP is to reduce the incidence and mortality of cervical cancer by detecting and treating pre-malignant and early invasive cervical abnormalities. The *Health of the Nation*[10] target is to reduce the incidence of cervical cancer by 20% to less than 12 cases per 100,000 women in the UK by the year 2000, as compared with the 1986 figures. Since 1991, the incidence of the disease has fallen year on year with the current number of new cases being approximately 3,500 per annum, with 1000 women dying from the disease.[4]

Cytology is an effective screening method with colposcopy an appropriate diagnostic tool for the evaluation of a woman with an abnormal smear. Cervical screening was initially introduced in a haphazard fashion in the UK. In 1988, a national programme was established and recent data reveal that at least 85% of women aged between 20–64 years resident in England have been screened at least once in the previous 5 years.[11] In 1996–1997, 3.8 million women were screened,[4] and an estimated 4.4 million smears were analysed. There is general agreement that the introduction of cytological screening has resulted in the fall in the incidence of invasive cervical cancer, although this is at a cost of £132 million per year.

With the huge amount of NHS resources, both in time and money, that this programme consumes, it is essential that a high quality service is provided and best use of resources made. It is an eminently suitable subject for audit and in the last few years the NHSCSP, in conjunction with the Royal Colleges and learned societies, has produced national guidelines for service quality.[12,13] These documents contain national recommendations and standards by which quality can be assessed. The NHSCSP has also in collaboration with the British Society for Colposcopy and Cervical Pathology (BSCCP) recently introduced recommendations on standards and quality in colposcopy.[14] This document has enabled colposcopy units to compare and audit their performance against national standards. The *Standards and Quality in Colposcopy* document is based on recommendations from a workshop of the BSCCP with revisions from a working group of the NHSCSP.[14] The document was published in January 1996. The recommendations are based on consensus opinion of the members of the working party and are, therefore, not evidenced-based. However, they recently have been re-endorsed by The Royal College of Obstetricians and Gynaecologists,[15] although others have questioned the practicality of some of the recommendations.[16,17]

The cervical screening programme involves smear-takers, general practitioners, cytology and histopathology services, the Family Health Service Association (FHSA) call and recall system, and both community and hospital colposcopy services. Close liaison between these groups is of paramount importance. The NHSCSP crosses the primary and secondary care interface, so if audit is to be successful and done properly, then it must be able to cross boundaries. It is, therefore, complicated, time consuming and can not be implemented regionally or nationally without incurring considerable cost.

## Cervical cytology

Cervical smears have been used to assess pre-cancerous cervical changes for over 30 years, but it has only been since 1988 that there has been a national call and re-call system. The cervical screening programme in the UK is thought to be one of the biggest, if not the biggest, in the world. Although the initial impact of the programme was questioned by some, it is now generally agreed that the programme has brought about the decline in invasive cervical cancer seen in the last few years.[18]

Many women find the thought of having a smear test or being referred for colposcopy stressful and frightening. Worries about cancer, future sexuality and fertility and about the actual procedure itself can be very real. The use of information leaflets have been shown by some to reduce patient anxiety levels.[19,20] In light of this evidence, the NHSCSP has produced guidelines for the presentation and content of information leaflets.[21,22] Information leaflets need to contain the correct information in an easy-to-read and understandable style. However, in a recent study,[23] information leaflets were found to be possibly harmful as they caused a greater degree of psychosexual dysfunction in those women who had received leaflets. The first person a woman may come in to contact with will be the GP's receptionist and they must be able to make the women feel reassured and at ease. Particular attention needs to be given to women from different ethnic groups and young women. Women need to be dealt with in an appropriate fashion in order that they will return for smears in the future. They must also be made aware of the limitations of the programme.

At present, about 75% of smears are taken by practice nurses[18] and they have a vital role in dealing with the women attending for smears. All women attending their GP's practice for a smear should be given a choice of who takes their smear. Many women will not mind being seen by a male doctor; but, if a female professional is available, the choice should be offered. The smear-taker is vital to the success of the programme. The guidance on training smear-takers recently published by the NHSCSP recommends best practice as well as other related issues.[24] It is important that smear-takers audit their own practice, including the percentage of inadequate smears. However, there are no national guidelines on the acceptable proportion of inadequate smears a taker should expect to get, but comparisons should be made between individuals.

Cytopathology laboratories are an integral component in the screening programme. Slides are first stained and then read by a cytological screener. A cytologist analyses a large number of slides per day and, with each slide containing between 100,000 and 300,000 cells – of which only a few may be abnormal – the highest levels of concentration are paramount. However, screeners are under paid, often working with poor equipment in facilities not designed for such purposes. They are expected to work to a very high standard and, on the whole, they achieve this.

Both internal and external quality initiatives must be in place for all laboratories reporting cervical smears. Internal quality mechanisms include rapid review[25] or re-screening[26] of cervical smears, although this has been shown to be possibly less effective than the use of the PAPNET system.[27,28] The PAPNET testing system is an interactive automated device, which uses neural networks, a type of artificial intelligence. Used as a supplement to rapid rescreening, it can reduce the rates of false negative smear reports. Other methods used by some laboratories are that of personal performance profiles[29] where the performance of each primary screener in the detection of both low and high-grade lesions is published on a quarterly basis in the laboratory. This method seems to help in identifying screeners with low detection rates and screeners who may require further training or who need to go on up-date courses. External quality mechanisms involve the comparison of reporting criteria between individual laboratories in order that they report smears to a uniformly high standard.[30,31] Proficiency testing has been mandatory for laboratory staff since 1988 and all laboratories now working in the NHSCSP must participate in the national proficiency testing scheme and demonstrate satisfactory performance levels.[32]

## Colposcopy

In 1925, Dr Hans Hinselmann developed an optical device to examine the cervix under magnification. Since then, developments in both the technology of optics and in the knowledge of the pathenogenesis of cervical cancer have resulted in colposcopy becoming an integral component in the diagnosis and management of pre-invasive cervical lesions. Around 266,000 women attended for colposcopy either as a new referral or as a follow-up attendance in 1996–1997 in England alone, at a total cost of £26 million, 20% of the NHSCSP budget.[4]

The cervix is initially examined using a low magnification and, if necessary, a cervical smear is taken at this stage. Solutions are applied to the cervix (normal saline, acetic acid and iodine) in order to identify any underlying abnormality. In the guidelines, colposcopists are expected to be able to diagnose over 70% of high grade lesions colposcopically.[14] For a satisfactory colposcopy, the squamo-columnar junction should be seen in its entirety together with the extent of the lesion. It is imperative that the colposcopist documents this in the records. Colposcopically directed punch biopsies should be taken for histological assessment if indicated.

The patient's history, colposcopy findings and details of treatment, smears, biopsies, etc. should be documented using specifically designed colposcopy pages, punch-cards. The gold standard would be a specially designed computer software programme, that would facilitate data analysis for prospective audit and research. It will soon be mandatory for all colposcopy clinics to provide annual data and, without the use of computer technology, this will be both expensive and time consuming. Many units still have inadequate data systems, often relying on written case notes and labour intensive retrospective data retrieval. The practicalities of any audit, whether retrospective or prospective, are huge when paper records continue to be used. With the increasing demands on doctors, they simply do not have time to pull case notes and extract complicated data by hand. The use of a colposcopy computer system has been shown to be beneficial with regard to audit.[33] The BSCCP is currently working on a minimum data set for colposcopy which will be of great value in directing audit in colposcopy at local, regional and national levels.

Waiting times for hospital appointments and treatment are easy to measure, but are considered by some[34] as a poor measurement of quality. Nonetheless, they are seen as important by both the government and patients. Most women referred for colposcopy have some degree of anxiety[35] and this will undoubtedly be heightened if they have a long wait from being told they have an abnormal smear and need referral to hospital for colposcopy.[36,37] The

NHSCSP quality recommendation for waiting times is that, overall, > 90% of women referred for colposcopy are seen within 8 weeks of referral, and that > 90% of women with high grade disease (moderate and severe dyskaryosis) are seen within 4 weeks of referral from their GP. In the first BSCCP national survey of colposcopy clinics carried out in 1988,[38] 89% of women were said to have been seen within 8 weeks of referral for colposcopy and this improved in the second survey in 1993.[39] In the initial survey, 83% of women with severe dyskaryosis were seen within 4 weeks of referral[38] and this actually fell to 51% in the 1993 survey.[39] However, national postal surveys are only a reflection of what clinicians think occur and this may be at variance with what actually happens.

More robust data are provided by a recent audit in Birmingham of 598 women who underwent large loop excision of the transformation zone (LLETZ) for various grades of cytological abnormality in 1995.[16] Only 57% of women were seen within 8 weeks of referral and only 22% of women with high-grade lesions on referral smear were seen within 4 weeks. This is in keeping with a regional audit of colposcopy services in the new North West region undertaken by the Royal College of Obstetricians and Gynaecologists Clinical Audit Unit. This study assessed 100 new referrals for colposcopy in the 29 gynaecological colposcopy units in the North West region. The study was performed in two stages. The first was carried out in 1996 identifying the 19 units in the former North Western region with data analysed from 1994 in order to get at least 2 years of follow-up data.[40] The second stage was undertaken in 1997 in the 10 units in the former Mersey region and data were assessed from 1995 again to get 2 years of follow-up data.[41] In total, 2796 sets of case notes were analysed, as in two units only 39 and 57 sets of notes were available for the time period of the study. The breakdown of the grade of abnormality on the referral smear is shown in Table 1. Overall, only 57% of women were seen within 8 weeks and only 18% of women with a moderate dyskaryotic smear and 31% with a severely dyskaryotic smear were seen within 4 weeks (Table 2). Out of the 29 units studied, only three met the overall waiting times criteria and no hospital met the criteria for high grade lesions. The data from the audit in Birmingham and from the RCOG Clinical Audit

**Table 1**   Grade of referral smears

| Grade of referral smear | North West Region (29 hospitals) Number (%) |
|---|---|
| Negative | 62 (2.2%) |
| Inadequate | 75 (2.7%) |
| Inflammatory/viral | 94 (3.4%) |
| Borderline | 217 (7.8%) |
| Mild dyskaryosis | 618 (22.1%) |
| Moderate dyskaryosis | 927 (33.1%) |
| Severe dyskaryosis | 685 (24.5%) |
| ? Invasion | 32 (1.1%) |
| Glandular | 55 (2%) |
| Missing | 31 (1.1%) |
| Total | 2796 (100%) |

**Table 2** Waiting times by grade of referral smear

| Grade of smear | % Seen within national standard | | | |
|---|---|---|---|---|
| | National standard | Mersey | N. Western | Overall |
| Mild dyskaryosis | > 90% in 8 weeks | 47% | 46% | 46% |
| Moderate dyskaryosis | > 90% in 4 weeks | 14% | 20% | 18% |
| Severe dyskaryosis | > 90% in 4 weeks | 42% | 26% | 31% |

Unit were taken from 1994 and 1995 before the quality standards were even published.[14] However, the situation has not improved. According to the National Audit Office Report,[4] only 50% of units reported that they met the overall waiting time standards and only 41% met the criteria for high grade disease. Even more worrying was that many units were unable to report data on waiting times at all.

Guidelines exist on the criteria for referral for colposcopy depending on the grade of cytological abnormality.[12,13] In a previous audit carried out by the RCOG Clinical Audit Unit,[42] which looked at all referrals for colposcopy for a 6 week period from 1 January 1994 in all 19 units of the former North Western region. The audit suggested a high compliance with referral criteria for colposcopy. In only 4.7% of referrals was colposcopy referral thought to be unnecessary. Referral may, however, have been initiated by patient request. This audit also highlighted the need for better communication between primary and secondary care, as 7.8% of referral letters did not contain any information about the referral smear.[42]

Only a relatively small number of consultants are contracted to undertake colposcopy, although they frequently perform colposcopy clinics or attend to supervise junior staff. This is vital for junior staff to gain expertise in colposcopy, which is even more relevant with the introduction of a programme of accreditation in colposcopy by the BSCCP. In the RCOG Clinical Audit Unit studies, consultants were only present in 40% of visits and trainees (SHOs and registrars) were only present in 10% of cases (Table 3). These figures are in keeping with the two published BSCCP surveys that showed consultants performing 50% of colposcopies in 1988 and 44% in 1993.[37,38] Of concern in the RCOG study was that only 10% of colposcopy was being performed by supervised or unsupervised trainees, which again is in keeping with the BSCCP national surveys which showed 16% of colposcopies in 1988 were

**Table 3** Most senior clinician at colposcopy in 29 hospitals in the North West Region

| Most senior clinician | Number (%) |
|---|---|
| Consultant | 1132 (40.5%) |
| Associate Specialist | 305 (10.9%) |
| Clinical Assistant | 704 (25.1%) |
| Staff Grade | 270 (9.7%) |
| Trainee | 289 (10.3%) |
| Others | 77 (2.8%) |
| Missing | 19 (0.7%) |
| Total | 2796 (100%) |

being performed by trainees which fell to 10% in 1993. In the RCOG study,[40,41] it was often impossible to determine the individual carrying out the colposcopy from the signature in the notes and, therefore, the name on the colposcopy clinic letter was taken as the most senior clinician. This may underestimate the involvement of trainees, as they may have been present in an observatory capacity or even performed the colposcopy but that the consultant signed the letter. Nonetheless, with the introduction of accreditation in colposcopy, it is essential that trainees are exposed to as much colposcopy as possible and that this is documented accordingly.

## Treatment

Treatment of cervical intra-epithelial neoplasia (CIN) the precursor of invasive cervical cancer can be divided broadly into two main categories. Firstly, there are destructive or ablative methods of treatment using laser, cold coagulation and diathermy or cautery. The second broad category is that of excisional treatment methods such as large loop excision of the transformation zone (LLETZ) and cone biopsy. The introduction of LLETZ as a treatment option has revolutionized colposcopy.[43] In the 1988 BSCCP national survey of colposcopic practice in the UK, LLETZ accounted for only 11% of treatments, but this had increased to 61% in the 1993 survey. In the most recent unpublished national survey looking at data from 1996,[44] the use of LLETZ had increased to 71%. The advantage of LLETZ is that it can be done as an out-patient, has low morbidity and provides a tissue sample for histology. In this way it can be both diagnostic and therapeutic. In the RCOG study, the breakdown of the various treatment methods is shown in Figure 1 with LLETZ accounting for 42%.

A 'see and treat' policy is so-called because patients have an excisional biopsy at their first visit without any prior histological diagnosis. The advantage to the patient is that she need only attend once for diagnosis and treatment. This alleviates clinic numbers and avoids the wait between the

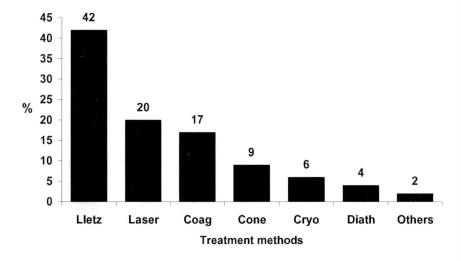

**Fig. 1** Overall methods of treatment (%). A total of 2796 cases were treated in 29 hospitals in the North West Region.

assessment clinic visit and the return for treatment. Destructive methods of treatment should not be used for 'see and treat' as the punch biopsy taken at the time may be equivocal. An underlying micro-invasive or invasive lesion can be missed and ablative treatment results in undertreatment. However, in the RCOG study, 47% of women who underwent 'see and treat' were treated using a destructive technique. This practice can not be justified, particularly when there is an appropriate alternative available.[17]

The national recommendation for evidence of CIN on all histology (either on punch biopsy or treatment biopsy) is that over 85% of all histology samples should have evidence of CIN. One of the concerns of the liberal use of a 'see and treat' policy is that of overtreatment. The national recommendation is that, for women who have treatment at their first visit, at least 90% should have evidence of CIN on histology.[14] Although some treatments will be performed for indications where CIN may not be present – such as persistent borderline smears or symptomatic cervical erosions – the standard of 90% does seem reasonable. However, only 78.8% of women undergoing treatment at their first visit in the colposcopy audit in Birmingham had evidence of CIN on histology.[16] This was not dependent on grade of the colposcopist performing the procedure. In the RCOG study, out of the 29 units assessed the use of 'see and treat' varied from 0% to 98%. Out of the 14 units which performed over 20% of treatments at the first visit, only two met the 90% standard for evidence of CIN on histology. This overtreatment results in unnecessary anxiety and morbidity for the women. Individual colposcopists must audit their own practice against these quality standards and review their practice. Audit of individuals is now mandatory by the BSCCP for training accreditation in colposcopy.

The national recommendation for use of anaesthesia for colposcopy treatments is that over 80% of patients undergoing treatment should have the treatment performed as an out-patient. Although a certain percentage of women will require or prefer a general anaesthetic, the vast majority of women will consent to out-patient treatment under local anaesthesia if the procedure is explained properly; again, the target does seem achievable. Local anaesthesia is safer, is quicker, carries a low morbidity and complication rate, frees theatre time and results can be communicated directly to patients.

Audit of the use of anaesthesia should be carried out in each unit. Where a treatment is carried out under general anaesthesia, the reason why should be documented in the case notes. If a unit exceeds the 20% level for general anaesthesia, then this should be reviewed and justified accordingly.

Although the smear is only a screening test, it is important for laboratories to compare the cytology results with the subsequent histology findings. To facilitate this, it is important that the colposcopist documents on a smear form that a biopsy has been taken so that they can be reported on together to avoid laboratory error. The national quality standard for the positive predictive value of moderately and severely dyskaryotic smears is that between 65–85% should have evidence of CIN 2 or worse.[12] The correlation between cytology and the subsequent histology in the RCOG study is shown in Table 4. In this survey, histology data were unavailable in 168 cases and, therefore, the total analysed was 2,628. Table 4 compares the referral smear cytology with histology taken from either a punch biopsy or excisional biopsy and, where both were available, the most severe histology was taken. Overall, the positive predictive

**Table 4** Correlation between referral smear and histology

| Histology | Neg | Inflam | Inad | Viral | B/line | Mild | Mod | Sev | ?Inv | Gland | Total |
|---|---|---|---|---|---|---|---|---|---|---|---|
| | | | | | Cytology | | | | | | |
| Negative | 4 | 2 | 3 | 3 | 16 | 13 | 25 | 5 | 1 | 4 | 76 |
| Inflammatory | 14 | 7 | 20 | 6 | 22 | 35 | 27 | 14 | | 7 | 152 |
| Inadequate | 3 | | | 3 | 8 | 13 | 9 | 2 | | | 38 |
| Viral | 4 | 4 | 5 | 4 | 24 | 69 | 43 | 21 | | 1 | 180 |
| CIN 1 | 15 | 2 | 12 | 2 | 66 | 191 | 128 | 37 | | 3 | 471 |
| CIN 2 | 5 | 6 | 7 | 6 | 32 | 158 | 322 | 139 | 2 | 6 | 693 |
| CIN 3 | | 1 | 8 | 1 | 35 | 99 | 319 | 428 | 20 | 13 | 935 |
| Microinvasion | | | | | | 1 | 7 | 8 | 1 | | 17 |
| Squamous cell Ca | | | 1 | | 1 | | 3 | 16 | 7 | 2 | 30 |
| CGIN | 2 | | | | 2 | 3 | 5 | 6 | | 6 | 24 |
| Adenocarcinoma | 1 | | | | | 1 | 1 | 5 | | 4 | 12 |
| Total | 48 | 22 | 56 | 22 | 206 | 583 | 889 | 681 | 31 | 46 | 2628 |

Histology data were available for 2628 of the 2796 (94%) cases reviewed.

value for a moderate and severely dyskaryotic smear in this survey was 80.4% (Table 5).

The aim of treatment of CIN is to remove the abnormality and to revert cervical epithelium back to normal. The recommended standard is that > 90% of women treated for confirmed CIN should have no residual dyskaryosis at 6 months on follow-up cytology. This was achieved in both the Birmingham audit and the RCOG Clinical Audit Unit study with only 9.5% and 9.2% of women having residual dyskaryosis at 6 months, respectively.

The national recommendation is that follow-up by cytology is essential after treatment for CIN, but that colposcopy is not essential, although this is not a consensus opinion. Colposcopy seems to increase the detection of persistent disease at 6 months[14,45] and may be particularly beneficial in follow-up if the lesion was large, excision appeared incomplete and if treatment was of a high-grade lesion. The RCOG study highlighted this variation in the use of colposcopy at the 29 hospitals studied. There was marked inter-hospital variation regarding the use of colposcopy at follow-up from less than 5% to over 90%. There is also no national consensus about how long women who have been CIN treated should be followed-up with annual smears before they can be returned to the national call and recall system. Should women treated for CIN be followed-up annually for 3 years, 5 years or 10 years? Should women treated for CIN 3 be followed-up for 10 years and those treated for CIN 1 for only 1 year? It would be helpful for audit and research if there was a national consensus both about the use of colposcopy at follow-up and also

**Table 5** Moderate dyskaryosis on cytology and subsequent histology

| Cytology result | Histology result CIN 2 or worse | Less than CIN 2 |
|---|---|---|
| Moderate dyskaryosis or worse | 1341 | 327 |
| Less than moderate dyskaryosis | 1711 | 917 |

The positive predictive value of a moderate or severe dyskaryotic smear having CIN 2 or worse on histology is 1341/1668 = 80.4.

how long close cytological surveillance should be carried out in women treated for CIN.

Patient satisfaction surveys are essential in order that consumers have a voice in what the health service provides. The government itself is due to introduce a national patient satisfaction survey[1] and it is essential that clinicians take a lead. Patient satisfaction surveys are fraught with many difficulties in setting them up, avoiding potential positive biases[46] and in the evaluation of the results.[47] It is essential, however, that clinicians find out what patients want and expect from the NHSCSP. The RCOG Clinical Audit Unit carried out a large patient satisfaction survey[48] in colposcopy in 26 out of the 29 gynaecological colposcopy units in the North West region in 1998. In general, women seem to be satisfied with the colposcopy service provided. Women felt that communication could be improved both from their GPs and practice nurses and also from hospital staff, in particular medical personnel. Other areas where it was felt improvements could be made were in the general facilities many colposcopy clinics provide, such as toilets, magazines and drinks machines. Many clinics were criticised for being too dark, gloomy and impersonal. A lack of privacy was also mentioned, with many clinics only having a curtain partition between the patient and the hospital staff. Significant improvements in these areas could easily be made in most hospitals at very little cost.

## CONCLUSIONS

While the UK cervical screening programme is one of the best in the world, clinicians should not be complacent but should constantly be looking for ways in which the quality of the service can be evaluated and improved. The introduction of regional quality assurance groups both for cervical screening and colposcopy is a beginning. Audit as an integral part of this quality agenda must be focused and directed at the areas of most concern. The services whether in general practice, GUM clinic[49,50] or in a gynaecological setting must be judged using the same quality criteria and it will soon be mandatory for all units to provide basic annual audit data. Without the use of modern information technology this will be both time consuming and expensive. The BSCCP is currently working on a minimum data set for colposcopy and this will be of great benefit in directing audit in colposcopy. This will allow clinics to be able to compare like with like. Audit is expensive and, therefore, needs to be directed and performed correctly. The RCOG Clinical Audit Unit currently has a database of audit activity in obstetrics and gynaecology in the UK and, at present, there are at least 80 audits on colposcopy on the database. Many of these audits contain tried and tested audit programmes, data collection sheets and results and this information is freely available to units wanting to undertake audit in colposcopy. With the establishment of supra-district quality assurance groups, it is hoped that they will be able to co-ordinate much of this work, possibly with the help of both local and regional audit clerks. The NHSCSP document on standards and quality in colposcopy is now over 4 years old. It could be argued that this document should be reviewed and updated in light of new evidence so that the targets are realistically achievable within the confines of NHS resources.

# References

1 Department of Health. A First Class Service. Quality in the new NHS. London: HMSO, 1998

2 Department of Health. Working for Patients. Working Paper 6: Medical Audit. London, HMSO, 1989

3 NHS Executive. Clinical Audit in the NHS. Using Clinical Audit in the NHS: a position statement. London: NHS Executive, October 1996

4. NHS Executive. National Audit Office Report by the Comptroller and Auditor General. The performance of the NHS Cervical Screening Programme in England. London: NHS Executive, April 1998

5 NHS Executive. South Thames Review of cervical screening services at Kent and Canterbury Hospitals: London: NHS Executive, 1997

6 Maxwell R. Dimensions of quality revisited: from thought to action. Qual Health Care 1992; 1: 171–177

7 Russell I T, Wilson B J. Audit: the third clinical science. Qual Health Care 1992; 1: 51–55

8 Farrel L. Audit my shorts. BMJ 1995; 311: 1171

9 Sherwood T. Exitus auditus – no fun. Lancet 1992; 340: 37–38

10 Department of Health. Health of the Nation. London: HMSO, 1992

11 Monitor; Population and Health; Office for National Statistics, MB1 96/2,1996.

12 NHSCSP. Achievable Standards, Benchmarks for Reporting & Criteria for Evaluating cervical Cytopathology. NHSCSP Publication No 1, October 1995.

13 NHSCSP. Quality Assurance Guidelines for the Cervical Screening Programme. NHSCSP Publication No 3, January 1996

14 NHSCSP. Standards and Quality in Colposcopy, NHSCSP Publication No 2, January 1996

15 Royal College of Obstetricians and Gynaecologists. Recommendations for Service Provision and Standards in Colposcopy. Report of a RCOG Working Party. London: RCOG, January 1999

16 Teale G, Etherington I, Luesley D et al. An audit of standards and quality in a teaching hospital colposcopy clinic. Br J Obstet Gynaecol 1999; 106: 83–86

17 Semple D, Saha A, Maresh M. Colposcopy and treatment of cervical intra-epithelial neoplasia: are national standards achievable? Br J Obstet Gynaecol 1999; 106: 351–355

18 NHSCSP. Cervical Screening Programme Annual Review 1998, London: NHSCSP 1998

19 Barsevick A M, Johnson J E. Preference for information and involvement, information seeking and emotional responses of women undergoing colposcopy. Res Nurs Health 1990; 13: 1–7

20 Marteau T M, Kidd J, Cuddeford L. Reducing anxiety in women referred for colposcopy using an information booklet. Br J Health Psychol 1996; 1: 181–189

21 NHSCSP. Improving the quality of the written information sent to women about cervical screening. Guidelines on the presentation and content of letters and leaflets. NHSCSP Publication No 5. April 1997

22 NHSCSP. Improving the quality of the written information sent to women about cervical screening. Part I: Evidence-based criteria for the content of letters and leaflets. Part II: Evaluation of the content of current letters and leaflets. NHSCSSP Publication No 6. April 1997

23 Howells R E J, Dunn P D J, Isasi T et al. Is the provision of information leaflets before colposcopy beneficial? A prospective randomised study. Br J Obstet Gynaecol 1999; 6: 528–534

24 NHSCSP. Resource Pack for Training Smear Takers. London: NHSCSP 1998

25. Shield P W, Cox N C. The sensitivity of rapid (partial) review of cervical smears. Cytopathology 1998; 9: 84–92

26 Cross PA. Internal quality assurance in cervical cytology one laboratory's experience. Cytopathology 1996; 7: 25–31

27 Mango L J. Reducing false negatives in clinical practice: the role of neural network technology. Am J Obstet Gynecol 1996; 175: 1114–1119

28 Halford J A, Wright R G, Ditchmen E J. Quality assurance in cervical cytology screening. Comparison of rapid rescreening and the PAPNET Testing System. Acta Cytol 1997; 41: 79–81

29 Houliston D C, Boyd C M, Nicholas D S et al. Personal performance profiles: a useful adjunct to quality assurance in cervical cytology. Cytopathology 1998; 9: 162–170

30 Sama D, Cotignoli T, Guerrini L et al. Intralaboratory reproducibility of cervical cytology diagnoses in the external quality assurance scheme of the Emilia-Romagna region of Italy. Gynecol Oncol 1996; 60: 404–408

31 Butland D, Herbert A. Comparison of cervical cytology reporting rates: a useful adjunct to external quality assurance. Cytopathology 1996; 7: 391–399

32 Kitchener H C, Mann E M F. Cervical cytology and colposcopy. In: Maresh M. (ed) Audit in Obstetrics and Gynaecology. Oxford: Blackwell, 1994; 162–185

33 Soutter W P. Computerization of a colposcopy clinic. Br J Obstet Gynaecol 1991; 98: 824–828

34 Sheldon T A, Quality: link with effectiveness. Qual Health Care 1994; 3 Suppl: S41–S45

35 Roberts R A, Blunt S M, The psychological reaction of women with an abnormal smear. Br J Obstet Gynaecol 1994; 101: 751–752

36 Marteau T M, Walker P, Giles J et al. Anxieties in women undergoing colposcopy. Br J Obstet Gynaecol 1990; 97: 859–860

37 Wilkinson C, Jones J K, McBride J. Anxiety caused by abnormal result of cervical smear test: a controlled trial. BMJ 1990; 300: 440

38 Kitchener H C. United Kingdom Colposcopy Survey, British Society for Colposcopy and Cervical Pathology. Br J Obstet Gynaecol 1991; 98: 1112–1116

39 Kitchener H C, Cruickshank M E, Farmery E. The 1993 British Society for Colposcopy and Cervical Pathology/National Coordinating Network United Kingdom Colposcopy Survey. Br J Obstet Gynaecol 1995; 102: 549–552

40 Maresh M, Semple D, Woodworth L. A report of the North West Regional Colposcopy Audit 1996–97. RCOG Clinical Audit Unit, June 1997

41 Maresh M J A, Semple D M. North West Regional Colposcopy Audit 1997–1998. Report 1: Mersey Region. RCOG Clinical Audit Unit, March 1998

42 Saha A, Woodman C B J, Cook G A, Maresh M. A report of the North West Regional Colposcopy Audit 1992–1994. RCOG Clinical Audit Unit, 1995

43 Prendiville W, Cullimore J, Normal S. Large loop excision of the transformation zone (LLETZ). A new method of management for women with cervical intraepithelial neoplasia. Br J Obstet Gynaecol 1989; 96: 1054–1060

44 Kitchener H C, Patnick J, Hicks D A. BSCCP/NHSCSP 1996 UK Colposcopy Survey. Unpublished data

45 Duncan I D. NHS Cervical Screening Programme: guidelines for clinical practice and programme management. Oxford: National Co-Ordinating Network, 1992

46 Fitzpatrick R. Scope and measurement of patient satisfaction. In: Fitzpatrick R, Hopkins A. (eds) Measurement of Patient's Satisfaction with their Care. London: RCP Publications, 1993; 1–17

47 Eccles M. Tailoring a questionnaire to your own practice. In: Baker R, Hearnshaw H, Cooper A, Eccles M, Soper J (eds) A Guide to Choosing and Using Patient Satisfaction Questionnaires in General Practice. London: Eli Lilly National Clinical Audit Centre, 1995, 25–32

48 Maresh M J A, Semple D M. North West Regional Colposcopy Audit 1997–1998. Report 2: Patient Satisfaction Survey and Assessment of Clinic Staffing, Facilities & Information Leaflets. RCOG Clinical Audit Unit, October 1998

49 Williams O, Bodha M, Hicks D et al. Survey of colposcopy services provided by genito-urinary medicine in England and Wales. Br J Obstet Gynaecol 1992; 99: 150–152

50 Shen R N, Hicks D A, Cruickshank M E. Colposcopy services provided by Genito-Urinary Medicine clinics in the United Kingdom. British Society for Colposcopy and Cervical Pathology/National Co-ordinating Network Survey, 1993. Int J STD AIDS 1996, 7: 98–101

**28**

*Diaa El-Mowafi  Michael P. Diamond*

# Adhesions and intestinal obstruction after gynaecological surgery

Intestinal obstruction is a broad term, which entails cessation of the normal progression of the intestinal contents. Intestinal obstruction can be segregated into complete and incomplete blockage, and be due to mechanical or functional etiologies.

Mechanical obstruction is a term usually applied when there is an actual physical barrier blocking the intestinal lumen, such as bands of adhesion, strangulated hernias, and pressure from pelvic tumors. In contrast, adynamic ileus is used to describe disorders of propulsive motility of the bowel.

## MECHANICAL INTESTINAL OBSTRUCTION

Intestinal obstruction is one of the more common and potentially fatal complications following gynecological surgery. Forty years ago, a mortality rate of 40–60% was not uncommon. Currently, the mortality rate has decreased but is still between 10–20% for all patients with obstruction of the small intestine.[1]

Adhesions, usually secondary to previous surgical procedures, are the most common cause of intestinal obstructions in the USA, and are responsible for 49–74% of small bowel obstruction in industrial countries.[2] Menzies and Ellis[3] reported that 93% of 210 patients, who had previously undergone abdominal operations, had substantial peritoneal adhesions at the time of re-operation. Gynecological procedures, appendectomies, and other intestinal operations are the three most common types of surgical procedures performed before

**Mr Diaa El-Mowafi** MD, Associate Professor, Obstetrics and Gynaecology Department, Benha Faculty of Medicine, Egypt; Lecturer and Researcher, Wayne State University, Detroit, Michigan, USA; and Fellow, Geneva University, Switzerland (Correspondence to: 4 Ghazza Street, El-Hossania, El-Mansoura 35111, Egypt)

**Prof. Michael P. Diamond** MD, Director, Division of Reproductive Endocrinology and Infertility, and Professor of the Department of Obstetrics and Gynecology, Wayne State University, Detroit, Michigan, USA

these occurrences.[4,5] Lo et al,[6] in 1966, reported a series in which 21% of patients with small bowel obstruction secondary to adhesions had had some form of gynecological surgery. Melody,[7] in 1957, reported that abdominal hysterectomy was the most common operation associated with postoperative intestinal obstruction among 487 gynecological surgeries. In 1983, Ratcliff et al[15] reviewed 59 cases of admitted women who underwent exploratory laparotomy for relief of small bowel obstruction. They found that 49 patients (83%) had previous abdominal surgery. Of these 49 patients, 38 (78%) had some type of obstetric or gynecological abdominal procedure, of which 33 of the 49 (67%) had previously undergone a total abdominal hysterectomy.

In 1994, Monk et al[8] reported that postoperative adhesions occur in 60–90% of patients undergoing major gynecological surgery. The incidence of adhesion-related intestinal obstruction after gynecological surgery for benign conditions without hysterectomy was approximately 0.3%, increased to 2–3% among patients who underwent hysterectomy, and was as high as 5% if a radical hysterectomy was performed.

## ADYNAMIC ILEUS

Some degree of adynamic ileus occurs after any intra-abdominal operation as well as in association with nearly all cases of intra-abdominal inflammation. The recovery of motor function of the intestines depends on many factors, including the length of the operation, the extent of handling of the bowel, the degree of chemical and bacterial peritonitis, and the underlying disease. After abdominal operations, the patient usually feels hungry and passes flatus within the first 3 postoperative days. If the patient is not interested in eating, denies flatus and the abdomen is distended and has inaudible intestinal sounds, further diagnostic procedure may be called for. Radiography of adynamic ileus shows distention of both the small and large bowel, with scattered air-fluid levels.

The treatment consists of correction of any electrolyte imbalance, if present, as low serum potassium or sodium as well as hypomagnesemia and severe protein depletion can cause bowel atony. Ambulation, systemic and localized intestinal stimulation by rectal suppositories may be helpful. Otherwise, nasogastric intubation for decompression may be needed.[1]

## PATHOPHYSIOLOGY OF INTESTINAL OBSTRUCTION

Obstruction of the small intestine causes collection of intestinal contents proximal to the obstruction leading to intestinal distention. Swallowed air, that represents over 70% of the air in the gastrointestinal tract, increases this distention. Because the veins and arteries enter the intestinal wall tangentially, the tension on them increases rapidly with distention. The veins, having the lower pressure, show the effect of the increase in tension first. As they are stretched, resistance in them increases, and flow slows down. Fluid rich in protein and salt begins to exude from the capillaries resulting in edema. Intraluminal fluid accumulation increases from both active secretion and decreased absorption. Subsequently, blood cells begin to escape from the capillaries, venous flow finally stops and, as arterial flow continues, blood accumulates in the wall and in the lumen of the bowel. If this process continues unabated. gangrene occurs, intestinal integrity is lost and peritonitis quickly follows.[1] Importantly, even in the absence of food and liquid ingestion, the volume within the gastrointestinal tract may continue to expand. The total volume of daily secretions into the normal gastrointestinal tract is estimated to be about 10 l. As much as 7–8 l of fluid can easily be sequestered in the bowel with intestinal obstruction.

Stagnant bowel contents in a distended loop of ileum show an increase in the number of bacteria. As long as the mucosa is intact and viable, the bacteria are harmless; however, increased intraluminal pressure for a sustained period will produce patchy areas of necrosis that allow some of the intestinal contents to escape into the peritoneal cavity. The main avenue of sepsis from intestinal obstruction is absorption from the peritoneal cavity and not the venous and lymphatic system.[9]

## PATHOPHYSIOLOGY OF ADHESION FORMATION

Following peritoneal injury, the microvasculature beneath the mesothelium becomes disrupted. This is followed by extravasation of serum and cellular elements. Within 3 h, this proteinaceous fluid coagulates, producing fibrinous bands between abutting surfaces.[10] Twelve hours later, polymorphonuclear cells are entangled in fibrin strands, which are subsequently replaced with a macrophage infiltrate. By 48 h after peritoneal injury, the wound surface is covered with a layer of macrophages.[8] In normal peritoneal healing, the fibrinolytic system is triggered to lyse these fibrinous strands within 72 h of the insult. Within the initial 5 days, re-epithelization of the peritoneal injury occurs. Interestingly, it appears that centripetal growth from the margin of peritoneal wounds contributes little to the healing process; the new mesothelium is derived from the metaplasia of subperitoneal perivascular connective tissue cells that resemble primitive mesenchymal cells.[11] Disruption of the existing equilibrium between fibrin deposition and fibrinolysis leads to persistence of the fibrinous strands, which then becomes infiltrated by proliferating fibroblasts. Subsequently, vascularization and cellular in-growth occur, and an adhesion is created.[10]

During mesothelial repair, macrophages and lymphocytes produce growth factors that modulate fibroblast proliferation and collagen synthesis, including platelet-derived growth factor, transforming growth factor-β, fibroblast growth factor, epidermal growth factor, interleukin-1, and tumor necrosis factor-α.[12,13] Prostaglandins, particularly prostaglandin $E_2$, are also involved in normal and abnormal mesothelial repair,[14,15] most likely through a separate mechanism not related to fibroblast proliferation.[16]

Adequate blood supply is critical for normal fibrinolysis to occur. Peritoneal injury associated with ischemia interferes with fibrinolysis and leads to organization rather than resolution of the fibrin–cellular matrix.[8] Ischemia may also induce adhesion formation by stimulating the growth of blood vessels form a non-ischemic to an ischemic site.[17] Ischemia may result from excessive handling, crushing, ligating, suturing, cauterizing, or stripping of the peritoneum.

Foreign body reaction causes excessive formation of the fibrin coagulum that stimulates the development of adhesions. Common foreign bodies include sutures as well as cornstarch powder and lint from drapes, caps, gown, masks, and laparotomy pads. It is interesting that foreign bodies in the absence of peritoneal injury are an infrequent cause of adhesion formation.[17]

The presence of intraperitoneal blood has also been proposed to play a role in adhesion formation, although its actual contribution is not clear. However, free blood in the peritoneal cavity generally does not lead to adhesions, except in the presence of tissue ischemia.[19]

Infection may result in the development of adhesions by causing the release of proteolytic enzymes, which lead to ischemia and tissue damage, resulting in the formation of adhesions.[5]

In summary, ischemia seems to play the central role in adhesion formation and factors that compromise blood flow within the area of tissue injury lead to the development of adhesions. Thermal injury,[20,21] infection,[22] foreign body reaction,[22,23] radiation induced endarteritis,[24] and impairment of the fibrinolytic activity, all probably act via inducing ischemia to enhance adhesion formation. The thermal effect on adhesion formation raises the question of the optimal method to achieve hemostasis: is it cautery or sutures? Both are incriminated in the etiology of development of adhesions.

## DIAGNOSIS OF INTESTINAL OBSTRUCTION

The initial symptom of intestinal obstruction is sudden onset of crampy abdominal pain. This pain is intermittent, with intervals devoid of it which are longer than the periods of pain. The pain is classically peri-umbilical for a mid-gut obstruction. Vomiting may accompany the onset of pain with the possibility of recurrence if obstruction persists.

Inspection of the abdomen usually shows distention in persistent obstruction. Loops of intestine with visible peristalsis may be seen beneath the abdominal wall in the very thin patient. High-pitched, tinkling, or metallic intestinal sounds are characteristic of obstruction and occasionally can be heard without a stethoscope. These sounds represent the existence of the air–fluid interface. Motility with violent bursts of peristalsis occurs proximal to the obstruction. The duration of quiet intervals between bursts of peristalsis may suggest the level of obstruction; in high obstruction the time may be 3–5 min, whereas in low obstruction it may be 10–15 min.[1] Palpation in the early stage of the disease may disclose no tenderness. As distention progresses, it is usual to find tenderness over the point of obstruction.

X-ray study demonstrating distended loop(s) of intestine with air–fluid levels, is suggestive of a mechanical obstruction, whereas grossly dilated loops of small bowel with gas in the colon is typically found is adynamic ileus.[7] Computed tomography (CT) was used recently to diagnose postoperative intestinal obstruction due to adhesions.[25] The CT findings that suggest strangulated obstruction are serrated beaks, mesenteric edema or vascular engorgement, and moderate to severe bowel wall thickening. In contrast, simple obstruction could be assumed when the beak is smooth, there are no mesenteric changes, and the bowel wall is normal or mildly thickened.

## PERITONEAL CLOSURE AND ADHESIVE INTESTINAL OBSTRUCTION

Suturing the parietal peritoneum of the anterior abdominal wall at completion of gynecological and obstetric surgery was always a tradition. Intuitive logic suggests that it will be of benefit to re-establish normal anatomical relationships and to prevent adhesion formation between the intestines and/or uterus and fascia. However, data supporting this hypothesis are lacking and, in fact, it may be incorrect. Importantly, reperitonalization also places pelvic and abdominal contents within the abdominal cavity, and possibly makes fascial closure easier.

Microscopic cellular studies in animals have demonstrated that the broad peritoneal reparative process is different from that of the edge-to-edge skin cicatrization.[26] When left undisturbed, peritoneal defects demonstrate mesothelial integrity (reperitonization) by 48 h and complete indistinguishable healing, i.e. without scaring, can be achieved by 5 days.[27,28]

Adhesions are caused by ischemia, inflammation, and infection rather than by open surfaces. Re-approximation of peritoneal edges or repair of defects via grafts, even with suture material considered to be minimally reactive, results in increased tissue ischemia and foreign-body tissue reaction, and may lead to increased adhesion formation at the site of reperitonization.[29]

Pietrantini and co-workers[30] compared 127 patient in whom the peritoneum was left unsutured after cesarean section with another 121 patients in whom it had been closed with a continuous 000 polyglactin suture. There were no postoperative differences between the two groups regarding the incidence of wound infection, dehiscence, endometritis, ileus, and length of hospital stay. They concluded that peritoneal closure at cesarean delivery provides no postoperative benefits, while unnecessarily lengthening surgical time, anesthesia exposure, and increasing patient costs. Finally, they advocated the elimination of closure of the parietal peritoneum from cesarean technique. However, they did actually evaluate the issue of the frequency of adhesion development as a function of peritoneal closure.

Hull and Varner[31] extended this modality to non-closure of the visceral and parietal peritoneum during lower segment cesarean section. In their randomized study on 113 patients, 59 patient were assigned to closure of both the visceral and parietal peritoneum with absorbable suture. The other 54 patients were left with no peritoneal closure. The incidence of postoperative fever, endometritis, or wound infection was not different between the two groups. The numbers of oral analgesic doses was significantly greater with closure of the peritoneum than without. The frequency with which postoperative lieus was diagnosed in each group was similar. Bowel stimulants were administered more frequently to the closure than to the non-closure patients. The average operating time was shorter for the open group than for the closure one.

Stricker et al[32] reviewed 100 cases of female intestinal obstruction where they found that postoperative adhesions was the most common cause being present (59%). Of those patients, 56% had a prior gynecological surgery, most commonly abdominal hysterectomy. From 11 patients who had records from their previous operation, 9 patients had peritoneal closure; among these patients,. adhesions were found always to the site of reperitonization. In the 2 patients in whom the peritoneum was left open, the adhesions causing the obstruction were found away form the site of reperitonization. In their study, Tulandi and others[33] confirmed that non-closure of the parietal peritoneum after gynecological surgery, as compared to closure using chromic cut gut suture, did not increase adhesion formation found at second-look laparoscopy (Table 1).

**Table 1** Different studies for closure versus non-closure of the peritoneum

| Reference | Type of study | Type of operation | No. of non-closure cases | Closure of visceral peritoneum | Closure of parietal peritoneum | Results |
|---|---|---|---|---|---|---|
| Tulandi et al 1988[33] | Controlled (n = 168) | Reproductive surgery | 165 | Yes | No | No difference in hospital stay, wound complications, adhesion formation, other postoperative complications |
| Pietrantoni et al 1991[30] | Controlled (n = 121, closure with 000 polyglactin) | Caesarean section | 127 | Yes | No | No difference in wound infection, dehiscence, endometritis, ileus, length of hospital stay |
| Hull & Varner 1991[31] | Controlled (n = 59) randomised | Caesarean section | 54 | No | No | No difference in postoperative fever ileus, endometritis, wound infection. Less oral analgesics, bowel stimulants and operative time in non-closure group |
| Nagele & Hussle 1991[34] | Retrospective | Abdominal hysterectomy | 80 | No | Yes | Low postoperative fever, no wound infection, no postoperative ileus in non-closure cases |
| Than et al 1994[35] | Controlled (n = 149) | Abdominal hysterectomy and Wertheim | 91 | No | – | No difference in hospital stay, but less postoperative need for pyelogram in non-closure group |
| Stark et al 1995[36] | Controlled | Caesarean section | – | No | No | Less postoperative fever, adhesion formation in non-closure group |
| Kadanali et al 1996[37] | Controlled (n = 50) | Hysterectomy + bil. Salpingoophrectomy + bil. Pelvic and peri-aortic lymphadenectomy, omentectomy, appendectomy | 52 | No | No | No difference in blood loss, transfusion rate, postoperative infectious and non-infectious complications, hospital stay; but less adhesion formation in non-closure group |
| Grundsell et al 1998[38] | Prospective randomised controlled (n = 182) | Caesarean section | 179 | No | No | No difference in wound dehiscence, urinary tract infection; but less postoperative fever, operating time, hospital stay and cost in non-closure group |

# MANAGEMENT OF INTESTINAL OBSTRUCTION

## Conservative management

Krebs and Goplerud[39] reviewed the management of intestinal obstruction associated with gynecological conditions in 368 patients. They found that gastro-intestinal intubation successfully relieved 81% of small bowel obstructions caused by postoperative adhesions. This success rate is similar to that reported by other authors.[40,41]

Carey and Fabri[1] recommended three circumstances in which non-operative treatment for intestinal obstruction should be considered. First, patients who had several operative procedures for intestinal obstruction and who are known to have dense intra-abdominal adhesions. Second, patients who develop obstructions in the early postoperative period are also candidates for a trial of non-surgical treatment. Lastly, intestinal obstruction due to known widespread intra-abdominal cancer may be successfully treated by intestinal tubes, such as the Miller-Abbott or Canter tube. It was claimed that postoperative intestinal obstruct-ions occurring less than 30 days after surgery has a better prognosis than that occurring more than 30 days after surgery.[44] It is also reported that partial small bowel obstruction is more likely to respond to tube suctioning than is complete obstruction.[40,42] Interestingly, in spite of their high resolution rate with intubation, Krebs and Goplerud[39] stated that tube suctioning is rarely successful when the obstruction is caused by neoplasm or strictures associated with radiation.

Meissner[43] described the technique of intestinal splinting for management of uncomplicated early postoperative small bowel obstruction. He concluded that this splinting rendered a significant reduction of early postoperative complications; the protective efficacy against early re-obstruction was clinically apparent but reached borderline significance only. In respect to late intestinal complications, splinting was not superior to simple enterolysis.

Intraluminal stenting of the small bowel has been advocated as a method of reducing the risk of recurrent adhesional obstruction in patients requiring adhesiolysis. This technique was reviewed in 25 patients in a recent study by DeFriend et al.[44] They reported that intraluminal stenting remains of unproven efficacy. They added that this technique may find a place as an adjunct to adhesiolysis in patients requiring repeated operations for the relief of obstruction due to extensive and dense adhesions; but, in view of the high rate of complications, careful case selection will be necessary.

Non-operative treatment of small bowel obstruction following operations on the ovary, tube or appendectomy was evaluated by Meagher and co-workers.[45] They clearly stated that a trial of conservative management of small bowel obstruction in such cases may be unsafe or not worthwhile.

We can conclude that patients with small bowel obstruction secondary to adhesions should be operated upon early, i.e. within 24 h, but may be treated non-operatively for 24–48 h, provided that no signs of strangulation are present or developed. Failure to show improvement during this 48 h usually requires immediate operative intervention. In general, those patients would have benefited if early operation were done routinely (Table 2).[1,46]

## Operative management

The laparotomy incision should be long enough to allow exploration of the

**Table 2** Different methods for management of adhesive intestinal obstruction

| Reference | Type of study | Method of management | n | Results |
|---|---|---|---|---|
| Hegedus et al 1988[48] | Retro-spective | 350 cm long intestinal tube with a balloon at its distal end | 24 | Success in 24/24 |
| Stordahl 1989[49] | Retro-spective | Ingestion of iohexol or Na diatrizoate (water-soluble media) | 25 | Success in 23/25 |
| Asbun et al 1989[50] | Retro-spective | Conservative (45%); surgical (55%) | 80 | Less hospital stay in conservative (8.5 ± 1.3 days versus 16.5 ± 1.8 days), less morbidity (5% versus 32%) |
| Mashev 1989[51] | Retro-spective | Conservative (21.7%); surgical (78.3%) | 23 | Conservative was effective in 100% of cases. 16.7% fatality in surgical |
| Diettrich et al 1989[52] | Retro-spective | Intestinal intubation with Miller-Abbott tube | 188 | No early recurrent obstruction, but late recurrence (1–5 yrs) in 4% of cases |
| Pickleman & Lee 1989[53] | Retro-spective | Conservative (77.2%); surgical (22.8%) | 101 | Mortality 5% in conservative, 13% in surgical |
| Manger & Winkler 1990[54] | Retro-spective | Miller-Abbott tube | 44 | Recurrent obstruction after 8 weeks in 2.2% |
| Chaib et al 1990[55] | Retro-spective | Surgical | 79 | Postoperative complications (15.7%), wound infection the most common. Operative mortality 9% |
| Mertens et al 1990[56] | Retro-spective | Medical treatment | 87 | 47% of episodes resolved, recur-rences not different between medical and surgical |
| Silva & Cogbill 1991[57] | Case report | Laparoscopic lysis of adhesions | 1 | Safely and effectively applied |
| Roscher et al 1991[58] | Retro-spective | Surgical resection, creation of stomata, or deviation anastomosis | 275 | Hospital mortality 7.6% |
| Bastug et al 1991[59] | Case report | Laparoscopic lysis of adhesions | 1 | Safely and effectively applied |
| Levard et al 1993[60] | Retro-spective | Laparoscopic lysis of adhesions | 25 | Succeeded in 9/25 cases, 16/25 had to be completed by laparotomy |
| Seror et al 1993[61] | Retro-spective | Conservative | 227 | 73% success, no increase in mortality or rate of strangulated bowel |

**Table 2** continued

| Reference | Type of study | Method of management | n | Results |
|---|---|---|---|---|
| Moiseev et al 1994[62] | Retro-spective | Splinting with a silicon catheter | 28 | Catheter removed prematurely in 2 cases due to stoma suppuration, re-operating in one patient 12 months later, doubtful results in another 3 cases |
| Francois et al 1994[63] | Retro-spective | Laparoscopic | 17 | Recurrence in 6 patients |
| Franklin et al 1994[64] | Prospective | Laparoscopic | 23 | Resolution in 20/23 |
| Federmann et al 1995[65] | Prospective | Laparoscopic | 15 | 25% of small bowel ileus could be treated |
| Finan et al 1995[66] | Controlled prospective | Water soluble, hyperosmolar, radiocontrast material via nasogastric tube | 57 | No difference regarding return of bowel function, day of oral intake, post-operative recovery, duration of hospital stay when compared to control group ($n = 58$) |
| Fleshner et al 1995[67] | Prospective randomised | Short nasogastric tube ($n = 28$) versus long nasointestinal tube ($n = 27$) | 55 | No advantage of one over the other |
| Ibrahim et al 1996[68] | Retro-spective | Laparoscopic | 25 | Success in 18/25 (72%) |
| DeFriend et al 1997[69] | Retro-spective | Intra-operative intraluminal stenting | 25 | Unproved efficacy |
| Mais & Eigler 1998[70] | Controlled retro-spective | Intra-operative intestinal splitting with a long nasointestinal tube left for ± 6.6 days | 95 | Recurrence rate was 3.9% in splinted group ($n = 52$) versus 18.6% in non-splinted group ($n = 43$) |

entire abdominal cavity. It is sometimes not advised to use the previous incision to get into the abdomen as this exposes the intestine, that might be attached to the anterior abdominal wall by adhesions, to injury.

The site of obstruction can be located by following the collapsed loop of intestine until the site of distension is identified. The distended bowel is highly susceptible to injury; fine scissors are usually utilized for dissection of the adhesion bands. Retractors, forceps, sponges, and laparotomy pads should be used particularly carefully during this time of the procedure.

Lysis of adhesions with postoperative splinting of the small intestine has usually been the extent of treatment for obstruction by adhesions, although it should be noted that there is little evidence that splinting reduces subsequent bowel obstruction. For obstructions caused by strictures or tumors, treatment usually consists of resection of the obstructed bowel segment and re-anastomosis of the healthy ends. Two techniques have been utilized to try to supplement clinical judgement in identifying sufficient blood supply in the segments of bowel to be anastomosed. Intra-operative use of Doppler ultrasound along the anti-mesenteric margin of the bowel allows recognition of areas of intact blood supply to support an intestinal anastomosis. Use of intra-operative intravenous fluoresceine has been recommended in patients in whom major segments of bowel must be resected; with the aid of a Wood's lamp, the fluorescence of the intact blood supply to the bowel can be detected.

While laparoscopic adhesiolysis in acute intestinal obstruction, was reported by Parent and colleagues,[47] we believe that it potentially carries an extremely high risk of intestinal perforation as well as other structures that may be included in the adhesion bands, and that this approach currently should only be undertaken as part of experimental investigative trials.

## COLONIC OBSTRUCTION

Postoperative adhesions are not a common cause of large bowel obstruction. Extrinsic compression from ovarian carcinoma, inflammatory strictures secondary to radiation therapy, fecal impaction, and intrinsic neoplasm are among the common etiologies of colon obstruction. Treatment of large bowel obstruction is primarily surgical, and decompression of a severely distended colon is achieved by performance of a proximal temporary colostomy, often of the transverse colon. Gastrointestinal intubation for evacuation of swallowed air may still be of value while the patient is being prepared for surgery. Unless there is distention of the small bowel due to an incompetent iliocecal valve, use of a nasogastric tube appears to be appropriate.[39]

## PREVENTION OF ADHESIONS

Postoperative intra-abdominal adhesions develop in over 90% of patients undergoing laparotomy.[48] Complete prevention of adhesion in those patients seems to be an unreached goal up till now. Meticulous adherence to the surgical principles for adhesion reduction, to the extent possible for the procedure being performed, gives good results. These principles include minimalization of tissue handling, avoidance of gauze and towels usage for hemostasis as this usually causes minute abrasions to the peritoneum, prevention of tissue desiccation, avoidance of introduction of foreign bodies such as talc into the operative field, the use of non-absorbable or delayed-absorbable sutures rather than the absorbable reactive cut gut, and meticulous hemostasis.

## DOES LAPAROSCOPIC SURGERY DECREASE THE INCIDENCE OF POSTOPERATIVE ADHESIONS?

In gynecology, laparoscopic surgery had been extended in the last two decades to involve not only the minor reproductive and gynecological surgery such as adhesiolysis, but also major one as adnexectomy, hysterectomy and even radical hysterectomy with lymphadenectomy. The advantage of endoscopic surgery is claimed to be reductions in patient's, morbidity, hospital stay, postoperative convalescence period, and costs.

One of the claimed benefits of laparoscopic surgery is a subsequent reduction in postoperative adhesion development. Such a conclusion is supported intuitively by the concepts of lack of use of retractors and packs at laparoscopy, maintenance of a closed abdomen with presumed reduction in peritoneal dryness, less likelihood of introduction of foreign bodies, a reduced likelihood of blind manual dissection of adhesions during abdominal exploration, and less tissue damage as assessed by the length of laparotomy versus laparoscopy incisions.

Luciano and co-workers[72] assessed this issue in rabbit horn studies. They demonstrated no intra-abdominal adhesions in those animals with the lesions created laparoscopically, whereas those lesions created at laparotomy were consistently followed by adhesion formation. Furthermore, the investigators then assigned these animals with adhesions to adhesiolysis at laparotomy or laparoscopy and demonstrated greater reduction in adhesion reformation following laparoscopic adhesiolysis. In a study in dogs, Tittel and colleagues[45] showed that laparoscopic operations were followed by significantly fewer adhesions; after conventional laparotomy operations, extensive adhesions to the abdominal incision and intestinal kinkings due to adhesive bands were found. In a retrospective chart study, Levrant and others[74] evaluated 215 women with previous laparotomy, laparoscopy(ies), or no surgery. They concluded that prior laparotomy, whether through a midline vertical or suprapubic transverse incision, significantly increased the frequency of anterior abdominal wall adhesions. Of the adhesions, 96% involved omentum and 29% included bowel. No anterior abdominal wall adhesions were found in patients with only previous laparoscopies or without prior abdominal surgery. Furthermore, Nezhat and co-workers[75] reported no *de novo* adhesion formation at the non-operated sites at a second-look laparoscopy done 4–18 months after laser laparoscopy for the treatment of endometriosis associated infertility in 157 patient who underwent laparoscopic adhesiolysis.

On the other hand, in a multicenter study, Diamond and co-workers[76] described a high (97%) incidence of adhesion formation seen at early (90 days) second-look laparoscopy following laparoscopic adhesiolysis. Moreover, adhesion reformation occurred regardless of the consistency or vascularity of the initial adhesion. This incidence is consistent with that previously reported following adhesiolysis at laparotomy. Therefore, they concluded that adhesion reformation would not be eliminated by utilization of endoscopic surgery *per se*. Their report also pointed to 12% incidence patients who developed *de novo* adhesions, (i.e. development of adhesions at sites without adhesion initially).

In summary, we can conclude that until now there is no clear and convincing evidence that laparoscopic adhesiolysis in humans is superior to surgical lysis of adhesions at laparotomy in terms of adhesion reformation and subsequent bowel obstruction.

## DOES LASER SURGERY DECREASE THE INCIDENCE OF ADHESION FORMATION?

Sutton[77] stated that $CO_2$ laser remains the most precise laser, especially in the ultrapulse mode, for the division of adhesions and the accurate and safe vaporization of deposits of endometriosis. Furthermore, it was claimed that the Nd:YAG laser is more suited to hysteroscopic surgery due to its great depth of penetration, while visible light lasers (e.g. argon and KTP-532) are more suitable for the management of ectopic pregnancies and ovarian endometriomas as the carbon dioxide beam is absorbed by the water molecule and becomes ineffective in the presence of blood.[77] The author concluded that the main advantage of the various lasers is that they allow fertility surgeons to perform operative surgery by the minimally invasive approach of laparoscopy rather than laparotomy.

In separate report, laser ovarian wedge resection was performed in 49 ovaries in 25 infertile patients with deep endometriosis or polycystic ovarian disease resistant to medical treatment. On second-look laparoscopy, McLaughlin[78] found that 36–37% of the ovaries had recurring adhesions. The actual pregnancy rate in this study was 60%, the majority of them occurred within the first 6 months postoperatively. The author concluded that laser ovarian surgery, coupled with second-look laparoscopy, appears efficacious in minimizing adhesion reformation and seems to have little adverse effect on subsequent conception.

In a multicenter prospective study, Diamond and co-workers[79] assessed tubal patency and adhesion formation by second-look laparoscopy within 12 weeks after intra-abdominal laser surgery by laparotomy. This surgery included adhesiolysis, neosalpingostomy, fimbrioplasty, vaporization of endometriosis and ovarian wedge resection. Their results were compared with those of another multicenter prospective study that utilized non-laser reconstructive pelvic surgery. Carbon dioxide laser was found to result in a higher tubal patency rate and adhesions were reduced from initial presentation at most sites. However, non-laser reproductive surgery appeared to also have efficacy in the prevention of adhesion formation, with no consistent benefit for laser or non-laser modalities. It was concluded that the $CO_2$ laser does not appear to be a panacea for the treatment of tuboperitoneal causes of infertility.

On the other hand, Dunn[80] examined 11 patients at second-look laparoscopy 12–21 days following laser laparoscopic adhesiolysis without intra-operative adjuvants for adhesion prevention. All patients had adhesion reformation in at least one site of 15 sites evaluated for adhesions. Of the available sites, 56% had adhesions at second-look laparoscopy, which was not a significant change from the 60% of the sites with adhesions at initial laparoscopy. De novo adhesions formed in seven of the patients at 23% of available sites.

In summary, it is our belief that laser endoscopic surgery can be beneficial in gynecological surgery when used by an experienced surgeon. However, it does not appear that use of a laser *per se* reduces postoperative adhesions or its subsequent complications, including intestinal obstruction, when compared to other surgical modalities.

As adhesion formation remains an unavoidable event, so the need for adjuvants for its prevention was called for. A multitude of agents with different mechanism of action have been developed, investigated and tried. Unfortunately, none of them proved to be absolutely effective in the prevention of postsurgical adhesions or getting a universal acceptance from surgeons.

The most commonly investigated and used agents are fibrinolytics, anticoagulants, anti-inflammatory agents, antibiotics, and mechanical separating agents (Table 3).

**Table 3** Classes of adhesion-reduction adjuvants and their proposed mechanism of action

| Class of adjuvant | Proposed mechanism of action |
|---|---|
| **I. Fibrinolytic agents** | Fibrinolysis |
| Fibrinolysin | Stimulation of plasminogen |
| Streptokinase | activators |
| Urokinase | |
| Hyaluronidase | |
| Chymotrypsin | |
| Trypsin | |
| Pepsin | |
| Plasminogen activators | |
| **II. Anticoagulants** | Prevention of clot and fibrin |
| Heparin | formation |
| Citrates | |
| Oxalates | |
| **III. Anti-inflammatory agents** | Reduce vascular permeability |
| Corticosteroids | Reduce histamine release |
| Non-steroidal anti-inflammatory agents | Stabilize lysozomes |
| Anti-histamines | |
| Progesterone | |
| Calcium channel blockers | |
| Colchicine | |
| **IV. Antibiotics** | Prevent infection |
| Tetracyclines | |
| Cephalosporins | |
| **V. Mechanical separation** | Surface separation |
| *Intra-abdominal instillates* | Hydroflotation |
| Crystalloid solutions | |
| Dextran | |
| Mineral oil | |
| Silicone | |
| Vaseline | |
| Carboxymethylcellulose | |
| Hyaluronic acid | |
| Chelated hyaluronic acid | |
| *Barriers* | |
| *Endogenous tissues* | |
| Omental grafts | |
| Peritoneal grafts | |
| Bladder strips | |
| Fetal membranes | |
| *Exogenous materials* | |
| Fibrin glue | |
| Polytetrafluoroethylene | |
| Oxidized cellulose | |
| Oxidized regenerated cellulose | |
| Gelatin | |
| Rubber sheets | |
| Metal foils | |
| Plastic hoods | |
| Modified hyaluronic acid & CMC | |
| Poloxamer 407 | |
| Repel | |

*Modified from* Diamond M P, DeCherney A H. Pathogenesis of adhesion formation/reformation: application to reproductive pelvic surgery. Microsurgery 1987: 8: 103 and Diamond M P, Hershlag A. Adhesion formation/reformation. In: *Treatment of Postsurgical Adhesions,* Wiley-Liss, 1990; 23–33.

Fibrinolytic agents act directly by reducing the fibrinous mass and indirectly by stimulating plasminogen activator activity.[81] These agents were promising in some animal studies,[82,83] and frustrating in others,[84] while it was even associated with hemorrhagic complication[85] and impairment of wound healing[86] in another reports.

Heparin is the most widely investigated anticoagulant for the purpose of prevention of adhesions. Heparin alone was found to be efficacious in two animal studies when added to peritoneal irrigants in high doses,[87,88] while another study did not confirm this result.[89] When added to local mechanical barriers, heparin enhances its anti-adhesive effects. This had been reported in experimental studies with amniotic membrane,[90] and Interceed (TC7).[89] However, these promising results with addition of heparin to Interceed were not confirmed in a clinical trial by Reid and co-workers.[91]

Anti-inflammatory agents were used to reduce the initial inflammatory response to tissue injury and, hence, subsequent adhesion formation. Most of the animal studies showed the effectiveness of non-steroidal anti-inflammatory drugs (NSAIDs) in prevention of adhesions.[92,93] In spite of that, other studies failed to prove any beneficial effect of intramuscular or intraperitoneal administration of ibuprofen in reduction of peritoneal adhesions in rat and rabbit models.[94,95] Unfortunately, no clinical trials with NSAIDs have been published up until now, although, several have been conducted.

The rationale behind the use of antibiotics is prophylaxis against infection, and hence the inflammatory response, that leads to adhesion development. Cephalosporines and tetracyclin[98] were among the widely used drugs for this purpose. Unfortunately, there are no well-designed clinical trial supporting this practice.

Mechanical separation of peritoneal surfaces of the pelvic organs during the most critical wound healing period of 1–5 days postoperative, is the practical and most accepted way nowadays to prevent postoperative adhesions. This separation, theoretically, may be accomplished by intra-abdominal instillates or barriers, whether endogenous tissue or exogenous materials. Crystalloid solutions, Dextran 70, carboxymethylcellulose, hyaluronic acid and endo-genous tissues such as omental grafts, peritoneal grafts, and fetal membranes were among the most commonly used agents for this purpose. Those currently in-use are the newer polymeric barrier films and tissue-protective polymer solutions or gels.

A gel-like, highly viscous, concentrated (1%) sodium hyaluronate solutions has been reported by Shushan et al[97] to inhibit postoperative adhesion in a rat uterine horn abrasion model. Another promising new jelly material is a chemically modified bioresorbable hyaluronic acid/carboxymethylcellulose (HA/CMC) gel (Sepragel, Genzyme Corp., Cambridge, MA, USA). Favorable adhesion prevention had been shown for this gel by Burns et al[98] in rat cecal abrasion and rabbit sidewall defect bowel abrasion models.

Interceed is composed of oxidized regenerated cellulose that has been shown to be efficacious in reduction of adhesion after ovarian surgery,[99–101] tubal surgery,[100] and adhesiolysis.[102,103] Interceed, which is an absorbable barrier, should be applied at the end of the surgical procedure just prior to closure. The most important instructions to maximize efficacy of Interceed are: (i) removal of intra-peritoneal irrigants, which usually requires aspiration of all residual fluid remaining in the cul-de-sac with the patient in the reverse Trendelenburg position; (ii) inspection to ensure that adequate hemostasis has been achieved as evidenced by Interceed not turning black; and (iii) use of a sufficiently large piece of Interceed to completely cover the area of interest leaving at least a 5 mm border.[104]

Gore-Tex is a barrier composed of a polytetrafluoroethylene (PTFE) which is non-toxic, non-reactive and antithrombogenic. It is non-absorbable and needs fixation by stitches; hence, its surgical removal. The results of a multicenter clinical study confirmed its efficacy in reducing adhesion.[105]

Seprafilm is a flexible membrane composed of modified hyaluronic acid and carboxymethylcellulose. It adheres well to moist tissue surfaces, and then turns into a gel within 24 h after placement. It is absorbed in the body, thereby omitting the need for a second operative procedure to remove it. Complete hemostasis is not mandatory for its use. Seprafilm was demonstrated to be efficacious in the reduction of adhesion development in a multicenter recent clinical study conducted by Diamond and co-workers.[106] In this study, 127 patients underwent myomectomy with at least one posterior uterine incision ≥1 cm in length. The use of Seprafilm in these patients significantly reduced the incidence of sites adherent to the uterus, as well as the severity, extent, and area of these postoperative adhesions. Additionally, Seprafilm application was not associated with an increase in postoperative complications.

## CONCLUSIONS

Postoperative adhesions are among the commonest causes of intestinal obstruction. The latter is a very serious condition, potentially exposing the patient to bowel perforation, peritonitis, and death within few hours in a considerable percentage of cases. Early diagnosis and treatment of these patients is the key to saving their life. Meticulous adherence to the surgical principles for adhesion reduction, as well as the use of adjuvants created for this purpose can, be of great help to decrease the incidence of subsequent postsurgical adhesions and, hopefully, bowel obstruction.

*References*

1  Carey L C, Fabri P J. The intestinal tract in relation to gynecology. In: Thompson J D, Rock J A. (eds) Te Linde's Operative Gynecology. Philadelphia: JB Lippincott, 1992; 1017–1047

2  Welch J P. Adhesions. In: Welch J P. (ed) Bowel Obstruction. Philadelphia: WE Saunders, 1990; 154–165

3  Menzies D, Ellis H. Intestinal obstruction from adhesions – how big is the problem? Ann R Coll Surg Engl 1990; 72: 60–63

4  Ulvik N M, Qvigstad E. Mechanical small bowel obstruction due to adhesions. Ann Chir Gynecol 1978; 62: 13–16

5  Ratcliff J B, Kapernick P, Brooks G G, Dunnihoo D R. Small bowel obstruction and previous gynecologic surgery. South Med J 1983; 76: 1349–1350

6  Lo A M, Evans W E, Carey L C. Review of small bowel obstruction in Milwaukee County General Hospital. Am J Surg 1966; 111: 884–892

7  Melody G F. Intestinal obstruction following gynecologic surgery. Obstet Gynecol 1958; 11: 139–147

8   Monk B J, Berman N L, Montz F J. Adhesions after extensive gynecologic surgery: clinical significance, etiology, and prevention. Am J Obstet Gynecol 1994; 170: 1396–1403

9   Wangensteen O H, Rea C E. The distention factor in simple intestinal obstruction: and experimental study with exclusion of swallowed air by cervical esophagestomy. Surgery 1939; 5: 327–332

10  diZerega G S. Contemporary adhesion prevention. Fertil Steril 1994; 61: 219–235

11  Raftery A T. Cellular events in peritoneal repair: a review. In: diZerega G S, DeCherney A H, Diamond M P (eds) Pelvic Surgery Adhesion Formation and Prevention. New York: Springer, 1997; 3–10

12  Kovacs E J. Fibrogenic cytokines: the role of immune mediators in the development of scar tissue. Immunol Today 1991; 12: 17–23

13  Kovacs E J, Brook B, Silber I A, Neuman J E. Production of fibrogenic cytokines by interleukin-2 treated peripheral blood leukocytes: expression of transforming growth factor-P and platelet derived growth factor P chain genes. Obstet Gynecol 1993; 82: 29–36

14  Montz F J, Shimaruki T, diZerega G S. Postsurgical mesothelial re-epithelization. In: DeCherney A H, Polan M L. (eds) Reproductive Surgery. Chicago: YearBook, 1987; 31–47

15  Golan A, Bernstein T, Wexter S, Neuman M, Bukovsky I, David M P. The effect of prostaglandins and aspirin an inhibitor of prostaglandin synthesis on adhesion formation in rats. Hum Reprod 1991; 6: 251–254

16  Golan A, Stolik A, Wexler S, Larger R, Eer A, David M P. Prostaglandins – a role in adhesion formation. Acta Obstet Gynecol Scand 1990; 69: 339–341

17  Gutmann J N, Diamond M P. Principles of laparoscopic microsurgery and adhesion prevention. In: Wallach E, Zacur H (eds) Practical Manual of Operative Laparoscopy and Hysteroscopy. New York: Springer, 1992; 55–64

18  Drollette C M, Badaway S Z A. Pathophysiology of pelvic adhesions. J Reprod Med 1992; 37: 107–121

19  diZerega G S. The peritoneum and its response to surgical injury. In: diZerega G S, Malinak L R, Diamond M P, Linsky C B. (eds) Treatment of Postsurgical Adhesions. Progress in Clinical and Biological Research, vol 358. New York: Wiley-Liss, 1989; 1–11

20  Luciano A A, Shitman G, Maier D B, Randolph J, Maenza R. A comparison of thermal injury, healing patterns, and postoperative adhesion formation following $CO_2$ laser and electromicrosurgery. Fertil Steril 1987; 48: 1025–1029

21  Mecke H, Schunke M, Schultz S, Semm K. Incidence of adhesions following thermal tissue damage. Res Exp Med 1991; 191: 405–411

22  O'Leary D P, Coakley J B. The influence of suturing and sepsis on the development of postoperative peritoneal adhesions. Ann R Coll Surg Engl 1992; 74: 134–137

23  Holtz G. Adhesion induction by suture of varying tissue reactivity and caliber. Int J Fertil 1992; 27: 134–135

24  Morgenstern L, Hart M, Lugo D, Friedman N E. Changing aspects of radiation enteropathy. Arch Surg 1985; 120: 1225–1228

25  Ha H K, Park C H, Kim S K et al. CT analysis of intestinal obstruction due to adhesions: early detection of strangulation. J Comp Assoc Tamogr 1993; 17: 386–389

26  Hubbard T B, Khan M Z, Carag V R, Albites V E, Hricko G M. The pathology of peritoneal repair: its relation to the formation of adhesion. Ann Surg 1967; 165: 908–916

27  Buckman Jr R F, Buckman P D, Hufinagel H V, Gervin A S. A physiologic basis for the adhesion-free healing of deperitonealized surfaces. J Surg Res 1976; 21: 67–76

28  Elkins T E, Stovall T G, Warren J, Ling F W, Meyer N L. A histological evaluation of peritoneal injury and repair: implication for adhesion formation. Obstet Gynecol 1987; 70: 225–228

29  Ellis H, Heddle R. Does the peritoneum need to be closed at laparotomy? Br J Surg 1977; 64: 733–737

30  Pietrantoni M, Parsons M T, O'Brien W F, Collins E, Knuppel R A, Spellacy W N. Peritoneal closure or non-closure at cesarean. Obstet Gynecol 1991; 77: 293–296

31  Hull D B, Varner M W. A randomized study of closure of the peritoneum at cesarean delivery. Obstet Gynecol 1991; 77: 818–820

32  Stricker B, Bianco J, Fox H E. The gynecologic contribution to intestinal obstruction in females. J Am Coll Surg 1994; 178: 617–620

33  Tulandi T, Hum H S, Gelfand M M. Closure of laparotomy incisions with or without peritoneal suturing and second-look laparoscopy. Am J Obstet Gynecol 1988; 158: 536–537

34  Nagele F, Husslein P. Visceral peritonealization after hysterectomy – a retrospective pilot study. Geburtshilfe Frauenheilkd 1991; 51: 925–928

35  Than G N, Arany A A, Schunk E, Vizer M, Krommer K F. Closure or non-closure of visceral peritoneums after abdominal hysterectomies and Wertheim-Meigs radical abdominal hysterectomies. Acta Chir Hung 1994; 34: 79–86

36  Stark M, Chavkin Y, Kupfersztain C, Guedj P, Finkel A R. Evaluation of combinations of procedures in caesarean section. Int J Gynaecol Obstet 1995; 48: 273–276

37  Kadanali S, Erten O, Kucukozkan T. Pelvic and periaortic peritoneal closure or non-closure at lymphadenectomy in ovarian cancer: effects on morbidity and adhesion formation. Eur J Surg Oncol 1996; 22: 282–285

38  Grundsell H S, Rizk D E, Kumar R M. Randomised study of non-closure of peritoneum in lower segment caesarean section. Acta Obstet Gynecol Scand 1998; 77: 110

39  Krebs H E, Goplerud D R. Mechanical intestinal obstruction in patients with gynecologic disease: a review of 368 patients. Am J Obstet Gynecol 1987; 157: 577–583

40  Helmkamp B F, Kimmel J. Conservative management of small bowel obstruction. Am J Obstet Gynecol 1985; 152: 677–682

41  Peetz D J, Gamelli R L, Pilcher D B. Intestinal intubation in acute, mechanical small bowel obstruction. Arch Surg 1982; 117: 334–339

42  Bolin R E. Partial small bowel obstruction. Surgery 1984; 95: 145–149

43  Meissner K. Intestinal splinting for uncomplicated early postoperative small bowel obstruction: is it worthwhile? Hepatogastroenterology 1996; 43: 813–818

44  DeFriend D J, Klimack O E, Humphrey C S, Schraibman I G. Intraluminal stenting in the management of adhesional intestinal obstruction: J R Soc Med 1997; 90: 132–135

45  Meagher A B, Moiler C, Hoffmann D C. Non-operative treatment of small bowel obstruction following appendicectomy or operation on the ovary or tube. Br J Surg 1993; 80: 1310–1311

46  Sosa J, Gardner B. Management of patients diagnosed as acute intestinal obstruction secondary to adhesions. Am Surg 1993; 59: 125–128

47  Parent S, Bresler L, Marchal F, Baissel P. Celioscopic treatment of acute obstructions caused by adhesions of the small intestine. Experience of 35 cases. J Chir 1995; 132: 382–385

48  Hegedus V, Poulsen P E, Mohammed S H. Management of obstructive small bowel lesions. Acta Chir Scand 1988; 154: 517–520

49  Stordahl A. Water-soluble contrast media in obstructed ischemic small intestine. A clinical and experimental study. J Oslo City Hosp 1989; 39: 22–30

50  Asbun H J, Pempinello C, Halasz N A. Small bowel obstruction and its management. Int Surg 1989; 74: 23–27

51  Mashev G. Early adhesive ileus. Khrurgiia (Sofiia) 1989; 25: 29–33

52  Diettrich H, Herrmann U, Hildebrandt J, Wundrich B. Intubation of the small intestine in ileus. Technique, results, complications. Gastroenterol J 1989; 49: 12–16

53  Pickleman J, Lee R M. The management of patients with suspected early postoperative small bowel obstruction. Ann Surg 1989; 55: 216–219

54  Manger T, Winkler H. Experience with intraluminal small intestinal intubation. Zentralbl Chir 1990; 115: 749–755

55  Chaib E, Toniolo C H, Figueira N C, Santana L L, Onofrio P L, de Mello J B. Surgical treatment of intestinal obstruction. Arch Gastroenterol 1990; 27: 182–186

56  Mertens R, Ocqueteau M, Guzman S et al. The medical treatment of intestinal obstruction due to adhesions and adherences. Rev Med Chil 1990; 118: 1085–1089

57  Silva P D, Cogbill T H. Laparoscopic treatment of recurrent small bowel obstruction. Wis Med J 1991; 90: 169–170

58  Roscher R, Frank R, Baumann A, Beger H G. Results of surgical treatment of mechanical ileus of the small intestine. Chirurgie 1991; 62: 614–619

59  Bastug D F, Trammell S W, Boland J P, Mantz E P, Tiley III E H. Laparoscopic adhesiolysis for small bowel obstruction. Surg Laparosc Endosc 1991; 1: 259–262

60  Levard H, Mouro J, Schiffino L, Karayel M, Berthelot G, Dubois F. Celioscopic treatment of acute obstruction of the small intestine. Immediate results in 25 patients. Ann Chir 1993; 47: 497–501

61 Seror D, Feigin E, Szold A et al. How conservatively can postoperative small bowel obstruction be treated? Am J Surg 1993; 165: 121–125

62 Moiseev A, Danilov A I, Dougov D L, Shulutko A M. Splinting in the treatment of small intestinal obstruction caused by adhesions. Khirurgia (Moscow) 1994; 6: 30–32

63 Francois Y, Mouret P, Tomaoglu K, Vignal J. Postoperative adhesive peritoneal disease. Laparoscopic treatment. Surg Endosc 1994; 8: 781–783

64 Franklin Jr M E, Dorman J P, Pharand D. Laparoscopic surgery in acute intestinal obstruction. 1994; 4: 289–296

65 Federmann G, Walenzyk J, Schneider A, Bauermeister G, Scheele C. Laparoscopic therapy of mechanical or adhesion ileus of the small intestine-preliminary results. Zentralbl Chir 1995; 120: 377–381

66 Finan M A, Barton D P, Fiorica J V et al. Ileus following gynaecological surgery: management with water-soluble hyperosmolar radiocontrast material. South Med J 1995; 88: 539–542

67 Fleshner P R, Siegman M G, Slater G I, Brolin R E, Chandler J C, Aufses Jr A H. A prospective, randomised trial of short versus long tubes in adhesive small bowel obstruction. Am J Surg 1995; 170: 366–370

68 Ibrahim I M, Wolodiger F, Sussman B, Kahn M, Silvestri F, Sabar A. Laparoscopic management of acute small bowel obstruction. Surg Endosc 1996; 10: 1012–1014

69 DeFriend D J, Klimack O E, Humphrey C S, Schraibman I G. Interaluminal stenting in the management of adhesional intestinal obstruction. J R Soc Med 1997; 90: 132–135

70 Mais J, Eigler F W. Can internal intestinal splinting prevent ileus recurrence? Results of a retrospective comparative study. Ann Surg 1998; 69: 168–173

71 Scott-Coombes C, Whawell S, Vipand M N, Thompson J. Human intraperitoneal fibrinolytic response to elective surgery. Br J Surg. 1995; 82: 414–417

72 Luciano A A, Maier D B, Kock E L et al. A comparative study of postoperative adhesions following laser surgery by laparoscopy versus laparotomy in the rabbit model. Obstet Gynecol 1989; 74: 220–225

73 Tittel A, Schippers E, Treutner K H et al. Laparoscopy versus laparotomy. An animal experiment study comparing adhesion formation in the dogs. Langenbeck's Arch Chir 1994; 379: 95–98

74 Levrant S G, Bieber E J, Barnes R E. Anterior abdominal wall adhesions after laparotomy or laparoscopy. J Am Assoc Gynecol Laparosc 1997; 4: 353–356

75 Nezhat C R, Nezhat F R, Metzger D A, Lucianb A A. Adhesion reformation after reproductive surgery by video laseroscopy. Fertil Steril 1990; 53: 1008–1013

76 Diamond M P, Daniell J F, Johns D A et al. Postoperative adhesion development after operative laparoscopy: evaluation at early second-look procedures. Fertil Steril 1991; 55: 700–708

77 Sutton C. Lasers in infertility. Hum Reprod 1993; 8: 133–140

78 McLaughlin D S. Evaluation of adhesion reformation by early second-look laparoscopy following micro laser ovarian wedge resection. Fertil Steril 1984; 42: 531–537

79 Diamond M P, Daniell J F, Martin D C, Feste J, Vaughn W K, McLaughlin D S. Tubal patency and pelvic adhesions at early second-look laparoscopy following intra-abdominal use of the carbon dioxide laser: initial report of the intra-abdominal laser study group. Fertil Steril 1984; 42: 717–721

80 Dunn R C. A longitudinal, observational study of adhesion reformation and *de novo* adhesion formation after laparoscopic adhesiolysis. 47th Annual Meeting of the AFS, 1991; 36

81 Daody K J, Dunn R C, Buttram V. Recombinant tissue plasminogen activator reduces adhesion formation in a rabbit uterine horn mode. Fertil Steril 1989; 51: 509–511

82 Vipond M N, Whawell S A, Scott-Coombes D M, Thompson J N, Dudley H A. Experimental adhesion prophylaxis with recombinant tissue plasminogen activator. Ann R Coll Surg Engl 1994; 76: 412–416

83 Le Grand E K, Rodgers K E, Girgis W, Campeau J D, diZerega G S. Comparative efficacy of non-steroidal anti-inflammatory drugs and anti-thomboxane agents in a rabbit adhesion prevention model. J Invest Surg 1995; 8: 187–189

84 Giehlbach D L, O'Hair K C, Parks A L, Rosa C L. Combined effects of tissue plasminogen activator and carboxymethylcellulose on adhesion reformation in rabbits. Int J Fertil Menopausal Stud 1994; 39: 172–177

85 Bothin C. Counteracting postsurgical adhesions, the effect of combining oxidized regenerated cellulose and tissue plasminogen activator. Int J Fertil Menopausal Stud 1995; 40: 102–105

86 Evans D M, McAfee K, Guyton D P, Hawkins N, Stakleff K. Dose dependency and wound healing aspects of the use of tissue plasminogen activator in the prevention of intra-abdominal adhesions. Am J Surg 1993; 155: 229–232

87 El-Chalabi H A, Otubo J A M. Value of a single intraperitoneal dose of heparin in prevention of adhesion formation: an experimental evaluation in rats. Int J Fertil 1987; 32: 332–338

88 Fukysawa M, Girgis W, diZerega G S. Inhibition of postsurgical adhesions in a standardized rabbit model: intraperitoneal treatment with heparin. Int J Fertil 1991; 46: 213–218

89 Diamond M P, Pines E, Linsky C B et al. Synergistic effects of Interceed (TC7) and heparin. J Gynecol Surg 1991; 7: 1–5

90 Tayyar M, Turan R, Ayata D. The use of amniotic membrane plus heparin to prevent postoperative adhesions in the rabbit. Tokai J Exp Clin Med 1993; 18: 57–59

91 Reid R L, Hahn P M, Spence J E H, Tulandi T, Yuepe A A, Wiseman D M. A randomized clinical trial of oxidized regenerated cellulose adhesion barrier (Interceed, TC7) alone or in combination with heparin: Fertil Steril 1997; 67: 23–29

92 Larsson B, Svanberg S G, Swolin K. Oxyphen-butazone, an adjuvant to be used in prevention of adhesion in operations for fertility. Fertil Steril 1977; 28: 807–809

93 DeSimone J M. Indomethacin decreases carrageenan induced peritoneal adhesions. Surgery 1988; 104: 788–792

94 Holtz G. Failure of a non-steroidal anti-inflammatory agent (Ibuprofen) to inhibit peritoneal adhesion reformation after lysis. Fertil Steril 1982; 37: 582–586

95 Luciano A A, Hauser K S, Benda J. Evaluation of commonly used adjuvants in the prevention of postoperative adhesions. Am J Obstet Gynecol 1983; 146: 88–91

96 Phillips R K S, Dudiey H A F. The effect of tetracycline lavage and trauma on visceral and parietal peritoneal ultrastructure and adhesion formation. Br J Surg 1984; 71: 537–541

97 Sushan A, Mor-Yosef S, Agvar A, Laufer N. Hyaluronic acid for prevention experimental postoperative intraperitoneal adhesions. J Reprod Med 1994; 39: 398–402

98 Burns J W, Skinner K, Colt M J, Burgess L, Rose R, Diamond M P. A hyaluronate based gel for the prevention of postsurgical adhesions: evaluation in two animal species. Fertil Steril 1996; 66: 814–821

99 Franklin R R, Diamond M P, Malinak R L et al. Reduction of ovarian adhesions by the use of Interceed. Obstet Gynecol 1995; 86: 335–340

100 Nordic Adhesion Prevention Study Group. The efficacy of Interceed (TC7) for prevention of reformation of postoperative adhesions on ovaries, fallopian tubes and fimbriae in microsurgical operations for fertility. Fertil Steril 1995; 63: 709–714

101 Van Geldorp H. Interceed absorbable adhesion barrier reduces the formation of postsurgical adhesions after ovarian surgery. Presented at the 50th Annual Meeting of the American Fertility Society, 1994; 273

102 Interceed (TC7) Adhesion Barrier Study Group. Prevention of postsurgical adhesions by Interceed (TC7), an absorbable adhesion barrier: a prospective randomized multicenter clinical study. Fertil Steril 1989; 51: 933–937

103 Azizz R, Interceed (TC7) Adhesion Barrier Study Group II. Microsurgery alone or with Interceed absorbable adhesion barrier for pelvic sidewall adhesion reformation. Surg Gynecol Obstet 1993; 177: 135–139

104 diZerega G S. Use of adhesion prevention barriers in pelvic reconstructive and gynecologic surgery. In: diZerega G S, De Cherney A H, Diamond M P (eds) Pelvic Surgery, Adhesion Formation and Prevention. New York: Springer, 1997; 188–209

105 Haney A F, Doty E. Expanded polytetrafluoroethylene (Gore-Tex surgical membrane) is superior to oxidized regenerated cellulose (Interceed TC7) in preventing adhesions. Fertil Steril 1995; 63: 1021–1028

106 Diamond M P, The Seprafilm Adhesion Study Group. Reduction of adhesions after uterine myomectomy by Seprafilm membrane (HAL-F): a blinded, prospective, randomized, multicenter clinical study. Fertil Steril 1996; 66: 906–910

# Index

# Progress in Obstetrics and Gynaecology
*Edited by John Studd*

*Contents of Volume 12*

ISBN 0 443 05307 3

# Progress in Obstetrics and Gynaecology
*Edited by John Studd*

*Contents of Volume 11*

ISBN 0443 05059 7

# Progress in Obstetrics and Gynaecology
*Edited by John Studd*

Contents of Volume 10

ISBN 0443 04754 5

# Progress in Obstetrics and Gynaecology
## Edited by John Studd

*Contents of Volume 9*

ISBN 0443 04412 0

# Progress in Obstetrics and Gynaecology
*Edited by John Studd*

*Contents of Volume 8*

ISBN 0443 04170 9

# Progress in Obstetrics and Gynaecology
*Edited by John Studd*

*Contents of Volume 7*

ISBN 0443 03885 6

# Progress in Obstetrics and Gynaecology
*Edited by John Studd*

*Contents of Volume 6*

ISBN 0443 03572 5

# Progress in Obstetrics and Gynaecology
*Edited by John Studd*

*Contents of Volume 5*

ISBN 0443 03268 8

# Progress in Obstetrics and Gynaecology
*Edited by John Studd*

Contents of Volume 4

ISBN 0443 03054 5

# Progress in Obstetrics and Gynaecology
*Edited by John Studd*

*Contents of Volume 3*

ISBN 0443 02665 3